Adolescent forensic psychiatry

Adolescent Forensic Psychiatry

Edited by

Susan Bailey OBE MD FRCPsych
Professor of Child and Adolescent
Forensic Mental Health,
University of Central Lancashire;
Consultant Child and Adolescent Psychiatrist,
Bolton, Salford and Trafford Mental Health Trust
Manchester, UK

and

Mairead Dolan MD
Senior Lecturer in Forensic Psychiatry,
University of Manchester;
Honorary Consultant Forensic Psychiatrist,
Bolton, Salford and Trafford Mental Health Trust,
Manchester, UK

ARNOLD

A member of the Hodder Headline Group

LONDON

First published in Great Britain in 2004 by
Arnold, a member of the Hodder Headline Group,
338 Euston Road, London NW1 3BH

http://www.arnoldpublishers.com

Distributed in the United States of America by
Oxford University Press Inc.,
198 Madison Avenue, New York, NY10016
Oxford is a registered trademark of Oxford University Press

Whilst the advice and information in this book are believed to be true and
accurate at the date of going to press, neither the author[s] nor the publisher
can accept any legal responsibility or liability for any errors or omissions
that may be made. In particular (but without limiting the generality of the
preceding disclaimer) every effort has been made to check drug dosages;
however it is still possible that errors have been missed. Furthermore,
dosage schedules are constantly being revised and new side-effects
recognized. For these reasons the reader is strongly urged to consult the
drug companies' printed instructions before administering any of the drugs
recommended in this book.

British Library Cataloguing in Publication Data
A catalogue record for this book is available from the British Library

Library of Congress Cataloging-in-Publication Data
A catalog record for this book is available from the Library of Congress

ISBN 0 340 76389 2

1 2 3 4 5 6 7 8 9 10

Commissioning Editor: Serena Bureau
Development Editor: Layla Vandenbergh
Project Editor: Zelah Pengilley
Production Controller: Deborah Smith
Cover Design: Stewart Larking
Cover photograph: Elizabeth Wewiora
Illustrations: Lynn P. Aulich

Typeset in 10/12 pt Minion by Charon Tec Pvt. Ltd, Chennai, India
Printed and bound in the UK by Butler & Tanner Ltd

What do you think about this book? Or any other Arnold title?
Please send your comments to **feedback.arnold@hodder.co.uk**

To our fathers,
Frank Bailey and Benny Dolan,
and our much missed and loved colleagues
Dave O'Callaghan and Richard Harrington

Contents

Foreword

This book provides a landmark in British psychiatry. It has always been a puzzle to me that the period in life of maximum disturbance, adolescence, is the one of the least interest to both psychiatrists and governments. Child psychiatry is neglected and under resourced, but compared to adolescent psychiatry, child psychiatrists seem like the rich relations.

Adolescence is the agonising period we all have experienced, of trying to adapt to an adult world that often seems uncomprehending and unsympathetic. In any case, we adolescents are too proud (for proud read insecure) to admit to problems and we certainly don't want to be labelled 'nuts'; death would be a better option. Thus, adolescence and adolescents require very skilled help.

Adolescence is the period of peak crime rates; stealing, fighting, drug taking, and binge drinking are all commonplace. An adolescent who is mishandled in such tricky situations can become a criminal and perhaps a prisoner after some years. The majority of the ghastly sadistic and violent characteristics of adult life begin in adolescence. Is it rational for a society allegedly concerned about high crime rates to neglect the psychiatry of this period of life? I think the neglect of adolescent psychiatry is a special form of self-harm undertaken by adult society.

Within the psychiatric profession there are voices (*sotto voce*), which want to see forensic psychiatry abolished and subsumed within general psychiatry. There are also voices that would like to see adolescent forensic psychiatry disappear as well. No suggestion for a special interest group has had a tougher time going through the council of the Royal College of Psychiatrists than the ultimately successful special interest group for adolescent forensic psychiatry.

Perhaps I am too harsh in my judgement, the chronology of 200 years set out at the beginning of this book shows that we have come a long way in care and understanding since 1800, even since 1950. The problem is that most of the improvements have been brought about (rightly) by penal reformers, social workers and teachers, largely without the assistance of the medical profession. Yet young people are prone to serious illnesses and malfunctions just as we all are at any age.

As this book also demonstrates, a few people, and Professor Bailey and Dr Dolan are leaders here, are determined to do something about it. The Gardener Unit in Manchester is a role model for the whole of Britain. It specialises in troublesome offending youngsters and helps them limp into adult life, and with a few assets, so they can grow away from the adult courts and prisons.

The title of this book may puzzle some non-British readers. 'Forensic', strictly, means 'law' or more particularly 'court' and there isn't a lot in this book about appearing in court, writing reports, and being a forensicist. This simply reflects that in Britain the term forensic psychiatry has developed an overwhelming emphasis on the treatment and management of offenders. Readers will find important law in the book (Chapter 30 by Anthony Harbour is a good example), but its place is just one part of the framework of care to be offered to adolescent offenders.

The readership of this book should not be confined to the growing but small group of people who practise as adolescent forensic psychiatrists. No psychiatrist in any subspecialty can understand his or her patients' needs without understanding adolescents. Non-psychiatrists who also deal with offending young people: psychologists, teachers, social workers, police officers and custody staff, should refer to and learn from this book. Psychiatry these days is a multi-professional world, as can be seen from the list of authors. Adult forensic psychiatrists have a very special need for this book; the behaviours described often go on into adult life, the techniques used to help youngsters can be helpful for adults stuck in a pattern of adolescent behaviour. Nobody who works with offenders can understand adult antisocial behaviour without analysing its origins in earlier life.

Some of us who have worked in British adult forensic psychiatry have long sought developments, recruitment and training for adolescent forensic psychiatry. I am convinced that when the chronology at the beginning of this volume is extended in a future book there will be a fully-fledged specialty doing much good work with younger offenders. Recruitment has begun, training schemes are being established. Over 40 expert writers have been brought together for this volume. As I mentioned there is now a Special Interest Group for Adolescent Forensic Psychiatry in the Royal College of Psychiatrists. Soon there will be a discreet and high status subspecialty in Britain and probably in the USA and Europe also. This textbook points us down that road.

It is always good to be at the beginning of something exciting and worthwhile. Trainee psychiatrists and psychologists thinking of which specialty to join should read this book and sign up for a fascinating and intensely rewarding career.

John Gunn CBE MD FRCPsych FMedSci
Emeritus Professor of Forensic Psychiatry
King's College, London

Preface and acknowledgements

Children and teenagers make up a quarter of the total population of the UK. We know that 50% of all offenders are under the age of 21 years and that rates of mental health problems are particularly high in children and young people who offend.

Forensic mental health encompasses the assessment and treatment of those who are both mentally disordered or whose behaviours have led or could lead to offending. Increasingly the specialism of forensic mental health has also involved direct work with victims. Traditionally, child and adolescent mental health practitioners have had to work as generalists but their workload often includes forensic work.

Mental illness among young offenders has become an ever-increasing concern. Diverse political and policy concerns range from those who are primarily interested in saving young people to those who are primarily interested in saving the public from young offenders. Public health policy has long recognized the government's obligation to attend to the basic health needs of prisoners and the importance of meeting the overall health, including mental health, needs of children.

Services surrounding the assessment and treatment of children and young people within forensic mental health services are influenced by professionals in many areas. People within those areas are often obligated to offer opinions on the reasons why children and young people break the law and what should be done with them. Changes in the law regarding culpability and capacity of children raise issues of whether to criminalize and punish or care and educate. The development of services, the methods of assessment and treatment of children and young people and issues surrounding future risk and rehabilitation are therefore central to the content of this book.

The variety of contributors reflects the mosaic of professionals that children and young people may meet, should they enter the criminal justice and/or social care system. In Part 1, assessment practices including needs assessment and assessment of risk are described. Child influences on psychopathology and an introduction to some major disorders and clinical syndromes are presented in Parts 2 and 3 respectively. Part 4 examines offenders and their offending behaviour. The core types of treatments currently available are outlined in Part 5. Part 6 describes the delivery of services. In Part 7, legal, social and healthcare systems and agencies are examined.

Whilst we hope this book will be of special interest to those people working with children and young people in secure care, it will also be of interest to people working with all looked-after children. It also provides a context in which to view secure care provision of adults. It will be of value to all those involved in the development of the needs of children and adolescents within educational, social, mental health and criminal justice services.

We acknowledge the time, patience and expertise given so generously by the authors and we thank them. Authors have written their contributions from their own unique and respected perspectives and as such this book will offer a wide range of comprehensive knowledge and opinion. Any overlap we believe captures the current state of both knowledge and opinion in this developing and exciting new field of mental health, juvenile justice work.

We wish to express a great debt of thanks to Paul Tarbuck, Service Director of Bolton, Salford and Trafford Mental Health Trust; James Millington and Nathan Whittle for their editorial assistance and for the support of mentors and pioneers in the field; Carol Sheldrick; Professor Pamela Taylor; Professor John Gunn; Mrs Dorothy Tonak; Joe Erulkar; and the late Barbara Kahan. We also wish to thank Deborah Rothwell, Nicola Tattersall, Iram Farooq and Hazel Flanagan for all the secretarial support they have provided in their own time.

Susan Bailey
Mairead Dolan

Contributors

Alex Apler MB BS LLB FRANZCP
Child and Adolescent Psychiatrist
Park House, Liverpool Hospital
Liverpool, NSW, Australia

Mark Ashford
Taylor Nichol Solicitors
Station Place
London, UK

Lynn P. Aulich BA(Hons) PG Dip ATh MA(Econ)
Clinical Specialist Art Therapist, FACTs Team
Adolescent Forensic Service
Bolton, Salford and Trafford Mental Health Trust
Manchester, UK

Susan Bailey OBE MD FRCPsych
Professor of Child and Adolescent Forensic Mental Health
University of Central Lancashire
Consultant Child and Adolescent Forensic Psychiatrist
Bolton, Salford and Trafford Mental Health Trust
Manchester, UK

Gillian Bell MB BS MRCPsych
Specialist Registrar
Northgate Hospital, Morpeth, UK

Deanne Bennett
Occupational Therapy Department
Rampton Hospital
Retford
Nottinghamshire, UK

Arnon Bentovim MB BS FRCPsych DPM
Consultant Psychiatrist
The London Child and Family Consultation Service
London, UK

Marie Boles
Clinical Nurse Manager
Adolescent Forensic Service
Gardener Unit
Manchester, UK

Roger Bullock MA PhD
Dartington Social Research Unit
Totnes, UK

Andrew Clark MA MB BS FRCPsych
Senior Lecturer and Honorary Consultant in
Adolescent Psychiatry
University of Manchester and
Bolton, Salford and Trafford Mental Health Trust
Manchester, UK

Christopher Cordess MA MBBCh MPhil FRCP FRCPsych
Honorary Professor of Forensic Psychiatry
University of Sheffield, Sheffield, UK

Marie Corran
Children Services Manager
CCRU
Rochdale, UK

Claire Dimond
Child and Adolescent Mental Health Service (CAMHS)
St George's Team
St George's Hospital
London, UK

Mairead Dolan MD
Senior Lecturer in Forensic Psychiatry
University of Manchester
Honorary Consultant Forensic Psychiatrist
Bolton, Salford and Trafford Mental Health Trust
Manchester, UK

Theo Doreleijers MD PhD
Child and Adolescent Psychiatrist
VU University Medical Center
Amsterdam-Duivendrecht
The Netherlands

Bernadka Dubicka BSc MB BS MRCPsych
Honorary Clinical Research Fellow in Child and
Adolescent Psychiatry
Royal Manchester Children's Hospital
Manchester, UK

Ian H. Dufton
Child and Adolescent Mental Health Service (CAMHS)
Royal Bolton Hospital
Bolton, UK

Kevin Epps PhD
Consultant Forensic Clinical Psychologist
Forensic CAMHS Team
Ardenleigh
Birmingham, UK

Simon G. Gowers BSc MB BS MPhil FRCPsych
Professor of Adolescent Psychiatry
University of Liverpool, and Honorary Consultant
Adolescent Psychiatrist, Academic Unit, Young Peoples
Centre, Chester, UK

Anthony Harbour
Solicitor, Scott-Moncrieff Harbour & Sinclair
London, UK

Richard Harrington (dec.) MB ChB MPhil FRCPsych MD(Hons)
Royal Manchester Children's Hospital
University of Manchester
Manchester, UK

Jane Holmes
Postgraduate student
School of Psychology, University of Queensland
Brisbane, Australia

Anthony James MB BS MRCP MPhil MA
Honorary Senior Lecturer
University of Oxford
Warneford Hospital
Oxford, UK

Anne Jasper MB ChB MRCPsych
Director of Forensic CAMHS, Birmingham and
Solihull Mental Health Trust,
Birmingham, UK

Leo Kroll MRCPsych MRCP(UK)
Consultant Child and Adolescent Psychiatrist
Department of Child Psychiatry and Psychology
Royal Manchester Children's Hospital
Salford, Manchester, UK

Cesar Lengua MB BCh MRCPsych
Consultant in Child and Adolescent Forensic Psychiatry
Kolvin Clinic
St Nicholas Hospital
Newcastle-upon-Tyne, UK

Michael Little BA PhD
Dartington Social Research Unit, Totnes, UK and
Chapin Hall Center for Children at the
University of Chicago
Chicago, US

Juliet Lyon
Prison Reform Trust
Northburgh Street
London, UK

Ruth E. Marshall MB ChB MSc MRCPsych
Consultant Child and Adolescent Psychiatrist
The Winnicott Centre
Manchester, UK

James Millington BSc Psych BST MHT
Adult Forensic Service
Edenfield Centre
Manchester, UK

Peter Misch
The Maudsley Hospital
London, UK

Gregory O'Brien MB ChB MA FRCPsych FRCPCH MD
Chair in Developmental Psychiatry
Northumbria University and
Lead Clinical and Consultant Psychiatrist
Forensic Division Northgate Hospital,
Morpeth, UK

David O'Callaghan (dec.) BA(Hons) CQSW
G-MAP
Sale, Cheshire, UK

Kenny Ross
The FACTS Team, Adolescent Forensic Service
Gardener Unit
Manchester, UK

Stephen Scott BSc FRCP FRCPsych
Reader in Child Health and Behaviour
Institute of Psychiatry and Consultant Child
and Adolescent Psychiatrist,
Maudsley Hospital,
London, UK

Parag Shah MRCPsych MBChB Dip(MHL)
Consultant in Child and Adolescent
Forensic Psychiatry
St Nicholas Hospital
Newcastle-upon-Tyne, UK

Carol Sheldrick MA MPhil MRCP FRCPsych
The Maudsley Hospital
London, UK

Carly Smith
Adolescent Forensic Service
Bolton, Salford and Trafford Mental Health Trust
Manchester, UK

David Smith MA BPhil
Professor of Criminology
Department of Applied Social Science
Lancaster University
Bailrigg
Lancaster, UK

Tracey Swaffer BSc PhD
Principal Forensic Psychologist
Rampton Hospital
Retford, UK

Anita Thapar MBBCh MRCPsych PhD
Professor of Child and Adolescent Psychiatry
University of Wales College of Medicine
Department of Psychological Medicine
Cardiff, UK

Eileen Vizard FRCPsych
NSPCC Young Abusers Project, London, UK

David Waplington
Juvenile Operational Management Group
Abell Street, London, UK

Nathan Whittle
Bolton, Salford and Trafford Mental Health Trust
Manchester, UK

Richard Williams TD MB ChB FRCPsych FRCPCH
DPM MHSM MInstD
Professor of Mental Health Strategy
Welsh Institute for Health and Social Care
University of Glamorgan and
Consultant Child and Adolescent Psychiatrist
Gwent Healthcare NHS Trust
South Wales, UK

Chronology of custodial options for young offenders, 1800–2000

Chronology of events	Custodial options for young offenders Key themes and events	Legislation/reports
Early 19th century	Punishment and retribution dominate the approach to young people and crime. No criminal/legal distinctions between adults and children over 7 years. Children tried and sentenced in adult courts. Adult penalties considered suitable for children, including the death penalty, imprisonment and transportation. No separate custodial provisions for children.	
1838–1842	The first penal institution reserved exclusively for male juvenile offenders was opened at Parkhurst on the Isle of Wight.	
Mid 19th century	The modern construction of childhood as a distinct social and legal category. The development of the separate treatment of young offenders. An emerging welfarist philosophy which recognizes the vulnerability and immaturity of children. Growing concerns about the imprisonment of children.	
1850–1870	The reformer Mary Carpenter and others establish a series of 'Reformatories' as an alternative to youth imprisonment. The new residential institutions combined the provision of education and skills training, taking both offenders and other children in need. Reformatories reduced the numbers of children in prison, but confirmed the place for institutional treatment of children and young people.	Youthful Offenders Act 1854
Late 19th century	Expansion in the use of reformatories and industrial schools.	Gladstone Report 1895
Early 20th century	The elements of welfare, punishment and treatment are all now contained within legislative and juvenile justice policy.	
1908	Legislation sets out a programme of reform for the treatment of young offenders and children in need. Amongst its key provisions, the Children Act created a distinct system of separate juvenile courts; abolished imprisonment for children under 14; restricted the use of imprisonment to those aged 14–16 who are deemed to be 'too unruly or depraved' to be sent to a place of detention; established a new short-term sentence of detention for up to one month to be served in a 'Remand Home' run by the police.	Children Act 1908 (Children's Charter)
1908	The introduction of borstal training for young offenders aged 16–20. The sentence was indeterminate between one and three years. Release was followed by a period of supervision in the community. 'Borstals' were distinct and separate institutions which incorporated a strict regime based on physical exercise, moral instruction, and industrial or agricultural training. Eventually half were open placement. The emphasis was on reforming young offenders through training and education.	Prevention of Crime Act 1908
1908–1920s	Numbers of children and young people in reformatories and industrial schools declined significantly. The approach to young people and crime became more firmly based on the 'welfare' of young offenders and the 'treatment' necessary to reform them.	Malony Committee Report 1927

(continued)

Chronology of events	Custodial options for young offenders Key themes and events	Legislation/reports
1930s	Strongly welfarist principles become enshrined in legislation. Reformatories and Industrial schools are abolished, and Home Office 'Approved Schools' run by local authorities or voluntary organizations are created. The age of criminal responsibility was raised from 7 to 8 years. Section 53 CYPA 1933 dealt with juveniles convicted of 'certain grave crimes' who should receive longer terms of detention.	Children and Young Persons Act 1933
1930s	The borstal regimes, which had become increasingly punitive during the 1920s, were reformed and modelled on the English public school system. The new distinctive regime based on the ideas of Alexander Paterson emphasized a detachment from penal origins. There was a significant expansion of borstal provision.	
1936	The age limit of young offenders eligible for borstal training was raised to 21.	
1938–1940s	A marked rise in recorded youth crime, and a changing emphasis towards the punishment of young offenders. The establishment of 'Detention Centres' to provide short custodial sentences for young offenders aged 14–21. The new regimes were to be based on punishment and deterrence (short sharp shock).	Departmental Committee on Corporal Punishment 1938
	Young offenders aged 14 to 17 could be detained for a maximum of six months in a 'Junior Detention Centre'. For those aged 17–21 there were separate 'Senior Detention Centres'. Detention centres were administered by the Prison Commission. Following a series of investigations, the regimes were later modified to be more educational, although the objectives remained inconsistent. The use of imprisonment for young offenders was further restricted to those aged over 16 in magistrates' Courts, and to those over 14 in the higher Courts.	Criminal Justice Act 1948
1948	Attempts were made to prevent the placement of neglected children alongside offenders in approved schools. Local authority children's departments were established with their own resources for residential care	Children Act 1948
1952	The first detention centre is actually opened.	
1950s–1960s	The numbers of young offenders sent to detention centres increased 5-fold. The approved schools were accommodating approximately 8000 children at any one time.	
1963	The age of criminal responsibility raised from 8 to 10 years.	Children and Young Persons Act 1963
Mid to late 1960s	A series of forward-looking (but ultimately inconclusive reports) return emphasis to welfare and treatment again and the connection between the 'deprived' and the 'depraved'. In 1964 the first of several 'Secure Units' is opened for children aged 10–18, and which, after 1969, are the responsibility of Social Services Departments.	White Paper 'Children in Trouble' 1968
	A 'Youth Treatment Service' with special secure provisions for distributed young people is formulated. Intermediate treatment is also introduced as an alternative to custody. Responsibility for local authorities (and therefore Approved Schools) passes from the Home Office to the DHSS (later Department of Health)	
1969	The approved school system was abolished and replaced by the establishment of 'Local Authority Community Homes with Education' (CHEs). These provided open and closed residential facilities for children and young people aged 10–18, including convicted offenders and other children in care. The new residential provisions set out to incorporate a child-centred regime appropriate to individual welfare and treatment needs.	Children and Young Persons Act 1969
1970s	A sharp decrease in the use of care orders, and the population of community homes declined significantly. At the same time there was a dramatic increase in the number of young people detained at borstals and detention centres.	

(continued)

Chronology of events	Custodial options for young offenders Key themes and events	Legislation/reports
	Overall the use of custodial sentences for juveniles increased from 3000 in 1970 to 7000 in 1978.	
	The number of secure provisions within child care establishments have been increasing since the late 1960s, to 300 beds. Two of four 'Youth Treatment Centres' had been opened – St Charles (Brentwood, Essex) and Glenthorne (Birmingham) – to provide special secure provisions for disturbed young people aged 10–18 (70 beds).	
Early 1980s	Approximately 6000 young people held in detention centres, and a further 1500 male young offenders are in borstals. Use of care orders for young offenders declining.	
	Further legislation imposes restrictions on the use of custody for young offenders aged over 15, and extends the range of non-custodial options.	Criminal Justice Act 1982
	The introduction of a new sentence of Youth Custody, fixed in length by the Courts, which replaced borstal and prison sentences for young people under 21. Borstals were abolished and replaced by 'Youth Custody Centres' for young offenders aged 15–21.	
Mid to late 1980s	Strong disillusionment with the use of custody for young offenders from magistrates and practitioners. Period of juvenile decarceration, diversion and decriminalization. The proportion of juveniles sentenced to custody decreased from 7700 in 1981 to 3200 in 1988. There was an emphasis on diversion from Court and custody and the expansion of Intermediate Treatment Programmes and Intensive Probation Initiatives.	
1988	Youth custody centres and detention centres are merged to form 'Young Offender Institutions'. The new sentence of Detention in a Young Offender Institution is applicable to young offenders aged 15–21.	Criminal Justice Act 1988
Early 1990s	The introduction of new Youth Courts. 17-year-olds are brought within the ambit of juvenile justice law and policy for the first time. Custodial sentences for young offenders are further restricted to categories of serious offences. The UK ratifies the UN Convention on the Rights of the Child (1991).	Criminal Justice Act 1991
Mid 1990s	Disillusionment with diversion from custody initiatives, as recorded youth crime continues to rise significantly. Period of particular concerns about 'persistent young offenders'. Other events, including the murder of James Bulger, lead to an intense debate about children and serious crime.	
	The juvenile justice system refocuses on the elements of punishment, retribution and deterrence.	
1994	The introduction of 'Secure Training Centres' for persistent young offenders aged 12–14. The maximum sentence to detention in a young-offender institution is increased to 24 months. The ambit of s53(2) of the CYPA 1933 is extended to include 10- to under 14-year-olds convicted of all 'certain grave crimes'.	Criminal Justice and Public Order Act 1994
	Increases in the use of custody for young offenders are noted.	
Late 1990s	Period of considerable restructuring and overhaul of the youth justice system, including: new statutory aim; the creation of the Youth Justice Board; the introduction of the Detention and Training Order (all custody for young offenders to include equal period of supervision in the community); replacement of the Secure Training Order; new range of non-custodial sentences; an increase in the extent of criminal responsibility by children; abolition of *doli incapax* for children aged 10–14.	Crime and Disorder Act 1998

Acknowledgement: The above is reproduced with the kind permission of its author, Ann Hagell, and the Home Office.

Assessment in adolescent forensic mental health services

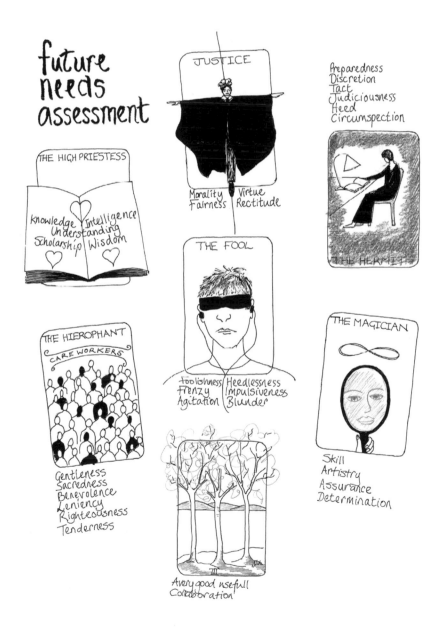

Assessing need in adolescent mental health

Assessing adolescent mental health

SIMON G. GOWERS

ADOLESCENT MENTAL HEALTH

Introduction

Adolescence is a transitional stage of development, between childhood and adulthood. The physical changes of puberty are generally seen as the starting point of adolescence, whilst the end is less clearly delineated. Adolescence ends with attainment of 'full maturity', and a range of social and cultural influences – including the legal age of majority – may influence this. In developed societies these tend to delay progression to adulthood. The extension of compulsory schooling and development of further education, with its economic consequences, generally contributes to a delay in reaching full independence. This may in turn lead to difficulties adjusting to the responsibilities of the next stage of life (Parry-Jones 1995).

The history of societies' concern with the mental health of adolescents – be it illness or adjustment – has been patchy. Whilst teenagers with mental disorder were frequently admitted to asylums and private madhouses 250 years ago, interest in the mental diseases of this age group increased in the mid nineteenth century. This followed a recognition of the physiological processes of puberty as potential contributors to the development of mental illness (Parry-Jones 1994). By the end of the nineteenth century this interest had flourished with the growing attention to the phenomenology of dementia praecox and manic depressive illness. With the development of the child guidance movement in the 1930s, the new multidisciplinary specialty of child psychiatry moved quickly into association with paediatrics. Whilst younger adolescents were generally accommodated within the new services,

those at the older end of the spectrum – and particularly those with severe mental illness – remained within the province of general psychiatry.

The growth of regional adolescent services in Britain in the late 1960s and early 1970s attempted to bridge the gap in services for adolescents, but these developments were generally in association with adult mental hospitals. This split between community provision contained in paediatric services and inpatient and older adolescent provision within general mental health services continued into the 1990s, though the development of Community NHS Trusts in Britain began to address this dislocation. More recently, Specialist Mental Health and 'Partnership' Trusts have attempted to provide continuity across the age spectrum by containing all mental health services for a population within one organization.

Influences on mental health

DEVELOPMENT

Given the transitional nature of adolescence, any assessment of mental health will involve a consideration of the presence or absence of illness or disorder, but also an evaluation of various components of development. Assessment of development encompasses personality, social and moral development, including such things as empathy and the ability to form relationships. It also includes physical and intellectual development, both of which have a considerable bearing on psychological development.

Not all aspects of development proceed at an even pace, and there are reasons to suppose that a mismatch between the various aspects of development is particularly potent at contributing to disorder. This mismatch may be between two aspects of intellectual functioning or between physical and emotional development. Specific reading retardation (a delay in reading later than two years beyond that which would be predicted by IQ), for example, seems to have a greater association with conduct disorder than a general retardation of equivalent magnitude. Similarly it is probable that a mismatch between physical and emotional development leads to comparable problems. The emotionally immature girl who is physically mature and looks older than her years may find herself involved in demanding relationships with which she feels ill-equipped to cope.

Traditionally, personality is thought of as malleable and in a process of evolution through adolescence, not becoming established until adulthood is reached. This view permits hope for apparent difficulties to be rectified before the door is closed on development, and also reduces the potential for the use of pejorative labels such as 'sociopath'.

Any judgement about the presence of disorder has to take account of the possibility of different presentations at different stages through development. Depressive symptoms, for example, may present differently at the age of 12 years from those presenting at 18. Later in adolescence, loss of libido may be a feature of depression, not present in pubescence. Where a presentation is abnormal, this may be either in terms of symptoms or behaviours which are within the bounds of normality at an earlier age (developmental delay), or symptoms or behaviours which are abnormal at any age (distorted or deviant development). Bed-wetting or fear of the dark provide examples of the former, whilst auditory hallucinations illustrate the latter.

PHYSICAL FACTORS

The relationship between physical development and disorder in adolescence is an important one. Psychological disorder can, on the one hand, influence physical development and on the other hand be influenced by it. Anorexia nervosa is an example of the former case; when it arises before linear growth and pubertal development are completed, it can result in stunting of growth and reversal or retardation of the process of puberty. Some of these physical effects are completely reversible, others only relatively so. Confidence and self-esteem, meanwhile, can be adversely affected by small stature or delayed pubertal development (particularly in boys), leading to anxiety or depression, sometimes mediated through bullying.

Finally, a degree of neuroendocrine maturity appears to be necessary for the development of psychotic illnesses such as bipolar affective disorder and schizophrenia, which become increasingly prevalent during the teenage years.

Genetic pre-disposition to a range of disorders confers additional risk. Genetic research is resulting in rapid advances. In general, polygenic inheritance seems to be more common than single gene effects, with the risk of psychiatric illness increasing with genetic fit to an affected relative.

RESILIENCE

The interplay between assessment of development and presence or absence of disorder is highlighted in the assessment of adjustment to a trauma, life event or change of social circumstance. For example, ability of an adolescent to cope with placement in a residential home will include presence of depression or anxiety, personality and social adjustment. The concepts of resilience and vulnerability are concerned with the factors that impinge on the ability to cope. Studies of the development of post-traumatic stress disorder in teenagers exposed to a common trauma have attempted to identify features which appear protective, but most are hampered by a lack of comprehensive assessment prior to the given disaster. Family support has long been recognized as one such variable (Garmezy 1984), and this almost certainly relates to healthy premorbid family functioning. The full range of family strengths and difficulties may be represented in a series of children exposed to an 'act of God' traumatic experience, but family difficulties are likely to be over-represented in those experiencing social traumatic experiences such as reception into care or parental divorce.

ILLNESS

Adolescence is a complex stage of development, when considering adjustment to physical disorder and adherence to treatment. Taylor and Eminson (1994) outline the possible ways in which children can fail to comply with the expectations of their medical attendants. These include screaming, struggling and vomiting, the demonstration of which may relate amongst other things to their attitudes to compliance with authority and resentment at intrusion on their autonomy.

Chronic physical disorders illustrate some of the issues in the interplay between adolescent development and disorder. In diabetes mellitus, metabolic control is dependent on adherence to a dietary and pharmacological routine. This requires a discipline and sense of responsibility, which mirror those being addressed by the adolescent in the rest of his or her life and in relationships with adults. It may be expected to result in some ambivalence. Compliance with any treatment regimen is a constraint upon autonomy (Taylor and Eminson 1994). In childhood, the parents are usually most affected by this constraint, but as responsibility passes to the adolescent they then share the burden with its attendant ambivalence. Each family has to negotiate the appropriate level of protectiveness and supervision. Concern about one's health may be offset by resentment at having to comply overly much, particularly in comparison with peers.

Experimentation with alcohol is just one aspect of normal adolescence which is more loaded with meaning in the diabetic, when drinking behind one's parents' back involves 'cheating' and putting one's health at risk. Failure of adherence results not only in a greater challenge to authority than that posed by peers, but also may result in being faced with parents' own worries about their illness. Frequently teenagers with such a disorder are faced with a choice between being overly protected and relatively lacking in independence, or 'super mature' and more responsible than their peers. This responsibility may include a burdensome responsibility for protecting parents from distress, by concealing fears and doubts.

There are suggestions that where metabolic control in adolescent diabetes is good, this may be at the expense of vulnerability to depressed mood and also a more rigid style of family functioning (Gowers *et al.* 1995). Gustafsson *et al.* (1987) have meanwhile also demonstrated links between family stress and poor diabetic control.

CLASSIFICATION OF ADOLESCENT PSYCHIATRIC DISORDER

Psychiatric disorders of adolescence

Psychiatric disorders in adolescence tend to fall into three developmental categories, namely continuing childhood disorder, mental illnesses typical of adulthood, and disorders which, although not confined exclusively to adolescence, seem characterised by difficulties surmounting this stage of development.

In the first category, a number of presentations, particularly developmental and conduct disorders, will continue from middle childhood into the teens. In the category of adult mental illnesses, schizophrenia and bipolar disorder are both extremely rare before the age of 12. Adolescence is a stage of growing cognitive sophistication and increasing social demand, both of which may play a part in the development of complex psychotic phenomena. It is possible that both are necessary to form, for example, a paranoid delusional belief. Most important, though, seem to be the neuroendocrine changes in the brain, signalled by puberty, which confer a risk for these disorders, in those genetically at risk. Psychoses precipitated by drugs also become more common as independence offers opportunity.

Disorders in the third category, which are typical of adolescence, can be seen as representing a difficulty in mastering the tasks of this developmental stage. Erikson (1965) identified the development of a personal identity as the main task of adolescence. The Group for Advancement of Psychiatry (1968) considered the following to be crucial supplementary tasks:

- proficiency in the adult sexual role
- the transition from being nurtured to being able to care for others
- learning to work and be self-supporting
- leaving home.

As well as arising from task failure, adolescent disorder usually interferes with satisfactory completion of these tasks. A clinical example will illustrate this point.

Claire was a 15-year-old girl who lived with her parents and elder brother. Claire had experienced bullying at school and suffered poor self-esteem consequent on her mild obesity. Her mother suffered with epilepsy. Following an occasion when her mother experienced a partial seizure whilst making a cup of tea and scalding herself, Claire stayed off school for a few days to help her mother with her housework. Very quickly her school refusal became entrenched, her school non-attendance being attributed by the family to bronchial asthma, which was never very evident at clinical assessment. Claire became, like her mother, socially isolated and the two of them spent little time apart. In this example, individual, family and social elements have come together to result in the presentation of school refusal. One can see that there are difficulties for Claire in achieving an identity for herself separate from that of her mother. In addition, the nurturing roles have become unclear through a mutual dependence of each on the other, in which both is carer and cared for. As social and academic aspirations become limited, the opportunities for Claire to attain further independence, or to form intimate relationships outside the family, are much reduced. In such a situation, the failure to move along a normal developmental trajectory generally results in a widening gulf between the subject's experience and that of her peers, thus compounding the above difficulties.

Formal classification systems

A system of classification is, in principle, an invaluable tool for both clinical practice and research. It may help in organizing one's thinking about an individual case as well as enabling comparison between clinical series. Classification also provides an aid to case management at a time when clinicians are increasingly encouraged to come to decisions on an evidence base. In the forensic field, where written communication between professionals from a range of discipline features high, a common language of reliable and valid diagnoses would appear to be highly desirable.

Graham (1982), however, has drawn attention to some of the problems with existing classification schemes. They tend to be viewed as flawed and many professionals working in adolescent mental health have reservations about a perceived medical bias, the negative consequences of 'labelling', and the lack of association between diagnosis and 'need'. Disciplines outside medicine tend to view adolescents in a different way. For example social services tend to view young people as at risk from their social circumstances, whilst educationalists classify pupils by the additional resources required to provide their education and the reason why those resources are necessary.

There are two main formal classification systems of psychiatric disorder in use, namely the World Health Organization's International Classification of Diseases 10th revision – ICD-10 (WHO 1992) – and the 4th revision of the Diagnostic and Statistical Manual of the American Psychiatric Association – DSM-IV (APA 1994). Both systems are subject to periodic revision. They each allow a multi-axial approach to classification; i.e. they permit different aspects of an adolescent's problems to be recorded separately without requiring an artificial judgement about the primacy of each.

In ICD-10, the first axis is concerned with clinical psychiatric syndromes, whilst axes two to four record developmental disorders, intellectual level and associated physical disorders. Axis five is concerned with abnormal psychosocial situations, whilst a final axis allows for a quantitative assessment of global psychosocial disability. DSM-IV's multi-axial system is similar, but axes 1–3 are effectively compressed into two, axis 1 including 'other conditions that may be a focus of clinical attention', whilst axis 2 is concerned with personality disorders and mental retardation. Both systems are for use across the whole lifespan, with a section for psychiatric disorders with onset usually occurring in childhood or adolescence.

In DSM-IV the section for psychiatric disorders with onset usually occurring in childhood or adolescence includes:

- mental retardation (coded on axis 2)
- learning disorders
- motor skills disorder
- communication disorders
- pervasive developmental disorders
- attention-deficit and disruptive-behaviour disorders
- feeding and eating disorders of infancy or early childhood
- tic disorders
- elimination disorders
- other disorders of infancy, childhood or adolescence (chiefly attachment and anxiety disorders).

In the ICD-10 system, mental and behavioural disorders are contained in Chapter V and given codes beginning with the prefix F. This chapter has two blocks of particular relevance: F80–89 consisting of disorders of psychological development and F90–98 consisting of behavioural and emotional disorders with onset usually occurring in childhood or adolescence. The main headings are:

- specific developmental disorders of speech and language
- specific developmental disorders of scholastic skills
- specific developmental disorders of motor function
- mixed specific developmental disorders
- pervasive developmental disorders
- hyperkinetic disorders

- conduct disorders
- mixed disorders of conduct and emotions
- emotional disorders with onset specific to childhood
- disorders of social functioning
- tic disorders
- other disorders
- unspecified.

In addition, Chapter XX comprises external causes of morbidity and mortality, which include intentional self-harm, coded X60–84.

Prevalence

The epidemiology of adolescent disorder reveals marked variation in rates in different sections of the population. Any estimate of the prevalence of disorder needs to take account of the threshold for a diagnosis, sex differences, differences between city and rural communities, and the possibility of changes in prevalence of certain disorders over time.

DIAGNOSTIC THRESHOLD

The relationship between symptoms, behaviours and disorders is a complex one. A number of disorders represent quantitative rather than qualitative differences from normality – e.g. *excessive* anxiety for a given situation. In determining caseness, it is usually helpful to consider the degree of associated, secondary difficulties a symptom, such as social avoidance confers. In both the ICD-10 and DSM-IV systems of classification, an essentially arbitrary issue of threshold must be addressed. ICD-10 offers guidelines to aid diagnostic decision-making, whilst DSM-IV operationalizes the process by specifying the number and type of symptoms or behaviours required. In conduct disorder, for example, three or more behaviours are required from section A, whilst criteria B and C must be satisfied. For most DSM diagnoses, significant impairment of social, academic or occupational function is required.

SEX DIFFERENCES

A number of disorders show marked sex differences, notably higher rates of internalizing disorders in girls and externalizing disorders in boys. Neurodevelopmental disorders are more common in boys and eating disorders in girls.

CHANGE OVER TIME

There is little evidence to support the notion of a change over time in the prevalence of disorders with a biological basis, such as schizophrenia and bipolar disorder. Whilst no disorders appear to have decreased in prevalence in

Table 1.1 *Percentage prevalence of adolescent psychiatric disorders*

Disorder	Prevalence	Group	Source
Nocturnal enuresis	1.0	14-year-old boys	WCCB
	0.5	14-year-old girls	WCCB
Encopresis	1.3	11- to 12-year-old boys	WCCB
	0.3	11- to 12-year-old girls	WCCB
Tic disorders	1.0	General population	WCCB
Reading backwardness	19	10-year-olds (Inner London)	WCCB
	8.3	10-year-olds (Isle of Wight)	WCCB
Specific reading retardation	9.9	10-year-olds (Inner London)	WCCB
	3.9	10-year-olds (Isle of Wight)	WCCB
Autism/autism spectrum	0.2	Young people	NHSE(T)
Hyperkinetic disorder	0.5	Adolescents	WCCB
Severe school phobia	0.1	10- to 16-year-olds	L&B
Emotional disorders	4.5	10-year-olds (small towns)	WCCB
Anxiety disorders	8.7		WCCB
Major depression	2–8	Adolescents	WCCB
Conduct disorder	10	10-year-old boys	WCCB
	2.5	10-year-old girls	WCCB
Obsessive–compulsive	1.9	Adolescents	WCCB
Anorexia nervosa	0.36–0.83	12- to 19-year-old girls	WCCB
	0.04–0.17	12- to 19-year-old boys	WCCB
Bulimia nervosa	2.5	12- to 19-year-old girls	WCCB
'Significant eating problems'	3.0	12- to 19-year-old girls	WCCB
	0.3	12- to 19-year-old boys	WCCB
Attempted suicide	2.0–4.0	Adolescents	WCCB
Completed suicide	0.0075	15- to 19-year-old boys	NHSE(T)
	0.0025	15- to 19-year-old girls	NHSE(T)
Adult-type psychoses	0.02	16-year-olds	L&B
	0.5	17- to 19-year-olds	L&B
Substance misuse:			
Alcohol (in previous week)	21	11- to 15-year-olds	WCCB
Solvents/illegal drugs	2.0	11-year-olds	NHSE(T)
	16	16-year-olds	WCCB
Regular drug use	8.0	15- and 16-year-olds	L&B
Heroin/cocaine	0.9	Adolescents	WCCB
Sexual abuse	7.0	3–16 year olds	L&B
With deviant behaviour	3.9	(=56%)	L&B
With serious emotional disorder	1.8	(=25%)	L&B

WCCB, Wallace, Crown, Cox and Berger (1997); L&B, Light and Bailey (1992); NHSE(T), NHS Executive (Trent Region) (Pearce and Holmes 1995).

recent years, there are suggestions of increases in eating disorders, disorders resulting from alcohol and substance misuse, and antisocial disorders of conduct. These are problems in which psychosocial factors are likely to play a considerable role. Delinquency, which may be one marker for conduct disorder, shows a marked gender bias, but one which has reduced over time. Rutter and Giller (1983), for example, reported a change in the ratio of male to female adolescent delinquency from 11:1 to 5:1 between 1957 and 1977.

Table 1.1 shows the best estimates of prevalence garnered from a range of sources. The total prevalence of all disorders in adolescence is considerably less than the total of these estimates owing to high rates of comorbidity.

The prevalence rates for selected groups at risk may significantly exceed the figures in the table. A study in Oxfordshire (McCann *et al.* 1996), for example, found that 67% of adolescents aged 13–17 who were 'looked after' by the local authority had a psychiatric disorder. This figure rose to 96% of those in residential accommodation.

ASSESSMENT IN ADOLESCENT PSYCHIATRY

Obstacles to assessment

Assessing an adolescent with a possible mental health problem is beset by a number of obstacles.

ADOLESCENT AS TARGET OF COMPLAINT

Whether or not there is a forensic issue, it is common for someone to be complaining about the adolescent. This is self-evident in conduct problems, but also true of a number of emotional disorders. In a number of these, the adolescent demonstrates ambivalence between the wish to be left alone and the wish to change. Obsessive–compulsive disorder is an example in which resistance to obsessional ruminations or performance of rituals is very variable. There may be a difference in this respect between the disorder presenting in adolescence and in adulthood, owing to the secondary gain of inappropriate power. Many adolescents seem able to control family members through an insistence that they comply with the obsessional ritual or face the consequences of an outburst of temper or sometimes physical aggression.

STIGMA OF MENTAL ILLNESS

Very few adolescents would wish their friends to know that they had been assessed or treated by a psychiatrist.

ARTICULATION

Many teenagers will lack confidence in their ability to put their ideas into words, particularly when an assessment may appear to recapitulate difficulties encountered in school.

RELATIONS WITH ADULTS OR AUTHORITY FIGURES

Many teenagers will have had poor relationships with parents, teachers, or the police and may see a psychiatrist in the same category. Some will have suffered abuse at the hands of adults.

> Steve was a 14-year-old boy with obsessive–compulsive disorder (OCD) who felt compelled to carry out a ritual which involved touching women's hair. This had got him into trouble, after first an adult and then the parents of an 11-year-old girl had complained to the police. Assessment of Steve exemplified many of the above issues. Parental and third-party concern had set up the assessment, rather than Steve himself. He merely hoped to convince the interviewer that nothing was wrong and be left alone. As is fairly typical in OCD, Steve had taken on a powerful position within the family, in which the parents were fearful of their son's temper when thwarted in carrying out his rituals, resulting in a situation where they accommodated a range of unreasonable demands. Steve's embarrassment and isolation as a result of this disorder led to a lack of confidence and self-esteem, so he did not feel easily able to express the nature of his predicament to an interviewer.

The result of these issues is that, more than in almost any patient group, the adolescent with a mental health problem – and one with a forensic component in particular – is at the outset very unlikely to fulfil the role of customer.

In any assessment, the interviewer needs to strike a balance between engagement, the need to elicit information, and examination. In some cases there is a conflict between these three elements, whilst the balance may vary according to whether the assessment is a one-off or the prelude to further treatment. One important consideration is ensuring adequate time for these processes, though account should be taken of the teenager's ability to tolerate a long session.

Engagement

Assessment will be facilitated by attention to the setting, outlining the length and remit of the assessment, and the information currently to hand. Thought should be given to the most helpful setting for the interview, in order that one's aims are achieved. An interview carried out in an adolescent outpatient clinic, in a police station, or behind a flimsy screen on a paediatric ward start from rather different positions.

It is usually helpful to explain the stages of the assessment, particularly that the adolescent will have an opportunity to be seen alone. Any unusual equipment, such as video or one-way screen, should be explained and appropriate consent obtained. This of course is likely to worry a suspicious or fearful subject particularly, and it may be helpful to let the teenager have a look at any video equipment and see behind a one-way screen.

Gathering information

Included here is the background information contained in the referral and in the history obtained at various stages of the assessment appointment, and other information collected subsequently. This may include reports from school and other third parties.

ORGANIZING THE INTERVIEWS

In order that the required information be obtained, thought should be given to who is invited to any appointment and in what order and combination they are seen. In a straightforward case, an adolescent will attend with parents or other carer. Clearly, different information may be obtained by seeing parents alone, adolescent alone and all together. Usually it is important to ensure that there is an opportunity for each of these, though there are different views on the order of them and some consideration should be given to the age of the subject. Many prefer to start with a joint interview, in order that the remit, the structure of the session and its aims can be discussed and any major misconceptions addressed. It is then often helpful to begin to obtain an account of the problem in general terms. This enables one to begin to see who is the spokesperson, who agrees with whom, who is party to what information and each's interpretation of it.

Many would advocate that the interview with the adolescent should come next in order not to alienate the individual and to respect his or her right to be seen as the customer. I prefer to see parents first, for a number of reasons.

The patient will usually accept that he or she will have their opportunity later. It ought to be possible to overcome any disgruntlement then. My main reasons for wishing to see parents first are to do with coherence and confidentiality. Parents are usually in the best position to set the child's difficulties in the context of a developmental and family history. Is this a child whose depressed mood has come on in the context of lifelong peer relationship difficulties or, for example, learning difficulty? It can be frustrating to see a sullen non-communicative adolescent and not know what is going on, only for the parental interview to clarify a potentially fruitful line of enquiry. An example might be: 'I expect he told you that it started when he was taunted in the school showers …'. The boundaries of confidentiality should be clarified at the outset. In general, teenagers can expect that information disclosed in their individual interview will be only disclosed with their consent unless there is a compelling reason. If the individual interview is followed by the parental interview, the adolescent may nevertheless believe that their confidences are being betrayed. If the adolescent is seen last, parents can then be brought in and the adolescent can witness the interviewer's ability to balance the parent's right to know against the adolescent's right to privacy. In some cases, the adolescent may not expect to have any privacy from parents. In this situation, demonstrating a contrary expectation may serve to have therapeutic benefit.

Adolescents sometimes wield inappropriate power in the family, as has been outlined above. It can be helpful to model to parents that this can be withstood. Once, when a girl was referred with anorexia nervosa, the parents were surprised that they were allowed to give their story before their daughter. 'You've done it now,' the father said, 'we only got her here under false pretences, saying that we were going to the seaside. She'll have run off by the time we finish.' In the event, the girl was sitting patiently in the waiting room half an hour later, demonstrating to the parents that they might not need to give in to all her demands and also that there might be a glimmer of motivation in the girl's mind to address her problem.

STRUCTURE OF THE ADOLESCENT PSYCHIATRIC HISTORY

The following are the main elements, which would be included in any general assessment:

- family composition
- present complaint
- history of complaint
- past medical history
- medication – therapeutic effects, unwanted effects
- drug, alcohol and substance use and abuse
- personality
- temperament
- family history and family psychiatric history
- developmental history
- social/peer relationships
- school – attendance, attainments, relationships.

INTERVIEW STYLE

A style which includes a number of open questions is more likely to encourage the young person to talk freely than are closed questions which invite brief responses. Leading questions should not be employed as suggestible subjects may acquiesce to a question, leaving the interviewer uncertain as to its reliability. Double and multiple questions should also be avoided as they either confuse the subject or leave the interviewer uncertain which part of the question has been answered.

EXAMINATION/INVESTIGATIONS

There are a number of forms of examination of relevance in adolescent psychiatry.

Mental state examination

This comprises an ordered series of observation and enquiry.

Appearance
The young person's facial expression may reveal clues about mood (whether happy, angry, anxious or sad). A number of abnormalities of motor functioning may have psychiatric implications. The most common manifestation is the restlessness and distractibility of hyperactivity, occasionally diagnosed for the first time in adolescence. This must be distinguished from the overactivity with grandiosity or irritability of hypomania. Depression may be accompanied by motor slowness, also seen in obsessive–compulsive disorder, where compulsive ruminations can be paralysing. Other abnormal movements include tics (usually facial or involving neck and shoulders, sometimes accompanied by vocalizations). Obsessive rituals sometimes include tapping movements of fingers or movements of the legs and feet. Those on medication should be observed for unwanted effects, such as akathisia and dystonias in those on major tranquillizers and the tremor of lithium intoxication.

Speech and language
Articulation defects or stuttering may benefit from specific therapeutic input. Other abnormalities of the form of speech include those of rate and volume. Depression and hypomania may respectively slow or increase the rate

of speech, whilst in the former, speech may be reduced to a nearly inaudible mumble. Vocal tics in Tourette syndrome may on occasion be present with motor accompaniment. The content of speech can be difficult to evaluate in adolescence, particularly when discussing beliefs and interests. Sometimes speech content will reveal the flight of ideas of hypomania, or in those with developmental disorders the echolalia or pronoun reversal of autism.

Thoughts

Assessment of mood always requires enquiry about thoughts of hopelessness, that life is not worth living and assessment of suicidality. Where suicidal ideas have been present, one must enquire about plans, such as storing tablets. In those suspected of psychotic disorder one should explore the presence of delusional ideas. Assessment of unusual beliefs, such as in the activities of aliens or the paranormal will need to take account of cultural norms in the young person's peer group. Sometimes a young person with a developing psychosis will retain a degree of insight and withhold delusional or overvalued ideas, which may be revealed only by a parent. Adolescents with obsessive ruminations or rituals sometimes express complex abnormal beliefs to explain their expression, which can sometimes be difficult to distinguish from delusional beliefs. Resistance to obsessive rituals is not universal, but enquiry will normally reveal that resistance leads to high anxiety, whilst the magical beliefs of obsessive–compulsive disorder are not usually held with the absolute conviction of delusions.

Abnormal perceptions

It is necessary to distinguish hallucinations from illusions (on the basis of presence or absence of a stimulus). Visual and tactile hallucinations are suggestive of organic (particularly drug-induced psychoses), whilst in schizophrenia auditory hallucinations often have the same quality as those seen in adults.

Social behaviour

A clinical interview can reveal much about social behaviour, both verbal and non-verbal. The interviewer can note shyness, disinhibition, aggressiveness or suspiciousness. How easy is it to develop a rapport? Is there normal reciprocal social communication? Is the young person overly friendly or socially inappropriate?

Mood

Shyness or sullenness is quite common at the outset of an interview with an adolescent, but after engagement, it is important to determine whether there is suggestion of mood disturbance. As well as looking out for depressed or elated mood, is the young person's mood appropriate to the areas being discussed? Is the individual able to show an appropriate range of affective responses? Is mood unusually labile? Is he or she able to enjoy life and look forward to planned activities? Clearly the assessment

in this area may be influenced by pending criminal proceedings. One should enquire about sleep and appetite, noting that the presentation of depression in young people may involve hypersomnia and increased appetite, more commonly than in adulthood. Loss of libido is a rare feature in adolescents.

Cognition

It is usually possible to make a brief assessment of orientation, concentration, attention and memory, whilst comprehensive developmental assessment requires trained standardized testing. A simple evaluation of developmental level can be achieved by testing reading, writing and mathematical ability. However, the subject may be sensitive about lack of academic attainment and the way such information is elicited requires careful attention.

Assessment of family relationships

Much may be gleaned from the initial meeting with all family members, or indeed from the waiting room. Parents may be sitting together whilst the adolescent stands apart. Alternatively one parent may be isolated, giving the impression that they have only come to provide the transport. An adolescent sitting between parents may demonstrate the family's support or closeness, or alternatively their position of power. When members of the family speak, are they critical, empathic or protective? Who agrees with whom and are disagreements expressed or not. Are they accepted or rejected? What are the alliances and identifications in the family? Frequently assessment of the family requires a more detailed assessment, sometimes as a prelude to family therapy, where indicated, whilst assessment instruments are mentioned below.

The physical examination

The importance of a physical examination may vary with the history and the type of presenting problem, but its potential importance should always be considered. A comprehensive assessment should include a physical assessment including measurement of height, weight and pubertal status with completion of appropriate centile charts. A brief general examination should be carried out, with focus on specific systems depending on the nature of the presenting problem. While the individual is dressing or undressing, one may note hand preference, any degree of clumsiness, incoordination or unsteadiness. Unusual facial appearance, asymmetrical physical development and pigmented or depigmented skin patches should be recorded, along with any bruising or scars. A patient with a psychotic illness or a learning disability will require a comprehensive neurological assessment. One with anorexia nervosa needs assessment of nutrition and haematological function.

A brief neurological assessment should be carried out, though there are few systematic population studies, with attention to accurate neurological assessment. The Isle of Wight study (Rutter and Tizard 1970) suggested that, although there was an association between neurological findings and behavioural abnormality, this was less close than had been previously assumed. The notion of neurological 'soft signs' is controversial and, it has been argued, a subterfuge for unscientific thinking. Soft signs have been described as being over-represented in autism, Tourette syndrome, borderline personality disorder, schizophrenia and anxiety-withdrawal (Pincus 1996). One explanation may be that these disorders do not constitute diseases in themselves, but expressions of a range of biological abnormality. A detailed review of neurological soft signs is provided by Pincus (1996). Asymmetrical physical or neurological findings are reliable indicators of pathology. Assessment should include assessment of coordination by observation of the young person's writing, drawing and copying of figures. Any tremor or abnormal movements should be noted. With the eyes closed, proprioception can be assessed by the finger–nose test. Walking heel to toe, on tip toes and in turn on the inner and outer edges of the feet – Fog's test (Fog and Fog 1963) may reveal asymmetry in and the extent of overflow movements, abnormal in post-pubertal children. Any mirroring of foot posture in the hands is also abnormal after the age of 11.

Physical investigations

Investigations are carried out for two main reasons: to examine for organic disorder and to check physical status before prescribing medication. Usually the history and mental state examination provide the main pointers to an organic contribution; a battery of investigations should not be routinely conducted in the hope of uncovering an unexpected condition. When a young person presents with a major change in behaviour or a psychotic illness, a remediable physical disorder may be present, or it may be difficult to assess the contribution of substance misuse. The initial investigation should include full blood count, ESR, serum urea and electrolytes, calcium and phosphate, liver function (including aspartate transaminase and albumin) and thyroid function. This latter is of particular importance where lithium therapy is considered. Urine analysis and urine toxicology screening should be conducted as young people may ingest a wider range of drugs than those volunteered (hallucinogens will not be detected by urinalysis, however).

An acute psychotic presentation merits an EEG and either a CT or MRI scan, though the pick-up rate is very low. It can be reassuring to parents that physical causes have been excluded.

CHECKLISTS, RATING SCALES, QUESTIONNAIRES AND SEMI-STRUCTURED INTERVIEWS

These have been devised to improve the reliability and validity of information and observation used in diagnostic assessment. They are primarily used for research but can be useful for screening populations or as a diagnostic aid in clinical settings. In general, adolescents report more reliably about *feelings* and parents about *behaviour*. These have been developed for a range of different purposes and for use in a specified context. Any interpretation of data yielded from them needs to take account of their original purpose (e.g. research or clinical), whether for example they are designed to measure change (or response to treatment), and the intended target population (e.g. cultural context). What degree of training (if any) is required for their use?

Screening instruments for normal samples

The recognition that a child's behaviour is abnormal can usually be achieved with sufficient accuracy for routine screening purposes by a brief symptom/behavioural checklist, such as the *Rutter A scale* (Rutter 1967) or the *Child Behaviour Checklist* (Achenbach and Edelbrock 1983). The *Strength and Difficulties Questionnaire* (Goodman 1997) is a newer instrument which has the merit of not focusing on problems alone. The *Conners' parent and teacher questionnaires* have shown particular value in evaluating response to pharmacological treatment of children and young adolescents with ADDH.

Assessment instruments for clinical samples

HIGHLY STRUCTURED INTERVIEWS

Diagnostic Interview for Children & Adolescents – DICA (Herjanic and Reich 1982)

This is suitable for children and young people aged 6–17. There are parent and child versions. It takes 60–90 minutes and requires no clinical judgement by the interviewer. The interview yields information on a wide range of symptoms, their onset and severity. ICD and DSM diagnoses can be yielded. The authors have demonstrated satisfactory inter-rater and test–retest reliability and validity using comparisons of referrals to paediatric and psychiatric clinics.

Diagnostic Interview Schedule for Children – DISC (Costello *et al.* 1985)

This takes 45–60 minutes and is suitable for children aged 6–18. Symptoms are coded on a three-point (0, 1, 2) scale. There are parent and child versions.

SEMI-STRUCTURED INSTRUMENTS

These require greater clinical interpretation and thus greater training to ensure reliability. The most widely used is the *Schedule for Affective Disorders and Schizophrenia for School Age Children – K-SADS* devised by Puig-Antich and Chambers and revised by Orvaschel and Puig-Antich (1982).

This interview is designed to be administered by clinically experienced interviewers. It starts with identification of all problems and symptoms, followed by a treatment history and observational assessment. Finally, the interviewer rates global functioning on a 1–100 scale the children's version of the Global Assessment of Functioning. It is designed to be administered to parents first. Inter-rater reliability for individual symptoms of major diagnostic syndromes range from 0.65 to 0.96.

Measurement of family functioning

There are a number of assessment aids for evaluating family functioning. The McMaster model (Epstein *et al.* 1978) is seeming particularly focused on areas pertinent to the adolescent stage of development. There is a self-rated version, the Family Assessment Device (FAD), and a clinician-rated version, the McMaster Structured Interview of Family Functioning (McSIFF) (Epstein *et al.* 1982, 1983). The ratings of family functioning provided by the McMaster model have been shown to be highly predictive of outcome of adolescent anorexia nervosa (North *et al.* 1997).

Instruments for rating clinical severity and change over time

Health of the Nation Outcome Scales for Children & Adolescents – HoNOSCA (Gowers *et al.* 1999a)

This is a brief outcome scale comprising 13 items rated on a five-point scale from 0 to 4, with a detailed glossary to guide ratings (Gowers *et al.* 1999b). It was developed as part of the Health of the Nation strategy to improve mental health within the population and is designed as a routine clinical measure. A small amount of training is required. An adolescent self-rated, guided questionnaire (HoNOSCA-SR) has recently been developed and shows promising features.

Strength & Difficulties Questionnaire (Goodman 1997)

This instrument also has self-rating and clinician-rated versions and is suitable for adolescents. The positive attention to areas of strength may make it particularly acceptable to patients and families.

Developmental and psychological tests

The following is a list of the more commonly used psychological and developmental tests used in the field of adolescent mental health, with an indication of their uses. Detailed description of their construction and performance is outside the scope of this chapter. Full references are not provided, but readers are directed to Racusin and Moss's (1996) overview of this area for further detail.

- *Wechsler Intelligence Scale for Children III (WISC-III).* Age up to 17 years. Yields performance, verbal and full-scale IQ.
- *Bruininks–Oseretsky Test of Motor Proficiency.* Age up to 14 years. Measures gross and fine motor performance (eight subtests).
- *Benton Visual Retention Test (BVRT).* Age up to adult. Tests visual perception.
- *Bender Visual Motor Gestalt Test.* Age up to adult. Assesses visual motor deficits and visual memory.
- *Peabody Picture Vocabulary – Revised (PPVT-R).* Age up to adult. A screening test for language.
- *Peabody Individual Achievement Test – Revised (PIAT-R).* Age up to 18 years. Tests educational knowledge and skills.
- *Trail Making Test (Reitan 1971).* Age up to adult. Tests attention. Useful in assessment of ADHD in adolescents.
- *Child Behaviour Checklist (CBCL) (Achenbach and Edelbrock).* School-age children. There are parent- and teacher-rating versions.
- *Conners' Teacher Rating Scale.* School-age children. Particularly useful for rating response to treatment in ADHD.
- *Wisconsin Card Sorting Test (Berg 1948).* Age up to adult. Tests attention.
- *Minnesota Multiphasic Personality Inventory – Adolescent (MMPI-A).* Age 14–18. Test of personality development.
- *Children's Appperception Test (CAT).* Age up to adult. Test of personality.
- *Vineland Adaptive Behaviour Scales – Survey Form.* Age up to adult. Measures social and adaptive behaviour.

CONCLUSIONS

The psychiatric assessment of an adolescent is likely to reveal a range of needs and also a number of risks. Health needs can be considered from the perspective of either the individual or a population. In essence, need can be thought of as the best that can be done for an individual in a particular setting (Wallace *et al.* 1997). Sometimes the need relates directly to a mental health problem, sometimes it is less direct and is concerned with the prevention of secondary handicaps, such as through the provision of special education.

Risk is part and parcel of assessment in adolescent psychiatry. It is usually considered in relation to the subject; e.g. risk from self-harm, substance use or anorexia. Sometimes the risk also encompasses others, most commonly through aggressive or other antisocial behaviour, such as firesetting or from acting on psychotic experiences.

The principles of assessment outlined above, and the assessment of need and risk, should encompass the same issues, whether in a forensic setting or not. The next chapters will amplify these points with particular reference to the forensic setting.

REFERENCES

Achenbach, T.M. and Edelbrock, C.S. 1983: *Manual for the Child Behaviour Checklist and Revised Child Behaviour Profile.* Burlington, VT: University of Vermont.

APA (American Psychiatric Association) 1994: *Diagnostic and Statistical Manual of Mental Disorders*, 4th edn. Washington, DC: APA.

Conners, C.K. 1971: Recent drug studies with hyperkinetic children. *Journal of Learning Disability* **4**: 467–83.

Costello, E.J., Edelbrook, C. and Costello, A.J. 1985: Validity of the NIMH Diagnostic Interview Schedule for Children: a comparison between psychiatric and paediatric referrals. *Journal of Abnormal Child Psychology* **13**: 579–95.

Erikson, E.H. 1965: *Childhood and Society*. London: Penguin.

Epstein, N.B., Bishop, D.S. and Levin, S. 1978: McMaster Model of Family Functioning. *Journal of Marriage and Family Counselling* **3**: 19–31.

Epstein, N.B., Baldwin, L.M. and Bishop, D.S. 1982: *McMaster Clinical Rating Scale*. Providence, RI: Brown University Family Research Program.

Epstein, N.B., Baldwin, L.M. and Bishop, D.S. 1983: The McMaster Family Assessment Device. *Journal of Marital and Family Therapy* **9**: 171–80.

Fog, E. and Fog, M. 1963: Cerebral inhibition examined by associated movements. In Bax, M. and MacKieth, R. (eds), *Minimal Cerebral Dysfunction*, Clinics in Developmental Medicine no. 10. London: Heinemann Medical Books.

Garmezy, N. 1984: Stress resistant children: the search for protective factors. In Stevenson, J.E. (ed.), *Recent Research in Developmental Psychopathology*. Oxford: Pergamon, 213–33.

Goodman, R. 1997: The Strength and Difficulties Questionnaire: a research note. *Journal of Child Psychology and Psychiatry* **38**: 581–6.

Gowers, S.G., Jones, J.C., Kiana, S., Price, D.A. and North, C.D. 1995: Family functioning; a correlate of diabetic control? *Journal of Child Psychology & Psychiatry* **36**: 993–1002.

Gowers, S.G., Harrington, R.C., Whitton, A. *et al.* 1999a: Brief scale for measuring the outcomes of emotional and behavioural disorders in children (HoNOSCA). *British Journal of Psychiatry* **174**: 413–16.

Gowers, S.G., Harrington, R.C., Whitton, A. *et al.* 1999b: Health of the Nation Outcome Scales for Children & Adolescents (HoNOSCA): glossary for HoNOSCA score sheet. *British Journal of Psychiatry* **174**: 428–31.

Graham, P. 1982: Child psychiatry in relation to primary health care. *Social Psychiatry* **17**: 109–16.

Group for the Advancement of Psychiatry 1968: Normal adolescence; its dynamics and impact. New York: GAP.

Gustafsson, P.A., Cederblad, M., Ludvigsson, J. *et al.* 1987: Family interaction and metabolic balance in juvenile diabetes mellitus: a prospective study. *Diabetes Research and Clinical Practice* **4**: 7–14.

Herjanic, B. and Reich, W. 1982: Development of a structured diagnostic interview for children: agreement between child and parent on individual symptoms. *Journal of Abnormal Child Psychology* **10**: 307–24.

Light, D.W. and Bailey, V. 1992: *A Needs Based Purchasing Plan for Child Based Mental Health Services*. London: NW Thames RHA.

McCann, J., James, A., Wilson, S. and Dunn, G. 1996: Prevalence of psychiatric disorders in young people in the care system. *British Medical Journal* **313**: 1529–30.

North, C.D., Gowers, S.G. and Byram, V. 1997: Family functioning and life events in the outcome of adolescent anorexia nervosa. *British Journal of Psychiatry* **171**: 545–9.

Orvaschel, H., Puig-Antich, J. *et al.* 1982: Retrospective assessment of pre-pubertal major depression with the Kiddie-SADS-E. *Journal of the American Academy of Child Psychiatry* **21**: 695–707.

Parry Jones, W. 1995: The future of adolescent psychiatry. *British Journal of Psychiatry* **166**: 299–305.

Parry Jones, W. 1994: History of child and adolescent psychiatry. In Rutter, M., Taylor, E. and Hersov, L. (eds) *Child and Adolescent Psychiatry: Modern Approaches*, 3rd edn. Oxford: Blackwell, 794–812.

Pearce, J. and Holmes, S.P. 1995: *Health Gain Investment Programme: Lead Document for People with Mental Health Problems*, part 4. Nottingham: NHS Executive (Trent).

Pincus, J.H. 1996: The neurological meaning of soft signs. In Lewis, M. (ed.), *Child and Adolescent Psychiatry: a Comprehensive Textbook*, 2nd edn. Baltimore: Williams & Wilkins, 479–84.

Racusin, G.R. and Moss, N.E. 1996: Psychological assessment of children and adolescents. In Lewis, M. (ed.), *Child and Adolescent Psychiatry: a Comprehensive Textbook*, 2nd edn. Baltimore: Williams & Wilkins, 465–78.

Rutter, M. 1967: A children's behaviour questionnaire for completion by teachers: preliminary findings. *Journal of Child Psychology and Psychiatry* **8**: 1–11.

Rutter, M. and Giller, H. 1983 *Juvenile Delinquency*. Harmondsworth: Penguin.

Rutter, M., Tizard, J. and Whitmore, K. (eds) 1970: *Education, Health and Behaviour*. London: Longman.

Taylor, D.C. and Eminson, D.M. 1994: Psychological aspects of chronic physical sickness. In Rutter, M., Taylor, E. and Hersov, L. (eds), *Child and Adolescent Psychiatry: Modern Approaches*, 3rd edn. Oxford: Blackwell, 737–48.

Wallace Crown, S., Cox, A. and Berger, M. 1997: *Health Care Needs Assessment: Child and Adolescent Mental Health*. Oxford: Radcliffe Medical Press.

WHO 1992: *The ICD10 Classification of Mental & Behavioural Disorders. Clinical Descriptions and Diagnostic Guidelines*. WHO: Geneva.

2

Needs assessment in adolescent offenders

LEO KROLL

INTRODUCTION

Professionals use the term 'needs assessment' to describe the population needs, the needs of an adolescent, a family, problems of an individual or a need for adolescent offenders to be punished or be treated. When used in these ways, needs assessment describes the demands or wants of individuals or a community. All of these uses are valid, the Oxford dictionary's initial definition of need being 'circumstances requiring some sort of action'. However, subsequent definitions include 'want, a time of difficulty or crisis, poverty, lack of necessaries'. Because of these different definitions, it is important for professionals to have an agreed understanding of terminology and theory of needs assessment.

A good review of these issues for professionals involved with adult mentally disordered offenders starts with a quote from Royse: 'Needs assessment is considered by experts to be an essential part of mental health planning; unfortunately, almost anything can pass for a needs assessment.' They suggest abandoning the term and substituting 'perspectives on need' which would more accurately describe the various valid perspectives of all concerned (Cohen and Eastman 1997).

This chapter will first describe the definitions and methodology of needs assessment. Second it will review some of the research conducted with adolescent offenders, and finally discuss how needs assessment might be used in research and service development for the care and treatment of adolescent offenders.

DEFINITIONS AND METHOD

Need for healthcare

A perspective of being in need depends on the values, beliefs and knowledge of the individuals involved, which in turn will be based in part on the culture and common views of groups of professionals or society. A need for healthcare should be distinguished from a general need. One definition is 'the ability to benefit in some way from (health) care' (Stevens and Raftery 1994). Another is 'a need is a cardinal (significant) problem that can benefit from an intervention that is not being offered' (Marshall *et al.* 1995).

Other definitions focus on who makes the judgement of need. The Department of Health (DoH 1991) states that 'need' is the requirements of individuals to enable them to achieve, maintain or restore an acceptable level of social independence or quality of life, as defined by the particular care agency or authority. This potentially puts the needs assessment firmly in the hands of professionals, rather than the users or consumers. Demands or wants therefore are not needs, and this distinction has been made in a number of reviews (e.g. Slade 1994). However, researchers have addressed this problem by refining both individual and population needs assessment methods to take into account the different perspectives of clients, carers and professionals (Marshall 1994). The DoH definition also broadens the scope of needs to include social independence, quality of life, and multiple agency involvement. Mental health needs thus become only one aspect of comprehensive needs assessment. This is particularly relevant not only for adults with long-term mental illnesses, but also for adolescents with similar problems or adolescent offenders who may have educational, social, physical and mental health needs.

Population needs assessment

Population-based needs assessment covers a number of areas and is viewed as a 'top-down' method. In a useful review of this area (Stevens and Raftery 1992), the requirements of purchasers and contracting agencies are set out. In particular, it details the areas needed to complete a population needs assessment. These include:

- incidence and prevalence of problems, as measured by diagnosis and severity
- resources, as described by services
- healthcare, quantity, quality and process
- health gain or outcome measures.

There are three main approaches to a population needs assessment: epidemiological, comparative and corporate. A frequently quoted example of the epidemiological approach is the Isle of Wight study by Rutter and colleagues. This, and other studies, demonstrated high rates of disorders but lower rates of families or individuals seeking help from psychiatric services. Many of these families did not see themselves as 'in need' and therefore did not seek help. Wallace et al. (1995) give a good review of an epidemiological approach.

The comparative approach compares areas or services, using various measures such as mortality and morbidity, service utilization, provision and processes, costs and outcomes. Some parts of the HAS review of Child and Adolescent Mental Health Services (HAS 1995), and the survey conducted by Kurtz et al. (1994), use this approach. Hospital comparative 'league' tables are another more controversial example, and need careful interpretation given the different socio-demographic and health characteristics of the populations utilizing services. The comparative approach can be a method to improve quality and quantity of services that have a marginal lack of resources, or where there is consensus that a core service should exist and services are absent or minimal. However, it can also be used to maintain the status quo, especially if the findings suggest a huge national shortfall in resources. A useful review (Hawe 1996) emphasized that needs assessment should be more focused on change, and before embarking on a survey the intentions of the key players should be explored.

The corporate approach integrates aspects of the epidemiological and comparative methods by gathering information from various groups such as purchasing teams, experts, local people in the community, healthcare professionals, other agencies and national executive bodies. There is often a focus on outcomes and effective treatments. Recent reviews emphasize that some children may be in contact with services but not receiving treatment that has been shown to work (Hibbs 1995; BAP 1997). This is particularly relevant in the USA with managed care services scrutinizing what treatments are offered to children and families. However, the effectiveness of treatments can depend on many factors. One review proposed a conceptual comprehensive outcome model that includes aspects of corporate needs assessment (Hoagwood et al. 1996; Jensen et al. 1996). Five domains were suggested: symptoms, functioning, consumer perspectives, environmental contexts, and systems. Using this model, a literature review was conducted of outcome research in children and adolescents. Only 38 studies met criteria that included all five factors. The studies were focused either on treatment trials for specific disorders, or on service evaluation. Studies of conduct disorder and services for adolescent offenders were among those selected. The authors emphasized that the two types of research are following parallel but independent paths, and that there is a need to integrate both types using the proposed model. This could then answer questions about policy and treatment as services become more accountable.

The Oregan initiative is an example of an attempt to put the corporate approach into practice (Ham 1998). Whilst welcomed by some, resources and resource pressures should be owned by all of those involved in the decision-making process. The Oregan study highlighted this as both a strength and weakness. For instance, the concept of ownership is open to misuse, where views of certain groups may be sought, but only as a token gesture by those with ultimate decision-making powers.

Individual needs assessment

Population-based needs assessment is the sum or composite of individual needs assessments. A population needs assessment may give broad information that will have planning and resource implications. However, for an individual with complex problems the clinical team will be more preoccupied in conducting an individual needs assessment. When conducted by a multi-professional team, this is one way of making a comprehensive assessment and treatment plan. This should lead to discussion and decisions between the teams over respective responsibilities, the views of the problems, and coordinated treatment planning. This does not always happen in child and adolescent services. Instead each profession focuses on its area of apparent responsibility. There is an opportunity for each agency to refer the individual to other agencies for problem management, in a belief that this will reduce the severity or resolve the problem faced by the referring agency. The clients may also experience this process, moving from one agency to another and seeking solutions to their problems, depending on their own beliefs and the information given to them by the various agencies. There is a risk that certain individuals will fall between services because of this process. The survey by Kurtz confirmed that this happens; it showed that service provision varied around the United Kingdom, and works in different ways. Although resources are extensive, there appears to be poor coordination, with overlap and isolation. Professionals expressed a good deal of frustration because of poor access to services (Kurtz *et al.* 1994, p. 57).

Adult mental health and associated services have taken steps towards individual needs-led services. A review article (McCrone and Strathdee 1994) suggests that needs rather than diagnoses should be the basis for service planning and resources. Such an approach has identified the many influences that determine individual requirements for services. Needs-related groups rather than diagnosis-related groups may be a more relevant measure to use when planning and assessing services. They also have the advantage of being used as outcome measures because the number of needs being met can be quantified and described. A subsequent study showed that some of the variation in costs incurred for adults with psychoses was due to certain factors, particularly a correlation with patient characteristics and social functioning (McCrone *et al.* 1998).

Risk assessment

Needs assessment and risk assessment are two separate but intertwined processes. A review noted, however, that assessment of dangerousness and the need to address this problem is at the centre of legislative and policy decision-making. In addition the perceptions of the public and media are focused on this area (Cohen and Eastman 1997).

Risk assessment has a theory and methodology separate from needs assessment. It combines statistical data with clinical information in a way that integrates historical variables, current clinical variables, and the contextual or environmental factors. Historical factors include areas such as an abusive or violent upbringing, past offences or violence. Clinical factors include moderating variables that increase or decrease the risk of dangerous behaviour, such as mood disorders, psychoses, drug or alcohol misuse and compliance with treatment. Contextual factors include problem areas such as social or family support, living situation or support from agencies. Some of these clinical and contextual factors are potential areas of need. Therefore needs assessment may both inform and be a response to the risk assessment process (Bailey 2002).

This reciprocal process can be termed 'risk management' where accurate information about the risk assessment, combined with recurrent needs assessment, leads to risk management procedures. For example, an adolescent or adult who has paranoid schizophrenia and is dangerous when untreated is at low risk if treated, housed, free of substance misuse, in contact with services and in a sheltered work placement. A change in need status for the person in one of these potential problem areas (such as losing their job) may affect other areas, thus starting a chain of events that results in the person losing contact with services and treatment. A recurrent needs assessment and risk assessment process should identify changes in problem areas, thus leading to monitoring or intervention as part of risk management.

Research interviews

Needs assessment interviews for individual assessments are based on the 'need for healthcare' assumption. For adults the main instruments were developed initially for those with chronic psychotic conditions living in residential establishments. In adults, the three common research instruments are: the MRC needs for care (Brewin *et al.* 1987), the Camberwell Assessment of Needs (CAN; Phelan *et al.* 1995), and the Cardinal Needs Schedule (Marshall *et al.* 1995). All three are based on first undertaking a comprehensive assessment of problem areas (usually about 20), and then evaluating what treatments or services are being offered to deal with the identified significant problems. The assessment procedures and decision algorithms vary, as do the classifications of need status. The differences are shown in Table 2.1 and include details of the Salford Needs Assessment Schedule for Adolescents (Kroll *et al.* 1999) for comparison.

The psychometric properties of these instruments vary from acceptable to good, and clinical versions of the CAN and Cardinal Needs Schedule have been developed. All three instruments require assessments of the client at interview, but the CAN and the Cardinal Needs Schedule specifically ask for the clients' view of their problems. The CAN allows the differing views of the client and carer to be measured as variation in numbers of needs perceived, whereas the Cardinal Needs Schedule incorporates these perceptions, cooperation with help offered, and carer stress into the algorithm that determines whether a significant problem exists (Marshall 1994). The CAN also includes satisfaction ratings, and asks whether the help is of the right type. The MRC schedule enquires about the right type of help in a more complex way in its nine rating categories. This includes appropriateness of help, and deferment of help because of clinical overload or priorities. The Cardinal Needs Schedule uses client cooperation criteria and ratings of help, such as categories of refused or inappropriate, to determine whether help is appropriate.

All the instruments involve value judgements when dealing with clinical decision-making processes. The Cardinal Needs Schedule limits the variation in value judgments by means of its software-dependent algorithms. All the research teams highlight the subjective aspects of

Table 2.1 *Comparison of assessment procedures*

	MRC need for care	Cardinal Needs Schedule	Camberwell Assessment of Need	Salford Needs Assessment Schedule
Assessment type and instruments	PSE 10 Mini-mental state SBS AIMS Educational attainment Medical questionnaire	Manchester scale REHAB scale Additional information (notes and main carer) Auxiliary questionnaires (drugs, alcohol, mini-mental state, literacy)	3-point severity scale for each problem area	5-point problem severity scale for client and carer interview
Treatments	Glossary of treatments for each area	Computerized glossary of treatments for each area	Ratings of help offered, type and amount, by family and professionals for each area	Computerized glossary of treatments for each area
Algorithms to determine significant problems	Thresholds set on instruments used	Thresholds on single or combinations of instruments used Three criteria used: cooperation, carer stress, severity	Definitions given with 3-point scale, clinical judgement	Thresholds set on client and carer interviews Four criteria used: client cooperation, perception, carer stress and severity
Method of rating	Manual and software algorithm	Software algorithm	Manual, but software for calculating scores	Software algorithm
Need algorithms and ratings made	1 Problems above threshold compared against treatment glossary 2 Nine possible ratings made 3 Algorithm 1 and 2 generates need status	1 Significant problems compared against treatment glossary 2 Five possible ratings made of help 3 Algorithm 1 and 2 generates need status	Needs ratings made on score of 3-point scale Ratings of help needed Effectiveness of help Satisfaction with help	1 Significant problems compared against treatment glossary 2 Five possible ratings made of help 3 Algorithm 1 and 2 generates needs
Need status terminology (equivalent terms given on each line)	1 No need 2 Unmet need (treatment) 3 Met needs (treatment worth continuing) 4 Unmet need (assessment) 5 Future needs 6 Possible needs 7 No need (no meetable need)	1 No need 2 Need 3 PDI (persistent despite intervention) 4 Suspended (assessment phase) 7 No need or in some cases PDI	1 No need 2 Need (unmet) 3 Partially met	1 No need 2 Need 3 PDI (persistent despite intervention) 4 Suspended (assessment phase) 7 No need, or in some cases PDI
Other information	Types of help offered or not offered	Types of help offered or not offered displayed	Help given Help needed Satisfaction with type of help Satisfaction with amount of help	Types of help offered or not offered displayed

PSE, Present State Examination; SBS, Social Behaviour Schedule; AIMS, Abnormal Involuntary Movement Scale.

needs assessments, and that needs vary over time and place; thus longitudinal needs assessments are relevant, both to researchers and clinicians. These instruments have been used in a number of adult groups and settings (Wiersma *et al.* 1998; Stansfeld *et al.* 1998; Hogg and Marshall 1992; Holloway 1991), and have been further developed to cover community samples (Bebbington *et al.* 1996), old age psychiatry (Reynolds *et al.* 2000) and more recently adolescent offenders (Kroll *et al.* 2002a).

RESEARCH WITH ADOLESCENT OFFENDERS

The epidemiological approach

Most needs assessment information is epidemiological, often grouped by type of offence, place of residence, gender, ethnicity and so on. There is much less information using comparative and corporate needs assessment methods at both population and individual levels. A selected summary of epidemiological research is shown in Table 2.2, and some of the studies are described in more detail later in the chapter.

The strategic approach

There are a number of published surveys, often combining instrument development with a survey of service provision. In such studies, details of the survey instrument and method are often scarce. The surveys often focus on specific issues, such as lack of resources, or poor standards of care.

For instance, one study described the healthcare provision in institutions for young offenders (Jameson 1989). They found that 20% had no medical care services, and 40% no medical screening. In addition 50% had no ongoing mental healthcare services. The authors commented that little progress had been made since an earlier study, but that agreed standards of care were to be drawn up by a coalition of 20 national healthcare organizations.

Another study (Brown 1993) reviewed the health needs of incarcerated youths, giving qualitative descriptions of health models adopted by such institutions. Such models include: on-site comprehensive primary and secondary care, on-site limited care, and off-site bought-in care. It describes the standards set by the National Commission on Correctional Healthcare (NCCHC) for institutions, and that accreditation can be sought under the NCCHC. The author also suggests a number of very reasonable views, including a need for detection of conditions (physical and mental health), the need to provide treatment in a consistent and comprehensive manner, and the need for continuity of care once the youth is discharged. An example of an initiative to do this was the awarding of start-up grants in 1990 to eight state–community partnerships

(community size 300,000 to 500,000 people) to develop systems of care to address the needs of youths with serious mental illnesses (England and Coe 1992). Common design features were used, while acknowledging the variation in local government organization in each area. The five main agencies (child welfare, mental health, public health, education, juvenile justice) were involved in this process as well as private health providers. Broadly the philosophy was to establish inter-agency steering committees and a commitment to long-term individualized case management. This case management ideally should coordinate the resources and strategies such as: clinical assessment and management, crises management, therapeutic foster placements and home services to support families directly. In Britain similar approaches have been proposed for child and adolescent mental health services (HAS 1995, p. 114).

Putting proposals into practice is rarely easy. In Britain considerable effort has been devoted to planning for the needs of children who are looked after by social services. A method has been developed (Bullock *et al.* 1995) to conduct some aspects of a corporate needs assessment in a locality. The assessment gives detail about why, how and when to conduct this assessment, as well as how the assessment could be fitted in with a Children's Service Plan. It also suggests that the other agencies – health and education – could conduct parallel surveys so informing and feeding into joint or respective planning of services. For a local authority, often serving a population of about 400,000 people, such an exercise is likely to be more meaningful than national guidlines, though the method clearly takes into account such guidelines and policy frameworks. This method could be applied more specifically for adolescent offenders, in both residential and community settings.

The comparative approach

The national survey by Kurtz *et al.* (1997) provides an overview of the mental health needs of adolescent offenders who are considered to require admission to a secure unit. This survey uses a comparative method focusing on resources, and estimates of numbers of adolescents seen at a national and local level. The postal questionnaires were sent to all services providing care for young offenders. These were CAMHS, forensic psychiatry, social services, youth justice teams, probation services, secure units and young offender institutions. The main areas covered were caseload and case mix, how mental health needs were assessed, what was the response to these needs, relationships between services, and desired availability of services.

Comparing services, there was a wide variation in referrals to secure units, and in the use of psychiatric services. Some services had not made any referrals to secure units, and 40% of CAMHS services had not received any referrals from criminal justice sources. Of more concern was that only 60% of those placed in secure care for more than one

Table 2.2 *Selected summary of epidemiological research*

Author	Location	Sample	Procedure	Findings
McManus et al. (1984)	Correctional residential schools, Michigan, USA	48 male, 36 female, mean age 16.2	Semi-structured interview and SADS DSM-3 diagnoses made	Principal diagnoses: psychoses 3%, schizotypal PD 6%, major affective disorder 15%, dysthymia 3%, borderline PD 37%, substance abuse 13%, conduct disorder 11%, mental retardation 4%
Curry et al. (1988)	North Carolina, USA, community sample	416 males aged 12–16 125 females aged 12–17	Achenbach CBCL compared with norms from mental health	Higher externalizing scores and hyperactivity scores in assaultive group, both males and females. Similar scores on other dimensions of CBCL Categorical comparisons made. Females over-represented in aggressive and cruel cluster
Eppright et al. (1993)	Juvenile detention centre, USA	79 male, 21 female, mean age 14.6	DICA-R, SCID II for personality disorders DSM-3R diagnoses	Conduct disorder in 87%; 9% of this group had no PD, 27% borderline PD (50% of female group), 75% antisocial PD
Gunn et al. (1991)	Nine young-offender institutions, Britain	406 sentenced males (5.3% of all sentenced youth)	CIS Clinical interview schedule ICD-9 diagnoses made	Personality disorders 11.4%, neuroses 4.5%, substance abuse 15.8%, psychoses 0.2%, any diagnosis 33.2%
Maden et al. (1995)	Four young-offender institutions, Britain	206 remanded males (10% of all remanded youth)	Structured clinical interview ICD-10 diagnoses made	Personality disorders 11.7%, neuroses 18.9%, substance abuse 36.4%, psychoses 1.9%, any diagnosis 53.4%
Milin et al. (1991)	Milwaukee Juvenile Court referrals	86 males, 25 females, mean age 15.5 57% repeat offenders	DICA, structured history, DSM-3R diagnoses	81% substance abusers. In this group: psychoses 7%, attention deficit 23%, major depression 18%, obsessive–compulsive disorder 12%, major depression 5%. In remainder, much lower rates of disorder
Kavoussi et al. (1988)	New York, USA, community sample	58 males aged 13–18, mean age 15.3 All sex offenders	SCID, KSADS DSM-3R diagnoses	No diagnosis in 19%, ADD 6.9%, depressed mood 8.6%, alcohol/substance abuse 18.9%
Timmons-Mitchell et al. (1997)	Ohio, USA, two institutions	121 males, mean age 15.9 52 females, mean aged 15.7	DISC in 50 cases SCL90-R in 169 cases MACI (Millon Adolescent Clinical Inventory) 164 cases DSM-3R diagnoses	Score for F > M for SCL90-R. Mental health needs in 24% males, 84% females using SCL90-R. Diagnoses: psychoses 14%, affective disorder 80%, substance abuse 72%, attention deficit 72%, anxiety disorder 62%. Average number of diagnoses per individual = 5

month had their needs assessed. Of this group, only 48% of assessment methods included some aspect of health and mental health assessment. Of individuals assessed, 22% had a mental health need identified. These findings clearly suggest not only a lack of assessment, but also an absence of health and mental health assessment. Overall only 28% of secure units had a health and mental health assessment process, this figure being somewhat worse than 40% receiving screening in the US study (Jameson 1989). In addition all services stated difficulties accessing mental health services, with a shortage of resources and a lack of a working agreement between social services and health in 22% of cases. Mental health expertise within secure units and young offender institutions was lacking, two-thirds of secure units, and just over a third of young offender institutions (YOIs) relying on limited guidelines on who and how to refer individuals to mental health services. Continuity of care into the community was poor.

Given that this was a postal survey with a response rate of 75% (though the response rate for some agencies was poor), the study highlights the gap between presumed need and resources, in terms of both people and organizational strategy. A more individual needs assessment of units and adolescents using a corporate approach would add to this information. This would help define how best to allocate scarce resources. This would be helpful, as the resource implications of this study are high. In addition more detail is required on the needs of a far greater number of adolescent offenders in the community.

The individual approach

INSTRUMENT DEVELOPMENT AND CONTENT

There is little specific literature about needs assessment instruments for adolescent offenders. The standards set by adult needs assessment instruments described in the first section should be considered. The instrument should include comprehensive measures of problem areas, as well as definitions of proposed treatments, and a method of rating whether or not the person is receiving them.

One study reviewed what methods were available to identify needs. It surveyed 50 states in British Columbia (Towberman 1992), asking whether needs assessment instruments had been developed, and what were the risks factors to high-risk offending. Unfortunately it did not give a definition of need, the paper suggesting that need equates with the presence of a problem. Sixteen states said they had formal needs assessment instruments, and 26 states had some method of assessing emotional or psychological problems. The author accumulated the results into nine theoretical factor groupings, which were:

- substance abuse
- emotional/psychological problems (including intellectual deficits)

- violent behaviour
- sexual abuse/deviance
- family problems (including parental substance abuse and criminality)
- peer problems
- educational deficits
- vocational deficits
- physical problems.

Another study describes the development of a questionnaire designed for teenagers with substance abuse and other related problems (McLaney et al. 1994; Knight et al. 2001). The POSIT questionnaire has 139 items and covers ten functional areas:

- substance abuse
- mental health
- physical health
- aggression/delinquency
- social skills
- family relations
- educational status
- vocational status
- peer relations
- leisure.

This was given to 170 males and 64 females, with a mean age of 15.6 in the original study. Convergent and divergent validity was measured against another more comprehensive questionnaire. Test–retest reliability data are available for various groups of teenagers (Knight et al. 2001).

More recently, a screening questionnaire has been developed specifically for use with youths in contact with the youth justice system – the Massachusetts Youth Screening Instrument (MAYSI-2; Grisso et al. 2001). It is a 52-item self-completion questionnaire that generates information about the last few months, in seven areas of functioning. These are:

- drug/alcohol abuse
- anger/irritability
- depression/anxiety
- somatic complaints
- suicidal ideation
- thought disturbance
- traumatic experience.

Its psychometric properties have been studied in a community and in an incarcerated sample of youths aged 12 to 17 (total 1279 youths). Psychometric data are available comparing the MAYSI-2 against other well-established questionnaires (the Achenbach Youth Self Report and the Millon Adolescent Clinical Inventory).

Questionnaire-based instruments do not usually collect sufficient information to conduct a comprehensive needs assessment. Developing a new interview-based assessment instrument and assessing its psychometric properties is a lengthy process. One approach to measure need, rather than presence of a problem or disorder, would be to adapt adult needs assessment instruments. The SNASA was developed in such a way (Kroll *et al.* 1999). It most closely follows the design of the Cardinal Needs Schedule (Marshall *et al.* 1995). It covers areas of functioning relevant to adolescents with each area independent, so that they can be omitted if not relevant. In a similar way, additional problem areas can be added, though the psychometric properties of the new areas would need to be ascertained. The psychometric properties (test–retest and inter-rater) have been studied in 40 adolescents and are acceptable to good. The problem areas covered are:

- self-care skills
- cooking and dietary skills
- physical/health problems
- educational attendance
- educational performance
- weekday occupation
- social relations
- family difficulties
- cultural identity
- destructive behaviour
- aggression to persons
- oppositional defiant behaviour
- sexually inappropriate behaviour
- substance/alcohol abuse
- depressed mood
- self-harm
- psychological problems (anxiety, obsessions, eating/anorexia, hyperactivity/attention problems)
- hallucinations, paranoid ideation
- leisure activities
- living situation
- benefits, money.

The process of rating need status is shown in Figure 2.1. This gives an outline of the assessment, the algorithmic decision-making process and the resulting need categories. A clinical version is available, as well as a shortened form (including a screening questionnaire) developed for use by Youth Offending Teams (Kroll *et al.* 2002b).

There are very few studies investigating teenage self-perception of need. One study (Post and McCoard 1994) surveyed adolescents at a shelter for teenage runaways. These teenagers were asked to develop the instrument in collaboration with professionals. A basic framework was offered drawn from the literature and those working in the area. Seventy-six youths were studied, the mean age being 15. Each of the 44 items developed was given a four-point rating scale. Factor analysis was conducted and three main factors emerged. The first covered external social deviance, including violence perpetrated or received, sexual problems, drugs and alcohol. The second factor was to do with feelings such as depression, fear or suicide, while the third factor focused on communication problems such as with parents, coping with stress, school-related work

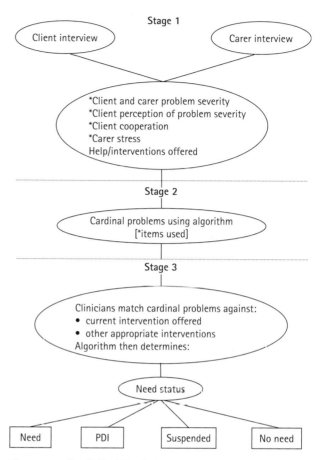

Figure 2.1 *The Salford Needs Assessment Schedule for adolescents.*

or understanding others. There are problems with this factor analysis, not least that the sample size is too small for the total numbers of items. The items themselves are interesting and cover perceived needs with peers, parents, education, sexual development, contraception, delinquency, drugs and alcohol, being victimized, depression, anxiety, fear, self-esteem and suicidal thoughts.

SOCIAL SERVICES ASSESSMENTS

In Britain, social services are required under the Children Act to assess and provide for children in need. The Children Act 1989 states that a child is in need if either (a) he or she is unlikely to maintain, or to have a opportunity of maintaining, a reasonable standard of health or development without provision of services by the local authority, or (b) his or her health is likely to be impaired, or further impaired, without the provision of services, or (c) he or she is disabled. Definitions of health, development and disability are given.

For children and adolescents 'looked after' by social services, assessment and planning is recorded and organized using LAC forms. This involves gathering information from the adolescents and carers. Adolescents may be fostered, be living in residential placements (open or secure), or remanded into custody. These LAC forms have not been developed as research instruments, but they do describe problems, ask what help has been given, and what action will be taken. Details can be collected on why it is not possible or appropriate to offer action at the present time. This would include lack of recognition and cooperation as well as resource pressures, or lack of access to other services. The forms for the adolescents cover: health, education, cultural identity, social relationships, family relationships, emotional problems, behavioural problems and self-care skills. These forms are used for adolescents with complex needs, some needing multi-agency assessment. Such teenagers are known to have high rates of psychiatric disorders (McCann et al. 1996) though this study did not describe their treatment needs. The LAC forms, though useful, do not collect much detail on possible psychiatric or psychological problems.

For young offenders, whether they are looked after or not, youth offending teams are required by the Youth Justice Board to use ASSETT forms. These cover similar areas, including drugs and alcohol, and offending histories past and present. The current version has only a limited mental health assessment. The YJB are considering incorporating an adaption of the Salford Needs Assessment Schedule in order to provide a comprehensive assessment (Kroll et al. 2002b).

The Framework for Assessment of Children in Need (DoH 2000) consists of a range of questionnaires, interviews and standards by which social services can assess children and families thought to be in need. This is particularly so for children under child protection procedures. Three broad domains are covered:

• the individual's needs
• parenting capacity
• environmental factors.

Each domain is then subdivided into particular categories. For example, individual's needs have categories such as emotional, education, and health. Parenting has safety, warmth, and stimulation. Environment has housing, income and community resources. Instruments to measure and assess each category are provided. This framework is applicable to some young offenders, but not to older offenders who are not in the 'looked after' category. These are more likely to be assessed using the ASSETT form by youth offending teams, and by other local agencies depending on their problem profile.

RESEARCH STUDIES

Many researchers use well-established instruments to assess problems, and then infer needs from the results (see Table 2.2). For severe disorders or problems this proxy method may be relatively accurate, especially in incarcerated or residential settings. However, there is little or no detail of psychological treatments offered. These treatments often depend on the person perceiving that he or she has a problem and wants treatment. These factors affect the pathways into and out of psychological services.

Young offenders in custody

Two studies in Britain focus specifically on mental health needs and treatments for males either sentenced or on remand (Maden et al. 1995; Gunn et al. 1991). A third study builds on these, using a similar methodology, but does not detail treatment needs (Lader et al. 2000).

The first two studies used the same methodology and had similar aims: to determine the nature and extent of mental disorders in prisoners or remand prisoners, and determine their treatment needs. Adult males and women were studied as well as young offenders. Because of the very small number of female young offenders, separate data were not given in the final reports. Information was collected via a structured interview, prison records, interviews with the staff, any health records, and previous convictions from the national Home Office index. The interview detailed developmental and childhood history, educational history, drug and alcohol use, gambling, physical problems and psychiatric disorders. ICD 10 diagnoses were made from the interviews. If the person had significant problems, a psychiatric history, a drug or alcohol history, or if the interviewee said he or she needed help, then further questions were asked about treatment. These included who had offered help, what had been done (medical or psychological treatments), the person's motivation for treatment, and expectations of treatment (e.g. unrealistic or realistic). Treatment needs were defined by the research team and grouped into seven categories.

By using this method, it was possible to interview 544 males, 245 females and 206 youths in young offender institutions. For the young offenders (all males), there were 110 who had a psychiatric diagnosis or serious symptoms; 27, however, were judged to not require treatment, and a further 25 required motivational interviewing for substance misuse problems. Six needed transfer to an inpatient hospital bed, and 11 to a therapeutic community. These needs were not being met at the time of the interview. The authors also described the resource implications of these results.

The interview and instruments are not comprehensive needs instruments. Nevertheless the results show the difference between rates of problems and rates of needs. The difference was largely determined by the person's insight and understanding about his or her problems, and the motivation to try deal with these problems. The research also highlights the different rates of disorders and needs in the prison compared to the remand population and has the advantage of using the same methodology and instruments. The results suggest that there are more needs in the remand group.

The third and most recent study used a similar methodology (Lader *et al.* 2000), but does not detail treatment needs. This study (conducted in 1997) reported on incarcerated teenagers aged 16–20. Five hundred and ninety of a possible 632 were interviewed (118 being females, the rest males). The interview covered comprehensive lifestyle (drugs/alcohol), educational and psychiatric problems (schizophrenia and severe depression) and neurotic disorders (anxiety, depression, PTSD, obsessions). Some 20% of this sample had an additional interview focusing on personality disorder and psychoses, 50% were convicted of acquisitive offences, and 20% of violent offences. In general, girls probably were more disturbed than boys; for instance 27% of girls accessed mental health services in the year prior to incarceration compared to 12% of males. The rate of admission to a mental hospital was double for females (9%), compared to males. Of those interviewed, neurotic scores were significantly higher in females.

For the total sample, 60% used drugs, and 25% drank heavily (four times a week). Antisocial personality disorder was found in 80% and paranoid personality disorder in 25%. Psychotic symptoms were present in 10%. Neurotic disorders were found in 52% of remand prisoners and 41% of sentenced offenders. The group had a lower IQ than the general population (quick score of 31 compared to a norm of 42). One-third to a quarter had a longstanding physical complaint. Academic qualifications were few, and only a third were in employment prior to incarceration.

These studies provide cross-sectional information about problems and needs. A longitudinal approach would describe changing needs over times, and be able to assess the effectiveness or treatment or resource provision. Using the Salford Needs Assessment for Adolescents, and other research instruments, the author's group studied the needs of offenders at three time points – entry into secure care, 3 months later, and 1–3 years after discharge. Information about time three is not yet available, but the time one and two data have been published (Kroll *et al.* 2002a). Briefly, 104 boys were studied aged 12–18. Needs were reassessed 3 months later in 97 cases. Some 26% had mild learning difficulties. Psychiatric need was high on admission, particularly with major depressive illness (26%) and generalized anxiety disorder (16%). There were high frequencies of aggression, substance abuse, self-harm, social, family and educational problems and associated needs. For instance, 70% were aggressive and 60% abused drugs or alcohol. Social needs were also prevalent, with 70% having significant problems with social relationships. Educational needs were often unmet, with more than two-thirds having serious educational problems, mainly because they had dropped out of school. The mean number of needs was 8.2 (SD 2.6) on admission, falling to 2.8 (SD 2.4) at 3 months. Domains where needs were met or mostly met after 3 months of admission were: education, substance abuse, self-care, and diet. Domains where the frequency of need fell substantially, but remained

high, were social and family problems, and aggressive behaviours. Psychological needs persisted, particularly depressed mood, anxiety problems, and post-traumatic stress symptoms. The commonest required interventions were psychological assessment, and cognitive behavioural work.

Community studies

Multi-systemic treatment (MST) studies evaluate multi-modal treatments on a more heterogeneous group of adolescents in contact with the service or research group. There are numerous studies now of MST, many with young offenders, though some with other categories of teenagers (Henggeler *et al.* 1998; Henggeler 1999). A brief summary of one such study is described here.

Borduin *et al.* (1995) evaluated MST against individual therapy (IT) in 176 offenders aged 12–17. Two hundred families were referred initially. Inclusion criteria were at least two arrests, living with one parent, and no evidence of psychoses or dementia. One hundred and forty completed treatment and 36 dropped out, an equal proportion from control and treatment groups. Post-treatment assessment was completed on 90% of the sample. The mean number of hours of treatment was 24 hours for the MST group and 29 for the IT group. The MST group received individual and systemic treatments (school, family, peers) in community settings in a flexible manner depending on the different presenting problems. Sessions were held at home or in a community setting. Services were time limited with an aim to empowering parents and adolescents with skills and resources. The research instruments used included the SCL90R, global severity index, revised behaviour problem checklist, perceived family functioning (FACES II), observed family functioning, peer relations inventory, and criminal activity from state records. The instruments were administered again soon after therapy completion. Criminal activity was measured at 4 years after treatment. The results showed significant instrumental changes in scores in the MST group over time in many areas, particularly individual functioning, family functioning (both reported and observed), but not for peer relations. Survival analysis was used (measure being not arrested). At 4 years the overall recidivism rate was 22.1% for the MST group, 71.4% for the IT group, 87.5% for those refusing treatment, and 46.6% for the MST dropouts. The number and type of crimes were also less frequent and serious in the MST group. Moderator variables such as age, sex, ethnic group and number of arrests before treatment did not affect the outcome.

The assessment used in MST is systemic, problem-orientated and goal-focused. It is not dissimilar from a needs assessment, though the researchers usually use questionnaires and other outcome measures to assess problem severity and change over time.

Another study conducted in community and residential psychiatric units described a treatment goal planning method to evaluate the outcome of 276 adolescents treated in four adolescent psychiatric units (Rothery *et al.* 1995). This also used a needs assessment approach. First the authors developed a new adolescent inpatient inventory consisting of two parts.

- The first part covered problems, diagnoses, history, and reason for admission, past treatments by health, education and social services, psychosocial functioning and a detailed statement of treatment goals. The treatment goals consisted of 16 areas divided into four sections: symptomatic improvement, relationship improvement, maturational task accomplishment, and intrapsychic restructuring. These goals are thus a mixture of symptom or behavioural change, and psychological changes, based on a psychodynamic developmental model. On average 7.7 goals were identified per admission (this is somewhat similar to the number of needs identified in adult needs assessment research).
- The second part, completed at discharge, rated outcomes for each of the treatment goals, and a method of coding all treatment interventions.

The treatments were described and consisted of 14 types that could be applied to any of the goals set depending on clinical judgement. No psychometric data are available on this inventory, though it seems to have good face and content validity. The researchers then describe the outcome of the study, and the types of treatments applied for each goal. Of interest is that no single treatment alone was considered a predominant reason for improvement, except for antidepressants and neuroleptic medication. The unit's therapeutic milieu was considered influential in between 18% and 50% of goal outcomes for all 16 areas.

CARE PLANNING AND FURTHER RESEARCH

The relationships between various needs assessment approaches, risk assessment and management are shown in Figure 2.2. Commissioners of services may require a population approach. If so the findings so far suggest that at a population level there is a lack of resources, of strategic planning and coordinated professional work. For agencies working with individuals the comparative may help service planning and development.

For instance, the study by Kurtz and colleagues indicates that services need a brief screening instrument to identify mental health needs in adolescents admitted to

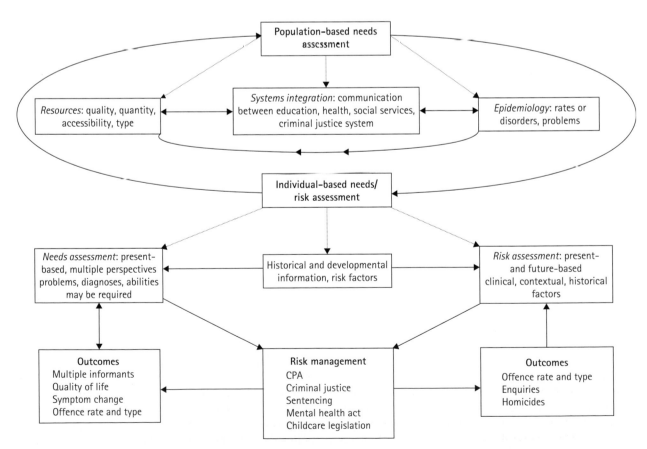

Figure 2.2 *Relationships between various need assessment approaches, risk assessment and management.*

a secure unit. In addition there seems to be a need to have a straightforward comprehensive needs assessment instrument that can be used in a variety of settings and by various professionals (Kroll *et al.* 2002b). Such an instrument could be used at an individual level. First it could be used to plan further detailed assessments and then treatments (e.g. psychiatric, educational and social). Second it could be integrated within risk assessment and management procedures. Third it could be used repeatedly to evaluate outcomes of either the needs assessment or risk management procedure. This type of process has been incorporated into the care plan approach in adult psychiatry (Kingdon 1994).

Some of the poor outcome results of treatment studies on offenders encourage a culture of therapeutic nihilism that is only slowly changing. These poor results may be due to not considering the factors set out in the review by Hoagwood and colleagues described in the first section of this chapter. Using a needs approach could lead to combined observational and intervention studies assessing services, treatments, and individual characteristics. Qualitative and quantitative methods should be used (Swales 1998). This type of programme and research has been proposed for violent adult offenders (Howells *et al.* 1997), particularly embedding psychological treatments within the system being studied, and collaborating closely with those involved directly with the offenders.

REFERENCES

Bailey S. 2002: Violent children: a framework for assessment. *Advances in Psychiatric Treatment* **8**: 97–106.

BAP 1997: British Association of Psychologists Consensus Statement. Child and learning disability psychopharmacology. *Journal of Psychopharmacology* **1**: 291–4.

Bebbington, P.E., Brewin, C.R., Marsden, L. *et al.* 1996: Measuring the need for psychiatric treatment in the general population: the community version of the MRC Needs for Care assessment. *Psychological Medicine* **26**: 229–36.

Borduin, C.M., Mann, B.J., Cone, L.T. *et al.* 1995: Multisystemic treatment of serious juvenile offenders: long-term prevention of criminality and violence. *Journal of Consulting and Clinical Psychology* **63**: 569–78.

Brewin, C.R., Wing, J.K., Mangen, S.P., Brugha, T.S. and MacCarthy, B. 1987: Principles and practice of measuring needs in the long-term mentally ill: the MRC Needs for Care assessment. *Psychological Medicine* **17**: 971–81.

Brown, R. 1993: Health needs of incarcerated youth. *Bulletin of the New York Academy of Medicine* **70**: 208–19.

Bullock, R., Little, M. and Mount, K. 1995: *Matching Needs and Services: The audit and Planning of Provision for Children looked after by Local Authorities.* Dartington Social Research Unit and Support Force for Children's Residential Care.

Cohen, A. and Eastman, N. 1997: Needs assessment for mentally disordered offenders and others requiring similar services. *British Journal of Psychiatry* **171**: 412–17.

Curry, J., Pellisier, B., Woodford, D. and Lochman, J. 1988: Violent or assaultative youth: dimensional and categorical comparisons with mental health samples. *Journal of the American Academy of Child Psychiatry* **27**: 226–32.

DoH (Department of Health, Social Services Inspectorate) 1991: *Care Management and Assessment: Summary of Practice Guidance.* London: HMSO.

DoH (Department of Health) 2000: Framework for Assessing Children in Need and their Families. London: HMSO.

England, M.J. and Cole, R.F. 1992: Building systems of care for youth with serious mental illness. *Hospital and Community Psychiatry* **43**: 630–2.

Eppright, T.D., Kashani, J.H., Robison, B.D. and Reid, J.C. 1993: Comorbidity of conduct disorder and personality disorders in an incarcerated juvenile population. *American Journal of Psychiatry* **150**: 1233–6.

Grisso, T., Barnum, R., Fletcher, K.E., Cauffman, E. and Peuschold, D. 2001: Massachusetts Youth Screening Instrument for mental health needs of juvenile justice youths. *Journal of the American Academy of Child and Adolescent Psychiatry* **40**: 541–8.

Gunn, J., Maden, T. and Swinton, M. 1991: *Mentally Disordered Prisoners.* London: Home Office.

Ham, C. 1998: Retracing the Oregan trail: the experience of rationing and the Oregan health plan. *British Medical Journal* **316**: 1965–70.

Hawe, P. 1996: Needs assessment must become more change-focused. *Australian and New Zealand Journal of Public Health* **20**: 473–9.

Health Advisory Service 1995: *Child and Adolescent Mental Health Services: Together We Stand.* London: HMSO.

Henggeler, S.W., Schoenwald, S.K., Borduin, C.M., Rowland, M.D. and Cunningham, P.B. 1998: *Multisystemic Treatment of Antisocial Behaviour in Children and Adolescents.* New York: Guildford Press.

Henggeler, S.W. 1999: Multisystemic therapy: an overview of clinical procedures, outcomes and policy implications. *Child Psychology and Psychiatry Review* **4**: 2–10.

Hibbs, E.D. 1995: Child and adolescent disorders: issues for psychosocial treatment research. *Journal of Abnormal Child Psychology* **23**: 1–11.

Hoagwood, K., Jensen, P.S., Petti, T. and Burns, B.J. 1996: Outcomes of mental health care for children and adolescents: I. A comprehensive conceptual model. *Journal of the American Academy Child and Adolescent Psychiatry* **35**: 1055–63.

Hogg, L.I. and Marshall, M. 1992: Can we measure need in the homeless mentally ill? Using the MRC Needs for Care assessment in hostels for the homeless. *Psychological Medicine* **22**: 1027–34.

Holloway, F. 1991: Day care in an inner city: II. Quality of services. *British Journal of Psychiatry* **158**: 810–16.

Howells, K., Watt, B., Hall, G. and Baldwing, S. 1997: Developing programmes for violent offenders. *Legal and Criminological Psychology* **2**: 117–28.

Jameson, E.J. 1989: Incarcerated adolescents. *Journal of Adolescent Healthcare* **10**: 490–9.

Jensen, P.S., Hoagwood, K. and Petti, T. 1996: Outcomes of mental health care for children and adolescents: II. Literature review and application of a comprehensive model. *Journal of the American Academy Child and Adolescent Psychiatry* **35**: 1064–77.

Kingdon, D. 1994: Making care programming work. *Advances in Psychiatric Treatment* **1**: 43–6.

Kavoussi, R.J., Kaplan, M. and Becker, J.V. 1988: Psychiatric diagnoses in adolescent sex offenders. *Journal of the American Academy of Child Psychiatry* **27**: 241–3.

Knight, J.R., Goodman, E., Pulerwitz, T. and DuRant, R.H. 2001: Reliability of the Problem Oriented Screening Instrument for Teenagers (POSIT) in adolescent medical practice. *Journal of Adolescent Health* **29**: 125–30.

Kroll, L., Woodham, A., Rothwell, J. *et al.* 1999: The reliability and validity of the Needs Assessment Schedule for Adolescents. *Psychological Medicine* **29**: 891–902.

Kroll, L., Rothwell, J., Bradley, D. *et al.* 2002a: Mental health needs of boys in secure care for serious or persistent offending: a prospective, longitudinal study. *Lancet* **359**: 1975–9.

Kroll, L., Bailey, S., Myatt, T. *et al.* 2002b: The Mental Health Screening Interview for Adolescents. The University of Manchester Child Psychiatry Department and The Adolescent Forensic Unit, Mental Health Services of Salford NHS Trust.

Kurtz, Z., Thornes, R. and Wolkind, S. 1994: *Services for the Mental Health of Children and Young People in England: National Review.* London: Department of Public Health, South Thames REA.

Kurtz, Z., Thornes, R. and Bailey, S. 1997: A study of the demand and needs for forensic child and adolescent mental health services in England and Wales. Mental Health Services of Salford.

Lader, D., Singleton, N. and Meltzer, H. 2000: Psychiatric morbidity among young offenders in England and Wales. London: Office for National Statistics.

Marshall, M. 1994: How should we measure need? Concept and practice in the development of a standardized assessment schedule. *Philosophy, Psychology and Psychiatry* **1**: 27–36.

Marshall, M., Hogg, L.I., Gath, D.H. and Lockwood, A. 1995: The Cardinal Needs Schedule: a modified version of the MRC Needs for Care assessment schedule. *Psychological Medicine* **25**: 605–17.

Maden, A., Taylor, C.J.A., Brooke, D. and Gunn, J. 1995: *Mental Disorder in Remand Prisoners.* Institute of Psychiatry, Home Office Research and Planning Unit.

McCann, J.B., James, A., Wilson, S. and Dunn, G. 1996: Prevalence of psychiatric disorders in young people in the care system. *British Medical Journal* **313**: 1529–30.

McCrone, P. and Strathdee, G. 1994: Needs not diagnosis: towards a more rational approach to community mental health resourcing in Britain. *International Journal of Social Psychiatry* **40**: 79–86.

McCrone, P., Thornicroft, G., Parkman, S., Nathaniel-James, D. and Ojurongbe, W. 1998: Predictors of mental health service costs for representative cases of psychosis in south London. *Psychological Medicine* **28**: 159–64.

McLaney, M.A., Del Boca, F. and Babor, T. 1994: A validation study of the problem oriented screening instrument for teenagers (POSIT). *Journal of Mental Health* **3**: 363–76.

McManus, M., Alessi, N.E., Grapentine, W.L. and Brickman, A. 1984: Psychiatric disturbance in serious delinquents. *Journal of the American Academy of Child Psychiatry* **23**: 602–16.

Milin, R., Halikas, J.A., Meller, J.E. and Morse, C. 1991: Psychopathology among substance abusing juvenile offenders. *Journal of the American Academy of Child Psychiatry* **30**: 569–75.

Phelan, M., Slade, M., Thornicroft, G. *et al.* 1995: The Camberwell Assessment Need (CAN): the validity and reliability of an instrument to assess the needs of people with severe mental illness. *British Journal of Psychiatry* **167**: 589–95.

Post, P. and McCoard, D. 1994: Needs and self-concept of runaway adolescents. *School Counsellor* **41**: 212–19.

Rothery, D., Wrate, R., McCabe, R., Aspin, J. and Bryce, G. 1995: Treatment goal-planning: outcome findings of a British prospective multicentre study of adolescent inpatient units. *European Child and Adolescent Psychiatry* **4**: 209–21.

Reynolds, T., Thornicroft, G., Woods, B. *et al.* 2000: The validity and reliability of the Camberwell Assessment of Need for the elderly. *British Journal of Psychiatry* **176**: 442–52.

Slade, M. 1994: Needs assessment: involvement of staff and users will help to meet needs. *British Journal of Psychiatry* **165**: 293–6.

Stansfeld, S., Orrell, M., Mason, R., Nicholls, D. and D'Ath, P. 1998: A pilot study of needs assessment in acute psychiatric inpatients. *Social Psychiatry, Psychiatry and Epidemiology* **33**: 136–9.

Stevens, A. and Raftery, J. 1992: The purchaser's information requirements on mental health needs and contracting for mental health services. In Thornicroft, G., Brewin, C.R. and Wing, J. (eds), *Measuring Mental Health Needs.* London: Gaskell Press.

Stevens, A. and Raftery, J. 1994: Introduction: concepts of need. In Stevens, A. and Raftery, J. (eds), *Healthcare Needs Assessment,* Vol. 1. Oxford: Radcliffe Medical Press, 13–14.

Swales, J. 1998: The National Health Service and the science of evaluation: two anniversaries. *Health Trends* **30**: 20–2.

Timmons-Mitchell, J., Brown, C., Schulz, C. *et al.* 1997: Comparing the mental health needs of female and male incarcerated juvenile delinquents. *Behavioural Sciences and the Law* **15**: 195–202.

Towberman, D. 1992: National survey of juvenile needs assessment. *Crime and Delinquency* **38**: 230–8.

Wallace, S.A., Crown, J.M., Cox, A.D. and Berger, M. 1995: *Healthcare Needs Assessment: Child and Adolescent Mental Health.* NHS Executive.

Wiersma, D., Nienhuis, F.J., Giel, R. and Slooff, C.J. 1998: Stability and change in needs of patients with schizophrenic disorders: a 15- and 17-year follow-up from first onset of psychosis, and a comparison between 'objective' and 'subjective' assessments of needs for care. *Social-Psychiatry Psychiatry Epidemiology* **33**: 49–56.

3

The assessment and management of risk

CAROL SHELDRICK

THEORETICAL AND CONCEPTUAL ISSUES

Definitions

The *Shorter Oxford English Dictionary* includes in its definition of risk 'danger, exposure to the possibility of loss, injury, or other adverse circumstances'. It also includes the concept of 'a person considered to be a liability or danger or a person exposed to risk'. The definition of danger is similar but also emphasizes the concepts of power and jurisdiction.

It will not be apparent from these definitions why most forensic psychiatrists consider that there has been an important shift, in recent years, in the thinking which used to underlie the assessment of dangerousness.

It is accepted that these concepts must be distinguished from fear (Gunn 1993) and worry (Grounds 1995). However, the main shift in thinking, clinically, has been from that of dangerousness to risk. Dangerousness is a subjective concept of a stable and consistent quality existing within individuals. Risk, on the other hand, is not a static entity, but a combination of factors each of which are not necessarily dangerous in themselves, which fluctuate over time and which may be modified or managed (Gunn 1993, 1996; Pollock and Webster 1990; Steadman *et al.* 1993).

The reconceptualization of risk

Steadman *et al.* (1993) have urged a reconceptualization to move the focus from dangerousness to that of risk. They suggest that the main points are:

- Move away from a focus on the legal concept of dangerousness to the decision-making concept of risk.

- Leading decision-makers and researchers to consider prediction issues as being on a continuum rather than simply being a dichotomy (yes/no).
- Shift from a focus on one-time predictions about dangerousness for the Court to ongoing, day-to-day decisions about the management and treatment of mentally disordered persons.
- Balance the seriousness of possible outcomes with the probabilities of their occurrence based on specific risk factors.

For practitioners the most important points are that predictions should not be on an all or none basis, and that these should cover the short term only, thereby allowing ongoing decisions about management and treatment.

It must be borne in mind that there is often pressure from professionals and the Courts to make long-term predictions of risk and this should be resisted. Carson (1996) usefully argues that psychiatrists should not make assessments or predictions of risk, for Court or other purposes, unless they can rely upon, or control, the following:

- the length of time over which their risk prediction is supposed to be based
- the conditions, such as the level of resources, that will be available to implement that risk decision
- the provisions for monitoring any risk decision that they have organized so that the decision can be put to an end at an early stage if that proves necessary.

Issues about prediction

The question usually asked is that of the risk that individuals pose to others. However, these individuals are also likely to be vulnerable to other forms of risk, for example self-harm, self-neglect or exploitation by others (RCP 1996).

Forensic psychiatrists are commonly asked to make assessments of risk, perhaps because they are trained to operate under mental health legislation. It should be borne in mind that these sorts of predictions also have to be made on a day-to-day basis by many other disciplines too, for example psychologists, social workers, probation officers, nurses and judges. The fact that so many different disciplines may be involved in this form of decision-making can be turned to advantage since different professionals can contribute in different ways, though it is important that any one professional sticks strictly to the limit of his or her skills.

Problems in the prediction of risk

A problem, often not emphasized in the literature, is the fact that professionals attempt to make predictions on the basis of sometimes one, at the best very few, incidents of extreme violent behaviour; i.e. low-frequency behaviour. There is a danger, therefore, that one cannot make a better prediction than that provided by chance (Steadman 1980). Practitioners are often not aware of higher frequency behaviours, whether or not they are severe because they do not come to their attention. The MacArthur Foundation (1996) have found, however, that if, in addition to arrest rates, information is obtained about violent incidents from self-reports, collateral informants and hospital records, there is a statistically significant increase in the number of violent incidents which can be recorded.

Studies looking for factors predictive of risk have been very restricted, usually involving hospitalized males with a history of previous violence or with those who have been institutionalized as patients for considerable periods of time and released into the community (Steadman and Keveles 1972; Steadman and Cocozza 1974). This is not only a limiting factor when assessing adults, but even more so for adolescents, on whom there has been no systematic risk research undertaken. The most difficult adolescents may have been placed in conditions of security, but usually within the childcare system, and not often within a hospital setting. However, the factors that appear to be significantly associated with future violence from these studies can also be assessed in adolescents.

In the large community study of Cocozza and Steadman (1976) it was also found that for every patient who met the cut-off point on their Legal Dangerousness Scale and who committed a violent offence, two did not. The best statistical strategy for predicting violence would be to assume that none of them is dangerous or, in order to reduce the total error rate (i.e. false positives and false negatives), to say that none of them would be violent again. Of course this assumes that all errors are of equal importance and there should be no attempt to weight or cost different kinds of

mistakes (Monahan 1981). The result of this is that, because of the responsibilities involved by professionals making judgements about risk, they tend to be cautious about their prediction and over-predict rather than under-predict the risk that any one individual poses.

The studies referred to have produced results of probability about populations. This does not really help when deciding whether or not an individual will behave violently, during a given period (Cocozza and Steadman 1974; MacArthur Foundation 1996). Actuarial statistics do not provide helpful guidance in this matter. In addition the studies focus on static, historical factors which limit the scope for taking into account such factors as changes over time and responses to treatment interventions.

New research

Having recognized these problems, Steadman *et al.* (1993, 1994) have set about designing a 'new generation of risk assessment research' – the MacArthur Risk Assessment Study. It is based on a study of adult patients who have been admitted to hospital, but not prison, for short periods and followed up in the community. As stated these factors put some limitations on its use for adolescents who have not been hospitalized. Another problem with this study is that emphasis is placed on risk factors which are thought to lead to untoward consequences, rather than looking at those that ameliorate harm, or even lead to a successful outcome. Clearly any assessment and management plan needs to take these possible factors into account too.

Although many of the results of the study are not yet in published form there are indications as to which aspects of the information are of predictive power (see the summary at the end of the section on a model of risk assessment). Of clinical use in an assessment is the summary of the cue domains in the study, which cover most of the factors that any thorough assessment should encompass. The 'dispositional' domain includes demographic, personality and neurological variables. The 'historical' domain includes significant events that have been experienced by the individual in the past, for example within the family, education and work situations, as well as the presence of a past history of psychiatric treatment and offending. The 'contextual' domain includes indices of current social supports, networks, and stress, as well as access to weapons. The final, 'clinical', domain includes diagnoses, psychiatric symptoms, drug and alcohol abuse and level of functioning.

Previously pessimistic views about the accuracy of risk prediction are changing to a more optimistic approach in which it is felt that some prediction of risk is possible. By using the principles of the decision-making concept of risk it is possible to conceptualize the risks that a person poses in specified circumstances, rather than simply asking if a person is dangerous.

Table 3.1 *Cue domains in the MacArthur risk assessment study*

Dispositional factors	Historical factors	Contextual factors	Clinical factors
Demographic	*Social history*	*Perceived stress*	*Axis I diagnosis*
Age	*Family history*	*Social support*	*Symptoms*
Gender	Child rearing	Living arrangements	Delusions
Race	Child abuse	Activities of daily living	Hallucinations
Social class	Family deviance	Perceived support	Symptom severity
Personality	*Work history*	Social networks	Violent fantasies
Personality style	Employment	*Means of violence* (e.g. guns)	*Axis II diagnosis*
Anger	Job perceptions		Functioning
Impulsiveness	*Educational history*		Substance abuse
Psychopathy	*Mental hospitalization history*		*Mental hospitalization history*
Cognitive	Prior hospitalizations		Prior hospitalizations
IQ	Treatment compliance		Alcohol
Neurological impairment	*History of crime and violence*		Other drugs
	Arrests		
	Incarcerations		
	Self-reported violence		
	Violence toward self		

Reproduced from Monahan, J. and Steadman, H.J. (eds) 1994: *Violence and Mental Disorder: Developments in Risk Assessment.* London: University of Chicago Press, 303; with permission from the editors and publishers.

In the case study at the end of this chapter, it would not have been predicted that X would become involved in instigating the index incident. However, even by the time he came to Court, having become increasingly out of control, he posed a risk in certain situations only. This was when his precise whereabouts were not known, when he was mixing with an alienated peer group, and when abusing alcohol and drugs. Identifying these factors then allowed decisions about his management and treatment.

Violence and psychosis

In practice very few adolescents assessed for the risk that they represent are psychotic. Probably more common phenomena are the possible presence of prodromal symptoms and the emergence of vague, poorly clarified psychotic symptoms, as well as a reluctance on the part of psychiatrists to make a diagnosis of psychosis in this young age group. In the case study X did not appear to be suffering from a psychotic illness, but the possibility of this developing in the future could not be totally ruled out. The importance of recognizing, or failing to recognize, psychotic illness is a major factor influencing risk management. There is a body of research looking at the links between violence and psychosis, some of it relatively recent, although most of it has been undertaken on adults.

Taylor and Parrott (1988) found that, in striking contrast to the indicators of general delinquency, evident in childhood and adolescence, a career of violence was most likely to have started after the onset of schizophrenia or other psychosis, the most usual pattern being for the violence to emerge 5–10 years after the first documentation of symptoms.

Wilkins (1993) studied the records of over 1000 children and teenagers admitted to the Bethlem Royal Hospital during the nineteenth century. Delusions were significantly more common in boys than girls. The unexpectedly high overall rate, compared with that which would be expected today, related more closely to the very high rate of dangerousness or suicidal ratings than with any other factor which offered an explanatory hypothesis.

Taylor (1985), in the Brixton Prison remand study, asking about motivation for violence found that one reason given was feeling 'driven'. 'Drive' was almost invariably related to delusions, although the men did not always recognize their beliefs as disordered. The delusions most likely to be associated with 'drive' and violent offending are a related cluster of passivity delusions, now known as the 'threat/control override' (TCO) symptoms (Link and Stueve 1994). These are, essentially, passivity delusions, thought insertion and persecutory delusions and have been found to be very significantly associated with violence (Link and Stueve 1994; Swanson *et al.* 1996). Taylor *et al.* (1994) have developed a scale to rate delusions in more detail, with particular reference to their potential for influencing action. The Maudsley Assessment of Delusions Schedule (MADS) measures delusions along nine dimensions. The factors associated with acting on a belief included the seeking of information to confirm or refute the belief, alleged finding of evidence to support the belief, the ability to accommodate hypothetical contradiction into the belief system, and sadness, anxiety or fear induced by the belief (Buchanan *et al.* 1993).

The literature appears to be consistent in refuting the importance of auditory hallucinations in relation to violence, although the situation may possibly be different for hallucinations of taste or smell when they occur in conjunction with delusions of being poisoned (Taylor 1995). Command hallucinations have attracted much interest but results about the significance of these are conflicting. Studies by Hellerstein *et al.* (1987) and McNiel (1994) show no association between command hallucinations and violence, although the MacArthur study (1996) did. Although it is not clear what the common feature of the 'command' is, it appears likely to be associated with an auditory hallucination instructing the individual to commit a violent act.

A MODEL FOR RISK ASSESSMENT

General issues

It is important to bear in mind that no one factor predicts that violent behaviour will occur and, as with the medical model of disease, the higher the loading of adverse factors the greater the likelihood of an adverse event occurring. As already indicated, the importance of ameliorating factors also needs to be taken into account. Assessments of risk in suicidal patients are common practice in child psychiatry and those concerning the risk that an individual may pose to others are similar, but with a slightly different emphasis.

Professionals must use their skills to get as much detailed information as possible. This need for detailed history-taking was emphasized by Scott (1977) and the necessity of collecting together many small pieces of evidence was made in the inquiry by Clothier *et al.* (1994) into the Beverly Allitt case. This clinical impression has been confirmed more objectively by the MacArthur study (1996), as already pointed out.

Unfortunately the practitioner is often asked to make an assessment of risk in a short period of time, because of pressures on other professionals to make quick decisions. This should be resisted where possible, or the limitations in any assessment such as this made clear. In fact detailed assessments of this kind usually take quite a long time and, if possible, the time is best divided between several interviews, since some conditions and information gained will change over time.

It is all too easy for a busy practitioner to minimize warning signals and signs of relapse. Bowden (1997) warns against ignoring these, arguing that this is an active, not neutral action, whilst Gunn (1996), in analysing some of the inquiries of cases that have ended in death, makes a similar point and warns of the dangers of re-diagnosing difficult patients, usually as having a personality disorder, and then rejecting them.

An approach to risk assessment

In setting about the task of data collection it is suggested that much of what needs to be collected is included in

Table 3.2 *Detailed analysis of the index offence and past offending*

Index offence	Past offending
Seriousness	Juvenile record
Nature and quality	Number of previous arrests
Victim characteristics	Convictions for violence
Intention and motive	Cautions
Role in offence	Self-reported offending
Behaviour after offence	Past behavioural problems:
Attitude to offence	Violence
Victim empathy	Self-harm
Compassion for others	Firesetting
	Cruelty to animals
	Cruelty to children

Look for: situations, triggers, frequency, severity, trends over time

Table 3.1, but that it will not necessarily be obtained, or organized, in that order in clinical practice.

It is of importance to make a detailed analysis of the index offence, as well as any past history of officially recorded offending and certain other behaviours of concern (Table 3.2). As in the assessment of suicidal behaviour, it is important to bear in mind that once an individual has moved from a position of thinking and talking about violence to one where the person has acted it out, the risk of doing so again in the future is greatly increased.

THE INDEX OFFENCE

It can be a subjective matter to assess the seriousness of an offence, but the Criminal Justice Act 1991 gives guidance as does the MacArthur Foundation Study (1996) which categorizes seriousness of violence into two main levels.

- Level 1 is the more serious and consists of violence where a weapon has been used; where a person has been threatened with a weapon in the hand; where sexual assault of the victim has taken place; and any other violence with injury, such as bruises, cuts, broken bones/teeth, stab/gunshot wounds, and/or death.
- Level 2 is less serious and includes the throwing of an object; pushing, grabbing or shoving; slapping; kicking; biting, or choking the victim; and hitting with a fist or object, but where there has been no injury to the victim.

It will be apparent, to practitioners, that even some of level 2 behaviours are serious in nature, but these two levels give a starting point for assessment.

For a further analysis of the nature of the offence there may be other aspects of concern. Bizarre aspects may suggest mental illness (Satten *et al.* 1960) or severe degrees of personality disorder (Britain 1970; MacCulloch *et al.* 1983). Caution needs to be applied when considering such personality characteristics in children and adolescents, however, since they may not be enduring and may not lead on to the development of a personality disorder (Scott

1977). In the case study later, the victim was subjected to both levels 1 and 2 of violence. In addition he was treated in a cruel manner, with threats to his life made over a lengthy period (48 hours).

Victim characteristics may indicate whether or not a perpetrator chooses a much more vulnerable individual to target. In the case study the victim, though of similar age, was of low intellectual ability and had been 'statemented' as having special educational needs. Another important aspect for consideration is whether a replacement victim is likely to be found. Listing potential future victim(s) can be usefully incorporated into the management plan, with a view to minimizing future risk.

Intent can be extremely difficult to assess (Briscoe 1990) but it is, nevertheless, an important issue to attempt to clarify, since it may link in with the attitude to the offence and empathy for the victim.

An individual's role in the offence can be considered with respect to that occurring during the offence as well as afterwards. It is useful to ascertain whether the individual being assessed took on the role of a follower or leader, and to what extent he or she was influenced by others. In the case study X was the leader, though it appeared that his two peers joined in willingly. In looking at the behaviour after the offence it is useful to ascertain whether humane feelings were shown – whether or not the individual tried to repair the damage, seek help, relieve suffering, or whether their own needs for escape or concealment were dominant. In the case study the victim made his own escape, but no attempt was made by X to deal with his distress during the 48 hours of captivity.

The common practice of looking for evidence of remorse in relation to the current offence is not a good criterion, for after a horrifying deed there are many protective mechanisms, including amnesia and denial, which may be mistaken for callous indifference. On the other hand, offenders, when being assessed, may make great efforts to impress the interviewer with an ability to show remorse for the victim, when it is not genuinely felt. The situation is more difficult in the case of young adolescents, where any assessment of victim empathy must occur in the context of their emotional and developmental status. It might be of more use to assess the capacity for an individual to show compassionate feelings for others, particularly those who may become a future victim. In the case study X showed no emotion throughout the interview, including discussion about the index incident; he could justify it, and only showed limited concern for the victim's feelings.

PAST OFFENDING

Three other factors can be elicited in the history taken from the individual (Cocozza and Steadman 1976):

- the presence of a juvenile record, suggesting an early age of onset of offending

- the number of previous arrests, giving an indication of the frequency of offending
- the presence of convictions for violent crimes.

It is essential that this history be corroborated by the police and/or the Central Criminal Records Office. These factors are useful in that they can add data which begins to build up a description of the situations in which offending occurs, elicit specific triggers, and quantify the frequency and trends over time.

Self-report studies show that much offending goes unrecorded (Sheldrick 1994). Ascertaining whether the young person has 'cautions' or other, self-reported, offending is important. X did not have a formal history of offending, but had received three cautions, as well as having a more extensive history of stealing and firesetting.

PAST BEHAVIOURAL PROBLEMS

It is important to ascertain whether there has been a history of behavioural disturbance at home, at school, or in the community. This may be ascertained from parents or other professionals and, if the indications are there, past records from schools or child psychiatric services should be obtained.

The MacArthur Foundation (1996) has found that a past history of violence is one of the most important factors in being associated with future violent behaviour, in group studies at least. So particular attention needs to be paid to this aspect of history-taking. As already stated, it is important to assess whether or not there is a history of violence/harm *towards* the individual. X had a history of cutting his arms and of jumping in front of a car.

Several authors, including Hellman and Blackburn (1966), reported finding that a combination of enuresis, firesetting and cruelty to animals may predict later violence. Whilst practitioners would not now put any weight on enuresis in predicting later violence, other behaviours such as firesetting, cruel or sadistic behaviour to animals and children would carry more clinical weight, particularly if seen in the context of severe behavioural disturbance of early onset. Children who are cruel to animals have often shown a prior history of an excessive interest in keeping and caring for animals, and likewise a premature interest in children and caring for them may precede cruelty to young infants and children. X had a history of behavioural problems, both at home and at school from his junior school years, including firesetting.

Other important areas to assess are the personal history, upbringing, and contextual, clinical and protective factors (Table 3.3).

PERSONAL HISTORY

It had been assumed that aggressive offending might be related to personality type, and show a higher heritability than non-aggressive offending, which was thought to be

crime, to desist, or reach significant turning points in their life (Farrington 1995; Sampson and Laub 1993). Important factors that have been identified are success in education and the workplace, as well as giving up delinquent peers and establishing a stable relationship with a partner. Hoge *et al.* (1996), looking specifically for risk and protective factors in adolescent offenders, also found relevant protective factors to include the effective use of leisure time and a positive response to authority.

At the time of initial assessment, X did not show any of the main protective factors. He had been offered some therapeutic input in the past, but had not felt able to continue with this and his first placement in care had not been a success. By the time of his trial, however, he was motivated to receive education and therapeutic help and an appropriate placement had been found so that moves to a secure, then open, structured child care placement allowed work to be undertaken on all of the areas identified above.

Summary

The assessment of risk is a detailed and lengthy process and there is no magic in assembling the data. There is no one factor that predicts future risk and the larger the constellation of the factors outlined the greater the likelihood of future risk. The most important single factors associated with future risk appear to be alcohol and drug use, and the personality traits of anger and psychopathy. Hyperactivity, if present as a comorbid feature, is important as is a past history of violence, of either high frequency and/or associated with cruelty or sadism. In the presence of a psychotic illness, TCO delusions are particularly important. Other factors of importance are factors which are related to resilience and which open up the possibility of creating 'turning points' in an individual's life, for example good school and vocational achievement, having positive peer relations, and having a stable relationship later in life. The more protective factors that can be identified the greater the resilience to other, adverse factors.

THE MANAGEMENT OF RISK

General principles

Risk is a matter of probability and cannot be eliminated. It can be thoroughly assessed and carefully managed, but outcomes can never be guaranteed. As stated already, assessments need to be undertaken on a short-term basis and be subject to frequent review if effective management is to occur.

In order to manage risk it is necessary to respond as rapidly as possible to concerns about individuals thought to represent a risk. These concerns may be raised by friends and family of the individual or by other professionals. It is, therefore, important to consult widely whilst undertaking the assessment and devising a management plan. Having identified the risk of dangerous behaviour there is then a professional responsibility to take decisions to ensure that the risk is reduced and managed effectively. Whilst it is essential to obtain information based on thorough history-taking, in emergencies it might be necessary to make immediate, short-term decisions based on limited information. In this situation it is better to err on the side of caution, bearing in mind that it is usually easier to reverse an over-cautious decision than an incautious one.

The management plan

Usually the first decision to be made is whether or not the adolescent can be managed safely in the community or requires to be admitted for residential input, either in an open or locked setting. Factors determining the decision about the level of security will include the seriousness of any previous violent behaviour, and the expected duration of risk from this behaviour. As already discussed, only a few adolescents will be considered to be psychotic or showing prodromal symptoms and in these cases resources within the health service will be required. For the majority of young people the resources of the childcare system will be more appropriate. However, factors which determine which sector to use are the type of psychiatric diagnosis made, its severity and prognosis, as well as the range of therapeutic services available. Although the legislation differs for the use of the two systems, principles are the same when considering the use of community, open and secure settings and whether on a voluntary or detained basis. The level of security applied should always be the minimum level compatible with safety and good management. Excessive caution – putting adolescents in greater degrees of security, or retaining them there for longer than is absolutely necessary – is bad practice, as is the case for adults (Gunn 1993).

Not only is the degree of security to be determined but also the level of supervision and support available. This should be considered for every level of security and is an essential element of management. Supervision depends on consent and its presence, or absence, respectively, may determine the level of security required. Support may come from family, friends and professionals and the appropriateness and level of this may also determine the level of security required.

In the case study later, it was appropriate that X should not be placed immediately within a secure setting as, although the index offence was serious in nature, it could not have been predicted with any accuracy that it, or anything similarly dangerous, would occur again. An open placement in the childcare system was not successful, however, since X's behaviours were not manageable and showed an escalation, particularly in terms of their bizarre presentation. It is not clear why a return home was agreed to, except that this was the wish of X and his mother. Although it then became known that X was breaching his curfew and was missing from home this did not, unfortunately, trigger a reassessment of the risk that he represented to himself and others and bring about a change of management/care plan to ensure that an adequate level of supervision and security was provided. This only occurred after X had put himself and others at an unacceptable level of risk and the Court had insisted that the local authority take a more active role in his care. The initial phase then necessitated placement within conditions of security but only for a relatively short period of time, helped because X was motivated to cooperate and because the next, open placement was well structured. Once the situation was stabilized it was then possible not only to reduce the risk that X represented to himself and others, but also for him to benefit from other aspects of the care programme, which addressed his care, educational and therapeutic needs.

The reduction of risk

A thorough assessment having been undertaken, and having ensured that the adolescent and any potential victims are safe, it is then necessary to formulate a treatment plan, which can be incorporated into the total management plan. It will be necessary to make a decision as to which of the various factors associated with future risk can be changed, bearing in mind those protective factors, or strengths, that can be built on too. Rather than just aiming to reduce offending behaviours, a broader and more positive approach to treatment and management can be achieved in this way. It is also important to consider the time between reassessments, setting up contingency plans to intervene earlier if things go wrong.

As stated in the introduction, rather than asking if a person is dangerous, one can conceptualize the risks that a person poses in specified circumstances. All-or-none decisions are avoided and a plan of management is drawn up to modify risks and build on strengths, thereby ensuring flexibility. Short-term predictions allow management by means of a series of steps. A single assessment is of initial use but a risk path involves taking small, rather than large, steps which can be retraced if necessary, thereby making management a continuous process.

Steadman *et al.* (1993) argue that, of the four domains in the risk assessment study (Table 3.1), only two – the contextual and clinical ones – are open to modification, and therefore to risk management. They argue that factors within the dispositional and historical domains cannot be changed. This is unduly pessimistic since most clinicians feel that they can tackle several of the factors subsumed in these domains. For example, psychological interventions can be offered for anger control; previously undiagnosed neurological impairments may be open to therapeutic intervention; work can be undertaken with the family and individual to address damage experienced from past rearing and abuse within the family; and educational and vocational opportunities should be open to intervention. In all of this it is important to capitalize on the potential for growth in adolescence.

Although X had been identified as having problems from junior school age (i.e. at 8 years) no specific intervention was offered to him or his family. He was offered input at the age of 13, after disclosing his sexual abuse, but only attended one session because he found the work too painful. It was only once X had been stabilized, after his trial, that it was possible to oversee his mental state, including acts of self-harm, though this did not require any specific psychiatric intervention. Monitoring of any return to substance or alcohol abuse was possible as well as ensuring that he was not keeping or carrying any weapons. He was offered good quality care that had been absent during his time at home. His school work had deteriorated from the time of junior school and he had received no education from the age of 13. Because X was motivated, it was possible to reintroduce him to education, initially in a small group setting, but with a view to being integrated into a college of further education. Because he was rarely absconding it proved possible to allow X increasing freedom in the community, on a graded basis, as well as to encourage the development of more normal peer relationships, with the aim of introducing him to local social activities for other kinds of adolescents living in the community. X was then introduced to sessions of anger management work, with subsequent cognitive therapy and counselling for his past abusive experiences at home. Longer term planning was to include appropriate college education and supportive accommodation in the community, if reviews showed that overall progress was being made.

Communication of information

In all cases both the assessment and the management plan must be adequately recorded. These should preferably be in typewritten form but, if handwritten, must be legible so that all professionals can work from them. If the resources considered necessary to fulfil the management plan are not available and a compromise plan is adopted, both plans must be recorded (RCP 1996). The management plan should include a clear record of the role and responsibilities of each professional involved, who is the key worker, and what the contingency plans should be if any concerns arise. Procedures for monitoring the plan and reviewing it should be recorded, including the date of review. Such procedures are well established in the field of child protection and are also probably better worked out for suicidal patients than for those representing a risk to others.

Outcomes should be shared with those who are concerned with the implementation of the plan and this may involve the establishment, and maintenance, of links with other agencies. It is important to share the right amount of information with those who need to know if multidisciplinary and interagency working is to function effectively. This is particularly important if a case is handed on to new workers. Where professionals from more than one agency are involved, the adolescent needs to be told that some sharing of information is necessary. Information can be shared with someone else with the individual's consent; on a 'need to know' basis, when the recipient will be involved with the individual's care or treatment; and, in some cases, if the need to protect the public outweighs the duty of confidence to the individual (DoH 1996; GMC 1993).

SUMMARY

There is no quick, easy answer to the assessment and management of risk and it is the attention to good, detailed clinical practice that is of overriding importance. Inquiries into the disasters that have occurred when adult mentally disordered offenders have been released into the community have emphasized this too, the findings being just as relevant to adolescents whether or not they are suffering from a psychotic illness. Important features to emerge from these inquiries include:

- a failure to respond to reported episodes of violence
- poor record-keeping and communication
- a tendency to take a cross-sectional, rather than a long-term view of the individual and his or her behaviours (Gunn 1996; Petch and Bradley 1997).

APPENDIX: CASE STUDY

The personal characteristics of this case have been changed to prevent identification. A 15-year-old boy (X) was charged, with two others, of kidnapping and actual bodily harm (ABH). He, together with his co-defendants, entered a guilty plea of ABH, only.

Assessment (as from Tables 3.1 and 3.2)

Background information was obtained by interviewing X and his mother, as well as from copies of the witness statements and reports of his first placement in care. He had not been receiving any education for three years and no school reports were available, nor was there any record available from the local clinic where he had been seen for treatment, on one occasion.

INDEX OFFENCE

X, together with three other boys, spent time away from home with money given to him by his mother. When in the house of a friend, the victim (to be) was thought by X to have stolen his money. X then initiated physical attacks on the victim intermittently over 48 hours, and was joined by his two other friends in these, before the victim finally escaped. During the index period, X held a knife to the victim's throat and fired an unloaded air rifle at his head. All three boys made threats to kill the victim in various ways, although there appear to have been lengthy periods when the victim was not threatened or hurt at all. The victim was of similar age to the three perpetrators, but was of low intellectual ability.

With regard to the index incident, X explained that the victim had stolen his money and that this 'was a good enough reason' for the assault, adding that the victim 'had wanted to stay – we were friends most of the time'. He felt that he could not remember everything clearly, saying that his mind 'goes blank' in a fight. Despite this the witness statements showed that he gave the police, as well as the assessor, full details of extreme violence perpetrated against the victim (without any show of emotion). He felt that the victim probably felt scared, and stupid 'to have done it, because he would get a beating up'. X said that he did not think that his victim deserved what he got and knew that he was afraid to go out of his house now. X was expecting to be a victim himself if he ended up in the prison service.

OTHER OFFENDING AND BEHAVIOURAL PROBLEMS

X had no official offending history but had received two cautions for stealing and one for criminal damage, for setting a fire at his school, at the age of 12½ years. At interview X admitted to a history of stealing and using the money for cigarettes. He described the fires that he had lit as accidents, despite having received a caution for one of them.

X did well until in junior school, until his father came out of prison and was violent to his wife. X became spiteful to his sister and started firesetting at home; he also began stealing from home and local shops and his school work deteriorated. At secondary school he was defiant, had difficulties with his peers and became violent to them, his mother and siblings, after disclosing his sexual abuse when aged 12 years. He was suspended from school several times before being excluded at the age of 13. He became increasingly out of control of his mother and ran away from home several times, staying at the home of a friend. From this time he was not sleeping well, was crying and talking of wanting to die. He cut his arms at night. At 13½ years his mother found a knife under his pillow.

PAST HISTORY

X was of average intelligence. After being excluded from school he received no further education.

X had lived at home for most of his life, claiming that his mother was violent (punching him). His father was violent towards the mother and is reported to have thrown X across the room when he was 3 years of age. He had served many custodial sentences for violent offences. The parents separated after eight years. Mother's next partner had a history of alcohol abuse and violence towards the mother, though this was less severe than that experienced in the first relationship. There was a 2-year-old son from this relationship and a 12-year-old sister from the first, who discovered X being sexually abused by his maternal grandfather. The abuse included anal intercourse between the ages of 5–12 years.

CONTEXTUAL AND CLINICAL FACTORS

Without adult supervision X increasingly began to mix with a delinquent peer group, though it was not until he was breaching his bail conditions that he began to abuse alcohol and drugs (see below). His mother removed the knife that he had under his pillow, but was unaware that he also had one in the bag that he regularly carried with him.

At interview X was pleasant but showed no sign of emotion. He was not hyperactive. He said that he had girl friends from the age of 12 years, only admitting to interests and fantasies that appeared to be within the normal range. He described, with some pressure, vivid symptoms of post-traumatic stress disorder (PTSD) for his own 'rape' and for the index incident. He admitted carrying a knife for a year in his bag and having one under his pillow in order to protect himself from his grandfather. X admitted that he was often low, with crying, and often thought about killing himself. He readily talked about his self-injurious behaviours and also said that he had once tried jumping in front of a car. He described hearing the voices, possibly of two males, from the age of 11. They would call him saying 'X, come here we're going to get you – you hurt someone, they're going to hurt you.' He said that they had made him run through the local shopping centre and knock into people. On two occasions he had seen a boy in a chair, who then appeared to jump to another one. He admitted to a past history of solvent abuse.

He had been offered therapeutic help locally, after his disclosure of sexual abuse at the age of 13 years, but only went once, because it was 'too painful'. He had not been offered any other input, with regards to his behavioural disturbance. At the time of his assessment interview he was wanting help for his past sexual abuse, especially his self-harming behaviours and symptoms of PTSD.

PROTECTIVE FACTORS

X wanted to go to boarding school and was wanting therapeutic input.

Management

Despite the assessor making her findings available to those responsible for X's care, it did not prove possible to influence the management plan after the first care placement, until the assessment report and an addendum were presented in Court. Attempts at telephone contact with the social worker were very limited since he was either about to leave the office on each occasion that he was contacted, or was not there at all. Letters to the social worker and his team leader, detailing concerns about the progress of X, were passed up to a more senior manager, who argued that there were no legal grounds for taking any action.

PROGRESS WHILST AWAITING TRIAL

After his first Court appearance X was accommodated by the local authority in a children's home. He was difficult to manage, was disruptive and aggressive, and showed bizarre, sexualized behaviours. He then went home to live and on an increasingly frequent basis breached the curfew that had been imposed by the Court. He went missing from home on nearly 20 occasions. During these episodes he began to abuse alcohol and illicit drugs, including heroin. He was known to have been involved in several fights leading to two further charges of ABH.

PROGRESS AFTER TRIAL

The outcome of the criminal proceedings was decided after great thought so that X's care and therapeutic needs could be addressed on a long-term basis, as well as taking into account his need for punishment. He was made the subject of a 3-year Supervision Order on condition that he and the local authority report back to the Court on a monthly basis. Following this he was placed in a secure unit for 3 months, where his behaviours stabilized. He then moved to an open, structured setting where he was offered education and therapeutic input, to which he made a good response. There have been a few short episodes of absconding, but no known substance abuse, offending or further violence.

Acknowledgements

This chapter was first published in the *Journal of Child Psychology and Psychiatry* (JCCP), Vol. 40, May 1999, and is reproduced with the permission of the publisher. Table 3.1 is reproduced with permission from John Monahan, Hank Steadman, the Editor of University of Chicago Press, Publications Editor of JCCP and the Permissions Controller of Cambridge University Press. Permission was obtained to use this table for both the original article in JCCP and to reproduce it in this chapter. The author is grateful to two anonymous referees for their comments.

REFERENCES

Andre, G., Kendall, K., Pease, K. and Boulton, A. 1994: Health and offence histories of young offenders in Saskatoon, Canada. *Criminal Behaviour and Mental Health* **4**: 163–80.

Bailey, S. 1997: Sadistic and violent acts in the young. *Child Psychology and Psychiatry Review* **2**: 92–102.

Bowden, P. 1997: Risk management: from patient to client. *Psychiatric Bulletin* **21**: 3–38.

Briscoe, O. 1990: Intent. In Bluglass, R. and Bowden, P. (eds), *Principles and Practice of Forensic Psychiatry.* London: Churchill Livingstone, 251–4.

Britain, R.P. 1970: The sadistic murderer. *Medicine, Science and the Law* **10**: 198–207.

Buchanan, A., Reed, A., Wessley, S. *et al.* 1993: Acting on delusions: 2. The phenomenological correlates of acting on delusions. *British Journal of Psychiatry* **163**: 77–82.

Carson, D. 1996: Developing models of risk to aid cooperation between law and psychiatry. *Criminal Behaviour and Mental Health* **6**: 6–10.

Chaiken, J.M. and Chaiken, M.R. 1990: Drugs and predatory crime. In Tonry, M. and Wilson, J.Q. (eds), *Drugs and Crime: Crime and Justice, a Review of Research,* Vol. 13. Chicago: University of Chicago Press, 203–40.

Christian, R.E., Frick, P.J., Hill, N.L., Tyler, L. and Frazer, D.R. 1997: Psychopathy and conduct problems in children: 11. Implications of subtyping children with conduct problems. *Journal of the American Academy of Child and Adolescent Psychiatry* **36**: 233–41.

Clothier, C., MacDonald, C.A. and Shaw, D.O. 1994: *The Allitt Inquiry: Independent inquiry relating to deaths and injuries on the children's ward at Grantham and Kesteven general hospital during the period February–April 1991.* London: HMSO.

Cocozza, J. and Steadman, H. 1976: The failure of psychiatric predictions of dangerousness: clear and convincing evidence. *Rutgers Law Review* **29**: 1084–101.

Crepault, C. and Couture, M. 1980: Men's erotic fantasies. *Archives of Sexual Behaviour* **9**: 565–81.

DoH (Department of Health) 1996: *The Protection and Use of Patient Information.* London: DoH.

Dodge, K.A., Bates, J.E. and Pettit, G.S. 1990: Mechanisms in the cycle of violence. *Science* **250**: 1678–83.

Farrington, D.P. 1994: Early developmental prevention of juvenile delinquency. *Criminal Behaviour and Mental Health* **4**: 209–77.

Farrington, D.P. 1995: The development of offending and antisocial behaviour from childhood: key findings from the Cambridge Study in Delinquent Development. *Journal of Child Psychology and Psychiatry* **36**: 929–64.

Feindler, E.L. and Ecton, R.B. 1986: *Adolescent Anger Control: Cognitive–Behavioural techniques.* Oxford: Pergamon.

GMC (General Medical Council) 1993: *Professional Conduct and Discipline: Fitness to Practise.* London: GMC.

Grounds, A. 1995: Risk assessment and management in clinical context. In Crichton, J. (ed.), *Psychiatric Patient Violence: Risk and Response.* London: Duckworth, 54–5.

Gunn, J. 1993: Dangerousness. In Gunn, J. and Taylor, P. (eds), *Forensic Psychiatry: Clinical, Legal and Ethical Issues.* Oxford: Butterworth–Heinemann, 624–45.

Gunn, J. 1996: Let's get serious about dangerousness. *Criminal Behaviour and Mental Health,* Supplement, 51–64.

Hare, R.D. 1991: *The Hare Psychopathy Checklist–Revised.* Toronto: Multi-Health Systems.

Hellerstein, D., Frosch, W. and Koeningsberg, H.W. 1987: The clinical significance of command hallucinations. *American Journal of Psychiatry* **144**: 219–21.

Hellman, D.S. and Blackburn, M. 1966: Enuresis, fire-setting and cruelty to animals: a triad predictive of adult crime. *American Journal of Psychiatry* **122**: 1431–5.

Hoge, R.D., Andrews, D.A. and Leschied, A.W. 1996: An investigation of risk and protective factors in a sample of youthful offenders. *Journal of Child Psychology and Psychiatry* **37**: 419–24.

Hotaling, G.T., Straus, M.A. and Lincoln, A.J. 1989: Intrafamily violence, and crime and violence outside the family. In Ohlin, L. and Tonry, M. (eds), *Family Violence.* Chicago, IL: University of Chicago Press, 315–75.

Kazdin, A.E. 1997: Psychosocial treatments for conduct disorder in children. *Journal of Child Psychology and Psychiatry* **38**: 161–78.

Klassen, D. and O'Connor, W. 1985: Predicting violence among ex-mental patients: preliminary research results. Paper given at the Annual Meeting of the American Society of Criminology, 643.

Lang, R. 1993: Alcohol related violence: psychological perspective. In Martin, S. (ed.), *Alcohol and Interpersonal Violence: Fostering Interdisciplinary Perspectives.* NIAA Research Monogram 24. Washington, DC: Department of Health and Human Services, 121–48.

Le Blanc, M. 1994: Family, school, delinquency and criminality, the predictive power of an elaborated social control theory for males. *Criminal Behaviour and Mental Health* **4**: 101–17.

Link, B.G. and Stueve, A. 1994: Psychotic symptoms and the violent/illegal behaviour of mental patients compared to community controls. In Monahan, J. and Steadman, H.J. (eds), *Violence and Mental Disorder: Developments in Risk Assessment.* London: University of Chicago Press, 137–59.

Loeber, R. and Hay, D.F. 1997: Key issues in the development of aggression and violence from childhood to early adulthood. *Annual Review of Psychology* **48**: 371–410.

MacArthur Foundation Research Network on Mental Health and the Law. 1996: Violence, competence and coercion: the pivotal issues in mental health law. Paper given at Wadham College, Oxford, 4 July 1996.

MacCulloch, M.D., Snowden, P.R., Wood, P.J.W. and Mills, H.E. 1983: Sadistic fantasy, sadistic behaviour and offending. *British Journal of Psychiatry* **143**: 20–9.

McNiel, D.E. 1994: Hallucinations and violence. In Monahan, J. and Steadman, H.J. (eds), *Violence and Mental Disorder: Developments in Risk Assessment.* London: University of Chicago Press, 183–202.

Magnusson, D. and Bergman, L.R. 1990: A pattern approach to the study of pathways from childhood to adulthood. In Robins, L. and Rutter, M. (eds), *Straight and Devious Pathways from Childhood to Adulthood.* Cambridge: Cambridge University Press, 101–15.

Monahan, J. 1981: *The Clinical Prediction of Violent Behaviour.* Rockville, MD: Government Printing Office and National Institute of Mental Health.

Novaco, R.W. 1975: *Anger Control: The Development and Evaluation of an Experimental Treatment.* Lexington, MA: Lexington Books.

Novaco, R.W. 1994: Anger as a risk factor for violence amongst the mentally disordered. In Monahan, J. and Steadman, H.J. (eds), *Violence and Mental Disorder: Developments in Risk Assessment.* London: University of Chicago Press, 21–59.

Petch, E. and Bradley, C. 1997: Learning the lessons from homicide inquiries: adding insult to injury? *Journal of Forensic Psychiatry* **8**: 161–84.

Pollock, N. and Webster, C. 1990: The clinical assessment of dangerousness. In Bluglass, R. and Bowden, P. (eds), *Principles and Practice of Forensic Psychiatry.* London: Churchill Livingstone, 489–97.

Raine, A., Brennan, P., Mednick, B. and Mednick, S.A. 1996: High rates of violence, crime, academic problems and behavioural problems in males with both early neuromotor deficits and unstable family environments. *Archives of General Psychiatry* **53**: 544–9.

Robins, L.N. 1978: Sturdy childhood predictors of adult antisocial behaviour: replications from longitudinal studies. *Psychological Medicine* **8**: 611–22.

Robins, L.N. and Price, R.K. 1991: Adult disorders predicted by childhood conduct problems: results from the NIMH Epidemiologic Catchment Area project. *Psychiatry* **54**: 116–32.

RCP (Royal College of Psychiatrists) 1996: *Assessment and Clinical Management of Risk of Harm to Other People.* Special Working Party in Clinical Assessment and Management of Risk, Council Report CR53. London: RCP.

Rutter, M. 1985: Resilience in the face of adversity: protective factors and resistance to psychiatric disorder. *British Journal of Psychiatry* **147**: 598–611.

Rutter, M. 1987: Psychosocial resilience and protective mechanisms. *American Journal of Orthopsychiatry* **5**: 316–31.

Rutter, M. 1996 (ed.): *Genetics of Criminal Behaviour and Antisocial Behaviour.* Chichester: John Wiley.

Sampson, R.J. and Laub, J.H. 1993: *Crime in the Making: Pathways and Turning Points Through Life.* Cambridge, MA: Harvard University Press.

Satten, J., Menninger, K., Rosen, I. and Mayman, M. 1960: Murder without apparent motive. *American Journal of Psychiatry* **117**: 48–53.

Scott, P.D. 1977: Assessing dangerousness in criminals. *British Journal of Psychiatry* **131**: 127–42.

Sheldrick, E.C. 1994: Treatment of delinquents. In Rutter, M., Taylor, E. and Hersov, L. (eds), *Child and Adolescent Psychiatry: Modern Approaches.* Oxford: Blackwell Scientific, 968–82.

Simon, F.H. 1971: *Prediction Methods in Criminology.* London: Home Office.

Smith, D.J. 1995: Youth crime and conduct disorders. In Rutter, M. and Smith, D.J. (eds), *Psychosocial Disorders in Young People: Time Trends and their Causes.* Chichester: John Wiley, 389–489.

Steadman, H.J. 1980: The right not to be a false positive: problems in the application of the dangerousness standard. *Psychiatric Quarterly* **32**: 84–99.

Steadman, H.J. 1982: A situational approach to violence. *International Journal of Law and Psychiatry* **5**: 171–86.

Steadman, H.J. and Cocozza, J. 1974: *Careers of the Criminally Insane.* Lexington, MA: Lexington Books.

Steadman, H.J. and Keveles, C. 1972: The community adjustment and criminal activity of the Baxtrom patients: 1966–70. *American Journal of Psychiatry* **129**: 304–10.

Steadman, H.J., Monahan, J., Robbins. P.C. *et al.* 1993: From dangerousness to risk assessment: implications for appropriate research strategies. In Hodgins, S. (ed.), *Crime and Mental Disorder.* Newbury Park, CA: Sage, 39–62.

Steadman, H.J., Monahan, J., Appelbaum, P.S. *et al.* 1994: Designing a new generation of risk assessment research. In Monahan, J. and Steadman, H.J. (eds), *Violence and Mental Disorder: Developments in Risk Assessment.* London: University of Chicago Press, 297–318.

Steadman, H.J., Mulvey, E.P., Monahan, J. *et al.* 1998: Violence by people discharged from acute psychiatric inpatient facilities and by others in the same neighbourhoods. *Archives of General Psychiatry* **55**: 393–402.

Swanson, J.W., Holzer, C.E., Ganju, V.K. and Jono, R.T. 1990: Violence and psychiatric disorder in the community: evidence from the Epidemiologic Catchment Area surveys. *Hospital and Community Psychiatry* **41**: 761–70.

Swanson, J.W., Borum, R., Swartz, M.S. and Monahan, J. 1996: Psychotic symptoms and disorders and the risk of violent behaviour in the community. *Criminal Behaviour and Mental Health* **6**: 309–29.

Taylor, P.J. 1985: Motives for offending among violent and psychotic men. *British Journal of Psychiatry* **147**: 491–8.

Taylor, P.J. 1995: Schizophrenia and the risk of violence. In Hirsch, S.R. and Weinberger, D.R. (eds), *Schizophrenia.* Oxford: Blackwell Science, 163–83.

Taylor, P.J. and Parrott, J.M. 1988: Elderly offenders. *British Journal of Psychiatry* **152**: 340–6.

Taylor, P.J., Garety, P., Buchanan, A. *et al.* 1994: Delusions and violence. In Monahan, J. and Steadman, H.J. (eds), *Violence and Mental Disorder: Developments in Risk Assessment.* London: University of Chicago Press, 161–82.

Tiihonen, J. 1995: Quantitative risk assessment of homicidal behaviour. *Journal of Forensic Psychiatry* **6**: 477–85.

Wilkins, R. 1993: Delusions in children and teenagers admitted to the Bethlem Royal Hospital in the 19th century. *British Journal of Psychiatry* **162**: 487–92.

4

The social and historical context

DAVID SMITH

INTRODUCTION

We should start from a position of scepticism about claims that 'young people today' are more of a problem, or have more problems, than their parents' generation or their more remote predecessors in some distant, imagined past. Pearson writes of the 'profound historical amnesia' which characterizes discussion of 'the youth question', particularly youth crime and related forms of misbehaviour. We are all familiar from the media and political rhetoric with the idea that the conduct of young people has deteriorated, in Britain and elsewhere, 'since the war', and the sense that the immediate post-war period marks an important watershed also has currency in academic circles: an authoritative and ambitious recent survey, drawing on a wide range of expertise from western Europe and the United States, treats the years from 1950 to the early 1990s as the relevant period over which to chart trends in time in 'psychosocial disorders in young people' (Rutter and Smith 1995a). The survey tests the validity of a number of claimed causes of the supposed deterioration in young people's behaviour and well-being, most of which have been widely canvassed in the popular media as well as by social scientists: they include social disadvantage and its apparent opposite, increased affluence; unemployment; poor physical health; a breakdown in family stability; the prolongation of adolescence and of dependence; the malign effects of the mass media; and changes (for the worse) in moral values. Pearson produces a rather similar list in summarizing the most common terms of the language used in popular discussion of what has caused the problems of today's young people:

> 'the "permissive society"; the break-up of the family and community; the dwindling power of parents, teachers, magistrates and policemen; the lack of respect among the young for authority in all its forms; and the incitements of demoralizing popular entertainments such as television violence and video nasties which lead to imitative "copy-cat" crimes' (Pearson 1994, p. 1163).

But Pearson has no difficulty in showing that a very similar catalogue of complaint could have been heard before the war, exactly in the period when, according to so many recent commentators, young people were much less of a problem. In the 1930s, people looked back nostalgically to the time before the First World War, when young people knew their place, respected their elders, and had no thought of flouting social conventions. They blamed, among other things, the decline of parental and official authority, the loss of religious faith, the absence of social restraints, the influence of the American cinema, and the breakdown of traditional communities, for the allegedly unprecedented problem behaviour of young people between the wars. Indeed, Pearson (1983) has traced this tendency to regard the youth of today, whenever 'today' is, as uniquely out of control, disrespectful, prone to crime and so on much further back in history, at least to the mid-nineteenth century, when official fears of the new urban working class first began directly to influence social policy, for example in the development of industrial and reformatory schools. Instead of a source of hope, the young became an object of dread, a threat to civil society and its traditions, rather than the rising generation which would carry forward a tale of progress and social and economic improvement.

Given that this historical perspective can help to set current concerns about young people in a context which reveals such concerns as less novel or uniquely a product of the present than they are often claimed to be, should we simply dismiss them as symptoms of the usual nostalgic yearning for an imaginary Golden Age, or of an older generation's typical fears of a future it will not control? Or should we treat seriously the evidence which suggests that, for instance, the rise since the Second World War in crime rates in all advanced capitalist societies (with the notable and important exception of Japan) represents a qualitatively new development which demands some theoretical explanation? The view taken here is that while we should always be sceptical of claims about young people's behaviour that may be little more than a rationalization of fear, envy and resentment, there are nevertheless strong theoretical and empirical grounds for believing that the incidence of 'psychosocial disorders' among young people has increased in the past few decades, and certainly in the last twenty years. Importantly, these disorders include not only the manifestations of misbehaviour which have traditionally aroused the wrath of the older generation – crime, various forms of anti-social behaviour, and drug and alcohol use or abuse – but the more private and less obviously disruptive problems of unhappiness and insecurity which are also covered by the contributors to Rutter and Smith's (1995a) survey: depression, eating disorders, and suicide and suicidal behaviour. The main conclusions of this study are summarized, with some commentary, in the next section; more detailed examination of alternative approaches is reserved until later in the chapter.

TRENDS IN TIME AND CAUSATION: A SUMMARY AND CRITIQUE

All the conditions listed above 'tend to rise or peak in frequency during the teenage years' (Smith and Rutter 1995a, p. 1), and all are more or less common, two reasons why they were chosen as the 'target disorders' for the study, and why schizophrenia, for example, was not included: it is less common, though still affecting around one per cent of the population at some time in their lives, and its onset tends to occur after the teenage years – only about ten per cent of people admitted to hospital with this diagnosis are under the age of 20 when admitted for the first time (Gottesman 1991). The study was concerned with 'time trends and their causes'. Reviewing the evidence, the editors are confident about concluding that,

with the exception of eating disorders where the evidence of an increase is not strong enough to conclude that it has really occurred, 'there is unmistakable evidence of a postwar increase' (Smith and Rutter 1995b, p. 771) in all their target disorders. In very summary form, their conclusions are as follows.

Recorded crime rates per head of population in developed capitalist countries typically increased between 1950 and 1990 by a factor of about five, with some sign of a levelling-off or even a decrease in some countries in the 1980s (and according to the most recent British victimization surveys, into the 1990s; Mirrlees-Black *et al.* 1996; MVA 1998). According to Rutter and Smith (and there is hardly room for doubt over this), these figures reflect a real increase in criminal behaviour, not merely changes in the rate of reporting by the public or recording by the police. Alcohol use increased markedly from 1950 to 1980, when it levelled off; and the use of drugs other than alcohol increased massively over the same period, and has probably continued to rise. Suicide rates among young people (aged 15–24) rose during the period, particularly among males, and particularly during the 1970s, but since 1980 the suicide rate among young females has declined in most countries; suicidal behaviour not resulting in death followed a similar pattern over time, declining more sharply among young females than among young males after about 1980. Depression among young people increased over the period, judging by a number of cross-sectional and longitudinal studies which found a higher risk among more recent birth cohorts. For eating disorders, it is not certain that the incidence of anorexia has increased over time, and bulimia, which was not recognized as a distinct disorder until the late 1970s, is relatively rare, and it is impossible to infer trends in time from a small number of cases.

These authors (Rutter and Smith 1995b) are notably cautious compared with many others – some of whose work will be discussed later – in drawing conclusions about the causes of the changes identified in their collaborative research. They consider a number of more or less widely canvassed ideas on what social and economic developments in the post-war period might explain the increased incidence of their selected disorders among young people. One type of explanation is essentially demographic: for example, Easterlin (1980) has argued that large birth cohorts face greater competition for limited resources, such as jobs and educational opportunities, and that the resultant stresses will lead to higher levels of disorder among young people. The basic difficulty with this kind of theory is that, as is well known, there is a long-term trend for the population of Britain, as of other broadly comparable countries, to become older, with young people forming a declining proportion of the total population. On the basis of Easterlin's theory and other demographic approaches, this should have produced a long-term decline in the rate of disorder, rather than the increase which is suggested by research. On the other hand, as Rutter and Smith (1995b) acknowledge, shorter-term changes in the age structure, such as that resulting from the post-war 'baby boom' in Britain and other European countries, can have a direct effect on the prevalence of some problems, notably crime. Field (1990) found a close link in England and Wales between crime rates and the number of young males in the population, and the apparent (though disputed) decline in youth crime since the early 1980s has been attributed to the decrease in the overall number of juveniles in the population over the same period (Pratt 1985). Contrary to what one would expect from this demographic approach, however, the numbers of known young offenders continued to decline well into the 1990s (NACRO Youth Crime Section 1998), when the total population in the relevant age group had increased.

Pointing to evidence of rapid economic growth in all the countries covered by their study, especially from 1950 to the oil crisis of 1973, Rutter and Smith (1995b) firmly reject any general explanation in terms of a decline in living standards, although, as they recognize (and the point will be considered in more detail later), relative deprivation and poverty, and even absolute poverty among particular social groups, could be associated with a higher local incidence of the disorders with which they are concerned. Rutter and Smith have more time for the alternative hypothesis, that increased affluence is an indirect cause of increased rates of disorder, an idea which has a venerable lineage in criminology, stretching back to the work of Durkheim in the late nineteenth century. The possible links between overall increases in affluence and increased rates of crime have been specified quite closely by, for example, environmental criminologists, in terms of greater opportunities for predatory crime (for a summary see Bottoms and Wiles (1997)). From an economic perspective Field (1990) has suggested that violent crime tends to increase in periods of increased consumption, the proposed causal mechanism being that young men with more money to spend go out more, drink more, and are more likely to get into fights; on the other hand, property crime tends to increase in periods of economic recession.

The latter finding suggests that poverty might be an important causal factor in higher rates of predatory crime, but Rutter and Smith (1995b, p. 790) conclude, following other studies, that there is 'only a weak relationship between crime or conduct disorders and social class', in contrast, for example, to the strong association between social class and life expectancy. There is, however, good evidence for a much stronger link between low social class and serious offending (Graham and Bowling 1995); and in relation to drug use Hough (1995, p. 8) similarly concludes that the weight of evidence strongly suggests that 'both in this country and in the USA, problem drug use tends to be concentrated amongst the urban poor, especially in inner cities'. As with offending, there are strong indications that the most serious problems of drug abuse are more common among those experiencing economic stress and social disadvantage. The links between class or socio-economic status and the other disorders considered in the Rutter and Smith volume are less clear, but Rutter and Smith (1995b) themselves acknowledge that poverty can lead to stress in family life and thus to a higher general risk of psychosocial disorders – a relationship to be discussed later in this chapter. It is also clear that the 1980s and 1990s saw widening disparities in income between the richest and poorest social groups in Britain (Hutton 1996); and while Rutter and Smith are sceptical about a possible causal link between growing inequality and psychosocial disorders, there is evidence for such a connection, at least in respect of violent crime, and this too will be discussed later in the chapter.

Other widely canvassed possible causes of disorder lie in major social and economic changes as industrialization, urbanization and migration. The first two have often been adduced by criminologists as high-level explanations for the post-war rise in crime, as (it is argued) they both erode the informal social controls characteristic of rural communities and increase opportunities for predatory crime. Increased stress on family relationships might also result from such changes in long-established ways of life: Hood (1992) cites research which suggests that the children of immigrants are particularly prone to delinquency, a cross-cultural finding which might be explained in terms of the difficulty their parents find in coping with new social circumstances while at the same time maintaining strong family ties. It is, however, clear that urbanization and industrialization cannot in themselves provide an adequate explanation for rising crime rates: if they could, one would expect to find a massive increase in crime in Japan since the war, since these processes have been massively accelerated with the development of the Japanese economy. In fact, Japan is unique among industrialized countries in having a relatively low and stable crime rate (Braithwaite 1989); nor, despite popular stereotypes, does it have an exceptionally high suicide rate among young people or any other age group (Masters 1996). The question of what we might learn from the Japanese experience is considered later in this chapter.

A notable trend over the period covered by their survey has been the rise in the overall educational level of the populations of developed countries, and Rutter and Smith (1995b, pp. 793–4) consider how this general trend might be associated with a rise in psychosocial disorders. Two possibilities are that education prolongs the period of dependent adolescence, which could be associated with greater stress and therefore vulnerability to disorder; and that it tends to encourage a rise in expectations, which, insofar as they cannot be met, might increase the risk of disorder. Both of these ideas have a lengthy lineage in social science and indeed in popular understandings: a longer period of dependence might make the achievement of a secure adult identity more difficult, and the institutionalization of adolescence as a distinct social status may have led to the emergence of a 'youth culture' (or cultures) relatively immune from adult influence, in which the values and behaviour of the peer group are more influential than those of the adult world. There are grounds for thinking that the 1950s saw the emergence for the first time of a large and distinct market in goods, especially clothes and music, specifically aimed at teenagers (see, for example, Furlong and Cartmel (1997)), and there is little doubt that subsequent youth cultural styles have been exploited and to an extent shaped by commercial interests. But this market grew precisely because in the 1950s and 1960s young people in employment had more disposable income than their pre-war counterparts; those who had the money were, in general, those who had not stayed on in education. The second possibility is essentially that originally proposed by the American sociologist Robert Merton (1957; but the idea was originally formulated in 1938), who argued that crime could be understood as an 'innovative' adaptation on the part of those whose legitimate aspirations could not be met by legitimate means, because of inequalities in the social structure. This 'strain' theory of delinquency has undergone various elaborations since then, some of which are considered later; but at least in its pure form it suffers from a lack of empirical support when applied to youthful delinquency: one of the best established criminological findings is that young people whose aspirations and expectations are low, who dislike school and are not strongly attached to it, and who perform poorly in academic terms, are more likely to become delinquent than those with high expectations and a strong commitment to educational success (for a summary, see Braithwaite (1989)). At least in respect of delinquency, therefore, it is difficult to argue that long-term trends in education, or rising expectations, provide an adequate causal account: those who are most likely to become delinquent are those who spend least time in education, and who expect least of it.

The last factor to be considered here of those discussed by Rutter and Smith (1995b) is that of moral values and family structure and function, which, insofar as parental values influence the values of their children, are likely to be linked. Using a number of surveys of attitudes, Rutter and Smith note a general trend toward greater tolerance and acceptance of difference, particularly in personal and sexual morality; but the clearest trend they identify is in the growth of individualism (p. 804), defined in the relevant chapter (Halpern 1995, p. 382) as 'emphasis of individual convictions rather than external models'. The processes associated with late modernity – globalization, detraditionalization, 'disorganized capitalism' (Lash and Urry 1987), 'risk society' (Beck 1992), the fragmentation of social institutions – are all likely to promote the growth of individualism in Halpern's sense, and may be associated with the loss of a secure sense of personal and social identity (Giddens 1991, 1992, 1994). In his later work Giddens has taken a relatively optimistic view of the possibilities of social and political change opened out by the availability, through global communication networks, of a wide range of conceivable identities and ways of life, but whether the changes are celebrated or lamented (for a conservative lament, see Dennis (1993)), it is more or less common ground for these commentators that traditional beliefs no longer are or can be uncritically accepted. Old certainties have disappeared with the unprecedented pace of social and technological change, to be replaced at worst with a moral vacuum, at best with the need to struggle to find meaning and value in activities formerly taken for granted.

The uses of such high-level analysis of social change in understanding the problems of young people in difficulties will be considered later; the point here is that there is a near-universal recognition that important changes have taken place, and for many conservative commentators who regret them responsibility is placed not on global processes of technological development but on changing patterns of family life. Rutter and Smith (1995b) are far more measured than, for example, Dennis (1993) or Morgan (1995) – both published by the neo liberal 'think-tank', the Institute of Economic Affairs – in their conclusions about the impact of changes in family structure and functioning on delinquency and other problem behaviours. They note, for example, that one of the most significant changes, the reduction in average family size, might, by reducing stress on parents and enabling them to give their children closer individual attention, be protective against the emergence of disorders. But another obvious change, the rise in the number of divorces, often followed by remarriage and reconstitution of the family, has undoubtedly increased the proportion of young people who have experienced disruption in the make-up of the family unit during their upbringing. Divorce and remarriage are of course compatible with perfectly good parental care, and the evidence on the connections between family disruption and delinquency is complicated, as it is on the links between single parenthood and delinquency, despite the blame often attached to single parents (i.e. mothers) for the creation of a criminal underclass (Murray 1990). Nevertheless, there is powerful evidence that the most persistent and serious young offenders have suffered disproportionately from unhappiness, neglect, abuse and abandonment in their early years, and in any effort to explain young people's criminality and other problems of social functioning it is inevitable that their experiences of growing up in a family (or in some substitute for one) will be important.

The approach of the contributors to the Rutter and Smith volume has important limitations. Its concentration on aggregate data means that it can say little about local, specific and temporary conditions; its broad historical sweep means that even trends detectable over a period of a few years are liable to be ignored; it relies heavily on officially collected data (which are often missing or partial for the pre-war period); at least in respect of crime and drug use, it tends to conflate the minor and trivial with the major and serious; and it tends to what Mills (1959) described as 'abstract empiricism', in which explanatory theory tends to be submerged in a sea of figures. The remainder of this chapter, then, will examine other approaches, looking first at what is known about the early experiences of young people who become identified as serious or persistent offenders, in family life and in their experiences of school. Moving outwards from their immediate environment, it will consider what part economic inequality and relative (and absolute) deprivation might play in increasing the risks of criminality. Finally, it will consider the value of theories of late or postmodernity in understanding young people's difficulties. Mills (1959) was as critical of what he called 'grand theory' as of atheoretical empiricism, and it will be argued that more recent versions of this sociological tendency, while drawing attention to real processes of social change, tend to exaggerate the uniqueness of the late modern experience, and understate the persistence of structural inequalities and deprivation (Furlong and Cartmel 1997; Smith 1999).

FAMILY AND SCHOOL

It is common for young people, especially young males, to break the law (Graham and Bowling 1995; Farrington 1997). The well-known Cambridge Study in Delinquent Development, a prospective longitudinal study of a sample of London working-class males from the age of 8 in 1958 to the age of 32, found that virtually all of them were willing to report having committed at least one of ten specified offences by the age of 32. This study found that the peak age for acceleration in the rate of offending was 14, and the peak age for deceleration was 23 (Farrington 1997, pp. 368–9); and while Graham and Bowling (1995) suggest that the developmental stages traditionally associated with desistance from crime (establishing a stable sexual relationship, settling into a job, having a child) may not operate on young men as effectively as has been assumed, in a context of prolonged adolescent dependence, it still appears from their study that serious (and especially violent) offending does tail off in the early twenties. It is also clear from their self-report data that serious and persistent offending remains virtually a male monopoly; we should never lose sight of the fact that 'gender is the single most important variable in criminality' (Heidensohn 1988, p. 91). Even among males, however, serious or persistent offending is rare: only 23 of the 400 boys in the Cambridge study became 'chronic' offenders. Persistent offending was

reasonably well (but by no means universally) predicted in the Cambridge study by the presence of a number of risk factors at the age of 8–10, including parental criminality, poor child-rearing, conflict between parents, and socio-economic stress. Poor parenting includes harsh and erratic discipline, a cruel, passive or neglectful attitude towards the child, poor supervision, and lack of interest in education. Impulsivity and low intelligence in the child also predicted delinquency, though there is a strong argument that the association between intelligence and delinquency virtually disappears when the variables of school failure and attachment to school are controlled for, and that the association between school failure and delinquency can be almost completely explained by institutional practices such as negative labelling (Braithwaite 1989).

The family factors associated with an increased risk of serious and persistent offending are, however, fairly well established and understood, and seem to be consistent over time (Sampson and Laub 1993); so it is no surprise to find that these risk factors are strongly in evidence in the early histories of the most serious young offenders. For example, Boswell (1991, 1998) has studied offenders sentenced under Section 53 of the 1933 Children and Young Persons Act. Section 53(1) covers murder and Section 53(2) other 'grave crimes', including homicides. In 1991 there were 615 such offenders in the prison and child care systems; by 1994 the number had grown to 781, 750 of them male, an increase which Boswell (1998) attributes to a rise in juvenile violence as well as a greater willingness by courts to use Section 53(2) to ensure long periods of detention. In Boswell's second study, the files of 200 Section 53 offenders were read for hard evidence of experiences of abuse – categorized as emotional, sexual, physical, and organized or ritual – and of loss, through either the death of 'someone important' – usually a parent or grandparent – or loss of contact with them (in practice, nearly all the recorded losses of contact were with a parent). An attempt was made to interview offenders whose case files were ambiguous about whether abuse or loss had occurred; such cases were not counted unless the interview corroborated a suggestion of abuse or loss in the file. The abuse categories were defined as in the official guidance on working together under the 1989 Children Act (Home Office et al. 1991).

The study found that a total of 72% of the sample had experienced at least one form of abuse in childhood, and that 27% had experienced more than one. Forty per cent had been physically abused, just under 30% had been emotionally or sexually abused, and 1.5% had been subject to organized or ritual abuse. The evidence suggested that many of the sample had experienced lasting 'significant harm' as a result of the abuse, and that some for whom abuse was not specifically recorded had almost certainly experienced, at the very least, serious distress, as a result of conflict and violence in the home. Similarly, bereavement and loss of contact with an important person were only counted if the file showed that in the judgement of at least one expert they had had a significant impact on the young person and his or her subsequent behaviour. On this basis, 57% of the sample had experienced a significant loss: in 10% of cases a parent had died, and in just under 40% the young person had lost contact with one or both parents. Overall, evidence of significant abuse or loss was absent in only 18 (9%) of the sample cases, and 35% had experienced both abuse and loss. Boswell (1998, p. 155) interprets the findings as indicating that abuse and loss, in the absence of any compensating life experiences, constitute 'unresolved trauma which is likely to manifest itself in some way at a later date'. This conclusion is broadly in line with Widom's (1989) finding from a prospective study that physical abuse and neglect (though not sexual abuse) in childhood were both significantly predictive of later violence. This is not, of course, to claim that violence inevitably begets violence; many protective factors can intervene, and childhood trauma may become manifest in ways other than violence. Nevertheless, Boswell (1998) suggests that the professionals in the field whom she interviewed for her earlier study would probably be surprised only that the percentage figure for known abuse was so low.

More general surveys of populations of known offenders tell much the same story in a less extreme form. Dodd and Hunter (1992), Stewart and Stewart (1993) and Mair and May (1997), for example, all found that at least a quarter of those surveyed in the prison population and on probation officers' caseloads had had some experience of local authority care, compared with about 2% of the general population. Qualitative evidence from interviews has provided detailed examples of experiences of deprivation, neglect and abuse in childhood and early adolescence among young people known to the probation service (Smith and Stewart, 1998); the experience of care, by no means always a result of offending, seemed often to contribute to the development of an offending career. The pattern that emerges from these recent surveys strongly suggests that the family factors which predict offending are relatively independent of changes over time in the socio-economic environment. Sampson and Laub (1993) re-analysed the data collected by Sheldon and Eleanor Glueck (1950) forty years on, and concluded that the family factors associated with delinquency were parental criminality or mental health problems, poor supervision and erratic child-rearing, parental disharmony, and rejection, neglect or abuse of the child. In addition, they identified early child-bearing, teenage pregnancy, substance use during pregnancy, low birthweight and other types of birth complications as independent risk factors – a list which points to the potential value of projects such as the Elmira Prenatal/Early Infancy Project (in effect, intensive health visiting) discussed by Karoly et al. (1998). It should be stressed, however, that the association between single parenthood and delinquency is much less clear-cut than some commentators have claimed: Utting et al. (1993, p. 20) note the 'contrast to be drawn between children who grow up in a loving one-parent family and children who grow up in two parent families and are neglected or abused'. It is the quality of care – family function rather than structure – that matters.

The experiences at school of young offenders are likely in many cases to follow from their experiences at home: parents who see little value in education and supervise their children poorly are unlikely to promote a positive attitude towards school. Research has consistently shown that school variables are among the important early risk factors for delinquency, which is strongly associated with not liking school, being weakly attached to school and to teachers, low educational and occupational aspirations, poor school performance, truancy and exclusion (Braithwaite 1989; Graham and Bowling 1995). Surveys of young offender populations consistently find that a far higher proportion of known offenders leave school with no qualifications than in the general population (Stewart and Stewart 1993; Mair and May 1997). Educational failure and lack of attachment to school are more strongly associated than intelligence with delinquency, and it is important to remember that the relevant variables are not all within the child: there is good evidence that schools themselves can make a difference, either increasing or reducing the risk of delinquency (Rutter et al. 1979; Mortimore et al. 1988). For example, schools which minimize exclusion also minimize the delinquency risk. But since no school excludes children at random, 'troublesomeness' and the restlessness and poor concentration associated with impulsivity (Farrington 1997) must be relevant to understanding the school experiences of young offenders; like the experience of local authority care, exclusion from school can be a response to offending which increases the likelihood that offending will persist (Graham and Bowling 1995).

FAMILY EXPERIENCE AND THE SOCIAL ENVIRONMENT

While the elements of early childhood experience associated with offending seem to be fairly stable over time, their prevalence may change as a result of changes in the economic, social and cultural environment. James (1995) and Currie (1997) suggest, for Britain and the United States respectively, ways in which these broader changes might impact on family and community life so as to increase the risk of violent crime. As a number of commentators have noted (e.g. Zimring and Hawkins 1997), what is distinctive about crime in the USA is not its overall volume but the prevalence of violence, and especially lethal violence; and while it may not be inevitable that European countries should follow the American pattern,

James (1995) argues that social policy (or its disappearance) and increased economic inequality contributed to a marked increase from 1987 in juvenile violence in England and Wales.

Using criminal statistics and demographic data on the decline in the total number of juveniles in the population, James calculates that the number of known offences of violence committed by juveniles per 100,000 in the population increased by over 40% between 1987 and 1993. The number of juveniles known to have committed a violent offence increased by 34% over the same period. Both trends were directly contrary to the overall decline in the same period in the number of offences known to have been committed by juveniles and the number of known juvenile offenders. James also argues that in the same period violent offences as a proportion of all known juvenile crime increased from 4% to 9% among 10- to 13-year-olds, and from 8% to 13% among 14- to 16-year-olds. In contrast, violence as a proportion of all crime committed by older age groups did not change significantly during the period, nor did violence as a proportion of all juvenile crime in the years 1980–87. James concludes that the male cohort who reached the age of 10 in 1987 were more violent than those who were 10 in 1980 – and the most recent figures from both the British Crime Survey and the official criminal statistics, which show that the amount of violent crime has continued to rise while other types of crime are relatively static or even decreasing (as in Scotland), suggest that James's analysis would hold good for later age cohorts too (Mirrlees-Black et al. 1996; Povey et al. 1998).

James's proposed explanation is in terms of the increased inequality which was a marked feature of British economic development in the 1980s, and of the concomitant erosion of social security and other welfare measures which had provided some protection against the effects of market forces (cf. Currie 1985; Taylor 1999). James (1995, pp. 63–4) notes that in general societies become less violent as they become more prosperous, but adds the important qualification that in respect of homicide there is a strong correlation at the level of nation states between high rates of homicide and inequalities in income (Braithwaite and Braithwaite 1980). A number of American studies (Blau and Blau 1982; Land et al. 1990; Sampson and Wilson 1995) have shown the same relationship between inequality and violence at the level of metropolitan areas. James shows that the number of children living in relative and sometimes absolute poverty in England and Wales increased from about 1.4 million to 4.1 million between 1979 and 1991/2, and argues that low income is associated with depression and irritability in mothers of young children. Thus the proportion of boys being brought up by depressed and irritable mothers increased along with the proportion of families in poverty, and James argues that maternal irritability is a cause of childhood aggression and of adult violence. Like Utting et al. (1993), James concludes that the association of delinquency with single parenthood as such is largely a mirage; the key variable is not lone motherhood but low income.

In trying to answer the question why violent crime began to rise only in 1987, and not before, when increased income inequality, higher unemployment, and the erosion of welfare benefits and services were already evident, James follows Currie (1985) in arguing that poverty in itself is not a cause of violence; it is the socially and culturally defined meanings of poverty that provide the explanatory link. By 1987, the media were full of images of conspicuous or spectacular (Townsend 1992) consumption, placed in dramatic contrast with stories of a contemptible 'underclass', their exclusion and marginalization blamed on their own fecklessness and dependency (Murray 1990). In such circumstances, a sense of rage and resentment at blatant and morally indefensible inequality could easily develop, in a society increasingly polarized into winners and losers. This could arise not so much from positive strain, as in Merton's classic formulation – a sense of thwarted legitimate aspiration – as from the negative strain (Agnew 1985) that could be produced by the inability to escape from social disadvantage and oppression – such as might be experienced in a depressed family environment, in local authority care (Stewart et al. 1994), or more collectively among the male youth of economically depressed localities suffering from industrial collapse and with no prospect of improvement in sight (Campbell 1993). Among the other social problems which may come to characterize such areas is a high level of problem drug use (Pearson 1987), which is likely to be facilitated by the collapse of a local labour market and a high level of chronic unemployment (Downes 1993), with consequent effects on rates of crime and violence, and accelerated neighbourhood decline (Hough 1995).

Elliott Currie (1985, 1996, 1997) has over several years developed an analysis of violence and homicide in the USA in terms of economic inequality, sharp social divisions, the run-down of welfare services, and the social exclusion of disadvantaged groups, notably African Americans. Currie (1997) argues that the USA should be understood not simply as a market economy but as a market society, in which the values of the marketplace dominate social and cultural life, without any of the mitigating features of the 'family model' capitalism of Japan. The results, according to Currie (1997, pp. 154–6), include an increasingly segmented labour market, in which both lack of work and (in low-wage sectors of the economy) overwork reduce parents' capacity to care effectively for their children; extreme and growing economic inequality and deprivation; the disappearance of public services, especially those which could support parents under stress; and the erosion of informal networks of mutual support, care and control. Currie notes the extremes of both poverty and wealth that distinguish the

USA from any European country, reviews the evidence on the connections between inequality and homicide, and argues that there are clear correlations between poverty and family homicide and abuse of children. Family poverty, even if not accompanied by abuse or neglect of children, is likely to have negative impacts on child development, increasing the likelihood of failure at school and consequent economic marginality. Competitive social relationships are rewarded over cooperative ones, productive work and craftsmanship – a potential source of self-esteem – are devalued, and social and political alternatives are lost with the weakening of organized labour – all consequences of 'our increasingly heedless global assault, in the name of the market, on the preconditions of a sustaining social life' (Currie 1997, p. 169).

Currie (1996) argues that it would be a mistake for other countries to follow the American example in the 'war on crime'. The American approach since the mid-1970s has essentially been repressive: the total incarcerated population in the USA was 1.6 million in 1996, twice the figure in 1987 and about five times the figure in 1970 – and about five times the current rate of incarceration in England and Wales. Currie has no difficulty in finding cases of cities where the homicide rate increased along with drastic increases in the incarceration rate: for instance, Phoenix saw an 85% increase in homicides between the early 1970s and 1994, during which time the incarceration rate in Arizona increased by 467%; and homicides increased by 329% in New Orleans, 'the city that starved its schools to pay for the nation's third highest incarceration rate' (Currie 1996, p. 9). But, if locking more and more people up, with inevitable negative effects on spending on education and welfare services, is not the answer, what is? According to Currie (1996, pp. 16–17), a key element of a strategy to reduce violence should be to 'invest serious resources in the prevention of child abuse and neglect' (one of the aims of the Elmira project mentioned above). Secondly, he argues for pre-school educational programmes for children at risk of school failure – his example is the Perry programme in Michigan, the second early intervention programme discussed (and judged successful) by Karoly et al. (1998). A third type of programme should aim to support vulnerable young people at school to increase their chances of success in further education and in the jobs market. Finally, Currie argues for investment in the kinds of programme that have demonstrated effectiveness with young people who have begun to offend (for evidence on what works in such programmes, see McGuire (1995) and Vennard et al. (1997)).

Although Currie's policy proposals emerge from a radical critique of American culture and politics, they are close to those implied by some of the most careful empirical work available on juvenile and adult crime. Sampson and Laub (1993, p. 255), for example, conclude their re-analysis of the Gluecks' data with a strong prediction that imprisonment will increase rather than reduce the risk of further offending, and with a summary that is similar to Currie's account of the roots of violent crime:

'we believe that the causes of crime across the life course are rooted not in race, and not simply in drugs, gangs and guns – today's policy obsessions – but rather in structural disadvantage, weakened informal bonds to family, school and work, and the disruption of social relations between individuals and institutions that provide social capital.'

According to Braithwaite (1989), the strikingly low crime rate in Japan can be attributed to the success of Japanese social institutions in maintaining these social bonds, through the expression in schools and other socializing agencies of the 'reintegrative shaming' which Braithwaite sees as characteristic of good parenting (Masters 1997). Sampson and Laub (1993) conclude from the Gluecks' data that reintegrative shaming is a good description of the kind of upbringing that is protective against delinquency: essentially, this means parenting that is loving but firm, that conveys disapproval of a child's antisocial act while not rejecting or outcasting the child. The child may be sent to his or her bedroom for misbehaviour, but this demonstration of disapproval of the act will end with a loving hug of reconciliation and reacceptance.

LATE MODERNITY, RISK AND IDENTITY

The changes in American society described by Currie reflect some of the processes recent social theorists have analysed in terms of 'late', or 'high', or 'post' modernity. At the level of the economy, for example, the decline of heavy traditional industry, and of the solidaristic community life associated with it, provides a clear example of the rapid social changes which theorists like Beck (1992) and Giddens (1991, 1992) regard as consequences of 'globalization' and the technological developments associated with it, particularly in the diffusion of information. The main strands in this kind of theory that are relevant here are its concern with the nature of identity and the experience of risk in a world where unprecedented knowledge is combined with unprecedented uncertainty. Changes in one's sense of self and the possibility of shaping one's identity could well have implications for the vulnerability of young people to various disorders: although writers on these high-level global changes rarely address problems of crime directly (Giddens (1994) is a partial exception), they have offered accounts of some other disorders that typically affect young people. For example, Giddens' interest in the reflexive construction of identity leads him (Giddens 1991) to treat eating disorders such as anorexia as a distinctively late modern phenomenon, arising from an effort to establish a unique 'self-identity' in an environment in which young people with little ability to control most of what happens to them seek to control what they can – their own body and the image of themselves it presents to others.

It is arguable (Furlong and Cartmel 1997) that theorists such as Beck and Giddens exaggerate the newness and difference of the experience of late modernity, and that in claiming that the traditional categories of social analysis have become irrelevant they deny the continuing importance of structural inequalities, particularly those of class and geography. For example, Giddens (1994) writes as if everyone in developed societies were equally in a position to decide what to eat, and what variety of alternative therapy to select; he writes (pp. 6–7) that the decision to get married 'has to be made in relation to an awareness that marriage has changed in basic ways over the past few decades', as if everyone is equally conscious of these changes, and the nature of the choice is the same for all (Smith 1999). In short, Giddens writes as if the capacity to make playfully reflexive choices about what identity and way of life to choose were equally available to all, while on the contrary it is surely clear that, for example, the choice of what to eat is far more limited for someone who has to shop daily at the corner shop than for someone who has the money and access to transport to shop weekly at the hypermarket (and the healthfood and complementary medicine store).

Nevertheless, theories of late modernity can illuminate some of the changes that may have increased young people's vulnerability to crime and other kinds of trouble. Giddens (1994), for example, argues that one reaction to the strains of rapid social change is 'fundamentalism', which might be expressed as racially motivated violence, for instance, or as male violence against women and children, or as aggressive defence of a territory, since the essence of fundamentalism is a defensive attempt to reassert the values and power relations of a form of social organization perceived as under threat. And, like Giddens, Beck (1992) argues that as the collective identities of class and community affiliation arc weakened so identity becomes more a matter of individual choice; value systems lose their internal coherence and allegiances to this or that social group become more provisional and pragmatic as people struggle to make sense of a world of risk and uncertainty. Such theorists may exaggerate the extent to which people – and perhaps especially the young – are free to construct their own identities, but their accounts of late modernity have undoubtedly shown how global processes of change have made the social world radically more unstable and unpredictable. It is difficult now to make sense of the idea that people 'know their place' in society; young people who can feel confident about the course their lives will take are in a minority, and are probably to be found only among the most and least advantaged social groups. This uncertainty may open up possibilities of positive social development (Giddens 1994), but it is also likely to promote strain and anxiety – and, for those conscious of their exclusion from social and economic goods, anger and resentment.

CONCLUSIONS

The aim of this chapter has been to draw together a wide range of theoretical and empirical approaches to understanding criminality and other problematic behaviour among young people. An emerging theme has been that, despite the tendency of both empirical investigators (Rutter and Smith 1995) and social theorists (Giddens 1991) to deny or minimize the importance of social disadvantage, poverty and marginalization in explaining crime and associated problems such as drug or alcohol misuse, these socio-economic factors keep reappearing as soon as the focus is on serious, and especially violent, crime rather than on offending in general (Boswell 1998). The work of James (1995) and Currie (1997) has been used to suggest that middle-range theories, more adventurous than the cautious empiricism of Rutter and Smith, less speculative than the high theory of Beck or Giddens, can supply some of the causal mechanisms linking social change with family stress and the kind of childhood experiences that are associated with serious offending in later life, without being an inevitable or invariable cause of it.

The prevalence of childhood neglect and abuse, and of disrupted and unhappy experiences of family relationships, in the early lives of serious and persistent young offenders, is clear from the present author's own current work on projects for such offenders in Scotland. From data on around 200 young offenders, the great majority of them male, who represent the majority of the most extreme juvenile offenders in three different areas, the same patterns emerge again and again: experiences of neglect and abuse throughout childhood, conflictual and often violent relations between their parents, abandonment by parents, time spent in institutional care, experiences of loss of caring and cared-for adults, school failure and rejection of and by the school, alcohol and drug abuse – against a background of poverty, deprivation, and sometimes deeply ingrained subcultural criminality. Of course, many of the parents of these young people do care for them, but it is rare for them to have been able to express that care effectively – for instance, by the consistent practice of reintegrative shaming. Given the chance by the project workers, some can translate emotions of care into practical support for their children; but for many, by the time the project intervenes, the parent–child relationship has been strained or damaged beyond repair. This does not mean that progression to a career of adult offending is inevitable; there are numerous cases where the young person has been helped to stop offending or offend less damagingly, and in some instances to approach the threshold of adulthood with new hope and confidence. But the characteristic pattern is one of unhappiness, deprivation, loss and, often, violence, and this is the background not just to persistent routine offences against property or relatively minor offences of violence but to homicide and serious sexual violence. Given the evidence for the success of early intervention to support the most vulnerable families (Currie 1996; Karoly *et al.* 1998), the policy implications are clear: educational enhancement for disadvantaged children and focused support for mothers under pressure, ante-natally and in the first two years of the child's life, can reduce the likelihood of serious criminal careers and generally improve the life chances and social functioning for the children most at risk.

In the context of Britain at the start of the twenty-first century, there are some encouraging signs that government policy is being shaped in a way that suggests that these implications are having at least some influence. While aspects of the Labour government's approach to criminal justice, and especially to youth justice, are simply repressive (and thus in line with the policies of its predecessor), others reflect a new interest in social inclusion and integration. For example, the Youth Inclusion Programme, part of the Home Office's Crime Reduction Programme, involves the provision of services for young people and their families on a selection of the most deprived public housing estates in England and Wales; and the 'On Track' programme is providing funding for family support and compensatory education for 4- to 12-year-olds at risk of a slide into criminality. There are indications that the prevention of crime and criminality is receiving greater and more coherent government support, and (through the creation of multi-agency Youth Offending Teams) becoming better integrated with the direct provision of support and supervision to known young offenders. The language of social inclusion and 'joined-up government' may sometimes amount, as critics have claimed, to little more than aspirational rhetoric, but initiatives such as those mentioned above at least provide an opportunity to link policies on youth crime with a broader social policy agenda aimed at reducing inequalities and disadvantage, and to develop a coherent inter-disciplinary strategy, informed by evidence, that aims to support, and not simply to repress and deter, vulnerable young people and their families and carers.

REFERENCES

Agnew, R. 1985: A revised strain theory of delinquency. *Social Forces* **64**: 151–67.

Beck, U. 1992: *Risk Society: Towards a New Modernity*. London: Sage.

Blau, J. and Blau, P.M. 1982: The cost of inequality: social mobility, status integration and structural effects. *American Sociological Review* **32**: 790–801.

Boswell, G.R. 1991: *Waiting for Change: an Exploration of the Experiences and Needs of Section 53 Offenders*. London: The Prince's Trust.

Boswell, G.R. 1998: Criminal justice and violent young offenders. *Howard Journal of Criminal Justice* **37**: 148–60.

Bottoms, A.E. and Wiles, P. 1997: Environmental criminology. In Maguire, M., Morgan R. and Reiner, R. (eds), *The Oxford Handbook of Criminology*. Oxford: Oxford University Press, 307–59.

Braithwaite, J. 1989: *Crime, Shame and Reintegration*. Cambridge University Press.

Braithwaite, J. and Braithwaite, V. 1980: The effects of income inequality and social democracy on homicide. *British Journal of Criminology* **20**: 45–53.

Campbell, B. 1993: *Goliath: Britain's Dangerous Places*. London: Methuen.

Currie, E. 1985: *Confronting Crime*. London: Pantheon.

Currie, E. 1996: *Is America Really Winning the War on Crime and Should Britain Follow its Example?* NACRO.

Currie, E. 1997: Market, crime and community: towards a mid-range theory of post-industrial violence. *Theoretical Criminology* **1**: 147–62.

Dennis, N. 1993: *Rising Crime and the Dismembered Family*. London: Institute of Economic Affairs.

Dodd, T. and Hunter, P. 1992: *The National Prison Survey 1991*. London: HMSO.

Downes, D. 1993: *Employment Opportunites for Offenders*. London: Home Office.

Easterlin, R.A. 1980: *Birth and Fortune: Impacts of Numbers on Personal Welfare*. New York: Basic Books.

Farrington, D.P. 1997: Human development and criminal careers. In Maguire, M., Morgan R. and Reiner, R. (eds), *The Oxford Handbook of Criminology*. Oxford: Oxford University Press, 361–408.

Field, S. 1990: *Trends in Crime and their Interpretation*. London: HMSO.

Furlong, A. and Cartmel, F. 1997: *Young People and Social Change: Individualization and Risk in Late Modernity*. Buckingham: Open University Press.

Giddens, A. 1991: *The Consequences of Modernity*. Cambridge: Polity Press.

Giddens, A. 1992: *Modernity and Self-Identity*. Cambridge: Polity Press.

Giddens, A. 1994: *Beyond Left and Right: the Future of Radical Politics*. Cambridge: Polity Press.

Glueck, S. and Glueck, E. 1950: *Unraveling Juvenile Delinquency*. Cambridge, MA: Harvard University Press.

Gottesman, I.I. 1991: *Schizophrenia Genesis: the Origins of Madness*. Basingstoke: W.H. Freeman.

Graham, J. and Bowling, B. 1995: *Young People and Crime*. London: Home Office.

Halpern, D. 1995: Values, morals and modernity: the values, constraints and norms of European youth. In Rutter, M. and Smith, D.J. (eds), *Psychosocial Disorders in Young People: Time Trends and their Causes*. Chichester: John Wiley, 324–87.

Heidensohn, F. 1988: *Crime and Society*. London: Macmillan.

Home Office, Department of Health, Department of Education and Science *et al.* 1991: *Working Together under the Children Act. A Guide to Arrangements for Inter-Agency Cooperation for the Protection of Children from Abuse*. London: HMSO.

Hood, R. 1992: *Race and Sentencing*. Oxford: Clarendon Press.

Hough, M. 1995: *Drugs Misuse and the Criminal Justice System*. London: Home Office.

Hutton, W. 1996: *The State We're In*. London: Vintage.

James, O. 1995: *Juvenile Violence in a Winner–Loser Culture*. Free Association Books.

Karoly, L.A., Greenwood, P.W., Everingham, S.S. *et al.* 1998: *Investing in Our Children: What We Know and Don't Know About the Costs and Benefits of Early Childhood Intervention*. RAND.

Land, K.C., McCall, P.L. and Cohen, L.E. 1990: Structural covariates of homicide rates: are there any invariances across time and social space? *American Journal of Sociology* **95**: 922–63.

Lash, S. and Urry, J. 1987: *The End of Organized Capitalism*. Cambridge: Polity Press.

McGuire, J. (ed.) 1995: *What Works? Reducing Reoffending*. Chichester: John Wiley.

Mair, G. and May, C. 1997: *Offenders on Probation*. London: Home Office.

Masters, G. 1996: Reintegrative shaming and restorative justice. *Forensic Update* **45**: 9–14.

Masters, G. 1997: I conflitti e la mediazione nelle scuole in Giappone. In Pisapia G. and Antonucci, D. (eds), *La Sfida della Mediazione*. Italy: CEDAM, 133–46.

Merton, R.K. 1957: *Social Theory and Social Structure*. New York: The Free Press.

Mills, C.W. 1959: *The Sociological Imagination*. Harmondsworth: Penguin.

Mirrlees-Black, C., Mayhew, P. and Percy, A. 1996: *The 1996 British Crime Survey: England and Wales*. Home Office Statistical Bulletin 19/96. London: Home Office.

Mortimore, P., Sammons, P., Stoll, L. *et al.* 1988: *School Matters: The Junior Years*. Open Books.

Morgan, P. 1995: *Farewell to the Family? Public Policy and Family Breakdown in Britain and the USA*. London: Institute of Economic Affairs.

Murray, C. 1990: *The Emerging British Underclass*. London: Insitute of Economic Affairs.

MVA 1998: *Main Findings from the 1996 Scottish Crime Survey*. London: Scottish Office.

NACRO Youth Crime Section 1998: *Facts about Young Offenders in 1996*. NACRO.

Pearson, G. 1983: *Hooligan: A History of Respectable Fears*. London: Macmillan.

Pearson, G. 1987: *The New Heroin Users*. Oxford: Blackwell.

Pearson, G. 1994: Youth, crime and society. In Maguire, M., Morgan R. and Reiner, R. (eds), *The Oxford Handbook of Criminology*. Oxford: Oxford University Press, 1161–206.

Povey, D., Prime, J. and Taylor, P. 1998: *Notifiable Offences: England and Wales, 1997*. Home Office Statistical Bulletin 7/98. London: Home Office.

Pratt, J. 1985: Delinquency as a scarce resource. *Howard Journal of Criminal Justice* **24**: 81–92.

Rutter, M. and Smith, D.J. (eds) 1995a: *Psychosocial Disorders in Young People: Time Trends and their Causes*. Chichester: John Wiley.

Rutter, M. and Smith, D.J. 1995b: Towards causal explanations of time trends in psychosocial disorders of youth. In Rutter, M. and Smith, D.J. (eds), *Psychosocial Disorders in Young People: Time Trends and their Causes*. Chichester: John Wiley, 782–808.

Rutter, M., Maughan, R., Mortimore, P. *et al.* 1979: *Fifteen Hundred Hours: Secondary Schools and their Effect on Children*. Open Books.

Sampson, R.J. and Laub, J.H. 1993: *Crime in the Making: Pathways and Turning Points through Life*. Cambridge, MA: Harvard University Press.

Sampson, R.J. and Wilson, W.J. 1995: Race, crime and urban inequality. In Hagan, J. and Paterson, R.D. (eds), *Crime and Inequality*. Stanford, CA: Stanford University Press.

Smith, D. 1999: Criminality, social environments and late modernity. In O'Brien, M., Penna, S. and Hay, C. (eds), *Theorising Modernity: Reflexivity, Identity and Environment in Giddens' Social Theory*. Harlow: Longman, 121–38.

Smith, D. and Stewart, J. 1998: Probation and social exclusion. In Jones Finer, C. and Nellis, M. (eds), *Crime and Social Exclusion*. Oxford: Blackwell, 96–115.

Smith, D.J. and Rutter, M. 1995a: Introduction. In Rutter, M. and Smith, D.J. (eds), *Psychosocial Disorders in Young People: Time Trends and their Causes*. Chichester: John Wiley, 1–6.

Smith, D.J. and Rutter, M. 1995b: Time trends in psychosocial disorders of youth. In Rutter, M. and Smith, D.J. (eds), *Psychosocial Disorders in Young People: Time Trends and their Causes*. Chichester: John Wiley, 763–81.

Stewart, J., Smith, D. and Stewart, G. 1994: *Understanding Offending Behaviour*. Harlow: Longman.

Stewart, G. and Stewart, J. 1993: *Social Circumstances of Younger Offenders under Supervision*. Association of Chief Officers of Probation.

Taylor, I. 1999: *Crime in Context: a Critical Criminology of Market Societies*. Cambridge: Polity Press.

Townsend, P. 1992: Speech to Annual Conference of the Howard League for Penal Reform, New College, Oxford.

Utting, D., Bright, J. and Henricson, C. 1993: *Crime and the Family: Improving Child-rearing and Preventing Delinquency*. Family Policy Studies Centre.

Vennard, J., Sugg, D. and Hedderman, C. 1997: *Changing Offenders' Attitudes and Behaviour: What Works?* London: Home Office.

Widom, C.S. 1989: The intergenerational transmission of violence. In Weiner N.A. and Wolfgang, M.E. (eds), *Pathways to Criminal Violence*. London: Sage.

Zimring, F.E. and Hawkins, G. 1997: *Crime is Not the Problem: Lethal Violence in America*. New York: Oxford University Press.

5

Moral understanding and criminal responsibility of children

ALEX APLER

INTRODUCTION

'No civilised society regards children as accountable for their actions to the same extent as adults. ... The wisdom of protecting young children against the full rigour of the criminal law is beyond argument. The difficulty lies in determining when and under what circumstances that protection should be removed.' [R (a child) v Whitty (1993) 66 A Crim R 462]

Courts have always had to deal with the dilemma presented by the criminal behaviour of children. On the one hand, breach of criminal laws made children liable to punishment. On the other hand, the Courts recognized the immaturity of children, and their need for nurture and protection.

Whereas there is little controversy in distinguishing the behaviour of small children from adults, there is considerable debate about older children and the circumstances in which the protection of childhood should be removed and adult criminal responsibility attributed to their behaviour. This debate has focused mainly on young adolescents and their right to childhood.

Complicating this debate is the progressive and variable maturation of children. Maturity of young adolescents, as of children in all age groups, is not only subject to biological and familial influence, but also cultural (Offer *et al.* 1996). Actual and perceived differences in their ability to take on adult roles and responsibilities

may be enormous. Against this background the criminal process struggles with the very real task of managing the risk of adolescent crime (Rutter *et al.* 1998).

Criminal law has not found an adequate answer to this problem. The *doli incapax* presumption provided a framework of considering individual maturity of child offenders when evaluating their capacity to be criminally responsible. However, perceived inadequacies of the presumption led to its abolition in the UK in the Crime and Disorder Act 1998 (s34). The current approach to adolescent crime in the UK takes into account only the chronological age of the offender in determining his or her capacity to be criminally responsible. No consideration is given to the individual capacities of a young adolescent to shoulder the responsibility for personal behaviour.

Psychology of moral development can assist with determining the criminal responsibility of young offenders by providing a way of assessing the child offender's capacity to comprehend the wrongfulness of his or her behaviour.

THE LEGAL CONTEXT

The notion of childhood as a distinct state is common to all societies. All societies recognize that children, because of their immaturity, need special nurturing and protection. They are not given full responsibilities. Rites of passage often mark the point at which the child is no longer perceived as a child but as an adult, capable of bearing responsibility.

Transition to adulthood brings with it new rights and responsibilities (Bandalli 1999). These rights include a right to drive, vote, and marry. They are usually acquired towards the end of one's teenage years. It is understood that by that age, the adolescent can appreciate the consequences of actions sufficiently to exercise judgement and give consent.

The process of acquiring responsibilities, as opposed to rights, and in particular a capacity for criminal responsibility, is subject to social attitudes different from the attitudes about rights. It may represent considerable ambivalence towards the nature of adolescence and ability of adolescents to take on adult roles. Thus, adolescents are often judged capable of being criminally responsible at a much younger age than the age at which they are judged capable of exercising their rights.

Being responsible means having to confront the consequences of one's behaviour. In the context of criminal law, if a defendant is considered responsible, then the finding of guilt will make him or her liable to the full punishment that law may dispense (Hart 1968). Attributing full responsibility to children would make them as liable for their crimes as adults.

A variety of justifications is available for exonerating children from responsibility for their acts. One justification is that this protects them from punishment for their juvenile conduct, an essentially humane argument:

> '[children] are harmed in their development by the stigma and traumatic interference with natural psychological dependencies that in some degree any regime of public correction must cause ...' (Gross 1979)

Exculpation of children has also been argued on the basis that children have a limited ability to:

> 'appreciate the risks of doing certain things and to appreciate the significance of the resulting harm. Knowing what the risks are, and having regard for the interests of others, requires a social intelligence that the young are only in the process of developing ...' (Gross 1979)

A further argument for not holding children responsible is that they do not possess free will in the same way as adults. Children, much more than adults, function within a deterministic framework, subject to familial, peer, social and biological influences. This is especially true of young offenders, who often come from disadvantaged backgrounds and who:

> 'operate within a very constrained realm of choices, ... their prospects are limited, ... and the external pressures on them, be it from peers, parents or others, severely limit their scope of free choice'. (Zedner 1998)

While this last point may also be made about some adult offenders, it may be argued that environmental and biological influences are more significant in children who have not yet developed the capacity for independent or free will.

There is clear support for the proposition that children should not be held as responsible for their crimes as adults. What is not clear is when and how to remove the protection from full responsibility afforded by childhood. Every society struggles with this question. And yet the answers found vary enormously. For instance, in Ireland, children as young as 7 years can be held criminally responsible, while in Sweden, the minimum age of criminal responsibility is 15.

In England, the minimum age of criminal responsibility is 10 (Children and Young Persons Act 1933, s50, as amended in 1963). Children below 10 cannot be found criminally responsible, while those above 10 carry full responsibility of an adult. However, as with any purely age-based distinction, the sharp boundary of responsibility thus created is not consistent with what is known about child development. Child development is progressive and variable. It is subject to biological and environmental determinants. The capacity of children to appreciate consequences of their behaviour and to act intentionally through an exercise of free choice is still developing at a rate different for each individual. The age-dependent basis for criminal responsibility does not consider individual variability in maturity. Nor does the sharp cut-off for criminal responsibility take into account the progressive nature of maturation.

Until its abolition in the UK, the *doli incapax* presumption provided a framework for considering the individual maturity of child defendants. It did so by focusing the Court's attention on the child's understanding of his or her behaviour. In this way, criminal responsibility was attributed not merely by reference to the chronological age of the child defendant but also to maturity (Bandalli 1998).

Doli incapax means 'incapable of crime'. A Court applying this doctrine presumes that individuals who are in the 'intermediate stage' between the criminal incapacity of a child and full criminal capacity of an adult are incapable of committing crime. The 'intermediate stage' to which the presumption applies is between the ages of 10 and 14 years. This presumption of incapacity can be rebutted by the prosecution adducing evidence which proves the criminal capacity of the child defendant beyond reasonable doubt (Williams 1961).

To prove the criminal capacity of the defendant the prosecution must show that the child knew at the time of the offence that his or her actions were 'seriously wrong' and not 'merely naughty or mischievous'. If it were established that the child knew this difference, the prosecution could then proceed to prove the necessary mental and physical elements of the crime.

Implicit in this presumption is a recognition that chronological age is an insufficient criterion by which to judge the culpability of children. Children in the age group to which the presumption applies exhibit a wide variation in maturity. William Blackstone, who articulated the test in 1769, noted:

> '... by the law, as it now stands, and has stood at least since the time of Edward the third, the capacity of doing ill, or contracting guilt, is not so much measured by years and days, as by the strength of the delinquent's understanding and judgment. For one lad of eleven years old may have as much cunning as another of fourteen...'
> (*Blackstone's Commentaries on the Laws of England*, Book IV, 1st edn (1769), pp. 23–24)

However, the application of the presumption has not been without difficulties and it is partly in recognition of these that the UK legislature abolished the presumption by statute. These difficulties have centred around the issue of how to apply the *doli incapax* presumption. The courts have constantly struggled with the meaning of 'seriously wrong' and 'merely naughty or mischievous'. In C (A Minor) *v* DPP (H.L.(E.) [1995] 2 W.L.R. 383) the House of Lords cited authorities which propose that 'wrong means gravely wrong, seriously wrong, evil or morally wrong', and that 'wrong' refers to moral wrong as opposed to legal wrong. Another authority proposed that wrong means wrong 'according to the principles of ordinary people' (Field and SA *v* Gent (1996) 87 A.Crim.R. 225, at 230). These propositions do not fully clarify the meaning of 'wrong' in the presumption.

There has also been uncertainty in determining how 'seriously wrong' the child judged his or her behaviour. In part this might be attributed to the failure to develop a direct way of assessing the child's understanding (Apler 2000). Instead, the Courts have relied on indirect evidence such as the extent of formal education, previous criminal convictions, or what the child did or said before or after the crime. Absence of direct evidence has required the Courts to infer the child's knowledge indirectly.

THE POLITICAL CONTEXT

The debate concerning the *doli incapax* presumption is set against shifting social and political attitudes towards child offenders. These attitudes have stemmed from increasing community concern about crime, fuelled by highly publicized murders committed by children (Newburn 1997).

Punishing the young for their crimes is now often perceived as just. As recently as 1990 the policy of the British government was that allowance should be made for the fact that 'children's understanding, knowledge and ability are still developing' (Home Office 1990). Its current policy is that '[W]e must stop making excuses for children who offend. ... As they develop, children must bear increasing responsibility for their actions ...'

(Home Office 1997). Bandalli (1999) argues that there has been a change 'in the concept of childhood, shifting the approach to one that is premised on personal responsibility'.

A result of this change in attitude and government policy has been the statutory abolition of the *doli incapax* presumption. A practical consequence of the abolition is that children are no longer protected from the full force of criminal law. The courts now determine a 10-year-old child's guilt in the same way as an adult's: by establishing the necessary elements of the crime (*actus reus* and *mens rea*). The only point of distinction between a child and an adult for the purposes of determining criminal responsibility is that of age (10 years being the lower limit).

The protection afforded to children by the *doli incapax* presumption is still available in some other jurisdictions. In Australia, for instance, the presumption is still part of the law (Bartholomew 1998), although recently it has been subject to renewed public debate. This followed a widely-publicized NSW trial of a 10-year-old boy who was charged with murder after drowning a 6-year-old, but was acquitted on the basis that the prosecution was unable to rebut the *doli incapax* presumption.

Despite the abolition of the *doli incapax* presumption in the UK and uncertain future of the presumption in other jurisdictions, the necessity of differentiating the criminal responsibility of children from adults remains. However, the use of a child's age to determine when responsibility should arise is simplistic and does not accord with the reality of children's maturation being progressive and variable.

Moral development of children over the age of 10 should still be a legally relevant basis for determining their responsibility. Psychology of moral understanding can explain how children develop an awareness of right and wrong, and how that awareness can be assessed.

THE PSYCHOLOGY OF MORAL UNDERSTANDING

Psychological literature reveals that the understanding of right and wrong begins early in life. It depends on interactions with caregivers, usually within the family. It is unlikely that this understanding evolves into a distinct moral sense. Rather, it consists of cognitive and emotional components which guide the child's appreciation of the wrongs or rights of certain behaviours.

As early as age 2 years children have a basic understanding of rights and wrongs. They are sensitive to adult standards and attempt to uphold these (Kagan 1981). They are aware that rules exist in relation to integrity of property, harm to others, toileting and cleanliness. Kagan argues that even in the second year of life children already have inner standards and are capable of self-evaluation.

There is debate regarding whether children's understanding of right and wrong evolves into a distinct moral sense. Turiel argues that young children have a distinct moral sense, which depends on their understanding of how others feel (Turiel 1983). They would know, for instance, that hurting another child in the playground is wrong, regardless of rules. He contrasts this with children's understanding that conventions, such as calling the teacher by their first name rather than the second name, depend on the rules which can be altered by agreement. Others have questioned the idea of children developing a distinct appreciation of morality (Gabennesch 1990). The distinction between morality and convention may be blurred, as conventions may be founded on moral principles such as respecting authority and laying down rules (Kohlberg 1981).

Turiel's work suggests, however, that there can be two types of morality: that based on feelings and that based on rules. Awareness of rules and feelings marks the beginning of moral understanding. It develops in the context of family interactions in the second year of life (Dunn and Munn 1985). The child begins to understand and anticipate others' feelings and intentions. The child learns that others can be provoked and teased. He or she becomes aware of how personal feelings and behaviour affect others and how others' feelings and behaviour affect the child. The child is alerted to social rules which govern family conflicts, routines and consequences for transgression.

The above findings suggest that awareness of rules and feelings forms the basis of the child's moral development. This awareness depends on both cognitive and emotional maturation. Emotional maturation involves a developing capacity for empathy and the ability to experience guilt and shame. These factors are necessary for the child to be able to understand that certain behaviours can be wrong.

Cognitive factors

With cognitive maturation the child learns that there are rules which govern conduct. He or she understands that the breach of those rules has consequences. There may be unpleasant consequences for the child, such as punishment and disapproval, as well as harm to the victim. Awareness of these consequences helps the child understand why certain forms of conduct may be prohibited.

Kohlberg elaborated Piaget's cognitive theory of moralization, providing a useful basis for evaluating the child's understanding of rules and consequences. He proposed that moral development passes through three levels consisting of six stages in all (Colby and Kohlberg 1987).

1 The first level (*preconventional*) is characterized by the individual's inability to construct a shared or social viewpoint. Moral judgement at this level is egocentric and derives moral constructs from individual needs. It consists of acting in one's own best interests and letting others do the same. The individual's desire not to break rules is based on avoidance of punishment and of physical damage to persons and property. Kohlberg ascribes the preconventional level to children under the age of 9.

2 The second level (*conventional*) is characterized by an awareness of shared norms and values that sustain relationships, groups, communities and societies. At this level the notions of right and good are equated with the maintenance of existing social norms and values. This morality consists of a desire to live up to the roles and expectations others place on the individual, and to be 'good'. It involves being loyal and concerned about others' welfare. These individuals uphold the duties they agreed to and they understand the importance of maintaining social institutions.

3 The third and highest level (*postconventional*), according to Kohlberg, is not reached before the age of 20. Moral judgement at this level adopts a reflective perspective on social values and constructs moral principles that are universal in application. Individuals are aware of and tolerate a variety of rules and opinions which they uphold in the interests of impartiality (Locke 1986).

Kohlberg's approach points to the cognitive factors which can be assessed when evaluating the child's understanding of his or her behaviour. The child appreciates that behaviour is wrong by understanding that rules were transgressed and that this has consequences. The child may be concerned with the punitive consequences, and may be concerned with being 'good' and living up to others' expectations. He or she may also be aware of the consequences for the victim. By questioning the child about awareness of rules and consequences in relation to his or her behaviour, it is possible to clarify the cognitive factors affecting the child's understanding.

Developing empathy

The child's appreciation of how others may think and feel helps him or her understand how they may be affected by behaviour. Empathy is necessary for this understanding. Knowing the emotional reactions of victims, together with the cognitive understanding of the consequences of conduct enhances the child's perception of why some behaviours are unacceptable.

Capacity for empathy emerges with the child's developing ability to grasp that others have their own intentions, feelings and desires. In the child this understanding evolves into a 'theory of mind' – an idea that others have minds of their own, which guide their behaviour (Baron-Cohen 1992). The child learns to imagine, or form 'mental representations' of, what the mental states of others are and on that basis anticipates their behaviour.

The infant's capacity to understand the minds of others evolves in the context of a secure relationship (Main 1991). In the presence of a secure relationship, children begin to consider others' emotions and wishes from the second year of life, and others' beliefs from the third (Perner *et al.* 1987). The development of the reflective part of the self capable of representing others' minds is associated with the emergence of empathy (Zahn-Waxler *et al.* 1992).

Empathy has cognitive and emotional components (Hoffman 1981). Cognitive elements include a capacity for role-taking and appraisal of the other's predicament. These processes involve a movement away from Piaget's 'egocentrism' to an awareness of perspectives other than one's own – a stage of 'social reciprocity' (Light 1987). The child begins to understand that the experience of others may be different. These elements complement the second level of moral development described by Kohlberg.

The emotional component of empathy can be defined as an affective tendency to respond to another person's emotional behaviour with a parallel emotional reaction (Hay *et al.* 1994). It relies on the ability to perceive how the other person is feeling and why. The capacity to identify one's own feelings (emotional insight) and express them appropriately enhances the empathic response and in turn is more likely to result in prosocial behaviour (Roberts and Strayer 1996). The relationship between emotional insight and empathy may be mediated by role taking, as an understanding of one's own emotional experience helps to understand that of others (Zahn-Waxler *et al.* 1979).

Empathy helps the child appreciate that behaviour that hurts others may be wrong. It can inhibit negative behaviour and motivate positive behaviour. Evaluating the child's potential for empathy and his or her understanding of the hurtful consequences of certain behaviours for the victim can help determine the extent to which the child appreciated that the behaviours were wrong.

The sense of guilt

Negative emotional reactions such as guilt and shame following wrongdoing can signal to the child the unacceptability of that behaviour. Guilt arises when an empathic awareness of another's plight is coupled with self-blame as a result of the realization that one has been the cause of it (Hoffman 1981). A child may feel guilty and ashamed knowing that he or she breached rules and hurt another person. Assessment of these feelings, together with the child's cognitive and empathic awareness of the consequences of acts, can contribute to the overall evaluation of how seriously wrong the child considered the behaviour to be.

Children under the age of 8 years experience guilt differently from older children. Younger children may not have an internalized sense of wrongdoing; their feelings of guilt may depend on the presence of authority, which is seen as the source of rules and punishment. Without such authority feelings of guilt may be absent or diminished (Piaget 1932).

Feelings of guilt in young children may not bear a direct relationship to the extent of their responsibility for events. Their understanding of causality may still be developing and they may attribute responsibility inappropriately (Stipek and DeCotis 1988). Inappropriate feelings of guilt may also result from the tendency of young children to judge actions on the basis of outcome rather than intention (Nunner-Winkler and Sodian 1988). In contrast, older children may experience guilt and shame in a similar way to adults.

The child's experience of guilt and shame may depend on his or her evaluation and its context. Guilt may occur in the context of one's own evaluation of oneself, and shame in the context of evaluation by others (Tangney 1998). Shame is characterized by feelings of 'being small', worthless and powerless, and a desire to escape and hide, while guilt is characterized by feelings of tension, remorse and regret.

Feelings of guilt and shame may therefore depend on the child's age and the context in which these feelings are evoked. Reflecting on the behaviour and correctly attributing its negative consequences is relevant to the child's experience of these feelings. Assessment of negative feelings following wrongdoing can give additional information about the child's understanding of his or her behaviour.

The cognitive and emotional factors described above demonstrate how the appreciation of rights and wrongs emerges in childhood. While considerable information is available about moral maturation of young children, much less is known about moral development in early adolescence, the period most relevant to the debate on criminal responsibility. The way adolescents understand rights and wrongs may be different from the understanding of children. Exploration of moral development in early childhood nevertheless points to the factors which may be relevant to the assessment of adolescents. These factors may help judge the maturity of adolescents and their capacity to understand the rights and wrongs of their behaviour as a way of determining their capacity to be criminally responsible.

MORAL UNDERSTANDING AND DELINQUENTS

Experience within the family environment is crucial to the child's developing sense of morality. Delinquents, however, may not have the benefit of family relationships which promote the development of moral understanding. Their emotional development may be compromised. As a result they may be less able than their peers to consider the consequences of their actions.

There is a strong association between delinquency and a history of growing up in a chaotic home environment (Farrington 1978). Adolescents who offend are likely to come from families characterized by: marital disruption; parental illness; deficient physical care; social dependence; poor housing conditions; and poor maternal capacity or coping skills (Kolvin *et al.* 1988). About 50 years ago Bowlby (1953) commented on the relationship between maternal deprivation and delinquency and the development of what he called 'affectionless character'.

Adolescents in these families may not experience the kinds of relationships with parents and siblings that encourage the exploration and understanding of social roles and rules and which provide consistent consequences for misdemeanours. They are unlikely to experience emotional stability which allows understanding of their own feelings and that of others. Their capacity to comprehend the mental worlds of others and to respond empathically may be limited.

Limited awareness of mental states may disable the child's normally aversive reaction to others' distress (Fonagy *et al.* 1997). It may permit the child to disregard or at least misinterpret the psychological consequences of a certain act on others. Absence of the painful psychic consequences of identifying with the victim's mental state including feelings of guilt may make crimes against people more likely.

Delinquents may have a reduced capacity for emotional awareness of right and wrong. They may not understand, or be concerned with, the emotional effect of their behaviour on the victim. They may not be able to experience or acknowledge feelings of guilt or shame. Angry adolescents who appear indifferent to the consequences of their behaviour can fall into this category.

Arguably for these adolescents, the means to understanding behaviour as wrong is cognitive. They may be aware that they are breaking rules and that there may be adverse consequences such as punishment, expulsion or alienation. Their capacity to contemplate these consequences, however, may be limited.

ASSESSING MORAL UNDERSTANDING

The factors described above can help assess the child's understanding of his or her delinquent behaviour. This understanding consists of cognitive and emotional awareness of the personal consequences and the consequences for the victim. The child's understanding of rules, feelings and emotional response to his or her behaviour have the potential to indicate to the interviewer the nature and extent of the child's knowledge.

Assessment of cognitive factors would include exploration of the child's awareness of rules and of consequences for breaching those rules such as punishment or disapproval. Similarly, the child's understanding of the emotional and physical consequences for the victim may be considered. Evaluation of the child's ability to put himself or herself into the shoes of the victim would also be relevant, as would be the presence of a negative emotional reaction to personal acts, which may indicate the extent of the child's appreciation of misbehaviour.

Assessment of the factors outlined above may be complicated where the behaviour has had mixed consequences. A child may be reprimanded by police, yet cheered by a gang of peers; may feel some degree of guilt, but also some pride for the success of the mischief; and, while being aware that the victim was hurt, may also feel pleased and justified in his or her acts. For the purpose of assessing the child's capacity to be criminally responsible, it is the awareness of the negative consequences of personal behaviour that is relevant. It is this awareness that may allow a degree of responsibility to be attributed to the child.

The above assessment would not, however, indicate whether the child should be held responsible for his or her behaviour. Instead, it would indicate on a continuum the child's understanding of the wrongfulness of certain mischief. Whether that understanding is sufficient for exculpation would be for the criminal process to determine.

One further difficulty in assessing the child's understanding is the distinction that needs to be made between the child's understanding at the time of the offence and his or her understanding at the time of the interview. Only the former should be relevant to attribution of responsibility for offending behaviour. The act of interviewing itself, either by police or expert witness, can suggest to the child the wrongfulness of certain behaviour and influence the outcome of the assessment. There is no easy way to eradicate this difficulty, although other evidence of the child's knowledge, such as past criminal convictions, can assist with interpretation of the responses.

CONCLUSIONS

The current legal approach in the UK to determining the capacity of children to be criminally responsible may be easy to apply but it remains simplistic and arbitrary. The age-based test does not consider the variable and progressive maturation of children. In contrast, while the *doli incapax* presumption does provide a framework for considering the maturity of individual child offenders, it has proved difficult to consistently apply and it continues to attract controversy in jurisdictions where it is still part of the law.

The psychology of moral development can assist with assessing the capacity of children to be criminally responsible. It does not exclude an age-based approach, but can deflect criticisms of that approach by allowing for individual variations among child offenders to be taken into account. It may provide a more relevant basis for differentiating the criminal responsiblity of children from that of adults.

Acknowledgement

This chapter is based on a dissertation submitted for section II of the Royal Australian and New Zealand College of Psychiatrists examination, and funded by a Fellowship in Adolescent Forensic Psychiatry from the NSW Institute of Psychiatry.

REFERENCES

Apler, A. 2000: Naughty or bad? The role of expert evidence in rebuttal of the *doli incapax* presumption. *Psychiatry, Psychology and Law* **7**(1): 206–11.

Bandalli, S. 1998: Abolition of the presumption of *doli incapax* and the criminalisation of children. *The Howard Journal* **37**(2): 114–22.

Bandalli, S. 1999: Children and the expanding role of the criminal law. *Child Psychology and Psychiatry Review* **4**(2): 85–90.

Baron-Cohen, S. 1992: The development of a theory of mind: where would we be without the intentional stance. In Rutter, M. and Hay, D. (eds), *Developmental Principles and Clinical Issues in Psychology and Psychiatry*. Oxford: Blackwell Scientific.

Bartholomew, T. 1998: Legal and clinical enactment of the *doli incapax* defence in the Supreme Court of Victoria, Australia. *Psychiatry, Psychology and Law* **5**(1): 95–105.

Bowlby, J. 1953: Maternal care and mental health. In Fry, M. (ed.), *Child Care and the Growth of Love*. London: Penguin.

Colby, A. and Kohlberg, L. 1987: *The Measurement of Moral Judgment: 1. Theoretical Foundations and Research Validation*. Cambridge: Cambridge University Press.

Dunn, J. and Munn, P. 1985: Becoming a family member: family conflict and the development of social understanding. *Child Development* **56**: 480–92.

Farrington, D.P. 1978: The family backgrounds of aggressive youths. In Hersov, L.A., Berger, M. and Shaffer, D. (eds), *Aggression and Antisocial Behaviour in Childhood and Adolescence*. Oxford: Pergamon, 73–93.

Fonagy, P., Target, M., Steele, M. and Steele, H. 1997: The development of violence and crime as it relates to security of attachment. In Osofsky, J.D. (ed.), *Children in a Violent Society*. New York: Guilford Press.

Gabennesch, H. 1990: The perception of social conventionality by children and adults. *Child Development* **61**: 2047–59.

Gross, H. 1979: *A Theory of Criminal Justice*. Oxford: Oxford University Press.

Hart, H.L.A. 1968: *Punishment and Responsibility: Essays in the Philosophy of Law*. Oxford: Clarendon Press.

Hay, D.F., Castle J. and Jewett J. 1994: Character development. In Rutter, M. and Hay, D.F. (eds), *Development Through Life: a Handbook for Clinicians*. Oxford: Blackwell Scientific, 319–49.

Hoffman, M.L. 1981: The development of empathy. In Rushton, J.P. and Sorrentino, R.M. (eds), *Altruism and Helping Behaviour: Social, Personality and Developmental Perspectives*. Hillsdale, NJ: Lawrence Erlbaum Associates, 41–63.

Home Office 1990: *Crime, Justice and Protecting the Public*. Cmnd 965. London: HMSO.

Home Office 1997: *No More Excuses – A New Approach to Tackling Youth Crime in England and Wales*. Cm 3809. London: HMSO.

Kagan, J. 1981: *The Second Year: the Emergence of Self Awareness*. Cambridge, MA: Harvard University Press.

Kohlberg, L. 1981: *Essays on Moral Development: 1: the Philosophy of Moral Development*. London: Harper & Row.

Kolvin, I., Miller, F.J.W., Fleeting, M. and Kolvin, P.A. 1988: Social and parenting factors affecting criminal-offence rates: findings from the Newcastle Thousand Family Study (1947–80). *British Journal of Psychiatry* **152**: 80–90.

Light, P. 1987: Taking roles. In Bruner, J. and Haste, H. (eds), *Making Sense: the Child's Construction of the World*. London: Methuen.

Locke, D. 1986: A psychologist among the philosophers: philosophical aspects of Kohlberg's theories. In Modgil, S. and Modgil, C. (eds), *Lawrence Kohlberg: Consensus and Controversy*. Brighton: Falmer Press.

Main, M. 1991: Metacognitive knowledge, metacognitive monitoring, and singular (coherent) vs (incoherent) models of attachment: findings and directions for future research. In Harris, P., Stevenson-Hinde, J. and Parkes, C (eds), *Attachment Across the Life Cycle*. New York: Routledge.

Newburn, T. 1997: Youth, crime and justice. In Maguire, M., Morgan, R. and Reiner, R. (eds), *The Oxford Handbook of Criminology*, 2nd edn. Oxford: Clarendon Press.

Nunner-Winkler, G. and Sodian, B. 1988: Children's understanding of moral emotions. *Child Development* **59**: 1323–38.

Offer, D. *et. al.* 1996: Normal adolescent development: empirical research findings. In Lewis, M. (ed.), *Child and Adolescent Psychiatry: A Comprehensive Textbook*. Baltimore: Williams & Wilkins, 382–93.

Perner, J., Leekam, S.R. and Wimmer, H. 1987: Three-year-olds' difficulty with false belief. *British Journal of Developmental Psychology* **5**: 125–37.

Piaget, J. 1932: *The Moral Development of the Child*. London: Penguin.

Roberts, W. and Strayer, J. 1996: Empathy, emotional expressiveness, and prosocial behaviour. *Child Development* **67**: 449–70.

Rutter, M., Giller, H. and Hagell, A. 1998: *Antisocial Behaviour by Young People*. Cambridge: Cambridge University Press.

Stipek, D.J. and DeCotis, K.M. 1988: Children's understanding of the implications of causal attributions for emotional experiences. *Child Development* **59**: 1601–16.

Tangney, J.P. 1998: How does guilt differ from shame? In Bybee, J. (ed.), *Guilt and Children*. London: Academic Press, 1–18.

Turiel, E. 1983: *The Development of Social Knowledge: Morality and Convention*. Cambridge: Cambridge University Press.

Williams, G. 1961: *Criminal Law: the General Part*, 2nd edn. London: Stevens and Sons Ltd.

Zahn-Waxler, C., Radke-Yarrow, M. and King, R. 1979: Child rearing and children's prosocial initiations towards victims of distress. *Child Development* **50**: 319–30.

Zahn-Waxler, C., Radke-Yarrow, M., Wagner E. and Chapman, M. 1992: Development of concern for others. *Developmental Psychology* **28**: 126–36.

Zedner, L. 1998: Sentencing young offenders. In Ashworth, A. and Wasik, M. (ed.), *Fundamentals of Sentencing Theory: Essays in Honour of Andrew von Hirsch*. Oxford: Clarendon Press, 165–86.

PART 2

Forensic behaviours: neurobiology, genetics and childhood antecedents

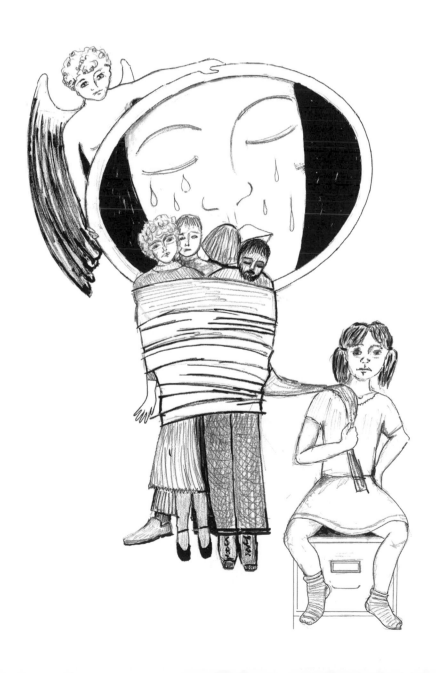

6

Neurobiological factors in aggressive children and adults

MAIREAD DOLAN

GENERAL ISSUES

Recent advances in our understanding of the biology of the brain allow us to postulate biological correlates of several personality traits and antisocial behaviours, particularly poor impulse control, aggression, affective lability and cognitive processing deficits (Kavoussi and Coccaro 1995; Coccaro 1989, 1992; Siever and Davis 1991; Van Pragg 1994). The methods used to investigate brain–behaviour relationships reflect those used in the study of major psychiatric syndromes such as schizophrenia. They include neurochemical, neuropsychological and neuroimaging techniques. Unfortunately, there is still considerable debate surrounding the issue of using categorical or dimensional approaches to examine the biological substrates of personality pathology and antisocial behaviour in children or adults.

From a biological perspective, however, both approaches may be necessary, although dimensional models allow for correlations with biological measures more readily than categorical models.

Reviews of the literature on empirical studies of relevance to aggression and antisocial behaviour in aggressive and violent subjects are compounded by the fact that different approaches to the assessment have been employed and there are relatively few truly replicative studies in any of the relevant domains. Nonetheless, it is possible to accumulate evidence of specific neurobiological deficits in relation to particular personality traits such as aggression

and impulsivity, and that is largely the focus of this review. The objective is to clarify some of the key issues surrounding neurobiological research in impulsive aggressive populations.

CONCEPTS OF IMPULSIVITY AND AGGRESSION

Impulsivity and aggression are complex concepts. Impulsivity is part of the defining characteristics of a number of psychiatric diagnosis – e.g. borderline and antisocial personality disorders, psychopathy, conduct disorder and disruptive behaviour disorders, and attention-deficit hyper-activity disorder (Stein et al. 1985, 1993). Traditionally, psychiatrists view impulsivity as an aspect of behavioural disorders and this is highlighted in the current psychiatric classification systems (Diagnostic and Statistical Manual, 4th edn [DSM-IV] or the International Classification of Diseases, 10th edn [ICD-10]) which rely on operational criteria to define specific categories. Psychological classification systems for personality dimensions such as impulsivity and aggression, however, generally rely on the identification of dimensions through factor analysis (e.g. Quay's behaviour classification dimensions), or the delineation of types through cluster analysis (e.g. Minnesota Multiphasic Personality Inventory (MMPI)).

Definitions of impulsivity also vary. In general, it is now accepted that impulsivity reflects a multidimensional concept which relates to behavioural restraint, rapid processing of information, novelty seeking, and inability to delay gratification (Barratt and Patton 1983; Barratt 1985). Although impulsivity is often confused with aggression, the differences from a theoretical and practical standpoint are important. Many studies use suicidal or aggressive behaviour as indices of impulsivity. This may be reasonable given the evidence that impulsivity measures correlate highly with pure aggression measures and account for about 30% of the variance in aggressive behaviour (Plutchik and Van Pragg 1995). Buss (1988) also emphasizes the fact that traits such as impulsivity do not occur in isolation, and that the combination of impulsivity with high levels of aggression contribute to delinquent/criminal and psychopathic behaviour.

Aggression also represents a complex set of behaviours displayed in almost all animal species in different conflict situations (Bevan 1989). It has been categorized as affective and predatory. The former is intra-species, associated with sympathetic arousal, and can be divided into offensive and defensive forms (Blanchard and Blanchard 1984). Predatory aggression occurs between species and is not associated with sympathetic arousal. The typology of aggressive symptoms is believed to relate to specific brain structures that mediate different forms of aggression. Ethnological research has further indicated that certain types of events (threats and challenges) increase aggressive impulses; but a number of modulating factors – such as access to weapons, personality structure and anxiety – may influence whether or not these impulses are translated to aggressive acts or violence.

Bond (1992) defined aggression, in humans, as 'behaviour directed by one individual against another individual (or object or self) with the aim of causing harm'. This definition encompasses both auto-aggression and outwardly directed aggression, although there is some debate as to whether auto-aggression should be allied with depressive symptomatology rather than aggression. The measurement of aggression largely focuses on outwardly directed aggression and concentrates on either trait aggression or overt acts. However, trait aggression, in itself, is a complex concept comprising several components including verbal and physical aggression, anger and hostility, all of which may be situation-specific to some degree.

NEUROBIOLOGICAL PERSPECTIVES ON IMPULSIVE AGGRESSIVE BEHAVIOUR

Although several psychosocial aetiological models have been proposed to explain the development of impulsive and aggressive styles of behaviour in criminal and delinquent antisocial populations, there is reasonable evidence, at a phenomenological level, that a neurobiological model may be a promising avenue of exploration. Early case studies provided some hypotheses about the nature of the brain structures involved in impulsive aggressive behaviour (Benson and Blumer 1975), but more recently attempts have been made to demonstrate subtle neurological impairments in patients who present with symptoms of aggression without frank brain injury.

In the following sections the neurobiology of impulsivity and aggression will be reviewed in terms of their anatomical and neurochemical substrates. The key empirical evidence supporting current theoretical models of antisocial behaviour will be reviewed.

Neuroanatomy of impulsive aggression

A number of authors have suggested that certain types of aggressive symptoms relate to specific brain structures which in turn mediate different forms of aggression (Weiger and Bear 1988; Bear 1989; Benson and Blumer 1975; Silver et al. 1992). Thus, structural lesions of the hypothalamus are associated with unprovoked and undirected aggression in response to physical contact. Temporolimbic lesions result in either enhanced or reduced aggression because of the modulatory function of the amygdala and the aggressive acts relate to emotional and environmental events. Prefrontal lesions produce a varying picture depending on the seat of dysfunction, but impulsive responses to environmental frustration point to dysfunction of the orbitofrontal cortex and associated structures (Weiger and Bear 1988; Stein et al. 1995). The frontal lobes have well-developed connections with limbic and subcortical areas via the dorsal medial nucleus of the thalamus to the orbitofrontal cortex or the convexity and the cingulofrontal pathways. Several functions have been identified as involving the frontal lobes, including conceptual ability, executive abilities, attention and arousal, perseverance, empathy and language functions (Gualtieri 1995). Cortical lesion studies examining damage to the frontal cortex have shown a pattern of changes, including shallowness, impulsive self-serving behaviour, disinhibition, irritability, aggression and a lack of concern for moral standards (Silver et al. 1992), which is reminiscent of those with antisocial or psychopathic personality traits. The site of damage, however, is believed to be a significant factor in the ultimate presentation and nature of deficits exposed (Damasio 1985; Luria 1973). Thus lesions of the dorsolateral convexity result in apathy, lack of reactivity, impairment in the formation of plans, reduction in intellectual functioning involving abstract reasoning and concept formation, and reduction in the ability to sustain attention, concentration and the ability to evaluate the consequences of one's own behaviour. Orbitofrontal lesions, on the other hand, result in impulsive behaviour, disinhibition and loss of guilt and remorse, but have no direct effect on higher cognitive functions.

Theoretically, the frontal lobes and their connections would provide a suitable anatomical substrate for the study of impulsive aggressive behaviour in antisocial populations. Psychophysiological, brain-imaging and neuropsychological techniques have been used to study relationships between frontal function and aggression; these will be reviewed later in the text.

Neurochemical theories of aggression

Both animal and human studies now point to a multiple neurotransmitter (NT) theory of aggression modulation, and support the notion that different types of aggressive behaviour have differing neurochemical and neuro-anatomical substrates. Three of the most significant NT systems implicated in aggression modulation are serotonin, noradrenaline (norepinephrine) and dopamine. To date, the serotonergic system has received most attention in clinical samples.

THE BEHAVIOURAL-DISINHIBITION/LOW-5-HT HYPOTHESIS OF AGGRESSIVE ANTISOCIAL BEHAVIOUR

This perspective suggests that antisocial and impulsive individuals are behaviourally disinhibited because of an imbalance of the behavioural activation system (BAS) and behavioural inhibition system (BIS) (Quay 1988; Fowles 1980). Some researchers argue that aggressive antisocial subjects have a hypersensitivity to reward – an overactive BAS relative to BIS (Scerbo et al. 1990); others suggest that an underactive BIS relative to BAS is the basic deficit (Fowles 1980; Newman 1987). Several studies have shown that criminal and delinquent psychopaths have difficulty avoiding responses leading to punishment, which has been interpreted as a deficiency in the BIS, when competing cues of reward and punishment are present (Newman et al. 1985; Newman and Kosson 1986). In addition, Fowles (1980) postulated, on the basis of reduced skin conductance responses when anticipating aversive stimuli, that an underactive BIS is related to disinhibited psychopathic behaviour.

Given that the septo-hippocampal-frontal (SHF) system is believed to be the anatomical substrate of the BIS and that serotonergic (5-HT) activity has a significant impact on the workings of the BIS, one would expect empirical evidence to support the suggestion that disinhibited individuals have reduced serotonergic activity. Much of the empirical research supports the notion that 5-HT shows an inverse relationship with disinhibited and impulsive aggressive behaviour, but largely in post-pubertal males (see Markowitz and Coccaro (1995) for a review). However, an underactive BIS would also be expected to result in reduced anxiety in punishable situations. As yet, there has only been limited investigation into the nature of anxiety in different populations of impulsive aggressive subjects, but there is some evidence on the basis of cortisol

output that aggressive/criminal subjects have reduced catecholamine output both at rest and in the face of punishable situations (Lidberg et al. 1978; Virkkunen 1985).

At present there are few published studies looking at the role of other neurotransmitters in impulsive aggressive behaviour. It is therefore difficult to clarify the proposed activities of the BAS. On the basis of Depue and Spoont's (1986) conceptualization of serotonin (5-HT) as a behavioural constraint mechanism, several studies have examined 5-HT function in aggressive populations. These will be reported later.

EMPIRICAL STUDIES OF 5-HT IN HUMANS: METHODOLOGICAL ISSUES

Unlike with animal studies, the techniques available for the study of brain dysfunction in humans, particularly at a biochemical level, remain restricted because of the invasive nature of many procedures. Studies of neurotransmitter (NT) function in man are limited to post-mortem (PM) studies, urinary and plasma sampling of NTs, cerebrospinal fluid (CSF) studies, and neuroendocrinological challenge techniques. Each method has specific limitations that contribute to the difficulties in interpreting conflicting results when they arise. Neuroendocrine challenges with selected psychopharmacological agents do, however, offer the advantage of allowing assessment of the responsivity of specific NT systems and therefore provide a more dynamic picture of neurotransmission (Van Praag et al. 1987).

Over the last 15 years, challenge agents have evolved from 5-HT precursor (5-HTP) challenges to stimulation with global release/re-uptake blockade, and stimulation with selective receptor agonists. Most measure plasma prolactin (PRL) and/or cortisol (CORT) responses as these are believed to be under serotonergic control, and 5-HT is believed to be predominantly stimulatory to PRL and CORT in human subjects (van der Klar and Bethea 1982; Lewis and Sherman 1985). Some of the more commonly used probes include indirect and direct agonists. Indirect agonists include the 5-HT precursors L-tryptophan and 5-hydroxytryptophan, the 5-HT releasing/uptake-inhibiting agent D,L-fenfluramine and D-fenfluramine, and the 5-HT uptake-inhibiting agent clomipramine. Direct agonists include the postsynaptic receptor agonists m-chlorophenyl-piperazine m-CPP, buspirone and ipsapirone (Coccaro and Kavoussi 1994; Coccaro et al. 1993). As yet, the specific receptor selectivities of many challenge agents remain unclear.

STUDIES OF CEREBROSPINAL FLUID 5-HIAA CONCENTRATION IN HUMANS (Table 6.1)

A substantial number of reports indicate that central nervous system (CNS) 5-HT may be altered in suicidal behaviour in humans (Van Praag 1983a,b; Coccaro and Astill 1990; Asberg et al. 1986, 1987; Marazziti et al. 1989) and in dependent on peripheral tryptophan metabolism and platelet physiology as well as being both state and trait dependent (Raleigh et al. 1984). Nevertheless, the direction of the relationship between 5-HT in blood and aggression is consistent with one report (McBride et al. 1987) that suggests whole-blood 5-HT is negatively correlated with levels of central serotonergic activity. Reduced numbers of imipramine binding sites on platelets, relative to controls, and significant inverse correlations between binding site measures and aggression on a parent-rated child behaviour checklist, have been found in pre-pubertal children with comorbid DSM-III conduct and attention-deficit disorders (Stoff et al. 1987). Platelet 5-HT uptake studies in aggression indicate evidence of an association between low serotonin platelet uptake and aggressive behaviour in schizophrenic adolescents (Modai et al. 1989), and impulsivity measures in male outpatients with episodic aggression (Brown et al. 1989). A reduction in $5-HT_2$ receptor platelet binding in delinquent adolescents has been reported (Blumensohn et al. 1995), suggesting a role for serotonin in general and $5-HT_2$ receptors in particular in aggressive behaviour. The direction of the association between the platelet measures and aggression suggest diminished presynaptic serotonergic activity, if the platelet findings can be extrapolated to 5-HT nerve terminals.

MONOAMINE OXIDASE ACTIVITY (Table 6.2)

In several studies, impulsive aggressive and disinhibited behaviour have been associated with low serotonergic activity (Linnoila and Virkkunen 1992), and the notion that platelet MAO activity reflects central serotonergic activity is supported by the findings of a positive correlation between CSF 5-HIAA and MAO activity (Oreland et al. 1981). The exact mechanism for the association is not known. A low or qualitatively weak serotonergic turnover, in several studies, has been found to be related to certain personality traits such as sensation seeking and impulsivity in both normal subjects and psychiatric patients (Zuckerman 1991). Accordingly, low platelet MAO activity has been used as a biological marker of vulnerability to disinhibitory psychopathology as evidenced by psychopathy, violent suicide attempts, hyperactivity and alcoholism (Oreland 1993). In addition, several reports suggest an association between low platelet activity and criminal behaviour (Lidberg et al. 1985; Belfrage et al. 1992).

Recently, Alm et al. (1994) showed that in men who had committed crimes before the age of 15 years those who had continued to offend displayed lower platelet MAO than those who had no continued criminality. They concluded that the link was probably secondary to the strong associations between low platelet MAO activity and personality traits such as sensation seeking and impulsiveness. Klinteberg and Oreland (1995) examined platelet MAO activity and found a positive relationship between

hyperactive behaviour and aggressiveness in childhood, and a negative association between hyperactive behaviour and adult platelet MAO activity. There was no significant interaction effect between aggressiveness and platelet MAO activity. Taken together with some of their previous reports, that hyperactivity in childhood correlated highly with an impulsive sensation-seeking psychopathy factor at age 27 years (Klinteberg et al. 1990), they suggested that the integrating factor was the relationship with trait impulsiveness, and that MAO activity and hyperactivity (impulsivity) could represent an underlying biological vulnerability in terms of low serotonergic turnover. Their findings also highlighted the importance of an interactional perspective, in which individual development is understood as an ongoing process involving psychological, biological and environmental factors.

Studies of platelet MAO (B) activity in non-psychiatric subjects indicate negative or inverse associations with a number of personality dimensions such as impulsivity (Schalling et al. 1987; Perris et al. 1980), sensation seeking (Fowler et al. 1980; Schooler et al. 1978; Von Knorring et al. 1984), psychopathy (Lidberg et al. 1985), suicidality (Buchsbaum et al. 1977; Gottfries et al. 1980), and substance abuse (Major and Murphy 1978). In Lidberg et al.'s (1985b) study of criminal offenders hospitalized for forensic assessments, the subgroup of psychopaths diagnosed according to Cleckley's criteria had lower mean MAO activity than controls. This was believed to relate primarily to poor impulse control. Others have shown that low platelet MAO measured in adulthood correlates with hyperactive behaviour (Klinteberg and Oreland 1995) and with criminal behaviour (Alm et al. 1994) in childhood, indicating a possible biological vulnerability to disinhibited behaviours.

Low platelet MAO, which is a marker of 5-HT function, appears to be reduced in a number of disorders characterized by impulsive, disinhibited behaviours. The findings appear more consistent in males and are consistent with other 5-HT studies reporting links between impulsive aggressive behaviour and reduced serotonergic function.

NEUROENDOCRINE CHALLENGES (Table 6.3)

The 5-HT receptor challenge paradigm more directly addresses the issue of 5-HT receptor sensitivity. Unfortunately, there are still relatively few studies in this area and the populations examined vary considerably. In addition, the challenge agents are disparate in nature, although the majority have used fenfluramine as the biochemical probe. Fenfluramine releases 5-HT, blocks reuptake, and acts post-synaptically through its metabolites. It is believed to act at $5-HT_{1A}$ and/or $5-HT_2$ receptors and, at the level of the hypothalamus, results in a dose-dependent increase in prolactin (DiRenzo et al. 1989; Goodall et al. 1993; Lewis and Sherman 1985).

Table 6.2 *Platelet MAO studies in aggression*

Authors	Group	Measure	Criteria	Results
Soloff *et al.* (1991)	BPD, females (72)	Platelet MAO	DIB, BIS HRSD, BDI	MAO correlates negatively with hostility/ trait impulsivity • Positively with state impulsivity • No relationship with depression
Yehuda *et al.* (1989)	15 male BPD/ASP	Platelet MAO	SADS DIB	Platelet MAO lower in BPD than normal controls BPD and ASP had lower MAO than controls No relationship with depression or history of substance abuse
Paykel *et al.* (1979)	10 female BPD depressed patients	Platelet MAO	Group comparisons	MAO greater in BPD compared with all depressed patients. MAO lower in BPD compared with secondary depression
Lahmeyer *et al.* (1988)	17 male/female BPD depressed patients	Platelet MAO	DIS DSM-IIIR: BPD	MAO lower in BPD than depressed patients
Lidberg *et al.* (1985)	Criminal offenders (psychopaths) Controls	Platelet MAO	Cleckley's criteria	MAO lower in criminal psychopaths than controls
Alm *et al.* (1994)	70 male criminals	Platelet MAO	Criminal careers	MAO in criminals less than controls. Mean platelet MAO activity in subjects with both early and late criminality was lower than in former delinquents without late criminality
Klinteberg and Oreland (1995)	75 male subjects assessed in adulthood Longitudinal study	Platelet MAO in adulthood	Teacher ratings of motor restlessness/ concentration difficulties/ aggressiveness Subjects aged 10–13 years	Hyperactive behaviour in childhood negatively correlates with MAO in adulthood
Schalling *et al.* (1988, 1987) Schalling (1978)	Normal males	Platelet MAO	Personality measures KSP	Low platelet MAO associated with extroverted, impulsive, sensation-seeking traits and low socialization
Belfrage *et al.* (1992)	59 offenders in forensic psychiatric facility	Platelet MAO	Classified according to: • crime • history of past • aggression	Lower MAO activity in violent offenders Lower MAO activity in aggressive offenders

MAO, monoamine oxidase; DBD, disruptive-behaviour disorder; DIB, Diagnostic Interview for Borderlines; BIS, Barratt Impulsivity Scale; HRSD, Hamilton Rating Scale for Depression; BDI, Beck Depression Inventory; SADS, Schedule for Affective Disorders and Schizophrenia; ASP, antisocial personality disorder; BPD, borderline personality disorder; DIS, Diagnostic Interview Schedule; KSP, Karolinska Scales of Personality.

The main studies of relevance to impulsive aggressive populations are shown in Table 6.3. The majority of studies in aggressive adults appear to show evidence of blunted prolactin responses to fenfluramine and/or significant negative correlations between prolactin response and measures of aggression, particularly, irritability and motor impulsivity (Coccaro *et al.* 1989; Siever *et al.* 1989; O'Keane *et al.* 1992; Dolan 1996; Dolan *et al.* 2001). Fishbein *et al.*'s (1989) study of substance abusers, however, found positive correlations between aggression and impulsivity and prolactin responses to D,L-fenfluramine which may relate to the impact of cocaine on the endocrine responsivity or increased post-synaptic sensitivity due to depletion of 5-HT by cocaine.

In children, the findings have largely been in the opposite direction. Stoff *et al.* (1992) found net D,L-fenfluramine-induced prolactin and cortisol release was not correlated with aggression rates in pubertal and adolescent disruptive-behaviour disordered (DBD) patients and did not differ significantly between adolescent DBD patients and normal controls. The methodology, however, was inconsistent. The pre-pubertal group – which comprised seven subjects

Table 6.3 *Neuroendocrine challenges in aggression*

Authors	Probe	Sample	Measure	Behavioural	Results
Meltzer et al. (1984)	5-HTP	Patients with affective disorder Normal controls	Cortisol	Suicide attempts HRSD SADS	Cortisol (5-HTP) in suicide-attempters Cortisol in affective disorder compared with controls Positive correlation between cortisol response and suicidality on HRSD SADS
Coccaro et al. (1989)	D$_L$-fenfluramine	Personality-disordered patients Normal controls Affective disorder	PRL (FEN)	Suicide-attempters BDHI rating BGA BIS	Reduced PRL (FEN) in suicide-attempters Strong inverse correlations with BDHI: assault and irritability in personality-disordered patients but not depressed
Lopez-Ibor et al. (1990)	D$_L$-fenfluramine	Suicidal but not depressed patients Normal controls	PRL (FEN)	Suicide-attempters	Reduced PRL (FEN) in suicide-attempters Suicide-attempters had higher self-reported aggression levels
Fishbein et al. (1989)	D$_L$-fenfluramine	Mixed substance abusers Normal controls	PRL (FEN)	Barratt rating scales of impulsivity BDHI	Elevated PRL (FEN) responses in impulsive aggressive substance abusers Positive correlations with BIS
Moss et al. (1990)	mCPP	Antisocial personality–disordered patients with history of substance abuse Normal controls	PRL (mCPP)	BDHI	PRL (mCPP) responses reduced in antisocial personality disordered patients compared with controls Inverse correlation with assault in whole sample
O'Keane and Dinan (1991)	D$_L$-fenfluramine (d-FEN)	Depressed patients Normal controls	PRL (d-FEN)	Suicide-attempters	PRL (d-FEN) blunted in depressive compared to controls Depressed suicide-attempters did not have reduced response compared to non-suicide-attempters
Coccaro et al. (1990)	Buspirone (BUSP)	Personality-disordered patients	PRL (BUSP)	BDHI	PRL (BUSP) correlated inversely with BDHI ratings in personality-disordered patients

Study	Drug	Subjects	Measure	Comparison	Findings
Coccaro et al. (1991)	Clonidine (CLON)	Personality-disordered patients Controls	GH (CLON)	BDHI	GH (CLON) correlated directly with irritability but not assault in whole sample
O'Keane et al. (1992)	D_L-fenfluramine	Violent offenders with ASP Normal controls	PRL (d-FEN)	ASP v Controls	PRL (d-FEN) responses in ASP subjects were significantly blunted compared with controls
Pitchot et al. (1992)	Apomorphine (APO)	Depressed suicide-attempters Depressed non-suicide-attempters	GH (APO)	Suicide attempts	GH (APO) depressed patients with suicide attempts had blunted response compared to depressed controls with no history of suicide attempts
Handelsman et al. (1993)	D_L-fenfluramine mCPP	Alcohol abusers Cocaine abusers	PRL (FEN) PRL (mCPP)	BDHI	Inverse correlations with BDHI scales in alcohol abusers Direct correlation with same scales in cocaine abusers
Botchin et al. (1993)	D_L-fenfluramine	Macaques	PRL (FEN)	Social affiliation and overt aggression ratings	Monkeys with reduced PRL (FEN) had higher ratings of overt aggression and lower ratings of social affiliation
Halperin et al. (1994)	D_L-fenfluramine	Children aged 7–10 with diagnosis of ADHD 15 non-aggressive 10 aggressive No controls	PRL (FEN)	Aggressive Non-aggressive	Aggressive group had greater PRL response than non-aggressive group
Stoff et al. (1992)	D_L-fenfluramine	15 prepubertal 9 adolescent patients with DBD Healthy controls	PRL (FEN) CORT (FEN)	DBD v normal controls Child parent ratings Aggression BDHI scales	No difference between DBD and controls (either prepubertal or adolescent) No correlation with any of the rating scales
Falk et al. (1995)	Ipsapirone (IPS)	9 personality-disordered patients 10 Normal controls	PRL (FEN) CORT (FEN) Temperature	BIS	IPS reduced temperature and increased cortisol in all subjects Temperature response to IPS correlated inversely with PRL (FEN) response and positively with Barratt impulsiveness

DBD, Disruptive Behaviour Disorder; BIS, Barratt Impulsivity Scale; HRSD, Hamilton Rating Scale for Depression: 5-HTP, 5-hydroxytryptamine; PRL, prolactin; FEN, fenfluramine; SADS, Schedule for Affective Disorders and Schizophrenia; ASP, antisocial personality disorder; mCPP, m-chlorophenylpiperazine; GH, growth hormone; CORT, cortisol; BGA, Brown Goodwin Lifetime History of Aggression.

Table 6.4 *Cortisol studies in aggression*

Authors	Group	Measure	Criteria	Results
Sapolsky and Ray (1989)	Male baboons	Plasma cortisol	Fighting in wild baboons	Dominant baboons have lower cortisol than subordinates Low cortisol in dominant group associated: • ability to differentiate threat • likelihood of initiating a fight • displacing aggression after leaving a fight • differentiating when wins/loses a fight
Higley et al. (1992)	Rhesus macaques	ACTH	Aggression measured by number of wounds	Increased ACTH in wounded and scarred
Lidberg et al. (1978)	Murderers	Plasma cortisol	Psychopaths	Psychopaths had reduced urinary free cortisol before trial compared with non-psychopaths
Virkkunen (1985)	90 male violent offenders 10 recidivist arsonists Healthy controls	24-h urinary free cortisol	Group comparisons	Habitually violent offenders with ASP had lower levels than: • other violent offenders • controls • arsonists • ASP alone
Virkkunen et al. (1994a)	Alcoholic forensic patients	CSF corticotrophin	KSP scales	CSF corticotrophin negatively correlates with psychic and somatic anxiety, irritability and indirect aggression
McBurnett et al. (1991)	8–13-year-old boys: • conduct disorder (CD) • anxiety disorder • mixed	Salivary cortisol	DSM-IIIR diagnosis	Children with anxiety disorder had higher levels of cortisol Children with both CD and anxiety disorder had higher levels of cortisol than CD without comorbid anxiety disorder
Lahey and Loeber (1991)	8–13-year-old boys: • conduct disorder (CD) • anxiety disorder • mixed	Salivary cortisol	DSM-IIIR diagnosis	Cortisol concentration correlates negatively with: • number of symptoms of aggression • Fights most/meanness by peers • No relationship with anxiety in whole sample, but positive relationship in CD youth

71

Study	Sample	Measure	Behaviour assessed	Findings
Kruesi et al. (1991)	Disruptive behaviour: • 19 disorders (ADHD/CD) • 19 controls	24-h urinary cortisol	Continuous performance task (CPT); Teacher ratings	No difference UFC between groups; UFC correlated negatively with performance on CPT
Kagan et al. (1988)	Anxious children	Salivary cortisol	Social behaviour	Cortisol correlates positively with inhibited social behaviour
Tennes et al. (1986)	Schoolchildren	UFC	Aggression to peers	Cortisol negatively correlates with inappropriate classroom behaviour
Vanyukov et al. (1992)	Conduct-disordered children; Preadolescent boys	Salivary cortisol	CD symptom counts in children; ASP and CD count in parents	Cortisol level in children was negatively associated with their CD symptom count and father's ASP count; Cortisol levels lower in sons of fathers with ASP than those with fathers without ASP
King et al. (1990)	Substance abusers; Normal controls	Plasma cortisol	Impulsivity EPI	Substance abusers had lower cortisol levels than controls; Cortisol negatively correlates with impulsivity in controls
Tennes and Kreye (1985)	School-grade children	UFC	IQ, popularity with peers, hostility to teachers; Cortisol on test/non-test days	Cortisol secretion higher on test days; High-IQ and low achievers had elevated cortisol; 68% variance in free cortisol secretion accounted for by popularity with peers/hostility to teachers and task behaviour
Scerbo and Kolko (1994)	Clinic-referred disruptive children 7–14 years	Salivary cortisol; Testosterone	Rated on aggression, inattention, over-activity, internalizing behaviour (parents, teachers, clinical)	Testosterone positively correlates with aggression; Cortisol negatively correlates with inattention/over-activity; No interaction between testosterone and cortisol

ASP, antisocial personality disorder; KSP, Karolinska Scales of Personality; ACTH, adrenocorticotrophic hormone; ADHD, attention-deficit hyperactivity disorder; EPI, Eysenck's Personality Inventory; UFC, urinary free cortisol.

with CD and ADHD, four with oppositional defiant disorder (ODD), and four with ODD plus ADHD – were allowed a low monoamine breakfast and lunch during the procedure; a matched group was not included. The adolescent group (which included four subjects with CD, two with CD plus ADHD, and two with ODD) fasted; this group was matched with a healthy control sample, and participated in fenfluramine and placebo challenges.

Subsequently, Halperin et al. (1994) also investigated prolactin responses to a similar dose of D,L-fenfluramine, plasma catecholamine metabolites and platelet 5-HT in non-aggressive and aggressive 7- to 11-year-olds with a diagnosis of ADHD. The aggressive group had a significantly greater prolactin response to fenfluramine than the non-aggressive group. The groups did not differ on peripheral measures of NT function. It would seem there are differences in central 5-HT responses in aggressive and non-aggressive children with ADHD, but in the absence of a normal control group it is impossible to ascertain the true significance of these differences in central 5-HT function in aggressive and non-aggressive subgroups. Further work by Halperin et al. (1997) using fenfluramine challenge in ADHD suggests that aggressive boys with a parental history of aggression have significantly lower prolactin responses than those without a parental history of aggression. The latter data suggests there may be an association between parental aggression and reduced 5-HT function in aggressive boys and that different neurochemical mechanisms operate in familial and non-familial aggressive children. Later work by Halperin et al. (1997) was unable to replicate the finding of enhanced 5-HT function in aggressive boys again using fenfluramine challenge, but found a significant inter-action bewteen age group and aggression, in which young aggressive boys had enhanced prolactin responses but older ones did not. These findings suggest there may be significant age-related changes in the association between 5-HT function and aggression, at least, in boys with ADHD. More recently Pine et al. (1998) reported on children at risk of aggressive behaviour (brothers of convicted delinquents) and found that boys with oppositional defiant or conduct disorder exhibited augmented prolactin responses to fenfluramine compared with other boys. However, adverse rearing circumstances that were conducive to the development of aggressive behaviour also correlated positively with prolactin response, highlighting the importance of evaluating environmental factors in the study of 5-HT and aggression.

Gender differences in prolactin response to fenfluramine challenge in children with disruptive behaviour disorders have been noted (Koda et al. 1996). In this study, girls showed greater prolactin responses to fenfluramine, but did not differ in plasma levels of catecholamine metabolites 3-methoxy-4-hydroxy-phenyl-glycol (MHPG) or HVA and they had lower levels of platelet 5-HT. This study suggests gender-associated differences in 5-HT responsivity are apparent before puberty. Their findings

were consistent with reports from adult cohorts which show enhanced prolactin responses in women compared to men (McBride et al. 1990). Future studies need to examine whether pre-pubertal girls and boys with aggressive/externalizing behaviours differ in central 5-HT function and whether these differences are accounted for by gender differences in neurochemistry.

The discrepancies between the results of the above studies relate partly to differences in the populations studied, the psychometric assessments used, and the variations in the challenge protocol including the presence/absence of a normal control group. Further work is required using samples who are well characterized and less heterogeneous clinically, environmentally and genetically.

CHALLENGES TO THE DOPAMINE AND NORADRENALINE SYSTEMS

To date, there are relatively few studies looking at the responsivity of other neurotransmitter systems with respect to impulsive aggressive behaviour, and all have been conducted in adults. Coccaro et al. (1991) reported a positive correlation between growth hormone (GH) response to clonidine challenge and the irritability scale on the BDHI in patients with DSM-III personality disorder and healthy controls. The GH (clonidine) responses did not correlate with PRL responses to fenfluramine in this sample, suggesting that the alpha-2 noradrenergic system may have a positive influence on irritability, while the serotonergic system relates inversely to this dimension. This finding is consistent with previous reports of elevated MHPG in aggressive men (Brown et al. 1982) and the notion that aggressivity is associated with increased noradrenergic function in animal data (Eichelman 1995).

In terms of dopaminergic challenges, the only published study relates to GH response to apomorphine in depressed age- and sex-matched subjects with and without a history of suicidal behaviour (Pichot et al. 1992). The data are consistent with reports that reduced CSF HVA is associated with suicidal behaviour in depressives (Roy et al. 1988). As yet, there are no available data on impulsive aggressive subjects undergoing challenge of both the serotonergic and dopaminergic systems in order to draw conclusions on the relationship of these neurotransmitter systems.

The roles of other hormones/factors

CORTISOL AND AGGRESSION (Table 6.4)

In primates, hypothalamic pituitary axis (HPA) function is related to social ranking and personality, and low cortisol levels within dominant groups are associated with a variety of 'personality and coping styles' which were beneficial in maintaining a dominant status (Sapolsky and Ray 1989).

In human studies, plasma cortisol levels in stress conditions were found to be low among habitually violent offenders with psychopathic personality (Lidberg et al. 1978). Virkkunen (1985) also reported reduced 24-hour excretion of urinary free cortisol in inmates with antisocial personality and a history of habitual violence. Among the habitually violent groups, those with a history of under-socialized aggressive conduct disorder, truancy and attentional difficulties at school had significantly lower cortisol than those without these characteristics. In a later study, Virkkunen et al. (1994a) again reported negative correlations between CSF corticotrophin concentrations and KSP scores for psychic and somatic anxiety, indirect aggression and irritability. Studies investigating cortisol levels and conduct disorder are inconsistent largely because of the heterogeneity of the samples and the lack of characterization of comorbid disorders, such as anxiety. However, there is some evidence of a negative correlation between cortisol level, regardless of how it is measured, and disruptive, distractible and aggressive behaviour (Scerbo and Kolko 1994; Tennes et al. 1986; Kruesi et al. 1989; Lahey and Loeber 1991). Several studies highlight the importance of examining the role of anxiety and social withdrawal in moderating the relationship between cortisol and aggressive disinhibited behaviour (McBurnett et al. 1991; Kagan et al. 1988). Work by McBurnett et al. (1996) indicates that the link between conduct disorder in children and cortisol appears to be a function of a more specific inverse relationship between cortisol level and aggression rather than conduct disorder per se. Studies of normal populations also suggest an inverse relationship between CSF cortisol and impulsivity, non-conformity, hostility and low fear on the KSP (Ballenger et al. 1983) and between plasma cortisol and impulsivity (King et al. 1990).

These results indicate that individuals with low cortisol tend to manifest a personality profile similar to that reported in groups showing non-conformity and disinhibitory psychopathology. Many factors influence cortisol level, but there is reasonable evidence that low cortisol secretion is related to unstable behaviours (e.g. impulsivity, reward-seeking, aggression, and lack of behavioural inhibition). Although plasma cortisol reflects activity of the hypothalamic–pituitary–adrenal (HPA) axis and arousal level, the link with 5-HT function and the contribution of other NT to cortisol secretion remains unclear, at least in humans.

It also remains unclear whether low cortisol in aggressive children represents a lower basal-tonic cortisol level or a blunted HPA response to stressors. Most investigators suggest that low tonic cortisol levels are associated with chronic aggressive and antisocial behaviour which begins in early life and persists into adulthood.

TESTOSTERONE AND AGGRESSION (Table 6.5)

A number of convergent findings strongly suggest that gonadal steroid hormones significantly shape some aspects of aggressive behaviour in primates. It has been shown, for example, that inter-male aggression relating to competition for females (after puberty) is more closely related to testosterone level than competitive aggression related to status. Castration results in a decrease in aggression which is reversed by testosterone administration (Huntingford and Turner 1987). Testosterone may raise the readiness to fight, but the fighting experience also elevates testosterone levels. After fighting, testosterone levels have been shown to remain high in the victor, but fall in the loser. In addition, testosterone levels are generally found to be higher in dominant than subordinate male primates (Huntingford and Turner 1987).

Human studies of subjects selected for violent behaviour indicate that plasma testosterone relates more to a history of violence in adolescence than current assaultative behaviour (Kruez and Rose 1972). Other studies indicate that subgroups of offenders who are characterized by violence or aggression have higher plasma testosterone than non-aggressive offenders, but there are no dimensional relationships between testosterone and aggression rating scales (Ehrenkranz et al. 1974; Rada et al. 1976).

Table 6.5 shows the main studies examining plasma and free testosterone (CSF and salivary testosterone) in human aggression. These studies seem to suggest that past or present aggressive behaviour may correlate with current plasma testosterone levels, while self-report measures of aggression, irritability and hostility seem to show a less significant relationship with endogenous testosterone, particularly, in large samples. Studies of free (salivary) testosterone also suggest that violent criminals have higher mean testosterone levels than non-violent criminals based on index offence or prison behaviour (Dabbs et al. 1987). More recently, Virkkunen et al. (1994a) demonstrated higher free CSF testosterone in alcoholic offenders with a diagnosis of antisocial personality (ASP) than in normal controls. Furthermore, in a discriminative analysis, in this study CSF testosterone correctly distinguished violent offenders from non-offenders. The authors interpreted the findings as indicating that testosterone was related to aggression and interpersonal violence; however, this conclusion is confounded by the fact that a history of alcoholism also discriminated between groups.

Studies of normal populations not selected for violent behaviour are also conflicting. Perskey et al. (1971) found that testosterone and its production rate correlated positively with Buss Durke Hostility Inventory (BDHI) score in young, but not older, groups of healthy subjects. Christiansen and Knussmann (1987) found positive correlations between self ratings of spontaneous aggression and several measures of testosterone in healthy young men, while Olweus et al. (1980, 1979) found plasma testosterone levels were associated with self-reports of verbal and physical aggression, but not with rated aggression, antisocial behaviour, body build, Eysenck Personality Questionnaire (EPQ) or the socialization scale in adolescents.

Table 6.5 *Testosterone in aggression*

Authors	Group	Measure	Aggression	Results
Kreuz and Rose (1972)	Prisoners	Plasma TEST	Aggression BDHI	No relationship between TEST and current assaultativeness on BDHI. Higher current TEST in those with a history of violence in adolescence
Ehrenkranz et al. (1974)	Prisoners	Plasma TEST	High/low aggression BDHI anxiety measures	TEST higher in prisoners with violent crimes. No relationship between TEST and BDHI. Negative correlation between TEST and anxiety
Bain et al. (1987)	Forensic patients	Plasma TEST	Murder (13) Assault (14) Property (14)	No difference in androgen levels between groups
Rada et al. (1976)	Sex offenders	Plasma TEST	Violent rapists (5) BDHI Other rapists (47) Child molesters (12)	Violent rapists higher testosterone levels than other groups No relationship with aggression ratings
Bain et al. (1988)	Offenders	Plasma TEST and other relevant assays	Sadistic sex offenders (20) Non-sadistic sex offenders (14) Prisoner controls (15)	No group differences
Dabbs et al. (1987)	Prisoners	Salivary TEST	Violent offence Non-violent offence	Higher TEST in violent offenders compared to non-violent
Virkkunen et al. (1994a)	Alcoholic forensic patients Controls	CSF TEST	Impulsive offenders Non-impulsive offenders ASP/IED	Antisocial PD higher in testosterone than controls
Perskey et al. (1971)	18 healthy young men 15 healthy older men 6 dysphoric male patients	Plasma TEST Testosterone production rate	BDHI	Testosterone production rates positively correlates with BDHI scores in young but not older men
Christiansen and Knussmann (1987)	117 healthy men (20–30 yrs)	DHT Salivary TEST Serum TEST	Self-report aggression scales, slides with sexual motifs	Serum TEST, salivary TEST and DHT correlate positively with spontaneous aggression subscale Serum TEST and DHT correlate positively with dominance DHT correlates negatively with restraint of aggression No relationship between aggressive sexuality and TEST or DHT
Olweus et al. (1980)	58 healthy adolescents	Plasma TEST	Self-report verbal/physical aggression, socialization Eysenck's personality questionnaire (EPQ)	Plasma TEST was associated with verbal and physical aggression (especially threat/provocation), but not with antisocial behaviour, body build, EPQ or socialization

ASP, antisocial personality disorder; IED, intermittent explosive disorder; BDHI, Buss Durkee Hostility Inventory; DHT, 5-dihydrotestosterone; TEST, testosterone.

The naturally occurring male hormone testosterone and its synthetic derivative (anabolic/androdrenic steroid AAS) have been implicated in several investigations of unexpected wins in athletes. AAS abuse among adolescent teenagers in the USA has been reported in several studies (Buckley *et al.* 1988; Terney and McLain 1990) and has been implicated in increased aggressive behaviour (Su *et al.* 1993). In the study by Melloni and Ferris (1996), hamsters exposed to AAS during adolescence showed increased aggressive behaviour and this predisposed to adult intensive aggressive outbursts. This work suggests that studies are required to investigate the impact of AAS exposure in adolescent populations.

Overall, the relationship between testosterone and aggression seems to be more consistent in subjects with high base rates of aggression and is probably strongest in younger subjects. Correlations between testosterone levels, particularly plasma testosterone and self-report aggression measures, are weak. In normal subjects the relationship is less clear. There is, however, some suggestion of an association between androgen levels and aggressive responses to threat or provocation. It appears that relatively simple measures of aggression based on reliable reports of overt behaviour are more robustly related to hormone levels than are self-report measures. Furthermore, testosterone levels are not static and it is difficult to draw firm conclusions from studies using single-specimen data.

AROUSAL THEORY

This theory argues that antisocial/impulsive–aggressive individuals are pathologically under-aroused physiologically, as indicated by low heart rate, low skin conductance, and excessive slow-wave electroencephalographic (EEG) activity (Raine 1989; Raine and Scerbo 1991; Hare 1978a, b). As a consequence, they engage in sensation-seeking activities whilst diminishing the perceived threat of, and response to, punishment (Zuckerman 1978). In a direct sense, under-arousal may make the individual less sensitive to the cues for prosocial learning, but also impair conditioning of emotional responses important for avoidance learning and conscience formation (Newman and Kossan 1986; Eysenck and Eysenck 1977).

AUTONOMIC NERVOUS SYSTEM AND ANTISOCIAL BEHAVIOUR

There are now several excellent reviews of the literature on the physiological correlates of antisocial behaviour (Raine 1993; Fowles 1993; McBurnett and Lahey 1994). These reviews seem to suggest that one of the most robust associations between physiological measures and antisocial behaviour is a low resting heart rate level (HRL). Raine (1993), in a review, reported effect sizes of 0.84 in the predicted direction in 14 studies of non-institutionalized conduct-disordered delinquents, children and adolescents. Studies using electrodermal correlates have been less conclusive, although the majority suggest evidence of an association between a reduction in non-specific fluctuations (NSF) at rest and antisocial behaviour in children.

Autonomic under-arousal appears to predispose to disinhibited temperament and behaviour (Snidman *et al.* 1991; Scerbo *et al.* 1993) and this temperamental pattern may itself predispose to antisocial behaviour in later life (Caspi *et al.* 1995). Studies assessing skin-conductance orienting responses (attentional allocation), particularly the frequency of skin conducting responses to orienting stimuli, suggest that antisocial children are characterized by a deficit in allocation of attentional responses to non-novel environmental events (Raine 1993; McBurnett and Lahey 1994). They do not, however, have deficits in attentional responses to all stimuli and may show exaggerated responses to rewarding stimuli (Scerbo *et al.* 1990; Quay 1993). Raine and Venables (1984) have also shown that orienting response deficits may particularly characterize those with schizoid or schizotypal features. Prospective studies are few, but work by Raine *et al.* (1995) suggest that low arousal and orienting, as assessed by skin conductance and heart rate, in 15-year-old school boys, predicted criminality at 24 years of age. Similarly, Raine *et al.* (1995) report that desistors (those who refrain from adult crime) have significantly higher heart rates and non-specific fluctuations (NSFs) than do non-desistors in adolescence. Social factors appear to influence interactions between physiological markers and criminal outcomes in that a number of studies suggest that physiological arousal and other biological factors have more impact on children from intact environmental backgrounds (Satterfield 1987; Raine and Venables 1984; Wadsworth 1976).

It remains unclear whether low arousal represents fearlessness or results in sensation-seeking and criminal behaviour. Future studies need to examine the role of multiple biological markers and brain dysfunction and the relationship to criminal outcomes in understanding aggressive behaviour in childhood and adulthood.

NEUROPSYCHOLOGY: THEORETICAL ISSUES

A number of theoretical models of antisocial behaviour have arisen from empirical studies of the neuropsychology of criminal and delinquent populations.

FRONTAL LOBE DYSFUNCTION/IMPULSIVITY THEORY

This theory suggests that prefrontal dysfunction predisposes to violent behaviour via loss of frontal inhibition on subcortical structures that facilitate aggression (Stuss and

Benson 1986; Gorenstein and Newman 1980) and impulsivity. In addition, the frontal dysfunction theory predicts that subjects would display poor judgement, loss of self-control (Luria 1973), behavioural changes such as emotional and aggressive outbursts (Damasio 1985), loss of intellectual flexibility and concept formation skills, and poor attention, concentration and reasoning ability (Lishman 1987). Empirical evidence to support this model on the basis of neuropsychological testing is limited, but there is some evidence of executive deficits in a variety of disorders characterized by behavioural disinhibition (Kandel and Freed 1989; Gorenstein 1982; Lapierre *et al.* 1995; Moffitt and Henry 1989). In addition, neuroimaging studies, particularly those employing functional rather than structural methods, seem to suggest clear evidence of frontal dysfunction in violent or personality disordered individuals (Raine *et al.* 1992, 1994; Goyer *et al.* 1994; Volkow *et al.* 1995).

LEFT HEMISPHERE DYSFUNCTION/REDUCED LATERALIZATION FOR LANGUAGE

Traditionally, the left-hemisphere dysfunction hypothesis, which is based on reports of impaired performance on language/verbal skills-related tasks (Mungas 1988; Hart 1987; Brickman *et al.* 1984; Moffitt 1990), postulated a role for structural damage to the left hemisphere. More recently, however, Nachshon (1988) argued for a generalized functional, as opposed to structural, disruption of the left hemisphere based on studies of skin conductance asymmetries (Hare 1978a), divided visual field studies (Hare and Jutai 1986) and dichotic listening studies (Nachshon 1983; Hare and McPherson 1984; Raine *et al.* 1990). There are, however, a number of problems with this theory, one of which is the lack of clarity on the exact significance, in terms of lateralization, of skin conductance responses and left-ear advantages on dichotic listening tasks. The possibility that antisocial individuals have reduced lateralization for speech processes has received some support from reports that psychopaths have abnormalities in speech processing such as increased non-semantic, language-related hand gestures (Gillstrom and Hare 1988) or 'unusual speech processing under conditions of distraction' on evoked potential studies (Jutai *et al.* 1987), and reduced lateralization for language on dichotic listening tasks (Hare and McPherson 1984).

The frontal, linguistic and disinhibition theories of antisocial behaviour are not necessarily mutually exclusive. Yeudall and Fromm-Auch (1979), for example, proposed that antisocial behaviour is caused by a deficit in a circuit involving left frontal and temporal regions, part of which may involve the SHF system. Although there is little empirical evidence to support this conclusion, it is unlikely that one specific region of the brain works in isolation to produce such a complex pattern of behaviour.

NEUROPSYCHOLOGY: EMPIRICAL STUDIES

Several authorities have demonstrated a relationship between antisocial behaviour and evidence of left-hemisphere anterior brain dysfunction on neuropsychological test batteries (Yeudall 1977; Fedora and Fedora 1983), particularly in assaultative offenders (Miller 1987, 1988). Much of the work has been conducted on incarcerated populations, particularly juvenile delinquents and criminal psychopaths, and these may represent a less able group in terms of intellectual function. Nonetheless, there is overwhelming empirical evidence to support a left frontotemporal dysfunction theory of psychopathy and antisocial behaviour.

Findings of delinquency-related cognitive deficits have been reported by most studies comparing delinquents with normal controls, and the majority indicate that both verbal language-based skills and executive (frontal lobe) functions are impaired. These will be reviewed in turn.

Verbal functioning in antisocial populations

Studies using Weschler intelligence quotient (IQ) scales in delinquents seem to support the notion of a verbal (VIQ)/performance (PIQ) discrepancy (PIQ > VIQ) in delinquency (Prentice and Kelly 1963; West and Farrington 1973). This has been taken as strongly supporting a specific deficit in language manipulation. Given that language functions are subserved by the left cerebral hemisphere in most subjects, the V–P deficit has also been interpreted as evidence of left hemisphere dysfunction. Confounds such as social disadvantage and reading ability, however, may have a significant impact on VIQ scores. Key studies are summarized in Table 6.6.

The majority of studies, using large sample sizes, report specific deficits in verbal/language skills and memory function and relatively normal performance on visuospatial tasks in delinquents compared with non-delinquent controls. Deficits in these areas were more prominent in those with a history of violence (Brickman *et al.* 1984) or ADHD (Moffitt and Henry 1991). The specific language-based impairments were seen on verbal learning tasks, verbal fluency and VIQ subtests of the Revised Weschler Intelligence Scale for Children (WISC-R).

Interaction effects have been observed between family adversity and verbal ability such that adolescents with both low verbal scores and disturbed family backgrounds had significantly higher mean aggression scores than any other group. Having a strong verbal ability, on the other hand, seemed to protect the individual from the development of aggressive behaviour even if he or she was reared in an adverse family environment (White *et al.* 1989). Although difficulties on verbal- or language-based tasks have been attributed to social and educational disadvantage, several studies have shown the delinquency-related verbal deficit to be robust when social class, family adversity or race are controlled for (Moffitt and Silva 1988a,b; Sobotowicz et al. 1987; Petee and Walsh 1987). Similarly, studies controlling for confounds such as reading ability suggest the verbal deficits remain significant in delinquent populations (Moffitt and Henry 1991; Sobotowicz et al. 1987) and therefore cannot be discounted by these confounds. Studies of incarcerated delinquents indicate that neuropsychological deficits in verbal/language function can discriminate violent from non-violent offenders (Spellacy 1977; Tarter et al. 1985) and that IQ influences the nature of offences committed. Thus, Walsh (1987) found that high-IQ delinquents showed less violent crime and more property offending than low-IQ delinquents. Petee and Walsh (1987) also demonstrated a relationship between PIQ/VIQ discrepancies and violent offending in juvenile probationers. Most of these studies are retrospective and the dichotomization of offenders into violent and non-violent was based on the index offence rather than the offending history. Given that juveniles are often only at the beginning of their criminal careers, this method of violence classification is probably spurious. Denno (1989), in one of the few published prospective studies of neurocognitive deficits in delinquency, was unable to support the contention that violent offenders (based on criminal career) had greater verbal deficits than non-violent offenders, but confirmed that delinquents were impaired in this area compared with non-arrested controls.

In adults, Spellacy (1978) found that verbal/executive deficits characterized adult violent offenders relative to adult property offenders. Yeudall (1977) also found that criminal psychopaths and depressed patients had significantly more anterior deficits than normal controls, but the dysfunction was predominantly left-sided in psychopathy and right-sided in depression. He concluded that, although the anterior deficits were not exclusive to psychopathy, the left-sided verbal deficits reflected dominant hemisphere dysfunction. In a later study, Yeudall et al. (1982) again demonstrated evidence of left-sided (verbal) anterior deficits in violent psychopaths compared with controls matched for age and handedness. Fedora and Fedora (1983), however, in a similar study found that both psychopathic and non-psychopathic criminals had this left frontotemporal pattern of deficits on testing, but impulsivity rather than psychopathy was a stronger correlate of this pattern of cognitive deficit.

Overall, the findings from studies on subgroups of delinquents with/without violence are mixed, but those studies of habitually violent adolescent and adult offenders do support the possibility of a violence-specific effect associated with verbal/left-hemisphere dysfunction (Moffitt 1990). The deficit is pervasive, affecting problem-solving, memory for verbal material and receptive listening.

Deficits in executive function

Extensive intellectual and neuropsychological test batteries suggest that delinquents (Krynicki 1978; Yeudall et al. 1979, 1982; Yeudall and Fromm-Auch 1979), criminal psychopaths (Yeudall 1977) and non-criminal psychopaths (Fedora and Fedora 1983) demonstrate deficit patterns implicating the left frontotemporal region of the brain. Other studies, while not focusing specifically on frontal lobe batteries, also suggest an association between delinquency and executive deficits. Thus, delinquency-related deficits were observed on the Category Test and Trails (Berman and Seigal 1976), verbal fluency and perseveration tasks (Kynricki 1978), sequencing (Miller et al. 1980; Brickman et al. 1984; Karniski et al. 1982), porteus mazes (Riddle and Roberts 1977), and go/no-go learning tasks (LeMarquand et al. 1998). Lueger and Gill (1990), in a study specific to the frontal lobe, found that conduct-disordered adolescents performed worse than matched controls on tasks sensitive to frontal function (conceptual perseveration, poorly sustained attention, impaired sequencing on memory and motor tasks), but not on non-frontal-specific measures – again supporting a role for disinhibition in antisocial behaviour.

Moffitt and Henry (1989) commented that delinquents with a past history of ADHD were more impaired on executive tasks than other delinquents, suggesting that attention deficits may be particularly related to frontal dysfunction. In support of this hypothesis, Lou et al. (1984) found focal hypoperfusion in the white matter tissues connecting the frontal to other brain regions in 11 ADHD patients compared with controls, an effect that was reversed by medication to control ADHD symptoms. Further evidence that attentional mechanisms may be involved in executive deficits comes from studies demonstrating impairment on the arithmetic scale of the WISC-R (Berman and Siegal 1976; Brickman et al. 1984).

In adult populations, studies of executive function deficits have concentrated largely on criminal psychopaths who are characterized by high levels of impulsive aggression. Gorenstein (1982) and Devonshire et al. (1988) reported evidence of frontal deficits on specific tasks in psychopaths compared with controls, while others (Hare 1984; Hoffman et al. 1987; Sutker and Allain 1987; Hart et al. 1990) did not find evidence to support a specific association between psychopathy and frontal dysfunction. The conflicting results may be partly explained by (a) the different populations studied, including prisoners (Hare 1984; Hart et al. 1990), psychiatric outpatients (Gorenstein 1982) and substance abusers (Hoffman et al. 1987; Sutker and Allain 1987), (b) the variation in diagnostic criteria, and (c) the lack of controls for confounds such as medication or substance misuse. Interestingly, Devonshire et al. (1988) noted differences on frontal performance measures in secondary psychopaths when patients were assessed using Blackburn's MMPI profiles rather than Hare's criteria.

Table 6.6 *Neuropsychological studies of delinquents and criminals*

Authors	Group	Test	Results
Brickman et al. (1984)	64 mixed-sex incarcerated delinquents Controls (standard scores)	Luria–Nebraska Neuropsychological Battery (LNNB)	Male delinquents showed reduced scores on all scales The expressive speech and memory scales discriminated between violent and non-violent
Spellacy (1977)	40 violent adolescents 40 non-violent adolescents (incarcerated)	Battery of neuropsychological tests Assault based on behaviour at school	Discriminant functional analyses using five test scores classified 83% of subjects correctly Delinquents: lower full-scale IQ score Delinquents: poor language-related tests when IQ taken into consideration
Lewis et al. (1979)	97 incarcerated boys dichotomized into high/low violence	Test battery	Impaired verbal/memory function in violent group
Denno (1989)	Longitudinal prospective study 987 blacks from low-income families	Test battery	Both violent and non-violent performed worse on verbal IQ and auditory memory compared with non-arrested controls
Kyrnicki (1978)	Male adolescent inpatients: • assaultative • non-assaultative • organic brain syndrome	Test battery	Non-assaultative group performed better than other two groups Assaultative had poor verbal fluency and more perseverative errors, suggesting left fronto-temporal dysfunction
Yeudall et al. (1977, 1982)	Delinquents and controls	Test battery	Delinquents have deficits in left fronto-temporal areas
Wolff et al. (1982)	56 adolescent male delinquents in low-security facility High-school boys	Test battery	Delinquents scored worse on reading, naming, vocabulary and receptive language Delinquents did not differ on spatial/perceptual measures
Karniski et al. (1982)	54 incarcerated delinquents 51 middle-class school boys	Test battery	Delinquents had deficits on visual processing and auditory/language function

Study	Sample/Design	Test	Findings
Berman and Siegal (1976)	45 delinquents Normal boys	Halstead–Reitan test battery	Delinquents deficient on most verbal skill tests Delinquents performed well on performance tasks except digit symbol (verbal task on other batteries)
Sobotowicz et al. (1987)	50 incarcerated delinquents 50 high-school boys (matched for age, race, class) • normal • juvenile delinquent (JD) • learning difficulties (LD) • JD + LD	Test battery	Controlling for learning difficulties, delinquents still performed worse on language, abstract concept formation and memory than all other groups The three problem groups scored better on performance tasks than non-delinquents
Moffitt and Henry (1991)	Longitudinal study, New Zealand All subjects born 1972 Comparison of delinquents and non-delinquents	Test battery Family factors	Delinquents performed worse on verbal/auditory verbal memory factors Subgroup with ADHD did worse Family adversity had interactive effect with verbal deficits in causing delinquency
Walsh et al. (1987)	256 18-year-old delinquents on probation • PIQ > VIQ • VIQ > PIQ • VIQ = PIQ	Intelligence test Andrews Violence Scale (AVS)	PIQ > VIQ and VIQ > PIQ groups had higher delinquency and aggression scores
Petee and Walsh (1987)	Same probationers as above Median split PIQ > VIQ score	Intelligence test Andrews Violence Scale	Subjects with high discrepancy scores (PIQ > VIQ) scored twice as high on AVS High IQ associated with less violent crime and more property offending Low IQ associated with impulsive violence

IQ, intelligence quotient; PIQ, performance intelligence quotient; VIQ, verbal intelligence quotient; ADHD attention-deficit hyperactivity disorder.

The lack of consistent findings may also relate to the variation in the specific tasks employed. This was highlighted in Lapierre *et al.*'s (1995) study which demonstrated deficits in ventral frontal function in psychopathic criminals, compared with non-psychopathic criminals, but no differences on measures of dorsolateral frontal and posterorolandic function – suggesting a specific dysfunction of the ventral frontal cortex.

Despite these criticisms, there seems to be reasonable evidence of left frontotemporal deficits in violent and antisocial populations and further empirical testing of this theory seems warranted. Deckel *et al.* (1996) confirmed the presence of frontal deficits in subjects with ASP on neuropsychological tests and observed an inverse relationship between a diagnosis of ASP and increased left frontal activation on EEG.

It has been hypothesized that intellectual ability may be a significant confound in studies comparing executive function in normal controls and incarcerated offenders (Hare 1984). Studies examining criminals and delinquents in community and custodial settings indicate that both groups show similar impairments on neuropsychological testing compared with controls, suggesting the incarcerated samples are no more intellectually challenged than the community samples (Denno 1989). In addition, Moffitt and Henry (1991) reported that tests of executive function successfully discriminated self-reported delinquents from non-delinquents even after statistically controlling for the effects of overall IQ. This suggests that subgroups of impulsive/aggressive/antisocial subjects demonstrate specific frontal deficits regardless of intellectual function.

CONCLUSIONS

Overall, evidence from neuropsychological tests suggests there is a relatively consistent relationship between antisocial behaviour in children and adults and deficits in verbal and executive (frontal lobe) function compared with normal control populations. In some cases neuropsychological tests were significant predictors of future antisocial behaviour independent of other appropriate control variables, but the causal process by which cognitive deficits result in antisocial behaviour remains unclear. The majority of neuropsychological studies suggest that individuals who display high rates of impulsive and aggressive behaviour are those with the specific frontal/verbal deficits, yet the nature of the relationship between dimensional measures of personality and cognitive dysfunction has not been extensively studied.

From the available neurochemical research in antisocial and criminal populations, there is mounting evidence that serotonergic function is altered in these groups. The relationship between 5-HT and aggression – particularly impulsive aggression – is inverse and most robust in white,

male, young offenders with personality disorders. In children, positive correlations between aggression and enhanced 5-HT activity have been reported. Sample sizes in these studies tend to be small, pubertal factors have not been controlled for, and many studies do not include healthy comparison groups or control for confounds such as comorbid psychiatric disorder. Studies employing dynamic assessments of 5-HT function are limited in number, disparate in the nature of the challenge agent, and variable in the population studied. In addition, although dimensional measures of impulsivity and aggression have been included in many of these studies, there has been little replication of the measures used, making data interpretation difficult. Problems in the assessment of complex concepts such as impulsivity and aggression no doubt contribute to the difficulty in drawing firm conclusions from the available data. To date, there are few published studies examining the relationship between biochemical and neurocognitive markers of impulsivity and aggression in children or adults. Future research needs to adopt a multimodal approach to unravel the biological basis of aggression, and efforts should be made to look at the interaction of biological and social factors in aggressive behaviour.

REFERENCES

Alm, P.O., Alm, M., Humble, K. *et al.* 1994: Criminality and platelet monoamine oxidase activity in former juvenile delinquents as adults. *Acta Psychiatrica Scandinavica* **89**: 41–5.

Asberg, M., Nordstrom, P. and Traskman-Bendz, L. 1986: Cerebrospinal fluid studies in suicide: an overview. In Mann, J.J., and Stanley, M. (eds), *Psychobiology of Suicide*. New York: New York Academy of Science, 168–73.

Asberg, M., Schalling, D., Traskman-Bendz, L. and Wagner, A. 1987: Psychobiology of suicide, impulsivity, and related phenomena. In Meltzer, H.Y. (ed.), *Psychopharmacology: the Third Generation of Progress*. New York: Raven Press, 655–88.

Bain, J., Langevin, R. and Dickey, R. 1987: Sex hormones in murderers and assaulters. *Behavioural Sciences and the Law* **5**: 95–101.

Bain, J., Langeuin, R., Dickey, R. *et al.* 1988: Hormones in sexually aggressive men: I. Baseline values for eight hormones. II. The ACTH test. *Annals of Sex Research* **1**: 63–78.

Ballenger, J.C., Post, R.M., Jimmerson, D.C. *et al.* 1983: Biochemical correlates of personality traits in normals. *Personality and Individual Differences* **4**: 615–25.

Barratt, E.S. 1985: Impulsiveness defined within a systems model of personality. In Speilberger, E.P. and Butcher, J.N. (eds), *Advances in Personality Assessment*. Hillsdale, NJ: Lawrence Erlbaum, 113–32.

Barratt, E.S. and Patton, J.H. 1983: Impulsivity: cognitive. behavioural, and psychophysiological correlates. In Zuckerman, M. (ed.), *Biological Bases of Sensation Seeking, Impulsivity, and Anxiety*. Hillsdale, NJ: Lawrence Erlbaum, 77–116.

Bear, D. 1989: Hierarchical neural regulation of aggression: some predictable patterns of violence. In Britzer, D.A. and Crowner, M. (eds), *Current Approaches to the Prediction of Violence*. Washington, DC: American Psychiatric Press, 85–100.

Belfrage, H., Lidberg, L. and Oreland, L. 1992: Platelet monoamine oxidase activity in mentally disordered violent offenders. *Acta Psychiatrica Scandinavica* **85**: 218–21.

Benson, D.F. and Blumer, D. 1975: Personality changes with frontal and temporal lobe lesions. In Benson, D.F. and Blumer, D. (eds), *Psychiatric Aspects of Neurological Disease*. New York: Grune & Stratton, 151–70.

Berman, A. and Siegal, A.W. 1976: Adaptive and learning skills in juvenile delinquents: a neuropsychological analysis. *Journal of Learning Disabilities* **9**: 51–8.

Bevan, P. 1989: 5-HT and aggression. In Bevan, P., Cools, A.R. and Archer, T. (eds), *Behavioural Pharmacology of 5-HT*. Hillsdale, NJ: Lawrence Erlbaum, 87–9.

Blanchard, D.C. and Blanchard, R.J. 1984: Affect and aggression: an animal model applied to human behaviour. In Blanchard, R.J. and Blanchard, D.C. (eds), *Advances in the study for aggression*. New York: Academic Press, 105.

Blumensohn, R., Ratzoni, G., Weizman, A. *et al.* 1995: Reduction in serotonin 5HT2 receptor binding on platelets of delinquent adolescents. *Psychopharmacology* (Berlin) **118**(3): 354–6.

Bond, A.J. 1992: Pharmacological manipulation of aggressiveness and impulsiveness in healthy volunteers. *Progress in Neuropsychopharmacological and Biological Psychiatry Research* **16**: 1–7.

Botchin, M.B., Kaplan, J.R., Manuck, S.B. and Mann, J.J. 1993: Low versus high prolactin responders to fenfluramine challenge: marker of behavioural differences in adult male cynmolgus macaques. *Neuropsychopharmacology* **9**: 93–9.

Brickman, A.S., McManus, M.M., Grapentine, W.L. and Alessi, N. 1984: Neuropsychological assessment of seriously delinquent adolescents. *Journal of the American Academy of Child Psychiatry* **23**: 453–7.

Brown, C.S., Kent, T.A., Bryant, S.G. *et al.* 1989: Blood platelet uptake of serotonin in episodic aggression. *Psychiatry Research* **27**: 5–12.

Brown, G.L. and Linnoila, M. 1990: CSF Serotonin metabolite (5-HIAA) studies in depression, impulsivity, and violence. *Journal of Clinical Psychiatry* **51**(suppl.): 31–41.

Brown, G.L., Goodwin, F.K., Ballenger, J.C., Goyer, P.F. and Major, L.F. 1979: Aggression in humans correlates with cerebrospinal fluid amine metabolites. *Psychiatry Research* **1**: 131–9.

Brown, G.L., Ebert, M.H., Goyer, P.F. *et al.* 1982: Aggression, suicide, and serotonin: relationships to CSF amine metabolites. *American Journal of Psychiatry* **139**: 741–6.

Brown, G.L., Kline, W.J., Goyer, P.F. *et al.* 1986: Relationship of childhood characteristics to cerebrospinal fluid 5-hydroxyindole acetic acid in aggressive adults. In Shagass, C. *et al.* (eds), *Proceedings of the 1985 Biological Psychiatry Congress*. Amsterdam: Elsevier Science, 171–9.

Buckley, W.E., Yesalis, C.E., Freidl, D.E. *et al.* 1988: Estimated prevalence of anabolic steroid use among male high school seniors. *Journal of the American Medical Association* **260**: 3441–5.

Buss, A.H. (ed.) 1988: *Personality: evolutionary heritage and human distinctiveness*. Hillsdale, NJ: Lawrence Erlbaum.

Caspi, A., Henry, B., McGee, R.O., Moffitt, T.E. and Silva, P.A. 1995: Temperamental origins of child and adolescent behaviour problems: from age three to thirteen *Child Development* **66**: 55–68.

Castellanos, F.X., Elia, J., Kruesi, M.J. *et al.* 1994: Cerebrospinal fluid monoamine metabolites in boys with attention-deficit hyperactivity disorder. *Psychiatry Research* **52**: 305–16.

Christiansen, K. and Knussmann, R. 1987: Androgen levels and components of aggressive behaviour in men. *Hormones and Behaviour* **21**: 170–80.

Cleare, A.J. and Bond, A.J. 1995: The effect of tryptophan depletion and enhancement on subjective and behavioural aggression. *Psychopharmacology* **118**: 72–81.

Coccaro, E.F. 1989: Central serotonin and impulsive aggression. *British Journal of Psychiatry* **155**(suppl. 8): 52–62.

Coccaro, E.F. 1992: Impulsive aggression and central serotonergic system function in humans: an example of a dimensional brain–behavioural relationship. *International Journal of Clinical Psychopharmacology* **7**: 3–12.

Coccaro, E.F. and Astill, J. 1990: Central serotonergic function parasuicide. *Progress in Neuro-Psychopharmacological and Biological Psychiatry* **14**: 663–74.

Coccaro, E.F. and Kavoussi, R.J. 1994: The neuropsychopharmacologic challenge in biological psychiatry. *Clinical Chemistry* **40**: 319–27.

Coccaro, E.F., Siever, L.J., Kavoussi, R. *et al.* 1989: Impulsive aggression in personality disorder: evidence for involvement of 5-HT-1 receptors. *Biological Psychiatry* **25**: 86–7.

Coccaro, E.F., Gabriel, S. and Siever, L.J. 1990: Buspirone challenge: preliminary evidence for a role for central 5-HT-IA receptor function in impulsive aggressive behaviour in humans. *Psychopharmacological Bulletin* **26**: 393–405.

Coccaro, E.F., Lawrence, T., Trestman, R. *et al.* 1991: Growth hormone responses to intravenous clonidine challenge correlates with behavioural irritability in psychiatric patients and in healthy volunteers. *Psychiatry Research* **39**: 129–39.

Coccaro, E.F., Kavoussi, R.J., Trestman, R.L. and Siever, L.J. 1993: 5-HT and aggression: assessment of pre- and postsynaptic indices of 5-HT. *Biological Psychiatry* **33**: 87 (abstract).

Dabbs, J., Frady, R. and Carr, T.S. 1987: Saliva testosterone and criminal violence in young adult prison inmates. *Psychosomatic Medicine* **49**: 174–82.

Damasio, A. 1985: The frontal lobes. In Heilman, K.M. and Valenstein, E. (eds), *Clinical Neuropsychology*. New York: Oxford University Press, 339–75.

Deckel, A.N., Vtesselbrock, V. and Bauer, L. 1996: Antisocial personality disorder, childhood delinquency and formal brain functioning: EEG and neuropsychological findings. *Journal of Clinical Psychology* **52**: 639–50.

Denno, D.J. (ed.) 1989: *Biology, Crime and Violence: New Evidence*. Cambridge: Cambridge University Press.

Depue, R.A. and Spoont, M.A. 1986: Conceptualizing a serotonin trait: a behavioural dimension of constraint. In Nemm, J. and Stanley, N. (eds), *Psychobiology of Suicidal Behaviour*. New York: New York Academy of Science, 47–62.

Devonshire, P.A., Howard, R.C. and Sellars, C. 1988: Frontal lobe functions and personality in mentally abnormal offenders. *Personality and Individual Differences* **9**: 339–44.

DiRenzo, C.T., Amoroso, S., Taglialatela, M., Canzoniero, L. and Basile, V. 1989: Pharmacological characterization of serotonin receptors involved in the control of prolactin secretion. *European Journal of Pharmacology* **162**: 371–3.

Dolan, M. 1996: Serotonergic function in personality disordered offenders. In Cooke, D., Forth, A.E., Newman, J. and Hare, R.D. (eds), *International Perspectives on Psychopathy: Proceedings of the NATO ASI on Psychopathy*. British Psychological Society, 30–5.

Dolan, M., Deakin, W.J.F., Roberts, M. and Anderson, I. 2001: Serotonergic and cognitive impairment in impulsive aggressive personality disordered offenders: are there implications for treatment? *Psychological Medicine* **32**: 105–17.

Ehrenkranz, J., Bliss, E. and Sheard, M.H. 1974: Plasma testosterone: correlation with aggressive behaviour and social dominance in man. *Psychosomatic Medicine* **36**: 469–75.

Eichelman, B. 1995: Animal and evolutionary models of impulsive aggression. In Hollander, E. and Stein, D. (eds), *Impulsivity and Aggression*. Chichester: John Wiley, 59–69.

Eysenck, S.B.G. and Eysenck, H.J. 1977: The place of impulsiveness in a dimensional system of personality description. *British Journal of Social and Clinical Psychology* **16**: 57–68.

Falk, J., Trestman, R., Katin, R. and Siever, L.J. 1995: Ipsapirone as a serotonergic probe in personality disordered patients. *Biological Psychiatry* **37**: 598 (abstract).

Fedora, O. and Fedora, D. 1983: Some neuropsychological and psychophysiological aspects of psychopathic and nonpsychopathic criminals. In Flor-Henry, P. and Gruzelier, J. (eds), *Laterality and Psychopathology*. New York: Elsevier Science, 141.

Fishbein, D.H., Lozovsky, D. and Jaffe, J.H. 1989: Impulsivity, aggression, and neuroendocrine responses to serotonergic stimulation in substance abusers. *Biological Psychiatry* **25**: 1049–66.

Fowler, C.S., Knorring, L. and Oreland, L. 1980: Platelet monoamine oxidase activity in sensation seekers. *Psychiatry Research* **3**: 273–9.

Fowles, D.C. 1980: The three arousal model: implications of Gray's two-factor learning theory for heart rate, electrodermal activity and psychopathy. *Psychophysiology* **17**: 87–104.

Fowles, D.C. 1993: Electrodermal activity and antisocial behaviour. In Roy, J.C., Boucsein, W., Fowles D. and Gruzelier, J. (eds), *Electrodermal Activity: From Physiology to Psychology*. New York: Plenum.

Gillstrom, B.J. and Hare, R.D. 1988: Language-related hand gestures in psychopaths. *Journal of Personality Disorders* **2**: 21–7.

Goodall, E.M., Cowen, P.J., Franklin, M. and Silverstone, T. 1993: Ritanserin attenuates anorectic, endocrine and thermic responses to D fenfluramine in human volunteers. *Psychopharmacology* (Berlin) **112**: 461–6.

Gorenstein, E.E. 1982: Frontal lobe functions in psychopaths. *Journal of Abnormal and Social Psychology* **91**: 368–79.

Gorenstein, E.E. and Newman, J. 1980: Disinhibitory psychopathology: a new perspective and a model for research. *Psychological Review* **87**: 301–15.

Goyer, P.F., Andreason, P., Semple, W.E. *et al.* 1994: Positron-emission tomography and personality disorders. *Neuropsychopharmacology* **10**: 21–8.

Greenberg, A.S. and Coleman, M. 1976: Depressed 5-hydroxylase levels associated with hyperactive and aggressive behaviour. *Archives of General Psychiatry* **33**: 331–6.

Gualtieri, C.T. 1995: The contribution of the frontal lobes to a theory of psychopathology. In Ratey, J.J. (ed.), *Neuropsychiatry of Personality Disorders*. Cambridge, MA: Blackwell Science, 149–72.

Halperin, J.M., Sharma, V., Siever, L.J. *et al.* 1994: Serotonergic function in aggressive and non aggressive boys with attention deficit hyperactivity disorder. *American Journal of Psychiatry* **151**: 243–8.

Halperin, J.M., Newcorn, J.H., Kopstein, I. *et al.* 1997: Serotonin, aggression, and parental psychopathology in children with attention-deficit hyperactivity disorder. *Journal of the American Academy of Child and Adolescent Psychiatry* **36**: 1391–8.

Handelsman, L., Kahn, R.S., Sturiano, C. *et al.* 1998: Hostility is associated with a heightened prolactin response to meta-chlorophenylpiperazine in abstinent cocaine addicts. *Psychiatry Research* **80**: 1–12.

Hare, R.D. 1978a: Electrodermal and cardiovascular correlates of psychopathy. In Hare, R.D. and Schalling, D. (eds), *Psychopathic Behaviour: Approaches to Research*. New York: John Wiley.

Hare, R.D. 1978b: Psychopathy and electrodermal responses to nonsignal stimulation. *Biological Psychiatry* **6**: 237–46.

Hare, R.D. 1984: Performance of psychopaths on cognitive tasks related to frontal lobe function. *Journal of Abnormal and Social Psychology* **93**: 133–40.

Hare, R.D. and Jutai, J.W. 1986: Psychopathy, stimulation seeking and stress. In Strelau, J., Farley, F.H. and Gale, A. (eds), *The Biological Basis of Personality and Behaviour*, Vol. 2. Washington, DC: Hemisphere, 175–84.

Hare, R.D. and McPherson, L.M. 1984: Psychopathy and perceptual asymmetry during verbal dichotic listening. *Journal of Abnormal and Social Psychology* **93**: 141–9.

Hart, C. 1987: The relevance of a test of speech comprehension deficit to persistent aggressiveness. *Personality and Individual Differences* **8**: 371–84.

Hart, S.D., Forth, A.E. and Hare, R.D. 1990: Performance of criminal psychopaths on selected neuropsychological tests. *Journal of Abnormal Behaviour* **99**: 374–9.

Higley, J.D., Mehlman, P.T., Taub, D.M. *et al.* 1992: Cerebrospinal fluid monoamine and adrenal correlates of aggression in free-ranging rhesus monkeys. *Archives of General Psychiatry* **49**: 436–41.

Hoffman, J.J., Hall, R.W. and Bartsch, T.W. 1987: On the relative importance of 'psychopathic' personality and alcoholism on neuropsychological measures of frontal lobe dysfunction. *Journal of Abnormal and Social Psychology* **96**: 158–60.

Huntingford, F.A. and Turner, A.K. (eds) 1987: *Animal Conflict*, 2nd edn. London: Chapman & Hall.

Jutai, J., Hare, R.D. and Connolly, J.F. 1987: Psychopathy and event-related brain potentials (ERPs) associated with attention to speech stimuli. *Personality and Individual Differences* **8**: 175–84.

Kagan, J., Resnick, J.S. and Snidman, N. 1988: Biological basis of childhood shyness. *Science* **240**: 167–71.

Kandel, E. and Freed, D. 1989: Frontal lobe dysfunction and antisocial behaviour: a review. *Journal of Clinical Psychology* **45**: 404–13.

Karniski, W.M., Levine, M.D., Clarke, S., Palfrey, J.S. and Meltzer, L.J. 1982: A study of neurodevelopmental findings in early adolescent delinquents. *Journal of Adolescent Healthcare* **3**: 151–9.

Kavoussi, R.J. and Coccaro, E.F. 1995: Neurobiological approaches to disorders of personality. In Ratey, J.J. (ed.), *Neuropsychiatry of Personality Disorders*. Cambridge, MA: Blackwell Science, 17–35.

Kavoussi, R., Armstead, P. and Coccaro, E.F. 1997: The neurobiology of impulsive aggression. *Psychiatric Clinics of North America* **20**: 395–403.

King, R.J., Jones, J., Scheuer, J.W., Curtis, D. and Zarcone, V. 1990: Plasma cortisol correlates of impulsivity and substance abuse. *Personality and Individual Differences* **11**: 281–91.

Klinteberg, B. and Oreland, L. 1995: Hyperactive and aggressive behaviours in childhood as related to low platelet monoamine oxidase (MAO) activity at adult age: a longitudinal study of male subjects. *Personality and Individual Differences* **19**: 373–83.

Klinteberg, B., Schalling, D. and Magnusson, D. 1990: Childhood behaviour and adult personality in male and female subjects. *European Journal of Personality* **4**: 57–71.

Koda, V.H., Halperin, J.M., Mewcorn, J.H. *et al.* 1996: Gender differences in prolactin responses to fenfluramine challenge in children with disruptive behaviour disorders. In *Understanding Aggressive Behaviour in Children.* New York: New York Academy of Sciences, 369–72.

Kruesi, M.J.P., Schmidt, M.E., Donnelly, M., Hibbs, E.D. and Hamburger, S.D. 1989: Urinary free cortisol output and disruptive behaviour in children. *Journal of the American Academy of Child Psychiatry* **28**: 441–3.

Kruesi, M.J.P., Rapoport, J.L., Hamburger, S.D. *et al.* 1990: Cerebrospinal fluid metabolites, aggression, and impulsivity in disruptive behavior disorders of children and adolescents. *Archives of General Psychiatry* **47**: 419–62.

Kreusi, M.J.P., Hibbs, E.D., Zahn, T.P. *et al.* 1992: A 2-year prospective follow-up study of children and adolescents with disruptive behaviour disorders: prediction by cerebrospinal fluid 5-hydroxyindoleacetic acid, homovanillic acid and autonomic measures. *Archives of General Psychiatry* **49**: 429–35.

Kreuz, L.E. and Rose, R.M. 1972: Assessment of aggressive behaviour and plasma testosterone in a young criminal population. *Psychosomatic Medicine* **34**: 321–32.

Krynicki, V.E. 1978: Cerebral dysfunction in repetitively assaultative offenders. *Journal of Nervous and Mental Disease* **166**: 59–67.

Lahey, B.B. and Loeber, R. (eds) 1991: A preliminary psychobiological model of conduct disorder. Paper presented at the annual meeting of the Society for Research in Child and Adolescent Psychopathology, Amsterdam, Netherlands.

Lahmeyer, H.W., Val, E., Gaviria, M. *et al.* 1988: EEG sleep, lithium transport, dexamethasone suppression, and monoamine oxidase activity in borderline personality disorder. *Psychiatry Research* **25**: 19–30.

Lapierre, D., Braun, C.M. and Hodgins, S. 1995: Ventral frontal deficits in psychopathy: neuropsychological test findings. *Neuropsychologia* **33**: 139–51.

LeMarquand, D.G., Pihl, R.O., Young, S.N. *et al.* 1998: Tryptophan depletion, executive functions, and disinhibition in aggressive adolescent males. *Neuropsychopharmacology* **19**(4): 333–41.

Lewis, D.A. and Sherman, B.M. 1985: Serotonergic regulation of prolactin and growth hormone secretion in man. *Acta Endocrinologica* **110**: 152–7.

Lewis, D.A., Shanok, S.S., Pincus, J.H. and Glaser, G.H. 1979: Violent juvenile delinquents: psychiatric, neurological and abuse factors. *Journal of the American Academy of Child Psychiatry* **2**: 307–19.

Lidberg, L., Levander, S.E., Schalling, D. *et al.* 1978: Urinary catecholamines, stress, and psychopathy: a study of arrested men awaiting trial. *Psychosomatic Medicine* **40**: 116–25.

Lidberg, L., Modin, I., Oreland, L., Tuck, J.R. and Gillner, A. 1985: Platelet monoamine oxidase activity and psychopathy. *Psychiatry Research* **16**: 339–43.

Linnoila, M. and Virkkunen, M. 1992: Aggression, suicidality and serotonin. *Journal of Clinical Psychiatry* **53**(10, suppl.): 46–51.

Linnoila, M., Virkkunen, M. and Roy, A. 1986: Biochemical aspects of aggression in man. *Clinical Neuropharmacology* **9**(suppl. 4): 377–9.

Linnoila, M., Virkkunen, M., Scheinin, M. *et al.* 1983: Low cerebrospinal fluid 5-hydroxyindoleacetic acid concentration differentiates impulsive from nonimpulsive violent behaviour. *Life Science* **33**: 2609–14.

Lishman, W.A. (ed.) 1987: *Organic Psychiatry*, 2nd edn. Oxford: Blackwell.

Lopez-Ibor, J.J., Lana, F. and Saiz-Ruiz, J. 1990: Conductas autoliticas impulsivas y serotonina. *Actas Luso-EsNeurol. Psiquiator* **18**: 316–25.

Lou, H.C., Henriksen, L. and Bruhn, 1984: Focal cerebral hypoperfusion in children with dysphasia and/or attention deficit disorder. *Archives of Neurology* **41**: 825–9.

Lueger, R.J. and Gill, K.J. 1990: Frontal lobe cognitive dysfunction in conduct disorder adolescents. *Journal of Clinical Psychology* **46**: 696–706.

Luria, A.R. (ed.) 1973: *The Working Brain: an Introduction to Neuropsychology.* New York: Basic Books.

Marazziti, D., De Leo, D. and Conti, L. 1989: Further evidence supporting the role of the serotonin system in suicidal behaviour: a preliminary study of suicide attempters. *Acta Psychiatrica Scandinavica* **80**: 322–4.

Markowitz, P.I. and Coccaro, E.F. 1995: Biological studies of impulsivity, aggression and suicidal behaviour. In Hollander, E. and Stein, D. (eds), *Impulsivity and Aggression.* Chichester: John Wiley, 71–91.

McBride, P.A., Mann, J.J., Polley, A., Wiley, J. and Sweeney, J. 1987: Assessment of binding indices and physiological responsiveness of the 5HT 2 receptor on human platelets. *Life Science* **40**: 1799–809.

McBride, P.A., Tierney, M., DeMeo, M., Chen, J.S. and Mann, J.J. 1990: Effects of age and gender on CNS serotonergic responsivity in normal adults. *Biological Psychiatry* **27**: 1143–55.

McBurnett, K., Lahey, B., Frick, P. *et al.* 1991: Anxiety, inhibition, and conduct disorder in children: II. Relation to salivary cortisol. *Journal of the American Academy of Child Psychiatry* **30**(2): 192–6.

McBurnett, K. and Lahey, B. 1994: Psychophysiological and neuroendocrine correlates of conduct disorder and antisocial behaviour in children and adolescents. In Fowles, D.C., Sutker, P. and Goodman, S. (eds), *Progress in Experimental Personality and Psychopathology Research.* New York: Springer, 199–232.

McBurnett, K., Lahey, B., Capasso, L. and Loeber, R. 1996: Aggressive symptoms and salivary cortisol in clinic referred boys with conduct disorder. In *Understanding Aggressive Behaviour in Children.* New York: New York Academy of Sciences, 169–79.

Melloni, R.H. and Ferris, C.F. 1996: Adolescent anabolic steroid use and aggressive behaviour in Golden hamsters. In *Understanding Aggressive Behaviour in Children.* New York: New York Academy of Sciences, 372–6.

Meltzer, H.Y., Perline, R., Tricou, B.J., Lowry, M.T. and Robertson, A. 1984: Effect of 5-hydroxytryptophan on serum cortisol levels in major affective disorders: II. Relation to suicide, psychosis, and depressive symptoms. *Archives of General Psychiatry* **41**: 379–87.

Miller, L. 1987: Neuropsychology of the aggressive psychopaths: an integrative review. *Aggressive Behaviour* **13**: 119–40.

Miller, L. 1988: Neuropsychological perspectives on delinquency. *Behavioural Sciences and the Law* **6**: 409–28.

Miller, L., Burdg, N.B. and Carpenter, D. 1980: Application of re-categorised WISC-R scores of adjudicated adolescents. *Perceptual and Motor Skills* **51**: 187–91.

Modai, I., Apter, A., Meltzer, H. *et al.* 1989: Serotonin by platelets of suicidal and aggressive adolescent psychiatric inpatients. *Neuropsychobiology* **21**: 9–13.

Moffitt, T.E. 1990: The neuropsychology of juvenile delinquency: a critical review. In Tonry, M. and Morris, N. (eds), *Crime and Justice: a Review of the Literature.* Chicago: University of Chicago Press, 76.

Moffitt, T.E. and Henry, B. 1991: Neuropsychological studies of juvenile delinquency and juvenile violence. In Milner, J.S. (ed.), *Neuropsychology of Aggression.* Boston: Klewer, 131–46.

Moffitt, T.E. and Henry, B.H. 1989: Neuropsychological assessment of executive function in self-reported delinquents. *Developmental Psychopathology* **1**: 105–18.

Moffitt, T.E. and Silva, P.A. 1988a: Neuropsychological deficit and self-reported delinquency in an unselected birth cohort. *Journal of the American Academy of Child Psychiatry* **27**: 233–40.

Moffitt, T.E. and Silva, P.A. 1988b: IQ and delinquency: a direct test of the differential detection hypothesis. *Journal of Abnormal and Social Psychology* **97**: 330–3.

Moss, H.B., Yao, Y.K. and Panzak, G.L. 1990: Serotonergic responsivity and behavioral dimensions in antisocial personality disorder with substance abuse. *Biological Psychiatry* **28**: 325–38.

Mungas, D. 1988: Psychometric correlates of episodic violent behaviour: a multidimensional neuropsychological approach. *British Journal of Psychiatry* **152**: 180–7.

Nachshon, I. 1983: Hemisphere dysfunction in psychopathy and behaviour disorders. In Myslobodsky, M. (ed.), *Hemisyndromes: Psychobiology, Neurology, Psychiatry.* New York: Academic Press, 389–414.

Nachshon, I. 1988: Hemisphere function in violent offenders. In Moffitt, T.E., Mednick, S.A. and Stack, S.A. (eds), *Biological Contributions to Crime Causation.* Dordrecht: Martinus Nijhoff, 55–67.

Newman, J. 1987: Reaction to punishment in extroverts and psychopaths: implications for the impulsive behaviour of disinherited individuals. *Journal of Research in Personality* **21**: 464–80.

Newman, J.P. and Kosson, D.S. 1986: Passive avoidance learning in psychopathic and nonpsychopathic offenders. *Journal of Abnormal and Social Psychology* **95**: 252–6.

Newman, J.P., Widom, C.S. and Nathan, S. 1985: Passive avoidance in syndromes of disinhibition: psychopathy and extroversion. *Journal of Social Psychology* **48**: 1316–27.

O'Keane, V. and Dinan, T.G. 1991: Prolactin and cortisol responses to D-fenfluramine in major depression: evidence for diminished responsivity of central serotonergic function. *American Journal of Psychiatry* **148**: 1009–15.

O'Keane, V., Maloney, E., O'Neill, H. *et al.* 1992: Blunted prolactin responses to D-fenfluramine in sociopathy: evidence for subsensitivity of central serotonergic function. *British Journal of Psychiatry* **160**: 643–6.

Olweus, D. 1979: Stability of aggressive reaction patterns in males: a review. *Psychological Bulletin* **86**: 852–75.

Olweus, D., Mattisson, A. and Schalling, D. 1980: Testosterone, aggression, physical, and personality dimensions in normal adolescent males. In Olweus, D., Mattisson, A. and Schalling, D. (eds), *Psychosomatic Medicine.* New York: Elsevier, 253–69.

Oreland, L. 1993: Monoamine oxidase in neuropsychiatric disorders. In Yasuhara, H. *et al.* (eds), *Monoamine Oxidase: Basic and Clinical Aspects.* New York: American Psychiatric Press, 8.

Oreland, L., Wiberg, A., Asberg, M. *et al.* 1981: Platelet MAO activity and monoamine metabolites in cerebrospinal fluid in depressed and suicidal patients and in healthy controls. *Psychiatry Research* **4**: 21–9.

Paykel, E.S., Panter, R.R. and Penrose, R.J. 1979: Depressive classification and prediction of response to phenelzine. *British Journal of Psychiatry* **134**: 572–81.

Perris, C., Jacobsson, L., VonKnorring, L. *et al.* 1980: Enzymes related to biogenic amine metabolism and personality characteristics in depressed patients. *Acta Psychiatrica Scandinavica* **61**, 477–84.

Persky, H., Smith, K.D. and Basu, G.K. 1971: Relation of psychological measures of aggression and hostility to testosterone production in man. *Psychosomatic Medicine* **33**: 265–77.

Petee, T.A. and Walsh, A. 1987: Violent delinquency, race, and the Wechsler performance–verbal discrepancy. *Journal of Social Psychology* **127**: 353–4.

Pitchot, W., Hansennes, M., Gonzalez-Moreno, A. and Asseau, M. 1992: Suicidal behaviour and growth hormone response to apomorphine test. *Biological Psychiatry* **31**: 1213–19.

Pine, D.S., Coplan, J.D., Wasserman, G.A. *et al.* 1998: Neuroendocrine response to fenfluramine challenge in boys: associations with aggressive behaviour and adverse rearing. *Archives of General Psychiatry* **55**: 625.

Pliszka, S.R., Rogeness, G.A., Renner, P. *et al.* 1988: Plasma neurochemistry in juvenile offenders. *Journal of the American Academy of Child Psychiatry* **27**: 588–94.

Plutchik, R. and Van Praag, H.M. 1995: The nature of impulsivity: definitions, ontology, genetics, and relations to aggression. In Hollander, E. and Stein, D. (eds), *Impulsivity and Aggression.* New York: John Wiley, 130.

Prentice, N.M. and Kelly, F.J. 1963: Intelligence and delinquency: a reconsideration. *Journal of Social Psychology* **60**: 327–37.

Quay, H.C. 1988: The behavioural reward and inhibition system in childhood behviour disorders. In Bloomingdale, L.M. (ed.), *Attention Deficit Disorder.* Oxford: Pergamon, 176–186.

Quay, H.C. 1993: The Psychophysiology of undersocialized aggressive conduct disorder. *Development and Psychophysiology* **5**: 165–80.

Rada, R.T., Laws, D.R. and Kellner, R. 1976: Plasma testosterone levels in the rapist. *Psychosomatic Medicine.* **38**: 257–68.

Raine, A. 1989: Evoked potential and psychopathy. *Psychophysiology* **8**: 1–16.

Raine, A. 1993: *The Psychopathology of Crime: Criminal Behavior as a Clinical Disorder.* San Diego: Academic Press.

Raine, A. and Scerbo, A. 1991: Biological theories of violence. In Milner, J.S. (ed.), *Neuropsychology of Aggression.* Boston: Kluwer, 1–26.

Raine, A. and Venables, P.H. 1984: Electrodermal non-reponding, schizoid tendencies, and antisocial behaviour in adolescents. *Psychophysiology* **21**: 424–33.

Raine, A., O'Brien, M., Smiley, N., Scerbo, A. and Chan, C.J. 1990: Reduced lateralisation in verbal dichotic listening in adolescent psychopaths. *Journal of Abnormal and Social Psychology* **99**: 272–7.

Raine, A., Sheard, C., Reynolds, G.P. and Lencz, T. 1992: Prefrontal structural and functional deficits associated with individual differences in schizotypal personality. *Schizophrenia Research* **7**: 237–47.

Raine, A., Buchsbaum, M., Stanley, J. *et al.* 1994: Selective reductions in prefrontal glucose metabolism in murderers. *Biological Psychiatry* **36**: 365–73.

Raine, A., Venables, P.H. and Williams, M. 1995: High autonomic arousal and electrodermal orienting at age 15 years as protective factors against criminal behaviour at age 29 years. *American Journal of Psychiatry* **152**: 1595–600.

Raleigh, M.J., McGuire, M.T., Brammer, G.L. and Yuviler, A. 1984: Social and environmental influences on blood serotonin in monkeys. *Archives of General Psychiatry* **41**: 405–10.

Riddle, M. and Roberts, A.H. 1977: Delinquency, delay in gratification recidivism and the proteus maze tests. *Psychological Bulletin* **84**: 417–25.

Roy, A., Pickar, D., De Jong, J. *et al.* 1988a: Norepinephrine and its metabolites in cerebrospinal fluid, plasma, and urine: relation to hypothalamic–pituitary–adrenal axis function in depression. *Archives of General Psychiatry* **45**: 849–57.

Salomon, R.M., Mazure, C.M., Delgado, P.L., Mendia, P. and Charney, D.S. 1994: Serotonin function in aggression: the effects of acute plasma tryptophan depletion in aggressive patients. *Biological Psychiatry* **35**: 570–2.

Sapolsky, B. and Ray, J. 1989: Styles of dominance and their physiological correlates among wild baboons. *American Journal of Primachology* **18**: 1–13.

Satterfield, J.H. 1987: Childhood diagnostic and neurophysiological predictors of teenage arrest rates: an eight-year prospective study. In Mednick, S.A., Moffitt, T.E. and Stack, S. (eds), *The Causes of Crime: New Biological Approaches.* Cambridge: Cambridge University Press.

Scerbo, A.S. and Kolko, D.J. 1994: Salivary testosterone and cortisol in disruptive children: relationship to aggressive, hyperactive, and internalising behaviours. *Journal of the American Academy of Child Psychiatry* **33**: 1174–84.

Scerbo, A., Raine, A., O'Brien, M. *et al.* 1990: Reward dominance and passive avoidance learning in adolescent psychopaths. *Journal of Abnormal Child Psychology* **18**: 451–63.

Scerbo, A., Raine, R., Venables, P.H. and Mednick, S.A. 1993: Relationships between autonomic arousal at age 3 and temperament at ages 8 to 11 years. *Journal of Abnormal Child Psychology* **18**: 451–63.

Schalling, D., Asberg, M., Edman, G. and Levander, S.E. 1984: Impulsivity, nonconformity and sensation seeking as related to biological markers for vulnerability. *Clinical Neuropharmacology* **7**(suppl. 1): 747–57.

Schalling, D., Asberg, M., Edman, G. and Oreland, L. 1987: Markers for vulnerability to psychopathology: temperament traits associated with platelet MAO activity. *Acta Psychiatrica Scandinavica* **76**: 172–82.

Schalling, D., Edman, G., Asberg, M. *et al.* 1988: Platelet MAO actually associated with impulsivity and aggressivity. *Personality and Individual Differences* **9**: 597–605.

Schooler, C., Zahn, T.P., Murphy, D. and Buchsbaum, M.S. 1978: Psychological correlates of monoamine oxidase activity in normals. *Journal of Nervous and Mental Disease* **166**: 177–86.

Siever, L.J. and Davis, K.L. 1991: A psychobiological perspective on the personality disorders. *American Journal of Psychiatry* **148**: 1647–58.

Siever, L.J., Murphy, D., Slater, S., De la Vega, E. and Lipper, S. 1989: Plasma prolactin changes following fenfluramine in depressed patients compared to controls: an evaluation of central serotoninergic response in depression. *Life Science* **34**: 1029–39.

Silver, J.M., Yudotsky, S.C. and Hales, R.E. 1992: Neuropsychiatric aspects of traumatic brain injury. In Hales, R.E. and Yudotsky, S.C. (eds), *Textbook of Neuropsychiatry.* Washington, DC: American Psychiatric Press, 363–95.

Simeon, D., Stanley, B., Frances, A. *et al.* 1992: Self-mutilation in personality disorders: psychologial and biological correlates. *American Journal of Psychiatry* **149**: 221–6.

Smith, S.E., Pihl, R.O., Young, S.N. and Ervin, F.R. 1986: Elevation and reduction of plasma tryptophan and their effects on aggression and perceptual sensitivity in normal males. *Aggressive Behaviour* **12**: 393–407.

Sobotowicz, W., Evans, J.R. and Laughlin, J. 1987: Neuropsychological function and social support in delinquency and learning disability. *International Journal of Clinical Neuropsychology* **9**: 178–86.

Soloff, P.H., Cornelius, J., Foglia, J., George, A. and Perer, J.M. 1991: Platelet MAO in borderline personality disorder. *Biological Psychiatry* **29**: 499–502.

Spellacy, F. 1977: Neuropsychological differences between violent and nonviolent adolescents. *Journal of Clinical Psychology* **33**: 966–9.

Spellacy, F. 1978: Neuropsychological discrimination between violent and nonviolent men. *Journal of Clinical Psychology* **34**: 49–52.

Stein, D.J., Hollander, E. and Liebowit, M.R. 1993: Neurobiology of impulsivity and the impulse control disorders. *Journal of Neuropsychiatry* **5**: 9–17.

Stein, D.J., Towney, J. and Hollander, E. 1995: The neuropsychiatry of impulsive aggression. In Hollander, E. and Stein, D. (eds), *Impulsivity and Aggression.* New York: John Wiley, 91–105.

Stoff, D.M., Pollock, L., Vitiello, B., Behar, D. and Bridger, W.H. 1987: Reduction of 3H-imipramine binding sites on platelets of conduct disordered children. *Neuropsychopharmacology* **1**: 55–62.

Stoff, D.M., Pastiempo, A.P., Yeung, J.H. *et al.* 1992: Neuroendocrine responses to challenge with D,L-fenfluramine and aggression in disruptive behavior disorders of children and adolescents. *Psychiatry Research* **43**: 263–76.

Stuss, D.T. and Benson, D.F. (eds) 1986: *The Frontal Lobe.* New York: Raven Press.

Su, T., Pagliaro, P.J., Schmidt, P.J. *etal.* 1993: Neuropsychiatric effects of anabolic steroids in male normal volunteers. *Journal of the American Medical Association* **269**: 2760–4.

Sutker, P.B. and Allain, A.N. 1987: Cognitive abstraction, shifting and control: clinical sample comparisons of psychopaths and non psychopaths. *Journal of Abnormal and Social Psychology* **96**: 73–5.

Tarter, R.E., Hegedus, A.M., Winsten, N.E. and Alterman, I. 1985: Intellectual profiles and violent behaviour in juvenile delinquents. *Journal of Clinical Psychology* **119**: 125–8.

Tennes, K. and Kreye, M. 1985: Children's adrenocortical responses to classroom activities and tests in elementary school. *Psychosomatic Medicine* **47**: 451–60.

Tennes, K., Kreye, M., Avitable, N. *et al.* 1986: Behavioural correlates of excreted catecholamines and cortisol in second-grade children. *Journal of the American Academy of Child Psychiatry* **25**: 764–70.

Terney, R. and McLain, L.G. 1990: The use of anabolic steroids in high school students. *American Journal of Disturbed Children* **144**(1): 99–103.

Traskman-Bendz, L., Asberg, M. and Schalling, D. 1986: Serotonergic function and suicidal behaviour in personality disorders. In Mann, J.J. and Stanley, M. (eds), *Psychobiology of Suicide*. New York: New York Academy of Science, 168–73.

Tuinier, S., Verhoevn, W.M.A. and Van Praag, H.M. 1995: Cerebrospinal fluid 5-hydroxindoleacetic acid and aggression: a critical appraisal of the clinical data. *International Journal of Clinical Psychopharmacology* **10**: 147–56.

Twitchell, G.R., Hanna, G.L., Cook, E.H. *et al.* 1998: Overt behaviour problems and serotonergic function in middle childhood among male and female offspring of alcoholic fathers. *Alcohol Clinical Experience Research* **22**: 1340–8.

Unis, A.S., Cook, E.H., Vincent, J.G. *et al.* 1997: Platelet serotonin measures in adolescents with conduct disorder. *Biological Psychiatry* **42**: 553–9.

Van der Klar, L.D. and Bethea, C.L. 1982: Pharmacological evidence that serotonergic stimulation of prolactin release is mediated via the dorsal raphe nucleus. *Neuroendocrinology* **35**: 225–30.

Van Praag, H.M. 1983a: Depression, suicide and the metabolism of serotonin in the brain. *Journal of Affective Disorders* **4**: 275–90.

Van Praag, H.M. 1983b: CSF 5-HIAA and suicide in non-depressed schizophrenics. *Lancet* **i**: 977–8.

Van Praag, H.M. 1994: 5-HT related anxiety and/or aggression driven depression. *International Journal of Clinical Psychopharmacology* **9**(suppl. 11): 5–6.

Van Praag, H.M., Lemus, C. and Kahn, R. 1987: Hormonal probes of central serotonergic activity: do they really exist? *Biological Psychiatry* **22**: 86–98.

Vanyukov, M.M., Moss, H.B., Plail, J.A. *et al.* 1992: Antisocial symptoms in preadolescent boys and in their parents: associates with cortisol. *Psychiatry Research* **46**: 9–17.

Virkkunen, M. 1985: Urinary free cortisol excretion in habitually violent offenders. *Acta Psychiatrica Scandinavica* **72**: 40–2.

Virkkunen, M., Nuutila, A., Goodwin, F.K. and Linnoila, M. 1987: Cerebrospinal fluid monoamine metabolite levels in male arsonists. *Archives of General Psychiatry* **44**: 241–7.

Virkkunen, M., Rawlings, R., Takola, R. *et al.* 1994a: CSF biochemistry, glucose metabolism and diurnal activity rhythms in alcoholic, violent offenders, firesetters and healthy volunteers. *Archives of General Psychiatry* **51**: 20–7.

Virkkunen, M., Kallio, E., Rawlings, R. *et al.* 1994b: Personality profiles and state aggressiveness in Finish alcoholic, violent offenders, firesetters and healthy volunteers. *Archives of General Psychiatry* **51**: 28–33.

Volkow, N.D., Trancredi, L., Grant, C. *et al.* 1995: Brain glucose metabolism in violent psychiatric patients: a preliminary study. *Psychiatry Research* **61**: 243–53.

Von Knorring, L., Oreland, L. and Winblad, B. 1984: Personality traits related to monoamine oxidase activity in platelets. *Psychiatry Research* **12**: 11–26.

Wadsworth, M.E.J. 1976: Delinquency, pulse rate and early emotional deprivation. *British Journal of Criminology* **16**: 245–56.

Walsh, A. 1987: Cognitive functioning and delinquency: property versus violent offenses. *Journal of Offender Therapy and Comparative Criminology* **31**(3): 285–9.

Walsh, A., Petee, T.A. and Beyer, J.A. 1987: Intellectual imbalance and delinquency: comparing high verbal and high performance IQ delinquents. *Criminal Justice and Behaviour* **14**: 370–9.

Weiger, W.E. and Bear, D.M. 1988: An approach to the neurology of aggression. *Journal of Psychiatry Research* **22**: 85–98.

West, D.J. and Farrington, D. (eds) 1973: *Who becomes Delinquent?* London: Heinemann.

White, J., Moffitt, T.E. and Silva, P.A. 1989: A prospective replication of the protective effects of IQ in subjects at high risk for juvenile delinquency. *Journal of Clinical Psychology* **57**: 719–24.

Wolff, P.H., Waber, D., Bauermeister, M., Cohen, C. and Ferber, R. 1982: The neuropsychological status of adolescent delinquent boys. *Journal of Child Psychology and Psychiatry* **23**: 267–79.

Yehuda, R., Southwick, S.M., Edell, W.S. and Giller, E.L. 1989: Low platelet monoamine oxidase activity in borderline personality disorders. *Psychiatry Research* **30**: 265–73.

Yeudall, L.T. 1977: Neuropsychological assessment of forensic disorders. *Canadian Mental Health* **25**: 7–15.

Yeudall, L.T. and Fromm-Auch, D. 1979: Neuropsychological impairments in various psychopathological populations. In Gruzelier, J. and Flor-Henry (eds), *Hemisphere Asymmetries of Function and Psychopathology*. New York: Elsevier, 257–65.

Yeudall, L.T., Fromm-Auch, D. and Davies, P. 1982: Neuropsychological impairments of persistent delinquency. *Journal of Nervous and Mental Disease* **170**: 257–65.

Zuckerman, M. 1978: Sensation seeing and psychopathy. In Hare, R.D. and Schalling, D. (eds), *Psychopathic Behavior: Approaches to Research*. New York: John Wiley, 165–85.

Zuckerman, M. (ed.) 1991: *Psychobiology of Personality*. Cambridge: Cambridge University Press.

7

Genetics and juvenile antisocial behaviour

JANE HOLMES AND ANITA THAPAR

INTRODUCTION

The genetic basis of antisocial behaviour has long been a topic of scientific interest as well as public controversy. In recent years, there have been enormous advances in genetics research and there now exists a considerable body of work, focusing on the role of genetic factors in antisocial behaviour. Twin and adoption studies have allowed us to examine whether genes contribute to antisocial behaviour. However, genetic epidemiological work is now moving beyond the basic task of quantifying the contribution of genes and environment. More recent research is beginning to focus on the much more interesting questions of how genes influence behaviours and disorders, and how these genetic influences interplay with environmental factors.

The advent of new molecular genetic techniques has enabled scientists to identify and locate an increasing number of genes for specific, albeit rare genetic syndromes. More recently, considerable effort has been channelled into unravelling the genetic basis of more common disorders, such as diabetes and psychiatric disorders, as well as continuous traits, such as personality and intelligence. These so-called 'complex' or 'multifactorial' conditions and traits are influenced by the action of multiple genes, in conjunction with environmental factors. Thus, it is increasingly apparent that the relationship between genes and environment is highly complex. Moreover, emerging research findings are revealing that even when a susceptibility gene for a complex disease is identified, the effects are variable. Even for relatively straightforward conditions, such as Alzheimer's disease, which is characterized by a distinct pathology, it is clear that susceptibility genes do not act in a deterministic fashion, but rather increase the probability of showing the disorder.

Despite the expanding interest in behavioural and psychiatric genetics, defining phenotypes remains a problem. There is no clear consensus on how best to define antisocial behaviour and related traits and categories. As a consequence, there has been much variation in the terminology used across studies, with some researchers focusing on psychiatric disorders such as conduct disorders, many examining the genetics of criminality and delinquency, and others investigating the influence of genes on continuous traits, such as antisocial personality and behavioural symptoms. For the purpose of this chapter, we have conceptualized antisocial behaviour in fairly broad terms, in order to encompass findings from these different studies.

We begin by examining the evidence for a genetic contribution to juvenile antisocial behaviour. We then move on to consider how genes might influence these behaviours, and how genetic factors interact with environmental influences. Finally, we consider the molecular basis of juvenile antisocial behaviour, review research strategies that are being used to unravel the molecular genetic basis of juvenile antisocial behaviour, and discuss emerging findings.

GENETIC AND ENVIRONMENTAL INFLUENCES ON JUVENILE ANTISOCIAL BEHAVIOUR

Does antisocial behaviour run in families?

The aetiology of antisocial behaviour is complex. Nevertheless there is overwhelming evidence that antisocial behaviour aggregates within families. Research indicates that criminality in parents is associated with a three- to four-fold increase in delinquency in offspring (Rutter *et al.* 1999). Similarly, family studies show that biological parents of children with conduct disorder are significantly more likely to be diagnosed with antisocial personality disorder than are parents of controls (Frick *et al.* 1992). The familial transmission of antisocial behaviour may of course be explained by shared environmental factors, such as social deprivation, as well as by genetic factors, or by a combination of both. Thus, twin and adoption studies are needed to enable us to distinguish whether this familiality is due to genes or to shared environmental effects.

Is juvenile antisocial behaviour heritable?

The methodological design of twin studies allows researchers to examine the extent to which traits and disorders are heritable, as well as estimate the contribution of environmental influences. Specifically, the basic premise underlying twin research is that MZ twins are genetically identical, whereas DZ twins share on average 50% of their segregating genes. Thus, for a genetically influenced trait or disorder, MZ twins will be more similar than DZ twins, assuming that MZ and DZ twins share environment to the same extent. In simple terms, we would expect the MZ correlation or concordance rate for a heritable trait or disorder to be greater than the DZ correlation.

A number of twin studies on antisocial behaviour have focused on juvenile delinquency, as defined by recorded transgressions of the law. Pooled data from early twin studies of delinquency yielded concordance rates of 87% for MZ twins and 72% for DZ twins (McGuffin and Gottesman 1985). Combined data from more recent twin studies of juvenile delinquency (Goldsmith and Gottesman 1996) also show high concordance rates for MZ twins (95%) and DZ twins (73%). These results again suggest that juvenile delinquency is highly familial. However, the small difference between MZ-DZ concordance rates suggests that this familiality is mainly accounted for by shared environmental effects, with only a modest genetic influence.

Other twin studies of juvenile antisocial behaviour have focused on a more clinically defined phenotype and used questionnaires to measure symptoms of conduct disorder. The findings from twin studies based on the Rutter A parents scale (Graham and Stevenson 1985; Thapar and McGuffin 1996; Eaves *et al.* 1997) and Child Behaviour Checklist (CBCL; Edelbrock *et al.* 1995; Gjone and Stevenson 1997) all suggest the importance of shared environmental influences on symptoms of conduct disorder. However, other studies have also reported some evidence for a genetic influence on juvenile antisocial behaviour (Eaves *et al.* 1997; Rowe 1983; Slutske *et al.* 1997).

Adoption studies provide another means of disentangling the effects of genes and environment. These studies compare the rate of disorder amongst biological relatives of affected individuals with that amongst adoptive relatives. Thus, for a genetically influenced disorder, we would expect an increased prevalence amongst biological relatives of probands, compared with adoptive relatives. Adoption study findings are very similar to those from twin studies, in that although genetic factors appear to contribute, shared environmental factors exert a greater influence on juvenile antisocial behaviour (Cloninger and Gottesman 1987; Cadoret *et al.* 1995).

The importance of environmental factors on antisocial behaviour is further supported by a wealth of epidemiological research, which shows that factors such as marital breakdown or discord, socio-economic disadvantage, large family size and poor parenting are associated with juvenile antisocial behaviour (McGuffin *et al.* 1994). However, two other important factors may also account for the finding that shared environment contributes to conduct disorder symptoms. First, there is some evidence to suggest that where one twin is involved in antisocial activity, this increases the likelihood that the other twin will become a 'partner in crime' (Rowe *et al.* 1992). Thus, the influence of one twin on another may account for the importance of shared environment effects detected in twin studies of juvenile antisocial behaviour. Second, assortative mating, in which parents choose to mate with others more similar to themselves than would be expected by chance (Plomin *et al.* 1997), can also result in an inflated shared environment component in the offspring (discussed further below).

Age effects

Despite differences in phenotypic measurement, data from several twin and adoption studies of juvenile delinquency and conduct disorder suggest that shared environment appears to account for much of the familiality of antisocial symptoms. This finding is striking given that research on adult criminality and antisocial personality disorder has consistently shown a substantial genetic component. (For a review, see McGuffin *et al.* 1994.) For instance, pooled twin data on adult criminality yield concordance rates of 52% for MZ twins and 23% for DZ twins (Goldsmith and Gottesman 1996).

These findings suggest that genetic factors may become more important as individuals mature, whereas the importance of shared environment may decrease with age. This type of developmental change in aetiology may also be important for less severe symptoms of conduct disorder. In a small sample of adolescent twins, McGuffin and Thapar (1997) found a substantial genetic influence on self-reported antisocial symptoms. These results differed markedly from their previous findings in younger children, where shared environmental influences were found to be of primary importance. A similar finding was found in a Norwegian sample of twins (Gjone and Stevenson 1997). Although shared environment was found to be important for externalizing symptoms, the effect was far stronger in the 5–9 years age group (47–50% of the total variance) than in the older age group (23–33% of the variance for 10–15 years).

Thus, genetic influences appear to be more important in older children, even for non-delinquent antisocial behaviour. This issue is more directly addressed in a twin study (Lyons *et al.* 1995) where juvenile and adult antisocial traits were examined in the same individuals. Additive genetic factors accounted for about six times more variance in adult antisocial traits (43%) than in juvenile traits (7%). The genetic determinants of juvenile antisocial behaviour overlapped entirely with the genetic influences on adult traits. These results are again consistent with the view that environmental factors are important for juvenile antisocial behaviour confined to the adolescent years, and that genetic effects are important for the persistence of antisocial behaviour into adulthood, such as antisocial personality disorder. This finding of an age effect is in keeping with results from twin studies for other traits, such as intelligence and personality, which also show a progressively increasing genetic aetiology throughout the lifespan.

What aspects of juvenile antisocial behaviour are heritable?

So far we have considered the influence of genes and environment on composite measures of juvenile antisocial behaviour (e.g. questionnaires, diagnostic interviews, court records). The results may be somewhat misleading, in so far as antisocial behaviour is highly heterogeneous. For instance, there has been some evidence to indicate that genetic factors may be important for certain components of antisocial behaviour. Thus, in a twin study based on the Child Behaviour Checklist, additive genetic factors accounted for 60% of the variance in aggressive behaviour, but for only 35% of the variance in non-aggressive delinquent behaviour (Edelbrock *et al.* 1995). These results suggest that aggressive behaviour in late childhood and adolescence may have a stronger genetic component than delinquent behaviour, for which shared environmental effects appear to be more important. Further evidence for the differential heritability of antisocial behaviour is provided by Lyons *et al.* (1995), who found that some

juvenile symptoms showed a substantial genetic component (e.g. truancy, fighting, weapon use) whereas other symptoms were influenced by shared environment (e.g. firesetting, damages property, stealing).

Comorbidity

The heritability of antisocial behaviour may also depend on the presence or absence of other types of symptoms. Epidemiological and clinical studies have demonstrated a high degree of comorbidity between symptoms of attention deficit hyperactivity disorder (ADHD) and conduct disorder, to the extent that some researchers have questioned whether these behaviours represent distinct diagnostic categories. There is also evidence to suggest that hyperactivity represents a significant risk factor for antisocial behaviour, and that first-degree relatives of probands with ADHD and comorbid conduct disorder show an increased prevalence rate of antisocial behaviours (Biederman *et al.* 1992; Rutter *et al.* 1997).

ADHD has consistently been shown to be highly heritable. (For a review, see Thapar *et al.* 1999.) Therefore, the genetic influence on conduct disorder symptoms reported in some studies may be mediated by comorbid symptoms of ADHD. Indeed results from the Virginia Twin Study suggest a high heritability for conduct disorder only when it is associated with hyperactivity symptoms (Silberg *et al.* 1996a). Further evidence indicates that hyperactivity and conduct disorder symptoms are influenced, to a substantial extent, by the same set of genes (Silberg *et al.* 1996b).

Overall the results from family, twin and adoption studies indicate that both genetic and environmental factors contribute to the development of antisocial behaviours. The next step is to consider how genes may influence behaviour via environmental factors, and to understand more about how genetic and environmental influences may interact.

THE INFLUENCE OF GENES ON BEHAVIOUR VIA ENVIRONMENTAL FACTORS

Behavioural geneticists are now moving beyond quantifying the contribution of genes and environment to antisocial behaviour, and beginning to examine what factors might mediate the influence of genes on behaviour. It is now apparent that the relationship between genetic and environmental influences for traits, such as juvenile antisocial behaviour, is highly complex and that the distinction between these influences is not necessarily clear-cut. Even where much of the variation in a disorder or disease is accounted for by genetic influences (e.g. lung cancer), the mediating factor may still be an environmental agent (e.g. cigarettes for lung cancer). Thus, potentially modifiable factors, such as negative parenting, that may be influenced by parental or child genotype, could mediate the pathway from genotype to antisocial behaviour. It is these sorts of questions that genetic studies are beginning to address.

The concept that there is some genetic control over exposure to the environment is known as *genotype–environment correlation*. There are three forms of genotype–environment correlation; namely passive, evocative and active (Plomin *et al.* 1997).

The passive genotype–environment correlation relates to the transmission of both genes and environment from parent to offspring. Scarr and McCartney (1983) refer to this transmission as a 'double whammy' effect, because parents who exhibit antisocial traits are more likely to provide their children with both genes and environments (e.g. marital discord or breakdown) which foster the development of antisocial behaviour. This example is supported by epidemiological studies which have shown that children with antisocial parents are more likely to be exposed to hostile parenting and marital discord (Rutter *et al.* 1997). There is a need to consider passive genotype–environment correlation as a possible mediating mechanism for antisocial behaviour in children and adolescents.

Evocative genotype–environment correlation occurs when an individual's genetically influenced behaviour evokes responses from other people. For instance, genetically influenced behaviours, such as aggression, may evoke negative reactions from an individual's parents or peers. In a recent adoption study (O'Connor *et al.* 1998), children and adolescents at genetic risk for antisocial behaviour (i.e. biological parent with reported or observed antisocial symptoms) were found to evoke more negative parenting from their adoptive parents, than adoptees not at genetic risk. Similarly, Ge *et al.* (1996) showed that the disciplinary practices of adoptive parents were significantly associated with comorbid antisocial and substance abuse problems amongst biological parents. This association with parenting style appeared to be mediated by antisocial behaviours in the child. Overall, these findings suggest that evocative genotype–environment correlations may partly mediate the relationship between childhood disruptive behaviours and negative parenting.

Finally, active genotype–environment correlation is another way genes may influence antisocial behaviour. Active genotype–environment correlation occurs when individuals seek out experiences that are correlated with their genetic propensities. One important example of active genotype–environment correlation that we have mentioned earlier in this chapter is assortative mating, in which people choose to mate with others more similar to themselves, than would be expected by chance.

It has consistently been shown that there is evidence of assortative mating for antisocial behaviour. For example, in a recent study, self-reported antisocial behaviour was found to be strongly correlated in couples (correlation coefficient of 0.54; Krueger *et al.* 1998). This propensity for antisocial individuals to select mates who engage in similar antisocial behaviours may be explained by the tendency for people to choose mates by geographical location or by institutions they frequent (e.g. rates of antisocial behaviour differ systematically for geographical areas, schools or workplaces).

Assortative mating has important implications for twin and adoption research. Positive assortative mating results in offspring sharing more genes in common than would be expected by random mating. With respect to twin studies, assortative mating elevates DZ correlations (i.e. DZ twins appear more similar) but has no effect on MZ correlations (i.e. MZ twins share all genes in common). Therefore genetic effects in twin studies of antisocial behaviour may be underestimated. Alternatively, assortative mating results in overestimates of heritability and shared environment in adoption studies. Positive assortment on the basis of antisocial behaviour in the biological parents would result in adopted away offspring receiving more antisocial trait-relevant genes. Similarly, assortative mating in adopted parents would result in greater environmental risks. Thus, research that fails to account for assortative mating may be misleading.

THE INTERACTION BETWEEN GENES AND ENVIRONMENTAL FACTORS

Gene–environment interaction refers to the non-additive interaction between genotype and varying environments that produce phenotypic differences (Simonoff *et al.* 1994). One of the best known studies of gene–environment interaction involved rats which were selectively bred for their performance on maze learning. By manipulating the rearing environments (restricted, normal or enriched) for 'maze-bright' and 'maze-dull rats', Cooper and Zubeck (1958) found that maze learning (as measured by number of maze errors) differed significantly depending upon genotype and environment. For instance, an enriched rearing environment greatly improved the performance of maze-dull rats but had little impact on the learning of maze-bright rats. Alternatively, a restricted rearing environment significantly impaired the learning of maze-bright rats but made little difference to the performance of maze-dull rats. This example illustrates how genotypes differentially respond to environments to produce changes in behaviour (Plomin *et al.* 1997). Considering how genetic and environmental factors may interact is vital in understanding the complex development and persistence of antisocial behaviour.

Adoption studies provide one design to detect gene–environment interactions. Several adoption studies of criminality have reported findings suggestive of gene–environment interaction. For instance, Mednick *et al.* (1984) found the highest rate of criminal behaviour amongst adoptees when both biological and adoptive parents had a history of court convictions. Similarly,

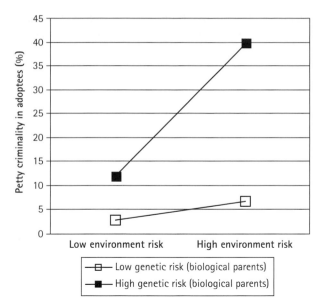

Figure 7.1 *Genotype–environment interaction for petty criminality in a cross-fostering study of Swedish adoptees (adapted from Bohman 1996).*

Bohman (1996) reported strong evidence for a gene–environment interaction in a cross-fostering analysis of petty criminality. These findings are displayed in Figure 7.1 and show that adoptees with a low genetic risk (e.g. biological parent has no criminal history) and low environmental risk (e.g. low social status) had a relatively low criminality rate of 2.9%. The criminality rate only marginally increased for adoptees with a high environmental risk (6.7%), but rose to 12.1% for adoptees at high genetic risk. However, the highest rate of criminality was reported at 40% for those adoptees with both genetic risk factors (e.g. biological parent has criminal history) and environmental risk factors (e.g. low social status). These findings are indicative of a non-additive interaction, given that when both genetic and environmental risk factors are present they account for a higher criminality rate than the combination of these two factors acting independently.

A number of adoption studies have also demonstrated the importance of gene–environment interaction in the genesis of more broadly defined behaviours, such as adolescent conduct disorder and aggression. These studies yield findings similar to those reported in adoption studies of criminality (Cadoret *et al.* 1983; Crowe 1974). For instance, Cadoret *et al.* (1995) reported an interaction between adverse home environment (e.g. marital discord) and genetic vulnerability (biological parent with alcoholism and/or antisocial personality disorder) which accounted for a greater rate of adolescent conduct disorder and aggression than that explained by genetic or environmental factors alone.

Thus, not only have adoption studies consistently provided evidence for the importance of gene–environment interaction for antisocial behaviour, but findings also suggest that environmental risks exert minimal influence on the development and persistence of antisocial behaviours, unless accompanied by a genetic vulnerability.

THE MOLECULAR BASIS OF ANTISOCIAL BEHAVIOUR

So far we have considered the influence of genes and environmental factors on juvenile antisocial behaviour and discussed the complexity of their interaction. The aetiology of antisocial behaviour has also been extensively examined by using strategies aimed at a molecular level. We now discuss the molecular basis of juvenile antisocial behaviour.

Investigating the molecular basis of a complex phenotype such as antisocial behaviour is a challenging proposition. Nevertheless new technologies and genetic strategies are increasingly being employed for this purpose. Here we consider three main types of research strategies; namely animal studies, research which has focused on serotonergic activity, and molecular genetic studies in humans.

Animal studies

Animal models are increasingly being used as a tool to dissect the molecular genetic basis of behaviour. Mice have provided particularly useful models, as the mouse genome has been extensively mapped and many genes are homologous with those in humans. Animal breeding experiments, in which animals are selected and bred to show extremes of behaviour, have been used to identify genes of small effect (quantitative trait loci; see later) for traits such as emotionality and hyperactivity. These genetic mapping studies of animal models look promising and may provide important leads for candidate genes involved in extremes of human behaviour.

More recently, it has been possible to examine the function of specific genes in animals using 'knockout' animals. In this type of experiment, a particular gene is targeted so that it is no longer functional and the behaviour of the animal subsequently studied. The function of genes has also been explored in animals by examining naturally occurring mutations, as well as by using transgenic experiments where mutant genes are introduced. There are now several examples of knockout mice which exhibit extreme aggression – for example, mice with targeted disruption of the 5-HT$_{1B}$ receptor gene (Sandou *et al.* 1994). Similarly, mice which lack the gene coding for monoamine oxidase A (MAOA), an enzyme which degrades catecholamines, also demonstrate increased aggression (Cases *et al.* 1995).

Disruption of other genes has also been shown to be associated with heightened aggression in mice. Neuronal nitric oxide synthase (nNOS) is an enzyme responsible for the synthesis of the biological messenger, nitric oxide, and disruption of this gene results in increased aggressive behaviour and inappropriate sexual persistence in mice (Nelson *et al.* 1995). Increased aggressive behaviour in both sexes is also exhibited in mice lacking the tailess gene. These results are undoubtedly exciting, although it is clearly implausible that aggression is caused by single gene defects. As yet, these types of animal experiments do not allow us to disentangle compensatory effects; and for that and many other reasons, caution is required in using the results to draw conclusions about the aetiology of human behaviour. Nevertheless, knockout models provide a novel and exciting tool for examining the genetic basis of behaviour and are likely to help shed light on the complex pathways leading to antisocial behaviour.

Serotonin and juvenile antisocial behaviour

The role of serotonin (5-HT) neurotransmission in antisocial behaviour has long excited debate, and this topic is comprehensively reviewed in Mitsis *et al.* (2000). Although much of this work has focused on adult behaviour, more recently there has been increasing interest in the role of serotonergic function in childhood antisocial behaviour.

Three main strategies have been used to determine serotonergic activity in humans. First, there are those studies that have relied on central measures of 5-HT activity, for example by examining cerebrospinal fluid (CSF). A second group of studies have utilized hormonal measures following neurochemical challenge as an indicator of neurotransmitter function, for example prolactin response to fenfluramine challenge. Finally, the least invasive, but most indirect method of measuring central serotonergic activity has been to use peripheral measures such as platelet binding and blood and urinary measures of 5-HT metabolites.

Overall for children and adolescents, there so far have been few such studies and findings have been conflicting. To date, there have been two studies of antisocial children which have utilized CSF measures of 5-HT. In the first study (Kruesi *et al.* 1992), low CSF 5-HIAA (5-hydroxyindoleacetic acid, a metabolite of 5-HT) was found to be associated with aggression in 29 children and adolescents with disruptive behaviour disorders. However, results have been inconsistent in that another group demonstrated a relationship between CSF 5-HIAA and aggression in the opposite direction (Castellanos *et al.* 1994). Similarly, findings from studies which have measured prolactin response to a fenfluramine challenge have been inconclusive, with one study failing to show an association with aggression (Stoff *et al.* 1992), and another demonstrating a positive association (Halperin *et al.* 1994).

Although peripheral indicators of 5-HT function provide a more indirect measure of central 5-HT function, some emerging results have been particularly interesting, as they suggest that environmental factors play an important role. There is now much to suggest that environmental adversity appears to produce changes in peripheral measures of 5-HT functioning in humans. More specifically, in studies of non-human primates, harsh rearing conditions appear to be associated with changes in 5-HT functioning. Thus, it is possible that the influence of 5-HT on antisocial behaviour is mediated by environmental factors. In one study of 38 boys who were selected for being at an increased familial risk of convicted delinquency (Pine *et al.* 1996), 5-HT$_{2A}$ platelet receptor density was negatively related to harsh parenting and family environments, characterized by frequent physical punishment and anger, rather than to disruptive behaviour. However, the finding of low platelet 5-HT$_{2A}$ receptor density in these children is in the opposite direction to that found in many adult studies.

Overall the role of 5-HT functioning in children and adolescents remains unclear. Studies using larger samples may help in resolving some of these discrepancies, and the use of genetic strategies may also be helpful. Nevertheless, on the basis of work so far, it is clear that the relationship between neurotransmitter functioning and antisocial behaviour is complex and that a neurobiological influence does not necessarily preclude the contribution of environmental risk factors.

THE MOLECULAR GENETIC BASIS OF ANTISOCIAL BEHAVIOUR

Earlier in this chapter we discussed the contribution of genetic factors to antisocial behaviour and concluded that these influences play an important role. This conclusion leads to the next question of whether we can identify specific genes that increase the risk of antisocial behaviour.

Previous enthusiasm for cytogenetic studies led to interest in the association of chromosomal abnormalities with antisocial behaviour. Early studies suggested an increased rate of the XYY syndrome in forensic units and prisons. However, it is now clear that most individuals with an XYY anomaly do not show criminal behaviour. Current attention is now focused on modern molecular genetics which has undoubtedly been remarkably successful in identifying and localizing genes responsible for single-gene conditions which show predictable Mendelian patterns of inheritance. It is possible, of course, that in some rare instances familial antisocial behaviour may be explained by an unknown single-gene mutation. An example of this was reported in an extended Dutch family where multiple members exhibited violent criminal behaviour which was found to be related to a mutation in the MAOA gene (Brunner *et al.* 1993). This is of particular interest, given the findings that MAOA knockout mice also exhibit marked aggression. However, isolated mutations of this type are rare and it is clearly not plausible to consider such defects as major determinants of antisocial behaviour. Even for highly heritable psychiatric conditions, such as schizophrenia and autism, although there was initial interest in the possibility of single gene subforms, it is becoming increasingly apparent that multiple genes are involved and that different strategies will be required to identify these types of susceptibility genes.

Identifying susceptibility genes

The success of modern molecular genetics has been based on two key technological advances. First, there are now a very large number of informative genetic markers available and these span the whole genome at increasingly close intervals providing a detailed genetic map. Genetic markers are informative when they involve variations or polymorphisms in DNA, and these variants are termed *alleles*. Second, improved and highly automated laboratory techniques allow for relatively rapid genotyping, that is the process of identifying which alleles are present for any given marker for a particular person.

The principle underlying all methods of identifying and localizing genes is illustrated in Figure 7.2. Here we have represented a stretch of chromosome along which there are five markers named A, B, C, D and E. Molecular genetic strategies essentially involve identifying where disease gene X is, by the process of finding that the disease gene is very near to marker C. The two main strategies which are being used to detect and localize genes are linkage studies and association studies.

Linkage studies

Linkage approaches involve collecting families where a number of members are affected with the disease (McGuffin *et al.* 1994). Markers along the genome are then genotyped for each person with the objective of finding out whether any of these markers are co-transmitted with the disorder. For Mendelian disorders, the collection of large families of multiply-affected members, and using a lod score method of linkage analysis (see McGuffin *et al.* 1994), has been fruitful. However this type of approach is not the most suitable for complex disorders, where we do not know the mode of inheritance and where we cannot reliably specify the boundaries of the phenotype to classify individuals as unaffected.

Affected-relative pair linkage methods overcome these problems in that it is not necessary to specify a mode of inheritance or include unaffected relatives. The approach is to collect relatives, usually siblings, where both siblings have the disorder being studied. Siblings inherit their genes from the same parents and we would expect them to share some, but not all, of the marker alleles in common. Affected-relative pair linkage analysis simply involves examining whether the affected siblings share marker alleles identical by descent, more often than would be expected. This type of strategy has been used successfully for mapping susceptibility loci for insulin-dependent diabetes. A major advantage of this approach is that linkage can be detected even when the susceptibility gene is at some distance from the marker. Thus it is relatively easy to search the whole genome using only about 300 markers. However, a drawback to this method is that the susceptibility gene needs to be of reasonably large effect to be detected, with realistically sized samples of affected relative pairs.

Association studies

Association studies are case–control studies, which involve examining whether a particular marker allele is more common in individuals with the disorder. Association studies are becoming increasingly attractive, given their sensitivity in locating genes of small effect. Positive association can arise for three main reasons.

- First, it may be that the marker allele is itself involved in susceptibility to the disorder.
- Second, the associated marker allele may lie extremely close to the susceptibility gene, and this is known as 'linkage disequilibrium'.
- Finally, positive association can also arise as a result of population stratification, when the control group and disease group differ in allele frequencies for spurious reasons.

False positive association, due to population stratification, has until recently been a major source of criticism of association studies. However, more recent statistical techniques (e.g. the transmission disequilibrium test (TDT) and haplotype relative risk method (HRR)) which use parental genotype information as an internal control group overcome this difficulty.

Although association approaches are appealing, in so far as they allow for the detection of genes of small effect, a major shortcoming has been that, unlike linkage, association will be only detected when the marker allele is extremely close to the disease susceptibility gene. Thus, so far association studies have focused on candidate genes, which are thought to be involved in the pathogenesis of the disorder. This of course is limiting when the pathophysiology of the disorder is not understood. Moving beyond a candidate gene approach and searching the whole genome for association would require the use of a very

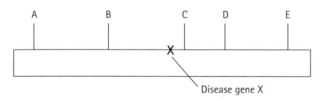

Figure 7.2 *The principle underlying all methods of identifying and localizing genes.*

dense map of markers, which until recently has not been feasible. However, recent laboratory techniques for pooling DNA greatly reduce the amount of genotyping and look very promising. Thus, whole-genome association studies may become a critical strategy in the future.

Molecular genetic studies of many psychiatric conditions – including disorders such as schizophrenia, bipolar affective disorder, alcoholism and autism – are now under way. However, so far there has been little in the way of molecular genetics research which has been directly relevant to the understanding of juvenile antisocial behaviour. Nevertheless, a recent population-based study showed evidence of association of childhood maltreatment with antisocial behaviour in males, the effects of which were moderated by a variant in the *MAO-A* gene (Caspi *et al.* 2002). Thus, there is a clear need to examine gene–environment interactions in future molecular genetic studies of antisocial behaviour. Current interest in the genetics of ADHD also promises to be of relevance to the field of juvenile forensic psychiatry. As mentioned previously, the genetic basis of ADHD is likely to be of importance in juvenile antisocial behaviour for at least two reasons.

- First, results from follow-up studies suggest that ADHD is an important risk factor for later conduct disorder and adult antisocial behaviour.
- Second, genetic epidemiological evidence suggests that when symptoms of ADHD and conduct disorder co-occur, this is primarily attributable to a shared genetic aetiology.

Thus, it seems reasonable to suppose that genetic influences on juvenile antisocial behaviour may, at least in part, be mediated via symptoms of ADHD.

Most published molecular genetic studies of ADHD have used a candidate-gene association approach with particular interest in genes involved in dopaminergic pathways. There is considerable appeal in focusing on these candidate genes, given that over 70% of children with ADHD show a rapid symptomatic improvement with stimulant medication. To date, the dopamine transporter gene DAT1 and the dopamine receptor gene DRD4 have been suggested as susceptibility loci for ADHD (Thapar *et al.* 1999).

DAT1 is a particularly attractive candidate gene, given that methylphenidate is known to inhibit the dopamine transporter, and DAT1 knockout mice show motor hyperactivity. There have been independent reports of a positive association for ADHD with the 480 base-pair allele of the DAT1 gene (e.g. Cook *et al.* 1995; Gill *et al.* 1997). Similarly, positive results for an association with the DRD4 7 repeat allele (Swanson *et al.* 1998) have now also been independently replicated (e.g. Smalley *et al.* 1998; Rowe *et al.* 1998), and shown is a meta-analysis (Faraone *et al.* 2001). Overall, the initial results from molecular

genetic studies of ADHD look promising, although the inconsistency in findings cannot be ignored. It is becoming increasingly clear in psychiatric genetics that, where susceptibility loci have been implicated (e.g. DAT1 and DRD4 for ADHD), the effect size of that gene is very small. Thus, large sample sizes are required to detect these effects and many negative findings may simply reflect a lack of statistical power. However, unravelling the molecular genetic basis of psychiatric disorders is clearly a complex task. Genetic researchers face the problems of phenotypic definition, dealing with aetiological and clinical heterogeneity, and taking into account the influence of other genes and environmental factors.

Quantitative trait loci

So far we have considered identifying susceptibility genes for disorders and categories. However, many behaviours including antisocial behaviour may be more easily viewed as continuous traits. An alternative approach to unravelling the molecular genetic basis of psychopathology may be to identify susceptibility genes for dimensional risk factors, such as personality traits or normal symptoms. These genes are known as 'quantitative trait loci' (QTLs).

QTL studies have already proved successful in plants and animals. Susceptibility genes for a wide range of quantitative characteristics, such as pH and mass of a tomato, and emotionality in mice have been successfully localized. QTL linkage studies in humans are likely to be of particular interest in the study of antisocial behaviour by either considering this or related behaviour as a continuous dimension itself, or by searching for susceptibility loci for risk dimensions such as impulsivity. There has been considerable recent interest in QTL studies of personality traits with two separate reports of an association with the dopamine receptor DRD4 7 repeat allele and novelty-seeking scores. Novelty seeking is characterized by excitable, exploratory behaviours that are very similar to some of the symptoms of ADHD. Thus, the replicated positive association findings for the DRD4 7 repeat allele with both novelty seeking and ADHD are of particular interest. Other studies have failed to replicate these results for novelty seeking and so it remains difficult to draw conclusions. Nevertheless, a QTL approach provides a promising method of identifying susceptibility genes for behavioural traits and risk factors related to juvenile antisocial behaviour.

CONCLUSIONS

We have considered the genetic basis of juvenile antisocial behaviour in detail. Family research has informed us that antisocial behaviour is a highly familial condition. Twin and adoption studies have yielded mixed findings, which illustrates the complex aetiology of antisocial behaviour. Overall, the results of these studies have indicated that both genetic and environmental factors contribute. However, it appears that shared environmental factors exert a stronger influence on antisocial behaviour in the childhood and adolescent years, and that genetic factors are of greater importance for the persistence of antisocial behaviour into adult life. Furthermore, there has been some research that suggests genetic factors are more important for certain aspects of antisocial behaviour, such as aggression.

Although twin and adoption studies have been important in quantifying the relative contributions of genes and environment, behavioural geneticists are now examining how these genetic and environmental factors influence psychopathology and how they interact with one another. There is evidence to suggest that environmental factors such as parenting style may mediate the influence of genes on juvenile antisocial behaviour. Findings from adoption studies (and now also molecular genetic studies) also suggest that environmental risks have a major influence on antisocial behaviour only when accompanied by genetic liability. Finally, technological advancements are enabling scientists to investigate the molecular basis of antisocial behaviour. Molecular genetic strategies, in conjunction with animal work, will help to identify risk factors at a molecular level. Nevertheless, the real challenge will be in attempting to understand the complex pathway from risk factors to behaviours.

REFERENCES

Biederman, J., Faraone, S.V., Keenan, K. *et al.* 1992: Further evidence for family–genetic risk factors in attention deficit hyperactivity disorder (ADHD): patterns of comorbidity in probands and relatives in psychiatrically and pediatrically referred samples. *Archives of General Psychiatry* **49**: 728–38.

Bohman, M. 1996: Predisposition to criminality: Swedish adoption studies in retrospect. In Bock G.R. and Goode J.A. (eds), *Genetics of Criminal and Antisocial Behaviour*. Chichester: John Wiley, 99–114.

Brunner, H.G., Nelen, M.R., Van Zandvoort, P. *et al.* 1993: X-linked borderline mental retardation with prominent behavioural disturbance: phenotype, genetic localisation and evidence for disturbed monoamine metabolism. *American Journal of Human Genetics* **52**: 1032–9.

Cadoret, R.J., Cain, C.A. and Crowe, R.R. 1983: Evidence for gene-environment interaction in the development of adolescent antisocial behaviour. *Behaviour Genetics* **13**: 301–10.

Cadoret, R.J., Yates, W.R., Troughton, E., Woodworth, G. and Stewart, M.A. 1995: Genetic–environmental interaction in the genesis of aggressivity and conduct disorders. *Archives of General Psychiatry* **52**: 916–24.

Cases, O., Seif, I., Grimsby, J. *et al.* 1995: Aggressive behaviour and altered amounts of brain serotonin and norepinephrine in mice lacking MAOA. *Science* **268**: 1763–6.

Caspi, A., McClay, J., Moffitt, T.E. *et al.* 2002: Role of genotype in the cycle of violence in maltreated children. *Science* **297**: 851–4.

Castellanos, F.X., Elia, J., Kreusi, M.J.P. *et al.* 1994: Cerebrospinal fluid monoamine metabolites in boys with attention deficit hyperactivity disorder. *Psychiatry Research* **52**: 305–16.

Cloninger, C.R. and Gottesman, I.I. 1987: Genetic and environmental factors in antisocial behavioural disorders. In Mednick, S.A., Moffit, T.E. and Stack, S.A. (eds), *Causes of Crime: New Biological Approaches*. Cambridge: Cambridge University Press, 92–109.

Cook, E.H., Stein, M.A., Krasowski, M.D. *et al.* 1995: Association of attention-deficit disorder and the dopamine transporter gene. *American Journal of Human Genetics* **56**: 993–8.

Cooper, R.M. and Zubek, J.P. 1958: Effects of enriched and restricted early environments on the learning ability of bright and dull rats. *Canadian Journal of Psychology* **12**: 159–64.

Crowe, R.R. 1974: An adoption study of antisocial personality. *Archives of General Psychiatry* **31**: 785–91.

Eaves, L.J., Silberg, J.L., Meyer, J.M. *et al.* 1997: Genetics and developmental psychopathology: 2. The main effects of genes and environment on behavioural problems in the Virginia Twin Study of Adolescent Behavioural Development. *Journal of Child Psychology and Psychiatry* **38**: 965–80.

Edelbrock, C., Rende, R., Plomin, R. and Thompson, L.A. 1995: A twin study of competence and problem behaviour in childhood and early adolescence. *Journal of Child Psychology and Psychiatry* **36**: 775–85.

Faraone, S.V., Doyle, A.E., Mick, E. and Biderman, J. 2001: Meta-analysis of the association between the 7-repeat allele of the dopamine D(4) receptor gene and attention deficit hyperactivity disorder. *American Journal of Psychiatry* **158**: 1052–7.

Frick, P., Lahey, B., Loeber, R. *et al.* 1992: Familial risk factors to oppositional defiant disorder and conduct disorder: parental psychopathology and maternal parenting. *Journal of Consulting and Clinical Psychology* **60**: 49–55.

Ge, X., Conger, R.D., Cadoret, R.J. *et al.* 1996: The developmental interface between nature and nurture: a mutual influence model of child antisocial behaviour and parenting. *Developmental Psychology* **32**: 574–89.

Gill, M., Daly, G., Heron, S., Hawi, Z. and Fitzgerald, M. 1997: Confirmation of association between attention deficit hyperactivity disorder and a dopamine transporter polymorphism. *Molecular Psychiatry* **2**: 311–13.

Gjone, H. and Stevenson, J. 1997: The association between internalising and externalising behaviour in childhood and early adolescence: genetic and environmental common influences. *Journal of Abnormal Child Psychology* **25**: 277–86.

Goldsmith, H.H. and Gottesman, I.I. 1996: Heritable variability and variable heritability in developmental psychopathology. In Lenzenwegger, M.F. and Haugaard, J.J. (eds), *Frontiers of Developmental Psychopathology*. New York: Oxford University Press, 5–43.

Graham, P. and Stevenson, J. 1985: A twin study of genetic influences on behavioural deviance. *Journal of the American Academy of Child and Adolescent Psychiatry* **24**: 33–41.

Halperin, J.M., Sharma, V., Sierer, L.J. *et al.* 1994: Serotonergic function in aggressive and non-aggressive boys with attention deficit hyperactivity disorder. *American Journal of Psychiatry* **151**: 243–8.

to the development and persistence of antisocial behaviour, and has led to the development of effective treatments. As yet these are not being widely used with the children and adolescents who need them. Therefore psychiatrists need to be able to contribute to the planning and delivery of an appropriate service.

THE HISTORY OF CONDUCT DISORDER

There have not been surveys in the same locations using the same methods in different decades to say reliably whether conduct disorder is becoming more common. However, there is better information about officially reported crime and self-reported criminal acts. Whilst crime reflects only one subset of antisocial behaviours, there is a strong overlap with adolescent conduct disorder as it covers non-aggressive acts such as theft, drug taking and deception, and aggressive acts such as fighting and mugging. From 1945 to 1985, crimes committed by all ages increased greatly in western and industrialized countries, by a factor of over 20 in Spain and Canada, by 10–15 in Sweden and Norway, and by 1–6 in Australia, England, France, Germany, Italy and the USA (Rutter *et al.* 1998). All the available evidence suggests that the juvenile component has risen in a similar way. Specific studies of conduct disorder across cohorts (Robins and Regier 1991) also suggest a rise over the last 40 years.

PREVALENCE OF CONDUCT DISORDER

Prevalence according to age
The prevalence of serious oppositional behaviour in preschool children has been found to range from 4 to 9% (Cohen *et al.* 1993; Richman *et al.* 1982).

In school-age children, oppositional disorders are found in 6–12%, whereas more severe conduct disorders are less frequent, occurring in 2–4% (Anderson *et al.* 1987; Rutter *et al.* 1970; Offord *et al.* 1991; Shaffer *et al.* 1996).

In adolescents, the rate of oppositional disorders has been assessed as being as high as 15% (Cohen *et al.* 1993), and that of severe conduct disorders 6–12%.

Early- versus adolescent-onset patterns
There are major differences between early and adolescent onset. Those with an early onset display defiant and aggressive behaviour before the age of 8 years, but it typically begins at around 3 years. These youngsters go on to accrue increasingly antisocial behaviours. However, not all young children with this early-onset pattern of problems progress to more severe difficulties later in childhood. Only about half persist; the remainder improve. Compared to the adolescent-onset group, the early-onset children already at age 3 show a more difficult temperament (restlessness, inattention, negativity, irritability, etc.). At school age this group have cognitive, language and motor deficits, reading difficulties, adverse family contexts and poor parenting. By 18 they have fewer friends and feel socially alienated, victimized, and are callous and suspicious. They continue behaving antisocially as adults. Some have called this group 'early-onset lifetime-persistent' (Moffitt *et al.* 1996).

More common by a ratio of about 3 to 1 are the adolescent-onset group who have not shown significant antisocial behaviour earlier in their lives. Moreover by their early twenties they have mostly stopped behaving antisocially, so some call them an 'adolescence-limited' group (Moffitt *et al.* 1996). The overall rate of arrests and convictions is somewhat lower than for the childhood-onset type, and there are more girls (about 2:1 instead of 4:1 for childhood onset). Their behaviour tends to be less aggressive and violent, and less impulsive. They have fewer cognitive and neuropsychological deficits, tend to come from less dysfunctional family environments, and tend to have more adaptive social qualities. Crucially, the adolescent-onset group are more likely to stop offending in early adulthood than are the early-onset group. There is only a small group of individuals who commence persistent antisocial activity in adulthood, less than 10% of the total.

GENDER DIFFERENCE

Conduct disorder is more common in boys at all ages, but the ratio of boys to girls depends of the type of disorder. In childhood, for oppositionality, boys outnumber girls by around 4 to 1. In adolescence the ratio narrows to around 2 to 1. However, for DSM-IV conduct disorder, which includes several violent offences, the ratio is up to 10 to 1. Definitions which include abuse of drugs and precocious sexual activity show a greater proportion of girls.

SOCIO-ECONOMIC STATUS

Conduct disorder is 3–4 times more common in children who are in socio-economically deprived families with low income, or who receive state welfare benefits, or who live in a poor neighbourhood. Each of these indices overlaps considerably, and is a marker for many of the aetiological factors discussed below.

GEOGRAPHICAL LOCATION

Rates found in surveys carried out in westernized countries such as Britain, the USA, France, New Zealand and Canada have found very similar rates when comparable methods have been used. Surveys in other locations such as Hong Kong and South America have found lower prevalences. Within countries, many but not all studies have found increased rates in urban compared to rural locations.

AETIOLOGY OF CONDUCT DISORDER

Nature and nurture

Conduct Disorder clusters in families. Until the 1980s most twin studies of antisocial behaviour showed a high concordance for monozygotic pairs at around 70–80%, but also high concordance for dizygotic pairs at around 60–70%, suggesting a major shared familial influence, a moderate unique environmental contribution for the individual, and only a limited genetic component (DiLalla and Gottesman 1989). However, the subjects were mostly in their late teens, when the adolescent-onset type outnumber the early-onset type by about 3 to 1. More recent twin studies of subtype conduct problems suggest that in older adolescents with pure conduct problems family environment indeed has the overwhelming effect; but in younger conduct-disordered children with comorbid hyperactivity and other problems, genetic influences predominate (Silberg *et al.* 1996). French and American adoption studies show 2–3 times higher rates of criminality in adolescence in infants adopted into families with lower socio-economic status. Danish and Swedish adoption studies have confirmed the effect of the socio-economic status of the rearing environment, but have also investigated the adoptee genetic potential for antisocial behaviour, as indicated by the birth parents' criminality. These studies show a marked genetic effect as well as the environmental one. What appears to be particularly damaging is the combination of a genetic predisposition plus an adverse upbringing, which interact to give a high rate of antisocial activity (Bohman 1996). Adoption studies are likely to underplay the importance of adverse environments, since adoption agencies select out prospective adoptive families who are notably dysfunctional and disadvantaged.

Genetic influences play a stronger role in the development of adult antisocial personality and criminality than in adolescent antisocial behaviour, in part owing to the greater proportion of early-onset types in this group. Cytogenetic and molecular genetic studies have not yet identified specific conditions associated with antisocial behaviour, except for the XYY karyotype where affected individuals show about three times the rate of criminal behaviour of controls or individuals with other chromosomal anomalies, such as XXY, even allowing for their reduced IQ.

Environment within the family

Parental rearing style
Conduct disorder is strongly associated with harsh, erratic discipline, hostility directed at the child, lack of warmth, and poor supervision (Farrington 1994). Follow-up and intervention studies show that these factors have a causal role in initiating and maintaining the child's disorder, and are not just a reaction to the child's behaviour. However, there is also good evidence that children with conduct problems elicit harsh negative parenting; both processes operate. In adolescence, supervision becomes a major factor, with parents of antisocial youths typically not knowing where they are for several hours in the day and at night. Discord between parents is also associated with persistent antisocial behaviour (Richman *et al.* 1982). The association of conduct disorder with large family size, and with broken homes (divorce, single parenthood, adoption) seems chiefly to be mediated by parenting practices and the previous characteristics of the individuals, rather than by the impact of a large family or broken home in themselves.

Moment-to-moment communication between parent and child
Fine-grained analysis by Patterson (1982) has shown that the moment-to-moment responses of parents towards children have a powerful effect on their behaviour. In families with a conduct-disordered child, the children are likely to be ignored when they are behaving reasonably, but criticized and shouted at when they are misbehaving. The consequence is that, to gain attention, they have to behave badly. What is perhaps surprising is that for these children who receive very little positive attention, they are prepared to elicit often unpleasant and frankly hostile reactions from their parents rather than be ignored. By contrast, children who receive a reasonable amount of positive attention within the family tend to avoid behaving in a way which elicits negative attention. All this can be summarized as the 'attention rule', which states that children will behave in whatever way necessary to gain a reasonable amount of attention.

Other behaviours by parents can unwittingly raise the probability of disruptive behaviour in the child. Giving up insisting that something the child finds unpleasant is carried out (e.g. tidying up the toys) unintentionally rewards the child for whining and refusing to do it, thus making the behaviour more likely next time a request is made (negative reinforcement). Giving in to demands and tantrums for what the child wants has similar effects (positive reinforcement for negative behaviour).

Most emphasis in social learning theory has been on the harmful effect of negative behaviour. However, other research (Gardner 1987) has made it clear that the presence of positive parental behaviour is equally important. Children with antisocial behaviour are ignored for a lot of the time by their parents, who do not respond to their overtures to join in activities, nor praise them when they are behaving well. Not only does this make quiet prosocial activity less likely, but also no models are provided for the child to learn social skills such as turn-taking, negotiating skills, etc.

The implications of the impact of the immediate interaction patterns on child antisocial behaviour are far-reaching. Rather than the child being seen as innately aggressive or with an antisocial type of personality that is unchangeable, he or she can be viewed as responding to the immediate context. Therefore changing the context offers the possibility of changing the behaviour of the child. This allows some therapeutic optimism if the response contingencies around the child can be altered, and has led to the development of effective treatments.

Physical maltreatment and sexual abuse

Serious abuse can lead to the emergence of conduct problems in girls or boys who were previously free of such problems. Kessler *et al.* (1997) found that physical aggression from the father was associated with more than doubling of rates of conduct disorder and quadrupling of rates of antisocial personality disorder. Trickett and McBride-Chang (1995) found sexual and physical abuse associated with a wide range of poor outcomes. The difficulty in ascertaining their effect arises because they are usually associated with multiple risk factors such as poor parenting and rejection, as well as genetic predisposition. Widom (1997), however, found that early childhood victimization raised later criminality by only 50%.

Parental mental illness

Depression features commonly in mothers, and alcoholism, drug abuse and psychoses are not infrequent in parents of children with severe conduct disorder. These disorders exert their effects in childhood through the quality of interaction and parenting practices, and by affecting the inherited characteristics of the child. There is no specific child psychiatric disorder which is more common, but conduct problems are more frequent as are emotional disorders (Rutter and Quinton 1984). Children of depressed mothers may have impaired cognitive and social development.

Paternal criminality

As an environmental influence, this is important and may be mediated through parent–child interactions and parenting practices as described above, plus an antisocial set of values and living in a deprived neighbourhood. It also represents an increased genetic risk.

Pregnancy and birth complications

These have no or extremely weak influence on antisocial behaviour. Raine (1997) has suggested they contribute to violent behaviour, but the evidence is unconvincing. There is more evidence that prenatal *in utero* exposure to alcohol and cocaine can impair brain development and lead to impulsivity and lower IQ, and hence antisocial behaviour (Streissguth 1993; Mayes and Bornstein 1997). Prenatal maternal smoking is associated with slightly higher levels of criminality in offspring, but is likely to be a marker for better known risk factors such as parenting style and impulsive child temperament (Gibson and Tibbetts 1998).

Environment outside the family

The peer group

Conduct disorder is more likely in children who associate with friends who have an antisocial attitude, value aggression, and commit destructive and rule-breaking acts. Associating with deviant peers increases conduct problems independently of the individual's level of aggression. In adolescence, quite a lot of antisocial behaviour is carried out with peers, sometimes in gangs. Together, conduct-disordered youths laugh and approve talk about antisocial activities and do not respond to talk about ordinary topics, so reinforcing the values put on delinquent acts (Dishion and Patterson 1997). If children are rejected by their peers, the chance of later conduct problems is increased. This seems to apply particularly to early-onset conduct disorder (Coie and Dodge 1997). Treatments which put antisocial youths together in groups often increase the level of antisocial behaviour.

Drugs and alcohol

Many of the risk factors which lead to alcohol and drug abuse are similar to those for antisocial behaviour. However, the relationship is more than just a passive overlap. Antisocial behaviour increases the chances of substance abuse, and vice versa. Longitudinal surveys show that antisocial behaviour in childhood and adolescence increase the risk of later alcohol- and drug-related problems, which peak in the twenties. ('Problems' refers to regular hard-drug or heavy alcohol use, with psychosocial impairment or medical complications as a result. This differs from occasional or 'recreational' use of marijuana or hallucinogens, which is far more widespread, or alcohol use without impairment.)

Heavy drinking of alcohol increases the chance of crime as it causes disinhibition and is associated with a range of disorderly and violent offences. With drugs, there is an increase in theft and non-violent offences to get money to buy drugs; those who deal in drugs may use violent methods to protect their business.

School

School organization has been shown to affect rates of antisocial behaviour independently of home background. Poorly organized, unfriendly schools with low staff morale, high staff turnover and poor contact with parents have higher conduct disorder rates even when catchment area characteristics have been allowed for (Rutter *et al.* 1979).

Locality

Conduct problems are associated with overcrowding, poor housing and poor neighbourhoods. How much these factors are causal or simply markers for other family or socio-economic variables is unclear. Multivariate analyses suggest that when factors such as poor parenting and maternal depression are accounted for, neighbourhood and poverty effects are not large. However, it is plausible that stressful living conditions with few amenities for children and many other demands on parents impair their ability to bring up their children constructively and responsively. Also, areas where there are closer relationships between neighbours with high perceived social cohesion by residents and informal social controls have less antisocial behaviour (Sampson *et al.* 1997). Moving out of a deprived area reduces rates of antisocial behaviour (Osborn 1980).

Child factors

Physiology

Physique has little influence on antisocial propensity. The relationship between testosterone (and other androgens) and antisocial behaviour is complex. Levels vary with age, type of antisocial behaviour and social rejection, so that no straightforward conclusion can be drawn (Tremblay *et al.* 1997); certainly to date no obvious relationship has been shown between higher levels and more aggression.

Serotonin is being investigated since reduced levels have been associated with suicidal, impulsive and aggressive behaviour in adults. However, samples have to be obtained through lumbar puncture, so studies are usually on small incarcerated samples, where reduced levels of metabolites in aggressive adults have been found. Moffitt *et al.* (1997) reported reduced blood levels (effect size 0.5 sd) in an epidemiological study of young adults, but the relationship between blood and brain levels has yet to be clarified. Studies in children are few and show no consistent picture.

Autonomic arousal has shown a consistent (albeit modest) association with persistent antisocial behaviour in young people. Their pulse rates are lower, their skin conductance is less, as is their adrenaline and cortisol excretion. Some have postulated that this leads to less anxiety when taking risks (Venables 1988); others see it as part of a wider picture of decreased central nervous system inhibition (Gray 1987). With all these physiological substrates and mechanisms, the direction of effect is unlikely to be only biology driving behaviour; equally, confrontative situations, social dominance, peer rejection and self-esteem influence physiological parameters.

Temperament

Infants with temperaments classified as 'difficult' at 3 years are more likely to be referred for aggressive problems later on (Thomas *et al.* 1968; Caspi *et al.* 1993). The dimensions involved are behavioural impulsivity (lack of restraint), short attention span and motor restlessness. Although not occurring at a clinical level, these are precisely the constituents of the hyperkinetic syndrome; together with the trait of negative emotionality (irritability, anger and bad moods) they have a clear modest effect in predicting later antisocial behaviour of the early-onset type. Social anxiety, on the other hand, is protective.

Intelligence

Children with early-onset lifetime-persistent conduct disorder have IQs that are 8–10 points below those of controls. The relationship with antisocial behaviour weakens after allowing for social class but is still present, although it accounts for only a few per cent of the variance. This is not just the effect of missed schooling, since it is present before these children go to school. Much of the association can be accounted for by the association with hyperactivity (Hinshaw 1992). It seems likely that low IQ alone does not confer much increased risk of antisocial behaviour, but in the presence of adverse parenting and other risks it has an interactive effect (Stattin *et al.* 1997).

Attitudes and beliefs

Significant cognitive attributional bias has been shown in aggressive children and youths. They are more likely to perceive neutral acts by others as hostile, and are more likely to believe conflicts can be satisfactorily resolved by aggression. As the individual gets more disliked and rejected by peers, the opportunity for seeing things this way increases (Dodge and Schwartz 1997). By their late teens these youths can have a highly suspicious attitude, and be quick to perceive disrespect from others and sometimes react explosively. Social skills are lacking. Emotional processes in antisocial children have been little studied, although self-esteem is often low and coexistent misery common. Youths with conduct disorder have been shown to plan their lives less than do controls, so that they are more driven by events than in control of them.

CLASSIFICATION

ICD-10

The ICD-10 classification has a category for conduct disorders – F91. The World Health Organization's clinical descriptions and diagnostic guidelines (WHO 1992) state:

> 'Examples of the behaviours on which the diagnosis is based include the following: excessive levels of fighting or bullying; cruelty to animals or other people; severe destructiveness to property; firesetting; stealing; repeated lying; truancy from school and running away from home; unusually frequent and severe temper tantrums; defiant provocative behaviour; and persistent severe disobedience. Any one of these categories, if marked, is sufficient for the diagnosis, but isolated dissocial acts are not.' (p. 267)

An enduring pattern of behaviour should be present, but no time frame is given and there is no impairment or impact criterion stated.

The ICD-10 diagnostic criteria for research (WHO 1993) differ, requiring symptoms to have been present for at least six months, and the introductory rubric indicates that impact upon others (in terms of violation of their basic rights), but not impairment of the child, can contribute to the diagnosis. The research criteria take a menu-driven approach whereby a certain number of symptoms have to be present. Fifteen behaviours are listed to consider for the diagnosis of *conduct disorder*, which usually but not exclusively apply to older children and teenagers. They can be grouped into four classes:

- aggression to people and animals
- destruction of property
- deceitfulness or theft
- serious violations of rules.

Aggression to people and animals

The criteria are:

1 often lies or breaks promises to obtain goods or favours or to avoid obligations
2 frequently initiates physical fights (this does not include fights with siblings)
3 has used a weapon that can cause serious physical harm to others (e.g. bat, brick, broken bottle, knife, gun)
4 often stays out after dark despite parenting prohibition (beginning before 13 years of age)
5 exhibits physical cruelty to other people (e.g. ties up, cuts or burns a victim)
6 exhibits physical cruelty to animals.

Destruction of property

The criteria are:

1 deliberately destroys the property of others (other than by firesetting)
2 deliberately sets fires with a risk or intention of causing serious damage).

Deceitfulness or theft

The criterion is:

1 steals objects of non-trivial value without confronting the victim, either within the home or outside (e.g. shoplifting, burglary, forgery).

Serious violations of rules

The criteria are:

1 is frequently truant from school, beginning before 13 years of age
2 has run away from parental or parental surrogate home at least twice or has run away once for more than a single night (this does not include leaving to avoid physical or sexual abuse)
3 commits a crime involving confrontation with the victim (including purse-snatching, extortion, mugging)
4 forces another person into sexual activity
5 frequently bullies others (e.g. deliberate infliction of pain or hurt, including persistent intimidation, tormenting, or molestation)
6 breaks into someone else's house, building or car.

DIAGNOSIS

To make a diagnosis of conduct disorder, three symptoms from this list have to be present, one for at least six months. There is no impairment criterion.

There are three subtypes:

- conduct disorder confined to the family context (F91.0)
- unsocialized conduct disorder, where the young person has no friends and is rejected by peers (F91.1)
- socialized conduct disorder, where peer relationships are normal (F91.2).

It is recommended that age of onset be specified, with childhood-onset type manifesting before the age of 10 years, and adolescent-onset type after. Severity should be categorized as mild, moderate or severe, according to the number of symptoms or their impact on others (e.g. causing severe physical injury; vandalism; theft).

SUBTYPES

For younger children, say up to 9 or 10 years old, there is a list of eight symptoms for the subtype known as *oppositional–defiant disorder* (F91.3):

1 has unusually frequent or severe temper tantrums for his or her developmental level
2 often argues with adults
3 often actively refuses adults' requests or defies rules
4 often, apparently deliberately, does things that annoy other people
5 often blames others for his or her own mistakes or misbehaviour
6 is often 'touchy' or easily annoyed by others
7 is often angry or resentful
8 is often spiteful or resentful.

To make a diagnosis of the oppositional–defiant type of conduct disorder, four symptoms from either this list or the main conduct-disorder 15-symptom list have to be present, but no more than two from the latter. Unlike the main variant, there is an impairment criterion: the symptoms must be maladaptive and inconsistent with the developmental level (p. 161).

Where there are sufficient symptoms of a comorbid disorder to meet diagnostic criteria, the ICD-10 system *discourages the application of a second diagnosis*. Instead it offers a single, combined category. There are two major kinds:

- mixed disorders of conduct and emotions, of which *depressive conduct disorder* (F92.0) is the best researched
- *hyperkinetic conduct disorder* (F90.1).

There is modest evidence to suggest that these combined conditions may differ somewhat from their constituent elements.

DSM–IV

The DSM-IV system (APA 1994) follows the ICD-10 research criteria very closely and does not have separate clinical guidelines. The same 15 behaviours are given for the diagnosis of *conduct disorder* (312.8), with almost identical wording. As for ICD-10, three symptoms need to be present for the diagnosis to be made. Severity, and childhood or adolescent onset, are specified in the same way.

However, unlike in ICD-10, there is no division into socialized/unsocialized, or family-context only types, and there is a requirement for the behaviour to cause clinically significant impairment in academic or social functioning (p. 91).

Comorbidity in DSM-IV is handled by giving as many separate diagnoses as necessary, rather than by having single, combined categories.

In DSM-IV, *oppositional–defiant disorder* is classified as a separate disorder on its own, and not as a subtype of conduct disorder. Its diagnosis requires four symptoms from a list of eight behaviours which are the same as for ICD-10; but unlike in ICD-10, all four behaviours have to be from the oppositional list, and none may come from the main conduct disorder list.

It is doubtful whether oppositional–defiant disorder differs substantially from conduct disorder in older children in any associated characteristics, and the value of designating it as a separate disorder is arguable (Lahey and Loeber 1994). In this chapter, the term 'conduct disorder' will henceforth be used as it is in ICD-10, to refer to all variants; oppositional–defiant disorder is included in this as a specific subtype.

DIFFERENTIAL DIAGNOSIS

Making a diagnosis of conduct disorder is usually straightforward since parents readily volunteer the symptoms, although it is essential to obtain an independent report from school so as not to overlook behaviour in that context. Sometimes the diagnosis may be inappropriate since antisocial behaviour may arise as part of other disorders such as autism or mania, or not be severe enough to warrant a diagnosis. More commonly the diagnosis is correct but comorbid conditions are missed.

HYPERKINETIC SYNDROME/ATTENTION–DEFICIT HYPERACTIVITY DISORDER

These are the names given by ICD-10 and DSM-IV, respectively, for very similar conditions. For convenience the term *hyperactivity* will be used here.

The condition is characterized by impulsivity, inattention and motor over-activity. Any of these three sets of symptoms can be misconstrued as antisocial, particularly impulsivity which is also present in conduct disorder. However, none of the symptoms of conduct disorder is a part of hyperactivity, so excluding conduct disorder should not be difficult.

A frequently made error, however, is to miss comorbid hyperactivity when conduct disorder is definitely present.

So much emphasis is placed on the irritating antisocial behaviour by parents and teachers that the clinician can easily fail to enquire properly about motor restlessness and inattention, which can be attributed to naughtiness. Standardized questionnaires are very helpful here, such as the Strengths and Difficulties Questionnaire (Goodman *et al.* 1998), which is brief, and just as effective at detecting hyperactivity as much longer alternatives (Goodman and Scott 1999).

ADJUSTMENT REACTION TO AN EXTERNAL STRESSOR

This can be diagnosed when onset occurs soon after exposure to an identifiable psychosocial stressor such as divorce, bereavement, trauma, abuse or adoption. The onset should be within one month for ICD-10, and three months for DSM-IV, and symptoms should not persist for more than six months after the cessation of the stress or its sequelae.

MOOD DISORDERS

Depression can present with irritability and oppositional symptoms but, unlike with typical conduct disorder, mood is usually clearly low and there are vegetative features; also more severe conduct problems are absent.

Early manic–depressive disorder can be harder to distinguish, as there is often considerable defiance and irritability combined with disregard for rules, and behaviour which violates the rights of others. Sometimes the mania becomes obvious only years later, but in retrospect was clearly driving the antisocial conduct.

The greater risk, however, is to miss depressive symptoms in young people with definite conduct disorder. Low self-esteem is the norm in conduct disorder, as is a lack of friends or constructive pastimes. Therefore it is easy to overlook more pronounced depressive symptoms, particularly as they are usually not complained of by the young person. Systematic surveys reveal that around a third of children with conduct disorder have depressive or other emotional symptoms severe enough to warrant a diagnosis.

AUTISTIC SPECTRUM DISORDERS

These are often accompanied by marked tantrums or destructiveness, which may be the reason for seeking a referral. Enquiring about other symptoms of autistic spectrum disorders should reveal their presence.

DISSOCIAL/ANTISOCIAL PERSONALITY DISORDER

In ICD-10, it is suggested a person should be aged at least 17 years before dissocial personality is considered. Since at age 18 most diagnoses specific to childhood and adolescence no longer apply, in practice there is seldom difficulty.

In DSM-IV, conduct disorder can be diagnosed in a person over 18, so there is potential overlap. A difference in emphasis is the severity and pervasiveness of the symptoms of those with personality disorder, whereby all the individual's relationships are affected by the behaviour pattern, and the individual's beliefs about his or her antisocial behaviour are characterized by callousness and lack of remorse.

SUBCULTURAL DEVIANCE

Some youths are antisocial and commit crimes but are not particularly aggressive or defiant. They are well adjusted within a deviant peer culture that approves of recreational drug use, shoplifting, etc. In some localities a third or more teenage males fit this description and would meet ICD-10 diagnostic guidelines for socialized conduct disorder. Some clinicians are unhappy to label such a large proportion of the population with a psychiatric disorder. Using DSM-IV criteria would preclude the diagnosis for most youths like this, owing to the classification's requirement for significant impairment.

MULTI-AXIAL ASSESSMENT

ICD-10 recommends that multiaxial assessment be carried out for children and adolescents, while DSM-IV suggests it for all ages. In both systems, *axis one* is used for psychiatric disorders which have been discussed above. The last three axes in both systems cover general medical conditions, psychosocial problems, and level of social functioning, respectively; these topics were covered above under 'aetiology'. In the middle are two axes in ICD-10, which cover specific (*axis two*) and general (*axis three*) learning disabilities, respectively; and one in DSM-IV (*axis two*) which covers personality disorders and general learning disabilities.

Both specific and general learning disabilities are essential to assess in individuals with conduct problems. Fully a third of children with conduct disorder also have specific reading retardation (Rutter *et al.* 1975), defined as having a reading level two standard deviations below that predicted by the person's IQ. While this may in part be due to lack of adequate schooling, there is good evidence that the cognitive deficits often precede the behavioural problems. General learning disability (mental retardation) is often missed in children with conduct disorder unless IQ testing is carried out. The rate of conduct disorder rises several-fold for IQs below 50 (Scott 1994).

CLINICAL FEATURES

Aggressive and defiant behaviour is an important part of normal child and adolescent development which ensures physical and social survival. Indeed, parents may express concern if a child is too acquiescent and unassertive.

The level of aggressive and defiant behaviour varies considerably amongst children, and it is probably most usefully seen as a continuously distributed trait. Empirical studies do not suggest a level at which symptoms become qualitatively different, nor is there a single cut-off point at which they become impairing for the child or a clear problem for others. There is no hump towards the end of the distribution curve of severity to suggest a categorically distinct group who might on these grounds warrant a diagnosis of conduct disorder.

Picking a particular level of antisocial behaviour to call 'conduct disorder' is therefore necessarily arbitrary. For all children, the expression of any particular behaviour also varies according to child age, so that for example physical hitting is at a maximum at around 2 years of age (Tremblay *et al.* 1999) but declines to a low level over the next few years. Therefore any judgement about the significance of the level of antisocial behaviour has to be made in the context of the child's age.

Before deciding that the behaviour is abnormal or a significant problem, a number of other clinical features have to be considered:

- the severity and frequency of antisocial acts, compared with children of the same age and gender
- the range of antisocial acts, and the number of settings in which they are carried out
- the duration over which the acts have continued to be carried out
- the impact, both in terms of the distress and social impairment, to the child of being antisocial, and the disruption and damage caused to others.

The type of behaviour seen will depend on the age and gender of the individual.

CHANGE IN CLINICAL FEATURES WITH AGE

Younger children, say from 3 to 7 years of age, usually present with general defiance of adults' wishes, disobedience of instructions, angry outbursts with temper tantrums, physical aggression to people especially siblings and peers, destruction of property, arguing, blaming others for things that have gone wrong, and a tendency to annoy and provoke others.

In middle childhood, say from 8 to 11 years, the above features are often still present; but as the child grows older, stronger, and spends more time out of the home, other behaviours are seen. They include: swearing, lying about what they have been doing, stealing of others' belongings outside the home, persistent breaking of rules, physical fights, bullying of other children, cruelty to animals, and setting of fires.

In adolescence, say from 12 to 17 years, more antisocial behaviours are often added: cruelty and hurting of other people, assault, robbery using force, vandalism, breaking and entering houses, stealing from cars, driving and taking away cars without permission, running away from home, truanting from school, and extensive use of narcotic drugs.

Not all children who start with the type of behaviours listed in early childhood progress on to the later, more severe forms. Only about half continue from those in early childhood to those in middle childhood (Lahey and Loeber 1994); likewise only about a further half of those with the behaviours in middle childhood progress to show the behaviours listed for adolescence. However, the early-onset group are important as they are far more likely to display the most severe symptoms in adolescence, and to persist in their antisocial tendencies into adulthood. Indeed, over 90% of severe, recurrent adolescent offenders showed marked antisocial behaviour in early childhood. In contrast, there is a large group who only start to be antisocial in adolescence, but whose behaviours are less extreme and who tend to desist by the time they are adults. These groupings are discussed more fully later.

GENDER DIFFERENCES

Severe antisocial behaviour is less common in girls but also has a different form. Girls are less likely to be physically aggressive and engage in criminal behaviour, but are more likely to show non-physical antisocial behaviours. These include spitefulness, emotional bullying (such as excluding children from groups, spreading rumours so others are rejected by their peers), frequent unprotected sex leading to sexually transmitted diseases and pregnancy, drug abuse, running way from home and truancy from school. Compared with boys, fewer girls show the early-onset pattern and more have an onset in adolescence.

PATTERN AND SETTING

No single behaviour carries special significance. The outlook is determined by the frequency and intensity of antisocial behaviours, the variety of types, the number of settings in which they occur, and their persistence. The main settings where antisocial behaviour in children and adolescents is manifested are home, school, and in public. For general populations of children, agreement about the presence of antisocial behaviour at home and at school is low – the correlation between parent and teacher ratings on the same measures is only 0.2–0.3. There are many children who are perceived to be mildly or moderately antisocial at home but well behaved at school, and vice versa. However, for more severe antisocial behaviour, there are usually manifestations both at home and at school. Concerns about antisocial behaviour in public occur more commonly in adolescents and often lead to police involvement.

PERSISTENCE

Many children go through phases of becoming more defiant and argumentative for a few weeks or months. Sometimes this may be a reaction to a change in circumstances such as settling into a new school, adjusting to a new step-parent, or losing a friend or loved one. Only when difficult behaviour has been present for, say, six months or more is it likely to indicate substantial problems.

IMPACT

At home the child often is subjected to high levels of criticism and hostility, and sometimes made a scapegoat for a catalogue of family misfortunes. Frequent punishments and physical abuse are not uncommon. The whole family atmosphere is often soured and siblings also affected. Maternal depression is often present, and families who are unable to cope may, as a last resort, give up the child to be cared for by the local authority. At school, teachers may take a range of measures to attempt to control the child and protect the other pupils, including sending the child out of the class, sometimes culminating in permanent exclusion from the school. This may lead to reduced opportunity to learn subjects on the curriculum and poor examination results. The child typically has few if any friends, who get fed up with the aggressive behaviour. This often leads to exclusion from many group activities, games, and trips, so restricting the child's quality of life and experiences. On leaving school the lack of social skills, low level of qualifications and presence of a police record make it harder to gain employment.

The experience of rejection and failure at home, at school and with peers usually leads to a negative self-image and low self-esteem, but is not usually described by the young person as actively distressing. In later adolescence intimate sexual relationships tend to be made with other young people who are also antisocial, and are frequently disruptive and violent.

OUTCOME AS YOUNG ADULTS

PREDICTION OF OUTCOMES

Studies of groups of children with early-onset conduct disorder indicate that a wide range of problems persist into adulthood, and these go well beyond antisocial behaviour. Outcomes are tabulated by domain in Table 8.1.

It is clear that there are substantially increased rates of antisocial acts, and that the general psychosocial functioning of children with conduct disorder is strikingly poor when they grow up. For most of the characteristics shown in Table 8.1, the increase compared to controls is at least double for community cases who were never referred, and three to four times for referred children (Robins 1996; Farrington 1995; Rutter et al. 1998).

Of those with early-onset conduct disorder (before the age of 8), about half persist with serious problems into adulthood. Of those with adolescent onset, the great majority (over 85%) desist in their antisocial behaviour by their early twenties.

Table 8.1 *Outcome as young adults*

Antisocial behaviour	More violent and non-violent crimes; e.g. mugging, grievous bodily harm, theft, car crimes, fraud
Psychiatric problems	Increased rates of antisocial personality, alcohol and drug abuse, anxiety, depression and somatic complaints, episodes of deliberate self-harm and completed suicide, time in psychiatric hospitals
Education and training	Poorer examination results, more truancy and early school leaving, fewer vocational qualifications
Work	More unemployment, jobs held for shorter time, jobs low status and income, increased claiming of benefits and welfare
Social network	Few if any significant friends, low involvement with relatives, neighbours, clubs and organizations
Intimate relationships	Increased rate of short-lived, violent cohabiting relationships; partners often also antisocial
Children	Increased rates of child abuse, conduct problems in offspring, children taken into care
Health	More medical problems, earlier death

Table 8.2 *Features associated with worse prognosis in young adulthood*

Onset	Early onset of severe problems, before age 8
Phenomenology	Antisocial acts which are severe, frequent and varied
Comorbidity	Hyperactivity and attention problems, thrill-seeking
Intelligence	Lower IQ
Family history	Paternal criminality; alcoholism in either parent
Parenting	Harsh, inconsistent parenting, with high criticism, low warmth, low involvement and low supervision
Wider environment	Low-income family in poor neighbourhood with ineffective schools

Many of the factors which predict poor outcome are associated with early onset (Table 8.2).

RESILIENCE

To detect protective factors, children who do well despite adverse risk factors have been studied. These so-called 'resilient' children, however, have been shown to have lower levels of risk factors – for example, a boy with antisocial behaviour and low IQ living in a rough neighbourhood but living with supportive, concerned parents. Protective factors are mostly the opposite end of the spectrum of the same risk factor; thus, good parenting and a high IQ are protective. Nonetheless there are factors which are associated with resilience independent of known adverse influences. These include a good relationship with at least one adult, who does not necessarily have to be the parent; a sense of pride and self-esteem; and skills or competencies.

PATHWAYS

The path from childhood conduct disorder to poor adult outcome is neither inevitable nor linear. Different sets of influences impinge as the individual grows up. Many of these can accentuate problems.

Thus a toddler with an irritable temperament and short attention span may not learn good social skills if raised in a family lacking them, and where he can get his way by behaving antisocially and grasping for what he needs. At school he may fall in with a deviant crowd of peers, where violence and other antisocial acts are talked up and give him a sense of esteem. His generally poor academic ability and difficult behaviour in class may lead him to truant increasingly, which in turn makes him fall further behind. He may then leave school with no qualifications and fail to find a job, and resort to drugs. To fund his drug habit he may resort to crime, and once convicted, find it even harder to get a job. From this example, it can be seen that adverse experiences do not only arise passively and independently of the young person's behaviour; rather, the behaviour predisposes the person to end up in risky and damaging environments. Consequently, the number of adverse life events experienced is greatly increased (Champion *et al.* 1995). The path from early hyperactivity into later conduct disorder is also not inevitable. In the presence of a warm supportive family atmosphere it is far less likely than if the parents are highly critical and hostile.

Other influences can steer the individual away from an antisocial path – for example, being separated from a deviant peer group; marrying a non-deviant partner; moving away from a poor neighbourhood; military service which imparts skills (but not harsh boot camps – see Henggeler (1999)).

SPECIFIC TREATMENT

Specific treatments for which there is good evidence of effectiveness include those which singly or in combination address parenting skills, family functioning, the child's interpersonal skills, difficulties at school, peer group influences, and medication for coexistent hyperactivity.

PARENTING SKILLS

Parent management training aims to improve parenting skills. There are scores of randomized controlled trials showing that it is effective for children up to about 10 years old (Kazdin 1997). They address the parenting practices identified in research as contributing to conduct problems. A more detailed account is given in Scott (1998). Typically, they include five elements.

1 *Promoting play and a positive relationship.* In order to cut into the cycle of defiant behaviour and recriminations, it is important to instil some positive experiences for both sides and begin to mend the relationship. Teaching parents the techniques of how to play in a constructive and non-hostile way with their children helps them recognize their needs and respond sensitively. The children in turn begin to like and respect their parents more, and become more secure in the relationship.

2 *Praise and rewards for sociable behaviour.* Parents are helped to reformulate difficult behaviour in terms of the positive behaviour they wish to see, so that they encourage wanted behaviour rather than criticize unwanted behaviour. For example, instead of shouting at the child not to run, they would praise him whenever he walks quietly; then he will do it more often. Through hundreds of such prosaic daily interactions, child behaviour can be substantially modified. Yet some parents find it hard to praise, and fail to recognize positive behaviour when it happens, with the result that it become less frequent.

3 *Clear rules and clear commands.* Rules need to be explicit and constant; commands need to be firm and brief. Thus shouting at a child to stop being naughty doesn't tell him what he should do, whereas for example telling him to play quietly gives a clear instruction which makes compliance easier.

4 *Consistent and calm consequences for unwanted behaviour.* Disobedience and aggression need to be responded to firmly and calmly, by for example putting the child in a room for a few minutes. This method of 'time out from positive reinforcement' sounds simple but requires considerable skill to administer effectively. More minor annoying behaviours such as whining and shouting often respond to being ignored, but again parents often find this hard to achieve in practice.

5 *Reorganizing the child's day to prevent trouble.* There are often trouble spots in the day which will respond to fairly simple measures. Examples are putting siblings in different rooms to prevent fights on getting home from school, or banning TV in the morning until the child is dressed.

Treatment can be given individually to the parent and child, which enables live feedback in light of the parent's progress and the child's response. Alternatively, group treatments with parents alone have been shown to be equally effective (Webster-Stratton 1984; Scott *et al.* 2001).

Trials show that parent management training is effective in reducing child antisocial behaviour in the short term,

with moderate to large effect sizes of 0.5–0.8 standard deviations, and there is little loss of effect at 1- or 3-year follow-up (Webster-Stratton *et al.* 1989).

Parenting skills interventions are chiefly used with younger children, although there is evidence for their successful use with delinquent boys (Bank *et al.* 1991).

FAMILY FUNCTIONING

Functional family therapy, multi-systemic therapy and *treatment foster care* aim to change a range of difficulties which impede effective functioning of teenagers with conduct disorder.

Functional family therapy addresses family processes which need to be present, such as improved communication between parent and young person, reducing interparental inconsistency, tightening up on supervision and monitoring, and negotiating rules and the sanctions to be applied for breaking them. Functional family therapy has been shown to reduce re-offending rates by around 50% (Alexander *et al.* 1994). Other varieties of family therapy have not been subjected to controlled trials for young people with conduct disorder or delinquency, so cannot be evaluated for their efficacy.

In multi-systemic therapy (Henggeler 1999), the young person's and family's needs are assessed in their own context at home and in their relations with other systems such as school and peers. Following the assessment, proven methods of intervention are used to address difficulties and promote strengths. Multi-systemic therapy differs from most types of family therapy – such as the Milan or systemic approach as usually practised – in a number of regards:

- Treatment is delivered in the situation where the young person lives (e.g. at home).
- The therapist has a low caseload (4–6 families) and the team is available 24 hours a day.
- The therapist is responsible for ensuring appointments are kept and for making change happen – families cannot be blamed for failing to attend or 'not being ready' to change.
- Regular written feedback on progress towards goals from multiple sources is gathered by the therapist and acted upon.
- There is a manual for the therapeutic approach and adherence is checked weekly by the supervisor.

Several randomized controlled trial attest to the effectiveness, with re-offending rates typically cut by half and time spent in psychiatric hospitalization reduced further.

Treatment foster care is another way to improve the quality of encouragement and supervision that teenagers with conduct disorder receive. The young person lives with a foster family specially trained in effective techniques; sometimes it is ordered as an alternative to jail. Outcome studies show useful reductions in re-offending.

CHILD INTERPERSONAL SKILLS

Most of the programmes to improve child interpersonal skills derive from cognitive behaviour therapy. Three of the most effective are *self-instructional training* (Kendall and Braswell 1985), the Anger Coping Program (Lochman and Wells 1996), and Promoting Alternative Thinking Strategies (PATHS) (Bierman and Greenberg 1996). These and other programs have in common training the young person to:

- slow down impulsive responses to challenging situations by stopping and thinking
- recognize the level of physiological arousal, and personal emotional state
- recognize and define problems
- develop several alternative responses
- choose the best alternative based on anticipation of consequences
- reinforce himself or herself for use of this approach.

Over the longer term they aim to increase positive social behaviour by teaching the young person to:

- learn skills to make and sustain friendships
- develop social interaction skills such as turn-taking and sharing
- express viewpoints in appropriate ways and listen to others.

Typically, given alone, treatment gains with interpersonal skills training are good within the treatment setting, but only generalize slightly to real-life situations such as the school playground. However, when they are part of a more comprehensive programme which has those outside the young person reinforcing the approach, they add to outcome gains.

DIFFICULTIES AT SCHOOL

These can be divided into learning problems and disruptive behaviour. There are proven programmes to deal with specific learning problems such as specific reading retardation – for example Reading Recovery. However, few of the programmes have been specifically evaluated for their ability to improve outcome in children with conduct disorder, although trials are in progress. Preschool education programmes for high-risk populations have been shown to reduce arrest rates and improve employment in adulthood (see below).

There are several schemes for improving classroom behaviour, which vary from those which stress improved communication such as 'circle time', and those which work on behavioural principles such as the 'good behaviour game' (Kellam and Rebok 1992), or are part of a multi-modal package. Many of these schemes have been shown to improve classroom behaviour, and some specifically target children with conduct disorder (Durlak 1995).

PEER GROUP INFLUENCES

A few interventions have aimed to reduce the bad influence of deviant peers. However, a number attempted this through group work with other conduct-disordered youths, but outcome studies showed a worsening of antisocial behaviour (Dishion and Andrews 1995). Current treatments therefore either see youths individually and try to steer them away from deviant peers, or work in small groups (say 3–5 youths) whereby the therapist can control the content of sessions. Some interventions place youths with conduct disorder in groups with well-functioning youths, and this has led to favourable outcomes (Feldman 1992).

MEDICATION FOR COEXISTENT HYPERACTIVITY

Where there is comorbid hyperactivity in addition to conduct disorder, several studies attest to a large reduction (effect size of 0.8 standard deviations or greater) in both overt and covert antisocial behaviour (Hinshaw 1992), both at home and at school (Pelham 1993). However, the impact on long-term outcome is unstudied.

TREATMENT RESISTANCE AND ITS MANAGEMENT

Engagement of the family is particularly important for this group of children and families, as the dropout from treatment is high at around 30–40%. Practical measures such as assisting with transport, providing childcare, holding sessions in the evening or at other times to suit the family will all help. Many of the parents of children with conduct disorder may themselves have difficulty with authority and officialdom and be very sensitive to criticism. Therefore the approach is more likely to succeed if it is respectful of their point of view, does not offer overly prescriptive solutions, and does not directly criticize parenting style. Practical homework tasks increase changes, as do problem-solving telephone calls from the therapist between sessions.

Parenting interventions may need to go beyond skill development to address more distal factors which prevent change. For example, drug or alcohol abuse in either parent, maternal depression, and a violent relationship with the partner are all common. Assistance in claiming welfare and benefits and help with financial planning may reduce stress from debts.

A multi-modal approach is likely to get larger changes. Therefore involving the school in treatment by visiting and offering strategies for managing the child in class is usually helpful, as is advocating for extra tuition where necessary. If the school seems unable to cope despite extra resources, consideration should be given to moving the child to a different school which specializes in the management of behavioural difficulties. Avoiding anti-social peers and building self-esteem may be helped by getting the child to attend after school clubs and holiday activities.

Where parents are not coping or a damaging abusive relationship is detected, it may be necessary to liaise with the social services department to arrange respite for the parents or a spell of foster care. It is important during this time to work with the family to increase their skills so the child can return to the family. Where there is permanent breakdown, long-term fostering or adoption may be recommended.

CONCLUSIONS AND FUTURE DIRECTIONS

There is now an enormous amount of knowledge about the causes and natural history of antisocial behaviour in childhood. The challenge for the future is to harness that knowledge to prevent early aggression turning into an antisocial adolescent lifestyle. Conduct disorder should offer good opportunities for prevention since (a) it can be detected early reasonably accurately; (b) early intervention is more effective than later; and (c) there are a number of effective early interventions.

In the USA a number of comprehensive interventions based on up-to-date empirical findings are being carried out. Perhaps the best known is Families and Schools Together (Conduct Problems Prevention Research Group 1992) – FasTrack. Here the most antisocial 10% of 5- to 6-year-olds in schools in disadvantaged areas were selected, as judged by teacher and parent reports. They were then offered intervention which was given for a whole year in the first instance and comprised:

- weekly parent training in groups with videotapes
- an interpersonal skills training programme for the whole class
- academic tutoring twice a week
- home visits from the parent trainer
- a pairing programme with sociable peers from the class.

Almost 1000 children were randomized to receive this condition or controls, and the project has cost over $50 million. However, so far, preliminary reports of outcome have been limited in effect size, with no improvement of antisocial behaviour at home on questionnaire measures and modest improvements in the classroom. There are a number of possible reasons for the smaller effects compared to those obtained in trials with clinically referred populations. The motivation of families may be less as they don't perceive they have a problem; starting levels of antisocial behaviour are lower, so there is not so far to go to reach normal levels; and keeping up the quality of the intervention across several sites is harder. It remains to be seen whether longer-term effects will be greater.

Preschool education programmes for disadvantaged children have also been evaluated in terms of adult outcomes, again chiefly in the USA. The best known is the Perry/Highscope project, where 2- to 4-year olds received intensive nursery education half-time for two years. Aged 27, the individuals fared better than controls on several psychosocial outcomes, including a third of the number of arrests for criminal offences, better jobs, higher income, and more stable marriages (Sylva 1994).

In the UK, in 1999 the government stressed the importance of helping parents of children in the first three years of life and put substantial resources (£540 million) into 'SureStart' centres in targeted high-risk neighbourhoods to support parenting. It is too early to evaluate outcome.

Separate from conduct disorder prevention (but related) is crime prevention, which can include reducing the opportunities for antisocial behaviour by tighter policing, reducing access to drugs and guns, and so on.

Much is known about the risk factors leading to conduct disorder, and effective treatments do exist. The challenge is to make these available on a wide scale, and to develop approaches to prevention which are effective and can be put into practice at a community level.

REFERENCES

Alexander, J.F., Holtzworth-Munroe, A. and Jameson, P.B. 1994: The process and outcome of marital and family therapy research: review and evaluation. In Bergin, A.E. and Garfield, S. (eds), *Handbook of Psychotherapy and Behavior Change*. New York: John Wiley, 595–630.

Anderson, J., Williams, S., McGee, R. and Silva, P. 1987: DSM–III disorders in preadolescent children. *Archives of General Psychiatry* **44**: 69–76.

APA (American Psychiatric Association) 1994: *Diagnostic and Statistical Manual of Mental Disorders – DSM IV*. Washington, DC: APA.

Bank, L., Marlowe, J.H., Reid, J.B., Patterson, G.R. and Weinrott, M.R. 1991: A comparative evaluation of parent-training interventions for families of chronic delinquents. *Journal of Abnormal Child Psychology* **19**: 15–33.

Bierman, K. and Greenberg, M. 1996: Social skills training in the FAST track program: preventing childhood disorders, substance abuse and delinquency. In Peters, R. and McMahon, R. (eds), *Preventing Childhood Disorders, Substance Abuse and Deliquency*. Thousand Oaks, CA: Sage, 65–89.

Bohman, M.I.E. 1996: Predisposition to criminality: Swedish adoption studies in retrospect. In *Genetics of Criminal and Antisocial Behaviour*, Ciba Foundation Symposium, 194.

Caspi, A., Lynam, D., Moffitt, T. and Silva, P. 1993: Unravelling girls' delinquency: biological, dispositional, and contextual contributions to adolescent misbehavior. *Developmental Psychopathology* **29**: 19–30.

Champion, L., Goodall, G. and Rutter, M. 1995: Behavioural problems in childhood and stressors in early adult life: a 20-year follow-up of London school children. *Psychological Medicine* **25**: 231–46.

Cohen, M.A. 1998: The monetary value of saving a high-risk youth. *Journal of Quantitative Criminology* **14**: 5–33.

Coie, J. and Dodge, K. 1997: Aggression and antisocial behavior. In Damon, W. and Eisenberg, N. (eds), *Handbook of Child Psychology: 3. Social, Emotional and Personality Development.* New York: John Wiley, 779–862.

Conduct Problems Prevention Research Group 1992: A developmental and clinical model for prevention of conduct disorder. *Development and Psychopathology* **4**: 509–27.

DiLalla, L.F. and Gottesman, I.I. 1989: Heterogeneity of causes for delinquency and criminality: lifespan perspectives. *Development and Psychopathology* **1**: 339–49.

Dishion, T. and Andrews, D. 1995: Preventing escalation in problem behaviors with high-risk young adolescents: immediate and 1-year outcomes. *Journal of Consulting and Clinical Psychology* **63**: 538–48.

Dishion, T. and Patterson, G. 1997: The timing and severity of antisocial behavior: three hypotheses within an ecological framework. In Stoff, D., Breiling, J. and Maser, J. (eds), *Handbook of Antisocial Behavior.* New York: John Wiley, 206–18.

Dodge, K. and Schwartz, D. 1997: Social information processing mechanisms in aggressive behavior. In Stoff, D., Breiling, J. and Maser, J. (eds), *Handbook of Antisocial Behavior.* New York: John Wiley, 171–80.

Durlak, J. 1995: *School-based Prevention Programs for Children and Adolescents.* Thousand Oaks, CA: Sage.

Farrington, D.P. 1994: Early developmental prevention of juvenile delinquency. *Criminal Behaviour and Mental Health* **4**: 209–27.

Farrington, D.P. 1995: The development of offending and antisocial behaviour from childhood: key findings from the Cambridge Study in Delinquent Development. *Journal of Child Psychology and Psychiatry* **36**: 929–64.

Feldman, R. 1992: The St Louis experiment: effective treatment of antisocial youths in prosocial peer groups. In McCord, J. and Tremblay, R. (eds), *Preventing Antisocial Behavior.* New York: Guilford Press, 233–52.

Gardner, F.M.E. 1987: Positive interaction between mothers and conduct-problem children: is there training for harmony as well as fighting? *Journal of Abnormal Child Psychology* **15**: 283–93.

Gibson, C.L. and Tibbetts, S.G. 1998: Interaction between maternal cigarette smoking and Apgar scores in predicting offending behaviour. *Psychological Reports* **83**: 579–86.

Goodman, R. 1997: *Child and Adolescent Mental Health Services: Reasoned Advice to Commissioners and Providers.* Maudsley Discussion Paper 4. London: Institute of Psychiatry.

Goodman, R. and Scott, S. 1999: Comparing the Strengths and Difficulties Questionnaire and the Child Behavior Checklist: is small beautiful? *Journal of Abnormal Child Psychology* **27**(1): 17–24.

Goodman, R., Meltzer, H. and Bailey, V. 1998: The strengths and difficulties questionnaire: a pilot study on the validity of the self-report version. *European Child and Adolescent Psychiatry* **7**: 125–30.

Gray, J. 1987: *The Psychology of Fear and Stress.* Cambridge: Cambridge University Press.

Henggeler, S.W. 1999: Multisystemic therapy: an overview of clinical procedures, outcomes and policy implications. *Child Psychology and Psychiatry Review* **4**(1): 2–10.

Hinshaw, S. 1992: Externalizing behaviour problems and academic under-achievement in childhood and adolescence: causal relationships and underlying mechanisms. *Psychological Bulletin* **111**: 127–55.

Hoare, P., Norton, B., Chisholm, D. and Parry-Jones, W. 1996: An audit of 7000 successive child and adolescent psychiatry referrals in Scotland. *Clinical Child Psychology and Psychiatry* **1**: 229–49.

Kazdin, A.E. 1995: *Conduct Disorders in Childhood and Adolescence.* Thousand Oaks, CA: Sage.

Kazdin, A.E. 1997: Psychosocial treatments for conduct disorder in children. *Journal of Child Psychology and Psychiatry* **38**: 161–78.

Kellam, S. and Rebok, G. 1992: Building developmental and etiological theory through epidemiologically based preventive intervention trials. In McCord, J. and Tremblay, R. (eds), *Preventing Antisocial Behavior: Interventions from Birth to Adolescence.* New York: Guilford Press, 162–95.

Kendall, P. and Braswell, L. 1985: *Cognitive–Behavioral Therapy for Impulsive Children.* New York: Guilford Press.

Kessler, R., Davis, C. and Kendler, K. 1997: Childhood adversity and adult psychiatric disorder in the US National Comorbidity Survey. *Psychological Medicine* **27**: 1101–09.

Lahey, B. and Loeber, R. 1994: Framework for a developmental model of oppositional defiant disorder and conduct disorder. In Routh, D. (ed.), *Disruptive Behaviour Disorders in Childhood: Essays in Honor of Herbert C. Quay.* New York: Plenum Press, 139–80.

Lochman, J. and Wells, K. 1996: A social–cognitive intervention with aggressive children: prevention effects and contextual implementation issues. In Peters, R. and McMahon, R. (eds), *Preventing Childhood Disorders, Substance Abuse and Delinquency.* Thousand Oaks, CA: Sage, 111–43.

Loeber, R. and Dishion, T.J. 1983: Early predictors of male delinquency: a review. *Psychological Bulletin* **94**: 68–99.

Mayes, L. and Bornstein, M. 1997: The development of children exposed to cocaine. In Luthar, S., Burack, J., Cicchetti, D. and Weisz, J. (eds), *Development Psychopathology: Perspectives on Adjustment, Risk and Disorder.* Cambridge: Cambridge University Press, 166–88.

Moffitt, T., Caspi, A., Dickson, N., Silva, P. and Stanton, W. 1996: Childhood-onset versus adolescent-onset antisocial conduct problems in males: natural history from ages 3 to 18 years. *Development and Psychopathology* **8**: 399–424.

Moffitt, T., Caspi, A., Fawcett, P. *et al.* 1997: Whole blood serotonin and family background relate to male violence. In Raine, A., Brenna, P., Farrington, D. and Mednick, S. (eds), *Biological Bases of Violence.* New York: Plenum Press, 231–50.

Offord, D., Boyle, M. and Racine, Y. 1991: The epidemiology of antisocial behavior. In Pepler, D. and Rubin, K. (eds), *The Development and Treatment of Childhood Aggression.* Hillsdale, NJ: Lawrence Erlbaum, 31–54.

Olweus, D. 1979: Stability of aggressive reaction patterns in males: a review. *Psychological Bulletin* **86**: 852–75.

Osborn, S. 1980: Moving home, leaving London and delinquent trends. *British Journal of Criminology* **20**: 54–61.

Patterson, G.R. 1982: *Coercive Family Process.* Eugene, OR: Castalia.

Pelham, W. 1993: Pharmacotherapy for children with attention-deficit hyperactivity disorder. *School Psychology Review* **22**: 199–227.

Raine, A. 1997: Antisocial behavior and psychopathology: a biosocial perspective and a prefrontal dysfunction hypothesis. In Stoff, D., Breiling, J. and Maser, J. (eds), *Handbook of Antisocial Behavior.* New York: John Wiley, 289–304.

Richman, N., Stevenson, J. and Graham, P. 1982: *Preschool to School: a Behavioural Study.* London: Academic Press.

Robins, L. 1966: *Deviant Children Grown Up*. Baltimore: Williams & Wilkins.

Robins, L. and Regier, D. (eds) 1991: *Psychiatric Disorders: the Epidemiological Catchment Area Study*. New York: Free Press.

Rutter, M. and Quinton D. 1984: Parental psychiatric disorder: effects on children. *Psychological Medicine* **14**: 853–80.

Rutter, M., Tizard, J. and Whitmore, K. (eds) 1970: *Education, Health and Behaviour*. London: Longman.

Rutter, M., Cox, A., Tupling, M., Berger, M. and Yule, W. 1975: Attainment and adjustment in two geographical areas. *British Journal of Psychiatry* **126**: 493–509.

Rutter, M., Maughan, B., Mortimore, P., Ouston, J. and Smith, A. 1979: *Fifteen Thousand Hours: Secondary Schools and their Effects on Children*. Cambridge, MA: Harvard University Press.

Rutter, M., Giller, H. and Hagell, A. 1998: *Antisocial Behavior by Young People*. Cambridge: Cambridge University Press.

Sampson, R., Raudenbush, S. and Earls, F. 1997: Neighborhoods and violent crime: a multilevel study of collective efficacy. *Science* **277**: 918–24.

Scott. S. 1994: Mental retardation. In Rutter, M., Taylor, E. and Hersov, L. (eds), *Child and Adolescent Psychiatry: Modern Approaches*, 3rd edn. Oxford: Blackwell Scientific, 616–46.

Scott, S. 1998: Aggressive behaviour in childhood. *British Medical Journal* **316**: 202–6.

Scott, S., Spender, Q., Doolan, M., Jacobs, B. and Aspland, H. 2001: Multicentre controlled trial of parenting groups for childhood antisocial behaviour in clinical practice. *British Medical Journal* **323**: 194–6.

Shaffer, D., Fisher, P., Dulcan, M. *et al.* 1996: The NIMH Diagnostic Interview Schedule for Children Version 2.3 (DISC 2.3): description, acceptability, prevalence rates, and performance in the MECA study. *Journal of the American Academy of Child and Adolescent Psychiatry* **35**: 865–78.

Silberg, J., Meyer, J., Pickles, A. *et al.* 1996: Heterogeneity among juvenile antisocial behaviours: findings from the Virginia Twin Study of Adolescent Behavioral Development. In Bock, G. and Goode, J. (eds), *Genetics of Criminal and Antisocial Behaviour*. Chichester: John Wiley, 76–85.

Stattin, H., Romelsjo, A. and Stenbacka, M. 1997: Personal resources as modifiers of the risk for future criminality: an analysis of protective factors in relation to 18-year-old boys. *British Journal of Criminology* **37**: 198–222.

Streissguth, A. 1993: Fetal alcohol syndrome in older patients. *Alcohol* **2**: 209–12.

Sylva, K. 1994: School influences on children's development. *Journal of Child Psychology and Psychiatry* **35**: 135–70.

Thomas, A., Chess, S. and Birch, H. 1968: Temperament and Behavior Disorders in Children. New York: New York University Press.

Tremblay, R., Schall, B., Boulerice, B. and Perusse, D. 1997: Male physical aggression, social dominance and testosterone levels at puberty: a developmental perspective. In Raine, A., Brennan, P., Farrington, D. and Mednick, S. (eds), *Biological Bases of Violence*. New York: Plenum Press, 271–92.

Tremblay, R., Japel, C., Pérusse, D. *et al.* 1999: The search for the age of 'onset' of physical aggression: Rousseau and Bandura revisited. *Criminal Behavior and Mental Health* **9**: 8–23.

Trickett, A. and McBride-Chang, C. 1995: The developmental impact of different forms of child abuse and neglect. *Developmental Review* **15**: 311–37.

Venables, P. 1988: Psychophysiology and crime: theory and data. In Moffitt, T. and Mednick, S. (eds), *Biological Contributions to Crime Causation*. Dordrecht: Martinus Nijhoff, 3–13.

Webster-Stratton, C. 1984: Randomized trial of two parent training programs for families with conduct-disordered children. *Journal of Consulting and Clinical Psychology* **52**: 666–78.

Webster-Stratton, C., Hollinsworth, T. and Kolpacoff, M. 1989: The long-term effectiveness and clinical significance of three cost-effective training programs for families with conduct-problem children. *Journal of Consulting and Clinical Psychology* **57**: 550–3.

Widom, C. 1997: Child abuse, neglect and witnessing violence. In Stoff, D., Breiling, J. and Maser, J. (eds), *Handbook of Antisocial Behavior*. New York: John Wiley, 159–70.

WHO (World Health Organization) 1992: *The ICD-10 Classification of Mental and Behavioural Disorders: Clinical Descriptions and Diagnostic Guidelines*. Geneva: WHO.

WHO (World Health Organization) 1993: *The ICD-10 Classification of Mental and Behavioural Disorders: Diagnostic Criteria for Research*. Geneva: WHO.

Linking disorders to forensic behaviours

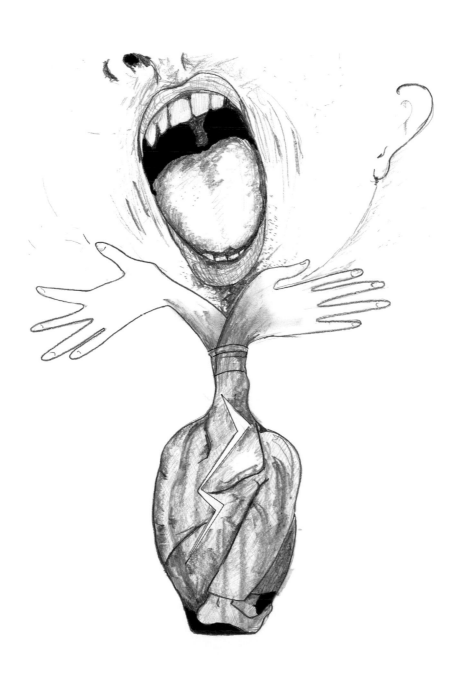

Eating disorders and obesity

9

Personality dysfunction and disorders in childhood and adolescents

MAIREAD DOLAN AND JAMES MILLINGTON

CONCEPTS OF PERSONALITY DYSFUNCTION AND DISORDER

Psychologists and psychiatrists define personality traits as consistent cognitive, emotional and behavioural patterns, which can be defined early in life and are stable over time.

Personality disorders are generally characterized by deeply ingrained, maladaptive and inflexible personality traits, which cause substantial distress or impairment. The International Classification of Diseases (ICD-10; WHO 1992) and Diagnostic and Statistical Manual (DSM-IV; APA 1994) have similar general definitions of personality disorder and they are categorized on a separate axis in the multi-axial diagnostic scheme. Table 9.1 lists the DSM-IV criteria for personality disorder.

DIMENSIONAL AND CATEGORICAL CONCEPTS OF PERSONALITY DISORDER

Paris (1996) described personality as a set of traits, each of which could be viewed as a dimension in space. Dimensional models of personality disorder view it as an exaggeration of normal traits, which are diagnosable at cut-off points beyond which the traits are maladaptive (Livesley *et al.* 1992). There are now several methods for assessing personality on a variety of dimensions and the key ones are shown in Table 9.2. Dimensional approaches

facilitate the handling of atypical cases and comorbidity and allow for the fact that personality traits occur on a continuum rather than as discreet entities. The difficulty with dimensional approaches, however, is knowing how many dimensions are required to adequately assess personality.

Table 9.1 *DSM-IV criteria for personality disorder state*

A An enduring pattern of inner experience and behaviour that deviates markedly from the expectations of the individual's culture. The pattern is manifested in two (or more) of the following areas:
  1 cognition (i.e. ways of perceiving and interpreting self, other people, and events)
  2 affectivity (i.e. the range, intensity, lability and appropriateness of emotional response)
  3 interpersonal functioning
  4 impulse control.
B The enduring pattern is inflexible and pervasive across a broad range of personal and social situations.
C The enduring pattern leads to clinically significant distress or impairment in social, occupational or other important areas of functioning.
D The pattern is stable and of long duration and its onset can be traced back to at least to adolescence or early adulthood.
E The enduring pattern is not better accounted for as a manifestation or consequence of another mental disorder.
F The enduring pattern is not due to physiological effects of a substance (e.g. drug) or general medical condition (e.g. head trauma).

Table 9.2 *Methods for assessing personality on a variety of dimensions*

Authors	Theoretical base	Dimensions
Eysenck	Neurophysiology	Extraversion Neuroticism Psychoticism
Buss and Plomin	Temperament	Emotionality Activity level Sociability
Cloninger	Neurochemistry	Novelty seeking Harm avoidance Reward dependence
Costa and McCrae	Empirical	Extraversion Neuroticism Openness to experience Agreeableness Conscientiousness
Siever and Davis	Neurochemistry	Cognitive–perceptual Impulsivity–aggression Affective instability Anxiety–inhibition
Wiggins	Interpersonal theory	Affiliation Dominance
Tyrer	Personality pathology	24 dimensions
Livesley	Personality pathology	18 dimensions
Torgersen	Personality pathology	18 dimensions

Categorical approaches to the diagnosis of personality disorder offer the advantage of highlighting the covariability of traits and the fact that traits can be adaptive or maladaptive by virtue of their associated traits (Millon 1996). However, categorical diagnoses as exemplified in ICD-10 and DSM-IV (Table 9.3) fail to recognize the continuous nature of personality pathology, and criteria for 'caseness' has not been adequately operationalized (Millon 1996).

A variety of structured-interview schedules and self-report assessment tools have been developed to assign DSM and ICD personality disagnoses. Unfortunately, studies examining diagnostic agreement between interview and self-report methods is generally low (median kappa 0.25) for individual personality disorder diagnosis (Perry 1992). There are several possible reasons for the discordant findings on measurement, including a lack of construct validity, rater inexperience, occasion variance, and state effects. Bronisch and Mombour (1994), using the International Personality Disorder Examination (IPDE) in a retest design, found that pairwise kappa agreements for the presence of personality disorder were 0.52 for DSM-III-R and 0.75 for ICD-10 diagnosis. The range for single personality disorder diagnoses varied considerably, particularly for DSM-III diagnoses, suggesting that a substantial proportion of the variance in personality disorder diagnosis could not be attributed to patients.

Table 9.3 *Comparison of DSM-IV and ICD-10 diagnoses*

DSM-IV diagnosis	Main clinical features	ICD-10 diagnosis
Schizoid	Detachment from social relations Restricted range of emotional expression	Schizoid
Paranoid	Distrust and suspiciousness	Paranoid
Borderline	Instability in interpersonal relationships Instability in self-image Instability in affects Impulsivity	Emotionally unstable, borderline subtype
Schizotypal	Acute discomfort in close relationships Cognitive or perceptual distortions Eccentricities of behaviour	Schizoid
Avoidant	Social inhibition Feeling of inadequacy Hypersensitivity to negative evaluation	Anxious Anxious
Compulsive	Preoccupation with orderliness, perfectionism, and control	Anankastic
Histrionic	Excessive emotionality and attention seeking	Histrionic
Dependent	Submissive, clinging Excessive need to be taken care of	Dependent
Antisocial	Disregard for and violation of the rights of others	Dissocial
Narcissistic	Grandiosity Need for admiration Lack of empathy	
Not otherwise specified	Meets general criteria for personality disorder but not any of above specific criteria	Unspecified or mixed

Overall, there is now a general acceptance that structured-interview schedules enhance the reliability of diagnosis in well-trained experienced raters.

STABILITY OF TEMPERAMENT AND PERSONALITY FROM CHILDHOOD TO ADULTHOOD

Reviews of longitudinal studies of temperament in children indicate that some personality traits and dispositions are relatively stable (Rothbart and Ahadi 1994). The New York longitudinal study (Chess and Thomas 1984) reported that of all nine dimensions of temperament measured, 'adaptability' and activity level were the most stable, while the shyness dimension (approach/avoidance, approach/withdrawal) showed greatest variability. In terms of later psychopathology, children with 'difficult' temperament (Maziade et al. 1990) and 'shyness' (Kagan 1994) were also the most stable predictors. Rutter and Rutter (1993) reported that there were critical periods in the development of personality that reflected the influences of genetic, family and environmental factors. Longitudinal studies indicate that adolescence is a high-risk period for the onset of personality disorder (Bernstein et al. 1993), and that age is a significant moderator in the development of personality dysfunction.

Bernstein et al. (1993), in a community-based sample of 733 adolescents (age range 9–19 years), found that the overall prevalence of personality disorders peaked at age 12 in boys and at age 11 in girls, and declined thereafter. In this study, obsessive–compulsive personality disorder was the most prevalent moderate axis II disorder, narcissistic personality the most prevalent severe personality disorder, and schizotypal the least prevalent axis II disorder-based on both moderate and severe diagnostic thresholds. At 2-year follow-up, although most axis II disorders did not persist, subjects with an axis II disorder identified earlier remained at elevated risk of receiving an axis II diagnosis again of follow-up.

The transition from adolescence to young adulthood appears to be the time when individual personality disorder diagnoses stabilize. In support of this notion, Grilo et al. (1998) showed that most DSM-III-R personality disorders were diagnosed with similar frequency in adolescents and young adults, although passive aggressive personality disorder (which has been dropped from DSM-IV) was more commonly diagnosed in adolescents while dependent personality disorder was reported to occur with higher frequency in the young adult population. Furthermore, Daley et al. (1999) demonstrated that personality pathology in adolescent females showed a moderately high degree of stability at 3-year follow-up, indicating the endurance of these traits in late adolescence.

PREDICTORS OF THE DEVELOPMENT OF PERSONALITY DISORDER

Bernstein et al. (1996) showed that childhood conduct problems were the most important independent predictor of personality disorder in adolescence regardless of cluster, but that childhood depressive symptoms were an independent predictor of cluster A personality disorder in boys, while childhood immaturity was an independent predictor of cluster B personality disorder in girls. This suggests that conduct problems in childhood are a non-specific predictor of later personality disorder, but that other childhood problems such as depression and immaturity are more discriminating in terms of the prediction of eventual personality disorder based on dimensional or cluster approaches. However, recent work by Kasen et al. (1999), examining the association between childhood psychopathology and young adult personality disorders, in a random sample of 551 youths (aged 9–16 years), indicated that the odds of young adult personality disorder increased when there was evidence of an adolescent personality disorder diagnosis in the same cluster at baseline. On the other hand, in this study there was also evidence that, prior to the development of personality disorder, anxiety disorders and major depression also significantly increased the odds of the development of personality disorder independent of an adolescent personality disorder. Furthermore, comorbidity of axis I and II disorders heightened the odds of a diagnosis of young adult personality disorder relative to the odds of a disorder on a single axis. Overall, these findings suggest that both childhood temperamental factors and adolescent psychopathology have an influence on the development of personality disorder in late adolescence and young adulthood.

PREVALENCE AND CORRELATES OF PERSONALITY DYSFUNCTION/DISORDER

Personality disorder is rarely diagnosed in children, but there are now an increasing number of studies examining the prevalence of personality disorder in adolescent populations. The lack of utility of personality disorder diagnoses in childhood may reflect the notion that specific personality disorder diagnoses may not be stable until adolescence. Indeed, DSM criteria generally suggest that a diagnosis of personality disorder can be applied only to children and adolescents whose maladaptive traits appear to be stable – with the exception of antisocial personality disorder which requires both conduct disorder symptoms in childhood and adult symptomatology. Wolff (1984) suggests that the reluctance in making a personality disorder diagnosis in children and adolescents may reflect a reticence in applying a theoretically pejorative label which may have negative consequences for the subject, including exclusion from treatment services.

Although there are eleven DSM-IV and ten ICD-10 personality disorder diagnoses, there is now considerable evidence of comorbidity in personality disorder diagnosis (Pfohl *et al.* 1986; Oldham *et al.* 1992; Perry 1992). To address this issue, Siever and Davis (1991) developed a multi-dimensional model for conceptualizing axis II personality disorders as a part of continuum from axis I disorders based on the psychobiological correlates of these dimensions. The model defines spectrums that range from axis I disorders through milder axis II disorders to subclinical presentations. Disturbances in four dimensions (i.e. cognitive/perceptual organization, impulsivity/aggression, affective instability, and anxiety/inhibition) are associated with specific phenomenological characteristic traits for a particular axis II personality disorder cluster. This provides a useful framework for understanding how personality dimensions and disorders operate from childhood through adolescence to adulthood.

Anxiety/inhibition: the anxious cluster

This largely corresponds to the anxious cluster (C) in DSM-IV, which includes avoidant, dependent and obsessive–compulsive disorder. Although both ICD and DSM have categories for avoidant personality disorders, most children and adolescents with extremes in this dimension of personality are characterized as having 'social sensitivity disorder of childhood' (ICD-10) or 'avoidant disorder of childhood or adolescence' (DSM-IV). This may account for the relatively low but similar prevalence rates of cluster C diagnosis in clinic samples of adolescents and young adults (12%: Rey *et al.* 1995) and community samples of adolescents (12.8%: Bernstein *et al.* 1996). It is likely that with the development of instruments to assess personality function in younger populations the prevalence rates of personality disorders within the anxious cluster will increase.

According to Siever and Davis (1991), individuals within the anxious cluster show evidence of autonomic arousal, fearfulness and inhibition and display avoidant, compulsive and dependent defensive coping strategies. These clusters of diagnoses are characterized largely by traits associated with anxiety. The importance of this anxiety dimension has been shown by studies demonstrating that children aged 2 years who were shy had greater autonomic arousal and that those who were on the extremes of this inhibition dimension remained physiologically overaroused on reassessment at age 13 (Kagan *et al.* 1988; Kagan 1994). While there may be a constitutional individual basis for the development and persistence of this trait, there is also evidence to suggest that parenting styles play a role in the development and persistence of avoidant (Arbel and Stravynski 1991) and dependent (Bornstein 1992) personality subtypes. Furthermore, there is some evidence

that an 'affectionless–controlling' family environment fosters the development of these disorders (Parker 1983; Head *et al.* 1991).

The specificity of the anxiety/inhibition trait in predicting later personality disorder diagnoses has come into question with Bernstein *et al.*'s (1996) study which suggests that anxiety/fear in childhood is not specifically predictive of cluster C personality disorder, but that conduct problems and depressive symptoms in childhood are stronger predictors of adolescent personality disorder in general. There is, however, at least some evidence for a heritable basis for avoidant and cluster A diagnoses, as the first-degree relatives of adolescents with avoidant personality disorder have increased prevalence of avoidant and other cluster A diagnoses (Johnson *et al.* 1995).

Perhaps some of the discordant findings reflect a lack of recognition that there may be gender differences in cluster A diagnoses and the anxiety/inhibition dimension (Bernstein *et al.* 1996; Grilo *et al.* 1996). This notion is supported to some degree by the finding that there are increased anxiety ratings in childhood in girls (Bernstein *et al.* 1996).

COGNITIVE/PERCEPTUAL ORGANIZATION: THE ODD CLUSTER

The odd cluster comprises schizotypal, schizoid and paranoid personality disorders. Subjects within this group tend to present with unusual or paranoid ideas, social isolation and odd styles of interacting with the environment. They are frequently also characterized by an inability to establish and maintain interpersonal relationships. While both DSM and ICD recognize paranoid and schizoid personality disorders, schizotypal personality disorder (DSM-IV) is classified amongst the psychoses in ICD-10.

In childhood and in adulthood there is some degree of overlap in the presentation of individuals who suffer from personality disorders within this cluster and those who suffer on the extreme of social withdrawal dimension – i.e. Asperger's syndrome or autistic spectrum disorders (Gillberg 1990). While there is some debate as to whether schizoid and schizotypal personality disorders are pervasive developmental disorders, Wolff (1993) recommends that, in children who do not manifest gross impairment, a personality disorder diagnosis may be more appropriate.

In general, schizoid and paranoid personality disorders are extremely rarely diagnosed in child and adolescent clinical settings (Pfohl *et al.* 1986) and this may reflect the impact of their detachment and guardedness in presenting to psychiatric services. In a sample of 145 adolescents with emotional and disruptive disorders, only 4% (six individuals) were diagnosed as having a cluster A diagnosis on Loranger *et al.*'s (1988) Personality Disorder Examination (Rey *et al.* 1995).

In terms of the stability of the odd cluster over time, there is evidence that schizoid personality disorders appear to be the most stable (Chick *et al.* 1979). Widiger *et al.* (1994) suggested that schizoid personality disorder should be viewed as an extreme on the dimension of introversion. Studies of children with schizoid personality indicate high rates of comorbid schizotypal personality disorder symptomatology (Wolff *et al.* 1991). Although studies of schizotypal personality disorder appear rare in the child and adolescent population, there is evidence from older cohorts that schizotypal personality disorder is also associated with an increased morbid risk of developing schizophrenia in adulthood (Battaglia *et al.* 1991; Schulz *et al.* 1989). It has also been found that the schizotypal personality disorder subjects demonstrate a variety of neuropsychological and neurochemical abnormalities (for a review, see Wainberg *et al.* (1995)) which are similar to those seen in individuals who develop schizophrenia in later life. The latter findings may explain why schizotypal personality disorder is classified under psychoses in ICD-10.

IMPULSIVE AGGRESSIVE DIMENSION: DRAMATIC CLUSTER

Impulsivity and aggression are dimensions of behaviour that reflect difficulty in inhibitory control, acting-out behaviours, lack of tolerance for frustration, sensation seeking and a tendency towards delinquent behaviours (Siever and Davis 1991). A number of personality disorders within the dramatic cluster (antisocial, borderline, narcissistic and histrionic) fall along the dimension of impulsivity/aggression. There is evidence to suggest there is a moderate genetic component to antisocial, borderline and other dramatic cluster diagnosis (Schulz *et al.* 1989; McGuffin and Thapar 1992). There is also evidence of familial aggregation of these disorders (Silverman *et al.* 1991) and this again probably operates through the impulsivity/aggression dimension. While family, peer group and community influences are important factors in the development of antisocial behaviour, including conduct disorder, antisocial personality and aggressive behaviour (Loeber and Farrington 1994), there is also emerging evidence that subjects on the extreme of the impulsivity–aggression dimension exhibit low levels of arousal, EEG abnormalities, reduced serotonergic function and fronto-temporal deficits on neuropsychological testing (for a review, see Dolan (1994)).

Temperamental traits that have been shown to be important in the development of conduct problems in childhood and antisocial personality in adolescence and young adulthood include impulsivity/thrill-seeking, fearlessness, aggression and high levels of activity. Richman *et al.* (1982) reported that overactivity at age 3 years predicted antisocial behaviour at age 8. Olweus (1979) also noted that aggression exhibited at age 3 years showed remarkable longitudinal stability, while Kagan *et al.* (1966) highlighted the importance of reflectiveness versus

impulsivity/aggression in the ultimate development of conduct problems and personality dysfunction in this domain. Hyperactivity and aggression appear to be fairly stable predictors of criminal and antisocial and aggressive behaviour in adolescence and adulthood (Magnusson 1988; Caspi *et al.* 1987) and there are moderately strong links between conduct disorder, hyperactivity, academic failure and familial/extrafamilial adversity and the progression to an adult diagnosis of antisocial personality disorder (Robins 1991; Loeber and Farrington 1994).

Studies examining the prevalence of the dramatic cluster (i.e. cluster B) diagnoses in community samples of adolescents report relatively low rates (6.6%: Bernstein *et al.* 1996; 7.1%: Johnson *et al.* 2000). In clinic samples of adolescents with emotional and behaviour disorders rates are higher (20%: Rey *et al.* 1997). Myers *et al.* (1998) found that antisocial personality disorder diagnosis were made in 61% of 137 cases four years after treatment for substance misuse in an inpatient unit for conduct-disordered adolescents. Eppright *et al.* (1993) found high rates of comorbid antisocial personality disorder in incarcerated conduct-disordered juvenile offenders. In suicidal populations of adolescents, borderline and emotionally unstable personality disorder were most prevalent (Braun-Scharm 1996), suggesting that limited emotional control, intolerance/frustration and impulsiveness were important factors in suicidal adolescence.

Antisocial personality disorder as a construct has been heavily criticized for its over-reliance on antisocial behaviour particularly in criminal populations (Blackburn 1988). This has led to the development of alternative measures which rely more on the interpersonal aspects of antisocial behaviour, such as the Psychopathy Checklist (Hare 1991).

PSYCHOPATHY IN CHILDREN AND ADOLESCENTS

Although antisocial/dissocial personality disorder and psychopathy are at times used as synonyms for the same disorder, there are significant differences in these concepts and their associated correlates. Psychopaths as described by Cleckley (1976) and Hare (1991) are individuals who are characterized by deficits in affective and interpersonal domains as well as the extent of their antisocial behaviour. Psychopathy is viewed as a higher-order construct, which captures Cleckley's notion of what constitutes the prototypical psychopath. The notion that 'psychopaths' are different from those with a diagnosis of antisocial personality disorder comes from research showing that there are high rates of antisocial personality disorder in prison populations, but only 20% of this group will meet the criteria for psychopathy based on Hare's 1991 criteria (Hare 1998).

Since the development of the Psychopathy Checklist Revised (PCL-R; Hare 1991), prototypical measures have been developed for the study of psychopathy in children (Frick 1998) and adolescents (Forth *et al.* 1990).

The Psychopathy Checklist: Youth Version (PCL:YV) will soon be published. This measure takes into account the restricted lifestyle of adolescents in terms of work and relationship experiences. Data from prevalence studies of incarcerated samples of juvenile offenders revealed moderately high rates (18–35%) of psychopathy using the traditional PCL cut-off scores of 30 (Laroche 1996; Forth *et al.* 1990). Rates were lower (9–15%) in probation settings (Kosson 1996; Bailey 1994). The PCL:YV, like the adult PCL-R, has a two-factor structure – one factor reflects the interpersonal and affective aspects of personality function, and the other reflects the chronic antisocial lifestyle. The validity of the PCL:YV has been demonstrated in studies which show relatively high correlations between PCL:YV total score and DSM-III-R conduct disorder symptoms (Forth 1995), particularly aggressive conduct symptoms.

Although there is relatively little published data on the utility of the PCL:YV, there is evidence that it has similar correlates to its parent adult assessment instrument. For example, Forth (1995) was able to demonstrate that the PCL:YV score correlates negatively with age of onset of violent and non-violent antisocial behaviours and positively with the frequency of violent and non-violent delinquent acts. In light of the fact that the adult PCL/PCL-R proved to be a valid risk predictor for future violence (Dolan and Doyle 2000), it is possible that the adolescent version will have similar predictive validity.

The childhood version of the PCL/PCL-R, known as the Psychopathy Screening Device (PSD; Frick 1998), is based on parent and teacher ratings rather than self-report or interview measures with the subject, because of concerns about the validity of children's accounts of their own emotional and behavioural difficulties (Kamphaus and Frick 1996). This instrument is not yet available for general use, but its validity appears sound as Frick *et al.* (1994) were able to demonstrate that the PSD has a similar two-factor structure to the adult and adolescent versions and it is able to distinguish interpersonal (callous–unemotional (CU) traits) from antisocial behaviours (impulsive-conduct problems (I-CP)) in children. The I-CP scale has been shown to correlate with traditional measures of conduct disorder (Frick *et al.* 1994). Furthermore, Barry *et al.* (2000) have also demonstrated that children with CU traits engage in more persistent antisocial behaviour, and the latter group exhibit an insensitivity to punishment cues irrespective of whether or not they have conduct problems (O'Brien and Frick 1996). These findings appear to fit with similar studies examining information and emotional processing deficits in adolescent and adult psychopaths assessed using similar measures (Newman 1998; Hare 1998), but they highlight the differences in the relationship between these correlates and the broader construct of antisocial personality disorder.

While the adult version of the Psychopathy Checklist has been shown to have reasonable construct and predictive validity in settings outside its development site, the instruments developed for use in child and adolescent populations require future validation in a variety of populations and settings before they can be accepted as appropriate measures of psychopathy in younger populations.

IMPACT OF PERSONALITY DISORDER ON OUTCOME

In general, there appears to be reasonable evidence that a diagnosis of personality disorder in adolescence is associated with a significant degree of impairment and poor outcome. Levy *et al.* (1999), for example, showed that hospitalized adolescents with a diagnosis of personality disorder were significantly more impaired than those without. At follow-up, personality-disordered adolescents had used significantly more drugs, required more inpatient treatment during the follow-up interval, and exhibited more impulsive aggressive and suicidal behaviours. Data from the longitudinal birth cohort study in Dunedin, New Zealand, suggest that 'high negative emotionality' at age 18 is associated with affective disorder, anxiety, substance dependence and antisocial personality disorder at age 21 when corresponding mental disorders at age 18 are controlled for (Moffitt *et al.* 2001). In the same study low 'constraint' which reflects impulsivity at age 18 was also linked with substance dependence and ASPD at age 21 if corresponding mental disorders at age 18 are controlled for (Krueger 1999). In clinic samples, having a personality disorder and poor family environment in adolescence is associated with poor functioning at follow-up (20 years) independent of adolescent diagnosis (Rey *et al.* 1997).

There also appear to be specific associations between borderline personality disorder in adolescence and suicidal behaviour (Martunnen *et al.* 1991; Brent *et al.* 1993), and between antisocial personality and criminal outcomes and poor work record and substance misuse (Rey *et al.* 1997; Myers *et al.* 1998). Cluster A and B traits in late-adolescence females appear also to predict interview rates of depression at 2-year follow-up (Daley *et al.* 1999). Johnson *et al.* (2000), in a longitudinal community study, found that cluster A personality disorder diagnoses in adolescence were more likely to be associated with acquisitive offences and threats to injure others. By contrast, cluster B diagnoses (not including antisocial personality disorder) were more likely to be associated with arson, vandalism and violence, with passive–aggressive, paranoid and narcissitic personality traits being particularly associated with violence to others. In Johnson *et al.*'s study, cluster C diagnoses were not associated with increased risk of committing violent acts.

The role and validity of psychopathy as a construct in the prediction of outcomes in child and adolescent populations remains to be investigated but appears to be a useful measure for studies examining the correlates of antisocial behaviour across age bands.

CONCLUSIONS

While there is some evidence to support the stability of temperamental traits in childhood, there is also evidence that the development of personality disorder peaks in early adolescence with specialization in the type of personality dysfunction/disorder occurring in later adolescence. Environmental, hormonal and genetic factors all probably contribute to this specialization and the relative contribution of each remains unknown.

Conduct problems in childhood appear to be a significant predictor of later personality dysfunction, but childhood depressive and immaturity problems may be more discriminating in the ultimate assignment of an eventual DSM cluster diagnosis. Personality dysfunction and disorder are probably best understood in child, adolescent and adult populations on a dimensional basis as this acknowledges the degree of comorbidity that exists between individual personality disorder diagnoses and DSM cluster diagnosis. Furthermore, dimensional approaches allow for a greater understanding of the psychobiological correlates of particular dimensions and how these might inform aetiological theories and possible future interventions.

There appears to be reasonable evidence that personality disorders can be traced to childhood emotional and behavioural disturbance and to suggest these problems have both general and specific relationships to adolescent personality functioning. Assessment of personality pathology before late adolescence may therefore be warranted and future studies need to focus on the mental health outcomes of those diagnosed with specific personality disorders in earlier life.

It would also appear important to note that childhood and adolescent axis I disorders may be associated with a set of maladaptive behaviours and environmental responses which foster more persistent psychopathology, including the development of personality disorder in later life.

For children and adolescents who appear to function on the extreme of the impulsivity–aggression dimension, a diagnosis of antisocial personality disorder may prove useful in predicting long-term outcome. Recent developments, however, suggest that the childhood and adolescence versions of the adult Psychopathy Checklist may prove more useful in identifying a core group of high-risk antisocial young people who are likely to have poor outcomes in terms of conventional treatments for conduct disorder or antisocial behaviour.

One concern, as in adults, will be the use of the label of 'psychopathy' to designate young people as high risk, given the current emphasis on risk reduction in personality-disordered offender and non-offender populations.

REFERENCES

APA (American Psychiatric Association) 1994: *Diagnostic and Statistical Manual of Mental Disorders*, 4th edn (DSM-IV). Washington, DC: APA.

Arbel, N. and Stravynski, A. 1991: A retrospective study of separation in the development of adult avoidant personality disorder. *Acta Psychiatrica Scandinavica* **83**: 174–8.

Bailey, D. 1994: Assessment of psychopathy in young offenders. Unpublished thesis, Carleton University, Ottawa, Canada.

Barry, C.T., Frick, P.J., DeShazo, T.M., McCoy, M.G., Ellis, M. and Loney, B.R. 2000: The importance of Callous-Unemotional traits for extending the concept of psychopathy to children. *Journal of Abnormal Psychology* **109**: 335–40.

Battaglia, M., Gasperini, M., Sciuto, G. *et al.* 1991: Psychiatric disorders in the families of schizotypal subjects. *Schizophrenia Bulletin* **17**: 659–65.

Bernstein, D.P., Cohen, P., Velez, C.N. *et al.* 1993: Prevalence and stability of DSM-III-R PD diagnosis in a community-based survey of adolescents. *American Journal of Psychiatry* **150**: 1237–43.

Bernstein, D.P., Cohen, P., Skodol, A., Bezirganian, S. and Brook, J.S. 1996: Childhood antecedents of adolescent personality disorders. *American Journal of Psychiatry* **153**: 907–13.

Blackburn, R. 1988: On moral judgements and personality disorders: the myth of psychopathic personality revisited. *British Journal of Psychiatry* **153**: 505–12.

Bornstein, R.F. 1992: The dependent personality: developmental, social and clinical perspectives. *Psychological Bulletin* **112**: 3–23.

Braun-Scharm, H. 1996: Suicidality and personality disorders in adolescents. *Crisis* **17**(2): 64–8.

Brent, D.A., Johnson, B., Bartle, S. *et al.* 1993: Personality disorder, leading to impulsive violence, and suicidal behaviour in adolescents. *Journal of the American Academy of Child and Adolescent Psychiatry* **32**: 69–75.

Brent, D.A., Johnson, B.A., Perper, J. *et al.* 1994: Personality disorder, personality traits, impulsive violence and completed suicide in adolescents. *Journal of the American Academy of Child and Adolescent Psychiatry* **33**: 1080–6.

Bronisch, T. and Mombour, W. 1994: Comparison of a diagnostic checklist with a structured interview for the assessment of DSM-III-R and ICD-10 personality disorders. *Psychopathology* **27**: 312–20.

Caspi, A., Elder, G.H. and Bem, D.J. 1987: Moving against the world: life course patterns of explosive children. *Developmental Psychology* **23**: 306–13.

Chess, S. and Thomas, A. 1984: *Origins and Evolution of Behaviour Disorders*. New York: Raven Press.

Chick, J., Waterhouse, L. and Wolff, S. 1979: Psychological construing in schizoid children grown up. *British Journal of Psychiatry* **135**: 425–30.

Cleckley, H. 1976: *The Mask of Sanity*, 5th edn. St Louis: C.V. Mosby.

Daley, S.E., Hammen, C., Burge, D. *et al.* 1999: Depression and axis II symptomatology in an adolescent community sample: concurrent and longitudinal associations. *Journal of Personality* **13**(1): 47–60.

Dolan, M.C. 1994: Psychopathy: a neurobiological perspective. *British Journal of Psychiatry* **165**: 151–9.

Dolan, M.C. and Doyle, M. 2000: Violence risk prediction and the role of the Psychopathy Checklist – Revised. *British Journal of Psychiatry* **177**: 303–11.

Eppright, T.D., Kashani, J.H., Robinson, B.D. and Reid, J.C. 1993: Comorbidity of conduct disorder and personality disorders in an incarcerated juvenile population. *American Journal of Psychiatry* **150**: 1233–6.

Frick, P.J. 1998: Callous–unemotional traits and conduct problems: applying the two-factor model of psychopathy to children. In Cooke, D.J., Forth, A.E. and Hare, R.D. (eds), *Psychopathy: Theory, Research, and Implications for Society*. Dordrecht: Kluwer, 161–87.

Frick, P., O'Brien, B., Wootton, J. and McBurnett, K. 1994: Psychopathy and conduct problems in children. *Journal of Abnormal Psychology* **103**: 700–7.

Forth, A.E. 1995: *Psychopathy and Young Offenders: Prevalence, Family Background, and Violence*. Unpublished report, Carleton University, Ottawa, Canada.

Forth, A.E., Hart, S.D. and Hare, R.D. 1990: Assessment of psychopathy in male young offenders. *Psychological Assessment: a Journal of Consulting and Clinical Psychology* **2**: 342–4.

Gillberg, C. 1990: Asperger syndrome in 23 Swedish children. *Developmental Medicine and Child Neurology* **31**: 520–31.

Grilo, C.M., Becker, D.F., Fehon, D.C. *et al.* 1996: Gender differences in personality disorders in psychiatrically hospitalized adolescents. *American Journal of Psychiatry* **153**: 1089–91.

Grilo, C.M., McGlashen, T.H., Quinlan, D.M. *et al.* 1998: Frequency of personality disorders in two age cohorts of psychiatric inpatients. *American Journal of Psychiatry* **155**: 140–2.

Hare, R.D. 1991: The Hare Psychopathy Checklist – Revised. Toronto: Multi-Health Systems.

Hare, R.D. 1998: The NATO Advanced Study Institute. In Cooke, D.J., Forth, A.E. and Hare, R.D. (eds), *Psychopathy: Theory, Research, and Implications for Society*. Dordrecht: Kluwer, 1–11.

Head, S.B., Baker, J.D. and Williamson, D.A. 1991: Family environment characteristics and dependent personality disorder. *Journal of Personality Disorders* **5**: 256–63.

Johnson, B.A., Brent, D.A., Connolly, J. *et al.* 1995: Familial aggregation of adolescent personality disorder. *Journal of the American Academy of Child and Adolescent Psychiatry* **34**: 798–804.

Johnson, J.G., Cohen, P., Smailes, E. *et al.* 2000: Adolescent personality disorders associated with violence and criminal behaviour during adolescence and early adulthood. *American Journal of Psychiatry* **157**: 1406–12.

Kagan, J. 1994: *Galen's Prophecy*. New York, Basic Books.

Kagan, J., Pearson, L. and Welch, L. 1966: Conceptual impulsivity and inductive reasoning. *Child Development* **37**: 583–94.

Kagan, J., Resnick, J.S. and Snidman, N. 1988: Biological basis of childhood shyness. *Science* **240**: 167–71.

Kamphaus, R.W. and Frick, P.J. 1996: *Clinical Assessment of Child and Adolescent Personality and Behaviour*. Boston: Allyn & Bacon.

Kasen, S., Cohen, P., Skodol, A.E., Johnson, J.G. and Brook, J.S. 1999: Influence of child and adolescent psychiatric disorders on young adult personality disorder. *American Journal of Psychiatry* **156**: 1529–35.

Kosson, D.S. 1996: Psychopathy and dual-task performance under focusing conditions. *Journal of Abnormal Psychology* **105**: 391–400.

Krueger, R.F. 1999: Personality traits in late adolescence predict mental disorders in early adulthood: a prospective-epidemiological study. *Journal of Personality* **67**: 39–65.

Laroche, I. 1996: Les composantes psychologiques et comportementales parentales associées à la psychopathie du contrevenant juvénile. Unpublished doctoral thesis, University of Montreal, Quebec.

Levy, K.N., Becker, D.F., Grilo, C.M. *et al.* 1999: Concurrent and predictive validity of the personality disorder diagnosis in adolescent inpatients. *American Journal of Psychiatry* **156**: 1522–8.

Livesley, W.J., Jackson, D.N. and Schroeder, M. 1992: Factorial structure of traits delineating personality disorders in clinical and general population samples. *Journal of Abnormal Psychology* **101**: 432–40.

Loeber, R. and Farrington, D.P. 1994: Problems and solutions in longitudinal and experimental treatment studies of child psychopathology and delinquency. *Journal of Consulting Clinical Psychology* **62**: 887–900.

Loranger, A.W., Lenzenweger, M.F., Gartner, A.F. *et al.* 1988: Trait–state artifacts and the diagnosis of personality disorders. *Archives of General Psychiatry* **48**: 720–8.

Magnussen, D. 1988: *Individual Development from an Interactional Perspective: a Longitudinal Study*. Hillsdale, NJ: Lawrence Erlbaum.

Martunnen, M.J., Aro, H.M., Henriksson, M.M. and Lönnquist, J.K. 1991: Mental disorders in adolescent suicide: DSM-III-R axes I and II diagnoses among 13- to 19-year-olds in Finland. *Archives of General Psychiatry* **48**: 834–9.

Maziade, M., Caron, C., Coté, R., Boutin, P. and Thivierge, J. 1990: Extreme temperament and diagnosis: a study in a psychiatric sample of consecutive children. *Archives of General Psychiatry* **47**: 477–84.

McGuffin, P. and Thapar, A. 1992: The genetics of personality disorder. *British Journal of Psychiatry* **160**: 12–23.

Millon, T. 1996: *Disorders of Personality: DSM-IV and Beyond*. New York: John Wiley.

Moffitt, T.E., Caspi, A., Rutter, M. and Silva, P.A. 2001: *Sex Differences in Antisocial Behaviour: Conduct Disorder, Delinquency, and Violence in the Dunedin Longitudinal Study*. Cambridge University Press.

Myers, M.G., Stewart, D.G. and Brown, S.A. 1998: Progression from conduct disorder to antisocial personality disorder following treatment for adolescent substance abuse. *American Journal of Psychiatry* **155**: 479–85.

Newman, J.P. 1998: Psychopathic behavior: an information processing perspective. In Cooke, D.J., Forth, A.E. and Hare, R.D. (eds), *Psychopathy: Theory, Research and Implications for Society*. Dordrecht: Kluwer, 81–104.

O'Brien, B.S. and Frick, P.J. 1996: Reward dominance: associations with anxiety, conduct problems, and psychopathy in children. *Journal of Abnormal Child Psychology* **24**: 223–40.

Oldham, J.M., Skodol, A.E., Kellman, H.D. *et al.* 1992: Diagnosis of DSM-III-R personality disorders by two structured interviews: patterns of comorbidity. *American Journal of Psychiatry* **153**: 543–53.

Olweus, D. 1979: Stability of aggressive reaction patterns in males: a review. *Psychological Bulletin* **86**: 852–75.

Paris, J. (ed.) 1996: *Social Factors in the Personality Disorders*. Cambridge: Cambridge University Press.

Parker, G. 1983: *Parental Overprotection: a Risk Factor in Psychosocial Development*. New York: Grune & Stratton.

Perry, J.C. 1992: Problems and considerations in the valid assessment of personality disorders. *American Journal of Psychiatry* **149**: 1645–53.

Pfohl, B., Coryell, W., Zimmerman, M. and Strangl, D.A. 1986: DSM-III personality disorders: diagnostic overlap and internal consistency of individual DSM-III criteria. *Comprehensive Psychiatry* **27**: 21–34.

Rey, J.M., Morris-Yates, A., Singh, M., Andrews, G. and Stewart, G.W. 1995: Continuities between psychiatric disorders and adolescents and personality disorders in young adults. *American Journal of Psychiatry* **152**: 895–900.

Rey, J.M., Singh, M. and Morris-Yates, A. 1997: Referred adolescents as young adults: the relationship between psychosocial functioning and personality disorder. *Australian and New Zealand Journal of Psychiatry* **31**(2): 219–26.

Richman, N., Stevenson, J. and Graham, P.J. 1982: *Preschool to School: A Behavioural Study.* London: Academic Press.

Robins, L.N. 1991: Conduct disorder. *Journal of Child Psychology and Psychiatry* **32**: 193–212.

Rothbart, M.K. and Ahadi, S.A. 1994: Temperament and the development of personality. *Journal of Abnormal Psychology* **103**: 55–66.

Rutter, M. and Rutter, M. 1993: *Developing Minds: Challenge and Continuity Across the Lifespan.* Harmondsworth: Penguin.

Schulz, P.M., Soloff, P.H., Kelly, T. *et al.* 1989: A family history of borderline subtypes. *Journal of Personality Disorders* **3**: 217–29.

Siever, L.J. and Davis, K. 1991: A psychobiological perspective on the personality disorders. In Frances, A.J. and Hales, R.E. (eds), *American Psychiatric Association Annual Review* **5**: 279–314.

Silverman, J.M., Pinkham, L., Horvath, T.B. *et al.* 1991: Affective and impulsive personality disorder traits in the relatives of patients with borderline personality disorder. *American Journal of Psychiatry* **148**: 1378–85.

Wainberg, M.L., Keefe, R.S.E. and Siever, L.J. 1995: The neuropsychiatry of schizotypal personality disorder. In Ratey, J.J. (ed.), *Neuropsychiatry of Personality Disorders.* Cambridge, MA: Blackwell Science.

Widiger, T.A. and Trull, T.J. 1994: Personality disorders and violence. In Monahan, J. and Steadman, H. (eds), *Violence and Mental Disorder: Developments in Risk Assessment.* Chicago: University of Chicago Press, 203–26.

Wolff, S. 1984: Annotation: the concept of personality disorder in childhood. *Journal of Child Psychology and Psychiatry* **25**: 5–13.

Wolff, S. 1993: Personality disorder in childhood. In Tyrer, P. and Stein, G. (eds), *Personality Disorder Reviewed.* London: Gaskell, 64–89.

Wolff, S., Townsend, R., Mcguire, R.J. and Weeks, D.J. 1991: 'Schizoid' personality in childhood and adult life: II. Adult adjustment and the continuity with schizotypal personality disorder. *British Journal of Psychiatry* **159**: 620–8.

WHO (World Health Organization) 1992: *The ICD-10 Classification of Mental and Behavioural Disorders.* Geneva: WHO.

10

Affective conduct disorder

BERNADKA DUBICKA AND RICHARD HARRINGTON

INTRODUCTION

Affective disorder is commonly found in the forensic adolescent population although it may often go unrecognized. This chapter focuses largely on depressive illness. However, since bipolar affective disorder is becoming increasingly recognized, that condition will be described separately at the end of the chapter.

Recognizing affective disorder in this group of young people is important for a number of reasons. Clinically, the comorbid condition can complicate the presenting symptomatology of conduct disorder (CD); it also has implications for course and outcome, the choice of treatment, and the level of functional impairment that can be expected. Recognizing comorbidity is also important as it can distort research findings.

The chapter begins with a description of the epidemiology of depressive conduct disorder (DCD), followed by a discussion of the causal mechanisms involved. The clinical implications of comorbid depression are outlined, and then there is a brief review of bipolar affective disorder. The chapter concludes with a review of clinical implications and future research, and some case studies.

PREVALENCE

Relative use of clinical and general population samples

Clinical samples are not representative of individuals with the disorder in the general population. Patients in clinical samples have more severe symptomatology, are more impaired and come from families that feel more burdened by their children's problems (Angold et al. 1998). Therefore clinical studies cannot provide unbiased prevalence or incidence rates, or estimates of risk factors. However, clinical samples can be useful in providing pointers towards potential risk factors and in examining potential aetiological mechanisms in defined risk groups (Angold et al. 1999).

Clinical samples

Studies that have examined the prevalence of depression in clinically referred youths with CD generally find rates of 15–31%. For example, Riggs et al. (1995) studied a substance-dependent group of 99 delinquent boys aged 13–19 years, all of whom had CD, and found 21% had major depression (MD) or dysthymia, or both.

Zoccolillo and Rogers (1991) studied 55 girls aged 13–16 years with CD, who were admitted to a locked psychiatric unit and re-evaluated 2–4 years later. At the time of admission, 24% had been arrested or had contact with the juvenile justice system. The lifetime prevalence rate of MD was 31%. Jasper et al. (1998) examined 100 consecutive referrals of girls in care aged 11–17 years to an adolescent forensic mental health service. The most common psychiatric diagnosis was a mixed disorder of conduct and emotions (22%).

Studies of the prevalence of CD in clinically referred depressed children and adolescents have also found much overlap between the two conditions. Kovacs and Devlin (1998) reviewed a number of studies encompassing

508 depressed referred patients aged 6–18 years and found an overall rate of CD of 16% (range 7–24%). Hammen *et al.* (1999) assessed 43 depressed 8- to 18-year-olds and found 43% had a diagnosis of either CD or oppositional defiant disorder (ODD). Goodyer *et al.* (1997a) studied 68 8- to 16-year-olds with MD and found 37% had CD and 44% had ODD at baseline assessment.

A study by King *et al.* (1996) examined adolescents with MD who were admitted to an inpatient unit (mean age 15.3 years). Of the 103 adolescents, more were found to have CD if they were also abusing substances or alcohol (47% versus 18%).

In summary, the evidence from clinical samples suggests that there is a high prevalence of depressive disorder in young people who present with conduct problems. A high proportion of adolescents who present with depression will also have conduct problems, particularly if there is concurrent alcohol or substance misuse.

Epidemiological samples

The association found between CD and depression in clinical studies has been supported by data from epidemiological studies. For example, in their meta-analysis of DSM population studies, Angold *et al.* (1999) found a highly significant association between the two disorders (odds ratio 6.6, confidence interval 4.4–11.0). Interestingly, the relationship between CD and anxiety was much weaker than that between CD and depression, suggesting a specific association and not just a generalized relationship between 'internalizing' and 'externalizing' disorders.

Rates found in epidemiological studies have varied widely. In the review by Angold *et al.* (1999), the rate of CD found in depression ranged from zero to 83%; the rate of depression in CD ranged from zero to 46%. The differences in rates are probably due to many factors. For example, there are differences between studies in sampling techniques, measurement, and type of informants. The age ranges used have varied, and in most studies the sample size has been too small to analyse different age groups separately.

Studies that have used the ICD classification system have also found a significant association between emotional and behavioural disorders. For example, the Isle of Wight and associated studies found that 'mixed disorder' was the third most common diagnosis in the 10- to 11-year age group (Rutter and Graham 1966), and also at ages 14–15 (Graham and Rutter 1973). There was a far higher frequency of this disorder than expected by chance.

Thus epidemiological studies suggest there is a substantial overlap between CD and depression, but rates found vary substantially across studies.

Developmental differences

AGE DIFFERENCES

Significant changes occur during childhood and adolescence in terms of cognitive capacity and social functioning. Thus a longitudinal perspective is particularly important in child and adolescent psychiatry to establish stability and continuity of disorders.

There is some evidence that conduct and depressive disorders are age dependent, but research is limited as most population studies lack sufficiently large sample sizes. A few longitudinal studies have, however, been able to examine age differences. The Dunedin cohort in New Zealand found that mood disorder tends to increase later in adolescence (prevalence at 11 years was 2%, whereas at 18 years it was 18%), whereas prevalence of CD peaks in late childhood/early adolescence and then declines (9% at 11 years versus 6% at 18 years; Anderson *et al.* 1987; Feehan *et al.* 1994). These findings are supported by the Oregon Adolescent Depression Project where the mean age of onset for externalizing disorder was 8 years, and that of MD was 14 years (Orvaschel *et al.* 1995).

These studies indicate that the high-risk period for onset of behaviour disorder is earlier than that for depressive disorder, which increases in prevalence with the start of adolescence. Kovacs and Devlin (1998) have noted that the developmental chronology of these disorders is consistent with the onset pattern of comorbid DCD that has been found in most studies. For example, Rohde *et al.* (1991) found disruptive behaviour disorder preceded depression for 72% of depressed adolescents. Kovacs and Devlin (1998) suggest that the changing structure and demands of the social environment are important developmental mediators for the onset of conduct disorder, whereas onset of depressive disorder is subject to even more complex biological, psychological and cognitive mediating processes.

In summary, adolescence is a particularly vulnerable period for the onset of depression which may frequently manifest itself for the first time in children with an already established history of CD.

SEX DIFFERENCES

Overall prevalence rates for CD tend to show higher rates for boys than girls. In the case of oppositional defiant disorder, rates tend to be similar for both sexes (Nottelmann and Jensen 1995), although some studies have shown higher rates for girls (e.g. Kashani *et al.* 1987). It has been argued that the defining features of CD in classification systems such as DSM are biased towards boys, whereas there are fewer sex-related features among the symptoms of ODD, and thus studies have underestimated the prevalence of girls with CD (Zoccolillo and Rogers 1991). However, studies which have not used DSM or ICD approaches have also found these sex-related differences (e.g. Achenbach *et al.* 1991).

With regard to depression, gender effects change with development. Rates tend to be similar in childhood or there is a male preponderance, but by adolescence the female preponderance found in adult depression becomes evident (Harrington 1994a).

With regard to DCD, studies have generally been too small to permit definite conclusions. Some studies have found no sex difference in prevalence, but others have found a higher incidence for boys (e.g. Steinhausen and Reitzle 1996). In his review, Zoccolillo (1992) found that conduct-disordered girls showed an increasing prevalence of emotional disorder with development, whereas conduct-disordered boys had the highest prevalence of emotional disorder in preadolescence, which then declined.

In summary, sample sizes from epidemiological studies are insufficient to draw firm conclusions regarding sex differences in prevalence of DCD. There are some data to suggest that prevalence may be higher in boys, but if there is a sex bias in the diagnosis of CD this could also under-estimate the prevalence of DCD in girls.

CAUSAL MECHANISMS: COMORBIDITY AS AN ARTEFACT

Explanations for comorbidity between two disorders can be divided into those due to artefact and those which reflect a real phenomenon (Caron and Rutter 1991; Angold *et al.* 1999). This section deals with the former, and the following section discusses possible true comorbidity.

There are numerous sources of artefact which may explain the co-occurrence between two disorders. These may be broadly divided into methodological and nosological artefacts.

Methodological artefacts

Possible methodological artefacts include referral bias in clinical samples, effect of rater expectancies (the halo effect), use of multiple informants, and single behaviours coding as multiple symptoms. However, there is little evidence to suggest that the co-occurrence of affective and conduct disorder is a result of a methodological problem (Angold *et al.* 1999).

Nosological artefacts

Even if comorbidity is not a result of methodological artefacts, the apparent overlap between depression and CD may not represent comorbidity because basic diagnostic concepts may themselves be mistaken.

OVERLAPPING DIAGNOSTIC CRITERIA

Comorbidity could be generated by non-specific symptoms that are shared by both diagnoses. For example, irritability is common in depressive symptoms and several symptoms of ODD could result from irritability, such as 'often loses temper'. However, Biederman *et al.* (1995) found that eliminating overlapping symptoms failed to eliminate comorbidity between oppositional defiant disorder and depression. Therefore, it is unlikely that overlapping diagnostic criteria could explain the co-occurrence between depression and CD.

DIAGNOSTIC CONCEPTUAL ISSUES: CATEGORIES OR DIMENSIONS?

There is a view that the concept of categories of disorder is fundamentally misconceived. Instead, psychopathology can best be seen as a mixture of extremes of various personality dimensions. Thus comorbidity arises only because current diagnostic approaches impose arbitrary cut-off points on a series of dimensional phenomena which may, in fact, be naturally linked, and thus artificial subdivisions are created. However, there has been little research to test this hypothesis.

IS ONE DISORDER PART OF THE OTHER?

In his review of depressive conduct disorder, Zoccolillo (1992) argued that the evidence suggested that DCD is not distinct from CD. In other words, depression is part of CD and the category of DCD is an artificial subdivision of CD. He argued that independent correlates of the mixed group are similar to those of the pure conduct-disordered group; the mixed group are no less antisocial than those with CD, and that these two groups are not distinct over time. In adults, an increasing number of CD symptoms in subjects with antisocial personality disorder or substance abuse has been shown to predict an increasing probability of non-externalizing disorder, and the majority of women with CD who persist with an adult externalizing disorder will also develop an internalizing disorder.

Thus Zoccolillo suggests that DCD is not distinct from pure CD and the distinction is meaningless. He has proposed a model of conduct disorder as a disorder of multiple dysfunction – in other words, a disorder with multiple symptoms – which would also explain the numerous other comorbid disorders associated with CD, such as hyperactivity.

There has been some subsequent evidence to support this idea. Steinhausen and Reitzle (1996), in a large retrospective study of clinic attenders, compared children with mixed disorder of conduct and emotion to those with a single disorder of either conduct or emotion. They looked at various correlates including age, sex, family background, premorbid behaviour, psychosocial situation and treatment. They concluded that children with the mixed disorder share many characteristics with those with pure CD, thus supporting the notion that the former is a subgroup of the latter. Likewise, in a longitudinal study of children with conduct, depressive or comorbid disorders, Renouf et al. (1997) found that by mid-adolescence the adolescents with either a history of conduct or comorbid disorder had lower social competence than did children with a history of depressive disorder. Further studies have shown a similar incidence of crime in relatives of children with both CD alone and with comorbid depression, and adult outcome studies found that the two groups have similar outcomes with regard to adult criminality and depression (Harrington 1994b).

Several longitudinal studies have found that externalizing disorders are predictive of both internalizing and externalizing disorders in adolescents, whereas internalizing disorders tend to show more specificity (Feehan et al. 1993; Ferdinand and Verhulst 1995). In fact, Ferdinand and Verhulst (1995) discovered that the risk of having an internalizing disorder at follow-up was three times greater if there had been an initial externalizing disorder rather than an internalizing disorder. Although these results could be interpreted to mean that both problems may be part of the same disorder, it has been suggested that there is an alternative explanation; namely that CD causes depression (Angold et al. 1999). However, the Oregon Adolescent Depression Project (Orvaschel et al. 1995), which is a longitudinal study of depression, did not find an increased predictive risk of depression with disruptive disorders.

Therefore, although there is some evidence to support the idea that depression is part of the natural history of CD, it is by no means clear-cut. Additional evidence will be presented later which suggests that the correlates of the comorbid condition and CD may in fact be different after all, indicating that these are two distinct disorders.

DOES ONE DISORDER REPRESENT AN EARLY MANIFESTATION OF THE OTHER?

As described earlier, epidemiological studies have shown that the high-risk period for the onset of behaviour disorder is earlier than that for depressive disorder, and most studies have found that comorbid depression tends to occur after the onset of CD (e.g. Riggs et al. 1995; Biederman et al. 1995; Rohde et al. 1991), although a few studies have found that the onset of depression precedes CD (e.g. Kovacs et al. 1988).

Since CD generally seems to precede depression, is there any evidence to suggest that CD is an early manifestation of depression? Studies have shown that CD predicts adult antisocial behaviour regardless of the presence or absence of other disorders, and that conduct disorder only predicts adult non-externalizing disorder in association

with externalizing disorders (Robins 1986; Robins and Price 1991). Conversely, there is no evidence to suggest that CD predicts emotional disorder in the absence of antisocial behaviour. Therefore it is unlikely that CD is an early manifestation of depressive disorder.

CAUSAL MECHANISMS: TRUE COMORBIDITY BETWEEN DEPRESSION AND CONDUCT DISORDER

Having ruled out various artefactual causes for the co-occurrence of depression and CD, what are the substantive explanations for this relationship?

Shared or correlated risk factors

One possible explanation for the co-occurrence of the two disorders is that they share the same risk factors. Many psychiatric disorders are multi-factorial in origin and many causal factors are not diagnosis specific. For example, child abuse, neglect and rejection are associated with a broad range of psychopathology, including conduct and personality disorder and depression (Brown et al. 1996; Maughan and McCarthy 1997). Late adoption has been found to predict both depression and antisocial personality disorder (Cadoret et al. 1990; Cloniger et al. 1982). Reiss et al. (1995) found that 60% of the variance in adolescent antisocial behaviour and 37% of the variance in depressive symptoms were a result of conflictual and negative parenting. Other examples of overlapping risk factors include peer rejection, poor social support, school failure, stressful life events, and socio-economic disadvantage (O'Connor et al. 1998). Studies have shown that it is the accumulation of risk factors that is important in the genesis of both CD (Kolvin et al. 1988) and depression (Beardslee et al. 1996).

There is some evidence to suggest that another shared risk factor may be a common genetic link for depressive and antisocial symptoms. In a three-year longitudinal study, O'Connor et al. (1998) followed 405 adolescents aged 10–18 years. The sample consisted of monozygotic and dizygotic twins, and full, half and unrelated siblings from non-divorced and step-families. Results indicated that the majority of the stability in, and co-occurrence between, antisocial and depressive symptoms was mediated by genetic factors. It is not yet clear which genetically influenced factors are responsible, but possible hypotheses are abnormalities in neurotransmitter systems common to both dimensions, or substrates that are involved in the stress reaction.

Environmental risk factors that were not shared by siblings also contributed to the stability of both symptoms. O'Connor et al. (1998) suggest that a possible candidate for this could be parental differential treatment between siblings which persists over time and may account for the stable differences in levels of depressive and antisocial symptoms between siblings. For antisocial symptoms only, risk factors shared between siblings also contributed to stability of symptoms. Possible candidates for these could be sibling conflict, marital discord and socio-economic disadvantage.

Even when risk factors for the two disorders are different, comorbidity may occur because the risk factors are associated. For example, Caron and Rutter (1991) suggested that comorbidity may arise between CD and depression through parental depression, which is associated with a genetic risk for depression in the offspring and an environmentally mediated risk through family discord for CD.

Another approach to assessing the extent to which comorbidity between the two disorders may be explained by shared or correlated risk factors was used by Fergusson et al. (1996a) in the Christchurch epidemiological study. They used a method called 'structural equation modelling' and found that more than two-thirds of the comorbidity between depression and CD arose because of common and correlated causal factors. Nevertheless, a substantial amount of the comorbidity was unexplained.

In summary, shared or correlated risk factors can explain much, but not all, of the comorbidity between depression and CD, and the risk factors involved are both environmental and genetic in origin. However, the shared risk-factor hypothesis cannot fully explain the longitudinal course of DCD, whereby CD precedes depression.

One disorder creating increased risk for another

Since antisocial behaviour tends to precede depressive symptoms, is it possible that CD is itself a risk factor for depression? The evidence cited by Zoccolillo (1992) to suggest that depression is part of CD can also be used to support this different hypothesis (Angold et al. 1999). His main arguments were as follows. The more severe the antisocial behaviour in adults, the greater the likelihood of comorbidity with non-antisocial disorders; CD only predicts adult affective disturbance in individuals who have persistent antisocial behaviour in adulthood; and CD is associated with an earlier onset of affective disturbances.

There are several possible mechanisms that could explain these links. Aggressive and conduct-disordered children often interpret others as hostile, are rejected by their peers, fail at school, are told they are bad, and often get into trouble with authority. Thus it is possible to understand how the presence of CD can result in these children becoming unhappy.

There has been some subsequent research with children and adolescents which has provided some indirect

evidence to support the idea that CD is a risk factor for depression. The Oregon Youth Study found that over a two-year period, boys with conduct problems showed a significant increase in depressive symptoms, whereas boys with depressive symptoms did not show a similar rise in conduct problems (Capaldi 1992). Also, epidemiological studies have shown that externalizing disorders in adolescence predict both internalizing and externalizing disorders, whereas internalizing disorders only predict internalizing disorders (e.g. Feehan et al. 1993; Ferdinand and Verhulst 1995).

However, the structural equation model by Fergusson et al. (1996a) found no evidence for a direct causal pathway between CD and depression. Therefore, further research is required in order to establish a definitive causal link.

Nosological distinctiveness of the comorbid condition

The last possible explanation for actual comorbidity is that the comorbid condition is not simply a co-occurrence of two separate disorders, but represents a meaningfully different condition that is distinctive from the two disorders when they occur separately.

Rutter (1997) has argued that there has been a reluctance to consider disorders in terms of their conceptual meanings, which has been exacerbated by the insistence of DSM-IV that comorbid patterns should not be separately recognized. He suggests that DCD is an example of a comorbid pattern of disorders which may be meaningfully distinctive. However, separate diagnostic categories for all co-occurring disorders would create difficulties in classification systems, and too many fine subdivisions may be clinically meaningless. Therefore, in order for a diagnostic category to be useful it must be shown to be valid with its own set of correlates. DCD has been listed in the ICD-10 classification system as a subdivision of CD, although it is acknowledged that more research is required for this category.

What evidence is there to suggest that DCD is a distinct condition from either depressive disorder or CD alone? A number of epidemiological studies found that the mixed condition has a worse outcome than either disorder alone. Marmorstein and Iacono (2001) report that female adolescent twins with both disorders were more likely to have particularly severe problems in some domains such as substance dependence and negative school events. In the Ontario Child Health Study, adolescents with depression and comorbid CD were more likely to abuse alcohol at four-year follow-up than those with either disorder alone (Fleming et al. 1993). Capaldi (1992) found that boys with both conduct problems and depressive symptoms were more likely to continue to have difficulties at two-year follow-up than boys with either conduct problems or depressive symptoms alone. Similarly, Verhulst and Ende (1993) compared anxious/depressed children to those with conduct problems and a mixed group, and again found that the mixed group had the worst outcome at six-year follow-up. In the Montreal School Study, Ledingham and Schwartzman (1984) found that children who were both aggressive and withdrawn did worse academically than those who were only aggressive or withdrawn.

Other studies have compared the independent correlates of either depression or CD alone to the comorbid condition.

DEPRESSIVE DISORDER COMPARED WITH DEPRESSIVE CONDUCT DISORDER

There is further evidence available to suggest that the comorbid pattern in childhood and adolescence does differ from pure depressive disorder on numerous different correlates. Depression has been shown to occur earlier in the presence of CD – the Dunedin epidemiological study in New Zealand found most cases of depression at 11 years had CD, compared to a third at 15 years, and only 7% at 18 years (Anderson et al. 1987; McGee et al. 1990; Feehan et al. 1994). In another epidemiological study, Lewinsohn et al. (1995a) found that depression comorbid with disruptive disorders had a significantly worse outcome in terms of global functioning and academic problems than did depression alone, but there was no difference between the groups for physical symptoms, and conflict with parents.

Clinical studies have found that, compared with depression alone, DCD has a worse short-term outcome (Goodyer et al. 1997a; Harrington et al. 1991; Puig-Antich 1982); results in lower social competence (Renouf et al. 1997; Riley et al. 1998); is associated with more adverse psychosocial circumstances (Simic and Fombonne 2001) and higher levels of critical expressed emotion in families (Asarnow et al. 1994); and is more likely to be associated with alcohol and other substance misuse, especially in girls (King et al. 1996). Alternatively, it has also been associated with less fatigue (Marriage et al. 1986; Puig-Antich et al. 1989) and less anxiety (Meller and Borchardt 1996; Simic and Fombonne 2001). Other studies have not shown any differences between the two groups with respect to cognitive distortions and depressed or angry affect (Kempton et al. 1994; Sanders et al. 1992).

With regard to duration of symptoms and severity of depression, the evidence is conflicting. Marriage et al. (1986) found that depression associated with CD lasted longer than in the single disorder alone. However, Kovacs et al. (1997b) did not find that externalizing disorder predicted duration of depression, but they did find an association with dysthymia. There has been some evidence to suggest that the depression associated with behaviour disorders is more severe (Carlson and Cantwell 1980), but other studies have either found no difference in severity of

depressive symptoms (Kovacs et al. 1988), or found fewer depressive symptoms (Simic and Fombonne 2001).

There have been few treatment studies comparing depression with DCD. One study reported that DCD had a higher response to placebo than depression alone (Hughes et al. 1990), but another study reported that a history of CD in depressed women had no effect on response to treatment (Rowe et al. 1996). Thus little is currently known about the treatment implications of the comorbid disorder.

Evidence for the intergenerational transmission of DCD is also conflicting. One study has found less depression in relatives of children with DCD suggesting that this may be a less familial subtype of depression (Puig-Antich et al. 1989). However, other family-history studies have found no difference in rates of depression in relatives of children and adolescents with either depression or DCD, but have found an increased prevalence of antisocial personality disorder in relatives of probands with the comorbid disorder (e.g. Kovacs et al. 1997a; Williamson et al. 1995).

Mood disorders have been shown to be associated with a particularly high risk of deliberate self-harm compared with other single disorders (e.g. Fergusson and Lynskey 1995). In addition, comorbidity is generally associated with a high risk of deliberate self-harm (e.g. Gould et al. 1998). Interestingly, there is evidence to suggest that the risk is higher still in co-occurring depression and CD. For example, in a large longitudinal study of comorbidity in adolescents, Lewinsohn et al. (1995a) found that the presence of a second disorder substantially increased the suicide attempt rate compared to the rate for those with a single disorder, but the combination of depression and disruptive behaviour made for a particularly 'lethal' mix. However, although the number of attempts in depression comorbid with disruptive disorders was significantly different from disruptive disorders alone, the difference between pure depression and the mixed condition did not reach significance. Nevertheless, the risk was still considerably elevated. Kovacs et al. (1993) found that affective disorders were significantly associated with higher rates of suicidal behaviours compared to non-depressive disorders, but if the affective disorder was comorbid with conduct and/or substance use disorder, the risk of suicide attempts increased even further (22% of children with an affective disorder had attempted suicide, versus 45% of those with the mixed disorder). Likewise, a longitudinal study by Fombonne et al. (2001a) found that their group of children and adolescents with DCD had higher rates of suicidal behaviour when followed into adulthood compared with the group with depression alone. However, not all studies have found this increased risk – in a retrospective study, Harrington et al. (1991) did not find any difference in suicidal ideation between children with depression alone and those with comorbid CD, although actual attempts were not measured.

With regard to completed suicide, affective disorder has generally been found to be the most important predictor (e.g. Groholt *et al.* 1998). In a large case–control study of suicides under the age of 20 years, Shaffer *et al.* (1996) found that mood disorder alone or in combination with disruptive and/or substance misuse disorders accounted for half of all subjects who committed suicide, and there was little difference between a mood disorder in isolation or comorbid with a disruptive disorder (mood disorder alone, 15%; mood and disruptive disorder, 13%; mood, disruptive and substance misuse disorders, 16%). Thus the risk of suicide was equally high with depression alone or in the comorbid disorder. However, in another case–control study, Brent *et al.* (1993) found that although major depression was the most significant risk factor for suicide (odds ratio 27.0), the risk was far less with an affective disorder and comorbid CD (odds ratio 2.5). In contrast, the more recent longitudinal study by Fombonne *et al.* (2001a) found that the annual incidence rate of suicide was substantially greater in the comorbid group, compared with the group with depression alone (261.4 per 100,000 versus 32.5 per 100,000). Therefore, there is some evidence to suggest that the risk of suicide is at least as great, if not greater for adolescents with DCD, compared to those with depression alone.

Outcome studies in adults suggest there may be a meaningful distinction between depression with and without CD, although findings have been conflicting with regard to the precise nature of these differences. One longitudinal study reported that the comorbid pattern carries a lower risk of recurrence of MD in adult life and a lower risk of attempted suicide, but a higher risk of personality disorder and criminality in adulthood (Harrington *et al.* 1991, 1994, 1996). Therefore, these adult outcomes suggest that the mixed group behaves more like pure CD than depression. However, the more recent findings of Fombonne *et al.* (2001a,b) have been largely contradictory, suggesting that the risk of depressive recurrence is similar in both groups, but the risk of suicide and attempted suicide is higher in DCD. A similarly elevated risk of personality disorder and criminality was found in the comorbid group. A cross-sectional study of depressed women (Rowe *et al.* 1996) also did not find a difference in the course of depression in those with a history of CD.

In summary, there is growing evidence that DCD is a different condition from depression alone on a number of correlates, although similarities remain between the two groups. Of particular importance is the finding from several studies that the risk of deliberate self-harm may be significantly elevated in these adolescents, and there is some evidence to suggest that the actual risk of suicide is at least as great, if not greater in DCD, compared with depression alone. In addition, studies have found worse outcomes on numerous other correlates both in the short- and long-term for DCD, thus indicating that this condition may have an overall worse prognosis than depression without conduct disorder.

CONDUCT DISORDER COMPARED WITH DEPRESSIVE CONDUCT DISORDER

Several epidemiological studies have found worse outcomes for the mixed condition than for CD alone (e.g. Capaldi 1992; Verhulst and Ende 1993). In the Ontario Child Health Study, Fleming *et al.* (1993) found that, at four-year follow up, adolescents with depression and comorbid CD had higher rates of MD, dysthymia, anxiety, as well as alcohol abuse and dependence than for CD alone, although levels of drug abuse were similar. However, a more recent epidemiological study reported the risk of substance dependency was greater in the mixed group, as was the risk of negative school events, and an inability to experience positive emotions (Marmorstein and Iacono 2001). Lewinsohn *et al.* (1995a) found that adolescents with comorbid depression and disruptive disorder had significantly worse outcomes for global functioning and suicide attempts than for disruptive disorder alone, but there was no difference between the groups for academic problems, conflict with parents and physical symptoms.

With regard to clinical studies, the data are sparse and contradictory. Riggs *et al.* (1995) studied 99 delinquent adolescent boys, all of whom had conduct and substance-use disorders, and 21 had MD and/or dysthymia. They found that the depressed boys were more likely to have attention deficit hyperactivity disorder, post-traumatic stress disorder, and anxiety disorders, compared with non-depressed boys, and they were more likely to develop conduct symptoms earlier. In addition, depressed boys had more substance-dependence diagnoses than the boys who were not depressed. Chiles *et al.* (1980) also found that depressed delinquents were more likely to have increased substance use compared to delinquents without depression, as well as a family history of depression. In contrast, a study of substance abusing juvenile offenders, found that comorbid substance misuse with externalizing disorders had the worst outcome, but the presence of an internalizing disorder had a buffering effect on criminal activity and drug use (Randall *et al.* 1999). With regard to other correlates, children and adolescents with CD have also been found to have lower levels of cognitive distortions and depressed affect, and higher levels of angry affect compared to those with depression and CD (Kempton *et al.* 1994; Sanders *et al.* 1992). Simic and Fombonne (2001) found that children and adolescents with DCD were more likely to have a history of abuse and loss, were less likely to be aggressive to others, but were more likely to have higher rates of self injurious behaviour than those with CD alone.

Other studies have similarly found high rates of deliberate self-harm in the mixed disorder compared to CD alone. Kovacs *et al.* (1993), in their longitudinal study, found that 45% of the mixed group attempted suicide compared to 10% of the group who were only conduct disordered. In the epidemiological study by Lewinsohn *et al.* (1995a), the risk of a suicide attempt was low with a disruptive disorder alone but increased substantially in the presence of a comorbid depressive disorder. Borst *et al.* (1991) investigated adolescent psychiatric inpatients and found that only 12% of the pure conduct-disordered group attempted suicide versus 55% of the mixed group, which was a similar result to that of the pure affective-disordered group (51%). These studies have also found an increased rate of suicide attempts in girls compared to boys, although the Lewinsohn *et al.* (1995a) study did not find this specific association for the mixed disorder.

With regard to completed suicide, the study by Shaffer *et al.* (1996) again found a higher incidence of suicide in adolescents with a comorbid mood and disruptive disorder compared to a disruptive disorder alone (13% versus 7%). Substance or alcohol abuse was also found to be a specific risk factor for boys but not girls. However, Brent *et al.* (1993) found that, although CD was a significant risk factor for suicide, its effect was greater in the *absence* of affective disorder, indicating that the two disorders are different, but the risk for suicide was lower for the comorbid condition. Renaud *et al.* (1999) compared adolescent suicide completers with community controls, all of whom had disruptive disorders. They did not find that comorbid mood disorder predicted suicide risk, however, a family history of mood disorder was significant, as was a current and family history of substance abuse, and a past history of deliberate self-harm. There was also a trend towards increased involvement with legal/disciplinary procedures in the suicide completers.

Other studies have found that there is no distinction between pure CD and the comorbid condition in terms of low levels of social competence (Renouf *et al.* 1997), adult outcomes of depression and criminality as well as a family history of crime (Harrington 1994b), and various other correlates (Steinhausen and Reitzle 1996; Zoccolillo 1992).

In summary, although there are fewer studies comparing the correlates of pure conduct disorder to the mixed disorder than for depression, there is evidence to suggest that the conditions are meaningfully different. The comorbid condition appears to have a worse prognosis than pure CD on a number of correlates, especially for deliberate self-harm, although, the evidence for suicide risk is conflicting. There is also evidence that the comorbid disorder has a higher risk of alcohol misuse, and a number of studies also suggest that the risk of substance misuse is greater. In addition, this group of adolescents is more likely to have additional comorbidity, poorer global functioning and an earlier onset of conduct symptoms, but display less aggression than adolescents with conduct problems alone. However, as with depression, similarities

between the two groups have also been found, for example, with regards to levels of social competence, adult outcomes of depression and crime, and family history of criminality and antisocial personality disorder.

Thus, overall there is growing evidence to show that comorbid depression and CD is a different condition from either disorder alone. Of particular significance are studies showing that each disorder begins earlier in the comorbid condition, which has been associated with a worse prognosis for conduct disorder (Lahey *et al.* 1999). The comorbid disorder also appears to have a worse outcome, in terms of poorer global functioning, a higher risk of deliberate self-harm, and alcohol and other substance misuse. This association is unsurprising in view of the fact that both depression and CD have been independently associated with substance misuse disorders (e.g. Boyle and Offord 1991; Rohde *et al.* 1996).

Further studies are required to substantiate the idea that depression comorbid with CD is a nosologically separate condition. In particular, longitudinal studies are needed which compare the correlates and outcomes of the individual disorders and the mixed condition.

CLINICAL IMPLICATIONS

An increased understanding of the relationship between depression and CD and the aetiological mechanisms involved is important in terms of recognizing depressive symptoms and informing treatment and management. As can be seen from the above review, this relationship is complex and requires a multidimensional approach to both assessment and treatment.

Implications for diagnosis

From the preceding discussion of causal mechanisms, it can be seen that there is still much uncertainty regarding the relationship between the two disorders. It is unclear at present whether depression is part of the natural history of CD as in Zoccolillo's 'disorder of multiple dysfunction' (Zoccolillo 1992); whether it should be classified as a subtype of CD as it currently appears in ICD-10; whether they should still be classified as two separate disorders which remain distinct as in DSM-IV; or whether there is sufficient evidence for a totally separate diagnostic category with its own natural history. Although the arguments over classification may appear largely academic, they are important as they can have an influence on further management.

Angold *et al.* (1999) illustrate this by their argument that perhaps depression with CD should in fact be a subcategory of depression rather than CD. They suggest that categorizing depression as a subtype of CD results in focusing attention where there exist fewer differences between the comorbid and non-comorbid disorder (i.e. conduct disorder symptoms); whereas if depression with comorbid conduct disorder were regarded as a subtype of depression, this would emphasize the relationship with affective disorder and focus attention on the differences between pure depression and its comorbid form. This approach may then result in more emphasis being placed on the treatment of the depressive disorder, and in particular, its relationship with suicidality, which is known to be more commonly associated with affective, rather than conduct, disorder.

Regardless of which classification system is currently used, the important issue for the clinician is to recognize the presence of affective disorder in disruptive youths, and consider the implications for outcome and management.

Assessment and engagement

As young people with disturbed behaviour often have a co-occurring depressive disorder, there should always be a high index of suspicion with regard to making this diagnosis. However, there are a number of reasons why depression may not be recognized in this group. Conduct problems tend to arise before the onset of depression, so symptoms which may be due to a depressive illness, such as irritability, could be attributed to the CD. These adolescents have poor interpersonal relationships generally and are likely to lack any confiding relationships, and thus others may not be aware of their problems. Depression is also associated with cognitive deficits in early childhood (e.g. Os et al. 1997) which, combined with the trajectory of school failure and learning problems seen in CD, will make the identification and verbal expression of feelings and experiences particularly difficult for these young people.

Engagement is often problematic, as the overt manifestation of adolescent depression is often hostility, boredom and irritability, which may mask the underlying mood disorder and impede diagnosis and engagement. Therefore, the assessment may have to occur over a number of sessions. It is vital to ensure that time is spent with the adolescent alone, as well as with parents or carers, particularly as there is likely to be a negative parent/child relationship, and the agreement between parents and child is generally low on depressive symptoms. Children usually give a better account of internalizing symptoms, whereas parents are more aware of overt behaviour (e.g. Barrett et al. 1991). In addition to interviewing the adolescent and parents or carers, it is important to obtain information from other sources such as teachers and social workers. As adolescents with comorbid depression and disruptive disorder have significantly higher deficits in global functioning compared with either disorder

alone (Lewinsohn et al. 1995a), a detailed assessment of the level of functioning in a variety of different settings is important.

A detailed assessment of the family environment is also required as there is likely to be a high level of critical expressed emotion (Asarnow et al. 1994), and negative and conflictual parenting (Reiss et al. 1995); and abuse is more likely than for adolescents who have conduct problems alone (Simic and Fombonne 2001). Inconsistent parenting and power-assertive punishment have also been shown to predict persistent depressive symptoms in children (Cohen et al. 1990). Differing environmental experiences between siblings are important contributory risk factors which continue to maintain both depressive and conduct symptoms (O'Connor et al. 1998), and the differential parenting of siblings may be one cause of this. Parental depression needs to be considered (Kovacs et al. 1997a; Williamson et al. 1995), as this may be adversely affecting the ability to parent.

Within the school setting, the adolescent with both depression and conduct problems will have academic problems that are likely to be as serious as those encountered with children with disruptive disorder alone (Lewinsohn et al. 1995a), if not more so, than either disorder alone (Ledingham and Schwartzman 1984). Therefore an adequate assessment of educational ability and behaviour in school is necessary, together with information about social competence and the peer group, particularly as there is evidence that poor friendships are associated with persistence of depression (Goodyer et al. 1997b).

Although each individual disorder is associated with substance misuse, there is some evidence that this risk is even higher in comorbid depression and conduct disorder, particularly for alcohol misuse, where girls may be at higher risk of misuse than boys (Riggs et al. 1995; King et al. 1996). Recognizing concurrent substance misuse is important as it can complicate treatment, and is associated with persistent depression (Sanford et al. 1995), and an elevated risk of deliberate self-harm (Kovacs et al. 1993). In addition, girls with early-onset conduct disorder are already at risk of teenage pregnancy (Kovacs et al. 1994), but it is possible to speculate that the higher rate of substance misuse makes these girls even more vulnerable to early sexual experiences, which may lead to pregnancy and/or sexually transmitted diseases.

The available evidence suggests that adolescents with depression and CD may be far more vulnerable to suicide attempts than those with a single disorder (Kovacs et al. 1993; Lewinsohn et al. 1995a), and the risk of actual suicide may also be greater (Fombonne et al. 2001a) so assessing this risk adequately is vital. Longitudinal studies have shown that adolescents suffering from depression remain at a protracted risk of suicide for some time, and furthermore, suicidality itself serves as a risk factor for the development of depression (Flisher 1999). Any involvement with legal or disciplinary proceedings may also heighten the risk of suicide attempts (Renaud *et al.* 1999).

A review of depressive symptoms should exclude the possibility of a bipolar affective disorder or psychosis, particularly if there is concurrent substance misuse. Also, consideration should be given to a physical examination if there is a possibility that a physical disorder may have given rise to affective symptoms.

As it is often difficult to recognize depression in these adolescents, a rating scale such as the Beck Depression Inventory (Marton *et al.* 1991) or the Child Depression Inventory (Kovacs 1992) may be used to ascertain depressive symptoms. However, because of their low specificity, these rating scales are not useful for diagnosing clinical depression. They can be used to screen for symptoms, assess the severity of depressive symptoms, and monitor improvement. In addition, a mood diary can be kept by the young person to identify triggers for the depression and aid assessment and engagement.

TREATMENT

General issues

The initial management of depression will depend on the nature of the problems identified in the assessment. If the depression is mild and relatively uncomplicated, then a brief, supportive, non-specific intervention may be all that is required. These sessions may consist of education and general advice about depression to parents and the adolescent, as well as simple interventions, such as school liaison, if appropriate. Around a third of mild to moderately depressed adolescents will remit with this kind of initial management (Harrington *et al.* 1998).

However, treatment will be potentially more difficult in this group than in adolescents with pure depression, for many reasons. Factors shown to be related to response to psychotherapy include age of onset and severity of depression, comorbid psychiatric disorders, lack of support, parental psychopathology, family conflict, stressful life events, motivation and socio-economic status (AACAP 1998). Adolescents with both depression and CD will be adversely affected by a number of these factors: depressive symptoms tend to start early in this group; they are likely to come from dysfunctional families with adverse psychosocial circumstances; there is a high risk of antisocial personality disorder and depression in the parents; and comorbidity with a behaviour disorder is in itself is a risk factor for poor response to treatment. Depressive conduct disorder is also associated with an increased risk of comorbid alcohol and substance abuse which may further adversely affect response to treatment. Both parental psychopathology and familial conflict have been shown to not only predict a poor response to treatment, but also to

increase the risk of recurrence of depression (e.g. Warner *et al.* 1992).

As depressive symptoms tend to start earlier in this group and may be harder to detect, the depressive disorder may have already been prolonged with significant impairment. There may have already been several episodes of depression which have resulted in neurobiological and psychosocial 'scarring' or 'sensitization' to further episodes (Post *et al.* 1996; Rohde *et al.* 1994). The level of global functioning will be poor and the person is likely to have substantial academic problems. Lastly, there may be numerous suicidal attempts which will precipitate crises, and heighten anxiety of both carers and therapists.

Therefore, complex cases of persistent depression which do not resolve with a brief initial intervention are likely to require multimodal and intensive treatment, as there are likely to be numerous impairments and problems in the adolescent's life. Treatment also needs to be prolonged as there is a high risk of recurrence of juvenile depression (Harrington 1994a), particularly in the presence of suicidality (Flischer 1999), as well as a risk of a switch to a bipolar illness (Kovacs 1996). The treatment setting chosen and the frequency of sessions will depend on the severity of the depressive illness, psychosocial circumstances, and the ability of the young person's parents to engage in the treatment plan, and keep the individual in a safe environment. Education of the adolescent and family about the disorder is critical early on, as this can aid engagement and compliance. It can also help remove parental blame towards the adolescent and allow for a more supportive parent/child relationship.

A variety of combined therapeutic interventions is usually required.

Psychotherapy

Individual psychotherapeutic techniques can be useful for the initial treatment of mild-to-moderate depression, and although group psychotherapy has been used for the treatment of depression, it is not generally helpful in CD (Dischion *et al.* 1999). Of the individual therapies, cognitive–behavioural therapy (CBT) is the most frequently evaluated therapy in depression, and there have been a number of randomized controlled trials demonstrating its efficacy for depressive symptoms and mild depressive disorder (Harrington *et al.* 1998). It focuses on the depressed individual's distorted negative cognitions, such as overgeneralization and personalization, which are also present with comorbid CD, and attempts to challenge and restructure these. Although clinical studies have shown CBT to be effective in depressed adolescents in the short term (e.g. Wood *et al.* 1996), there has been a high rate of relapse on follow-up, which suggests the need for continuation treatment (see below). Cognitively based treatments have also been shown to reduce aggressive and antisocial behaviour in conduct-disordered children and adolescents (Kazdin 2001) and therefore this may be a useful treatment modality for the comorbid condition.

There is some evidence to suggest that interpersonal therapy (IPT) may be useful for the acute treatment of adolescent depression. IPT focuses on grief, transitions, and interpersonal roles and difficulties, which could be potentially useful in adolescents with comorbid CD, as they will have poorer social role functioning than those with depression alone (Renouf et al. 1997). One randomized controlled trial compared outcomes for IPT and clinical monitoring over a 12-week period, and found a significantly greater improvement in the group of adolescents receiving IPT (Mufson et al. 1999). There has also been one randomized controlled trial which has compared IPT with CBT and a waiting list control group in depressed adolescents (Rossello and Bernal 1999). Results showed that both IPT and CBT were effective in reducing depressive symptoms, but IPT was more effective in increasing self-esteem and social adaptation when compared to the control group. Therefore these preliminary studies show that IPT is a promising treatment for depression, and may be particularly useful in improving the poor social functioning seen in depressive conduct disorder.

Family interventions need to be considered in order to address the home environment, as this has been shown to have particularly high levels of critical expressed emotion in comorbid depression and CD (Asarnow et al. 1994). Parenting issues should be explored, as negative and conflictual parenting has been shown to be a prominent risk factor in both depression and conduct problems (Reiss et al. 1995), and differential treatment of siblings may be involved in the maintenance of both sets of symptoms. However, despite the strong association between family malfunction and adolescent depression, the results of early randomized controlled trials of family interventions have so far failed to find any significant benefit of family treatment (Harrington 2002), although there is some evidence from controlled studies that functional family therapy can improve family communication and interactions in difficult to treat adolescent populations, such as multiple offenders (Kazdin 2001). Likewise, multisystemic therapy is a family-based, multimodal intervention which has been shown to improve family functioning, behavioural problems, reduce alcohol and substance abuse and also reduce psychiatric symptomatology in youths with serious clinical problems (Henggeler 1999). Therefore, family interventions may be of some benefit in adolescents with the comorbid disorder, but further studies of family treatments in adolescent depression are needed, particularly targeting negative parenting.

Lastly, parental depression should be recognized and treated, but it can be difficult to persuade depressed parents to take up treatment for their own depressive illness (Brent et al. 1997).

Pharmacological treatment

If the depression is severe, or has not improved with psychotherapy interventions, antidepressant medication may be indicated. Selective serotonin reuptake inhibitors (SSRIs) are the antidepressants of choice because of their safety, side-effects profile, ease of use and recent evidence base. There have been three randomized controlled trials of SSRIs in depressed adolescents. Two studies found that fluoxetine was superior to placebo (Emslie et al. 1997, 2002), and one study reported that paroxetine demonstrated significantly greater improvement compared to both placebo and imipramine (Keller et al. 2001). Numerous placebo-controlled trials of the tricyclic antidepressants have not found them to be any more efficacious than placebo, despite evidence for their efficacy in adult depression (Hazell et al. 1995). SSRIs for under-18 year olds are under ongoing review by the Commission on Safety of Medicine (in England), reinforcing that medication is not a first-line treatment for childhood depressions, but may be indicated if the depression is severe.

Research on the pharmacological treatment of comorbid depression with CD is scant. One double-blind clinical trial compared the effects of imipramine and placebo in 31 prepubertal patients, and found that children with pure depression, or depression and anxiety, had a higher drug response rate and lower placebo response rate, when compared to children with depression and comorbid conduct problems (Hughes et al. 1990). In contrast, another small, uncontrolled study of 13 boys with depression and CD found that the depression abated in all 13 when they were treated with imipramine, and the conduct symptoms were seen to improve in 11 of these boys with the improvement of the depressive symptoms (Puig-Antich 1982). Also, Rowe et al. (1996) found that a history of CD in depressed women did not have an effect on response to treatment. None of the studies of the SSRIs in depressed adolescents examined the outcomes of comorbid behaviour disorder, therefore it is unclear at present what the effect of comorbidity may be on response to pharmacological treatment. However, in view of the relative efficacy of the SSRIs and their safer side-effect profile, compared to the tricyclic antidepressants, they remain the drugs of first choice.

Continuation treatment

Depression is a highly recurrent disorder, so continuation treatment is recommended for at least 6 months. There have been no randomized trials of continuation treatment in juvenile depression, but a non-randomized study (Kroll et al. 1996) suggests that monthly CBT sessions may be efficacious in preventing relapses of depression in adolescents. Adult studies have found that both psychotherapy and pharmacotherapy have been helpful in preventing relapses of MDD (AACAP 1998). At the end of the continuation phase, if maintenance treatment is not required, medication should be discontinued over a six-week period or more to avoid withdrawal effects (AACAP 1998).

Maintenance treatment

Once the patient has been asymptomatic for 6–12 months, consideration should be given as to whether maintenance treatment is required, particularly as MDD has also been shown to recur even after successful treatment (e.g. Wood *et al.* 1996). There are no published data regarding maintenance treatment in children and adolescents, but the available guidelines for adults have been used as a basis for recommendations in children and adolescents (AACAP 1998). It has been suggested that youths with two or three episodes of MD should receive maintenance treatment for at least 1 year. Patients with second episodes accompanied by psychosis, severe impairment, severe suicidality, and treatment resistance, as well as patients with more than three episodes, should be considered for longer treatment.

Other factors which need to be considered include willingness to comply with further treatment, the severity of the episode, chronicity, other comorbidity, environmental factors, and contraindications to treatment. In the case of DCD, there are likely to be numerous complicating environmental factors and additional comorbidity which will make the adolescent vulnerable to relapse, so the threshold for considering maintenance treatment should be low.

Compliance may be difficult to obtain over a prolonged period, so efforts should be made to explain the rationale for continuing treatment, and difficulties with treatment such as drug side effects should be explored.

Treatment–resistant depression

If there is treatment failure, consideration should be given to whether an adequate drug trial and dosage has been given, as well as an adequate duration of psychotherapy with a skilled therapist, who has been able to engage the patient. Other relevant factors which should be reviewed include lack of compliance, other comorbidity, especially substance abuse, medical illnesses, undetected bipolar illness, and chronic or severe life events, such as abuse or parental mental illness.

Where there has been a lack of response to an adequate trial of one SSRI, then current recommendations are a further trial of a different SSRI, on the grounds that the SSRIs are chemically distinct (Hughes *et al.* 1999). If the young person then fails to respond to a second SSRI, then another antidepressant with stronger noradrenergic action, such as venlafaxine, should be considered. Brent (2001) reported that in an open trial around 50% of those who failed to respond to an adequate trial with an SSRI responded to venlafaxine.

Risk management

The most important risk to address in adolescents with depression and conduct problems is that of deliberate self-harm. As the risk is particularly high in this group, the early recognition and effective treatment of depressive symptoms is important. If the risk of suicide is deemed to be especially high and the adolescent cannot be managed safely in the community, then an inpatient admission may need to be considered. If the adolescent remains in the community, an adequate safety plan should be discussed with the parents or carers.

During a risk assessment, the possibility of physical and sexual abuse has to be excluded because of their strong association with suicidal behaviour (Fergusson *et al.* 1996b). Other factors which need to be considered as they have been found to be associated with deliberate self harm, include being female, juvenile offending, police contact, substance use, school dropout, low self-esteem, socially disadvantaged or dysfunctional family circumstances, parental substance abuse or offending, marital conflict, compromised child-rearing, and high residential mobility (Fergusson *et al.* 1995). There is some evidence that depression may actually protect against aggression and criminal activity compared with youths with behaviour problems alone (Randall *et al.* 1999; Simic and Fombonne 2001). However, the risk of substance misuse may be increased and therefore this is an important risk factor to target because of its strong association with suicidality.

COMORBIDITY BETWEEN BIPOLAR AFFECTIVE DISORDER AND CONDUCT DISORDER

Prevalence

Bipolar affective disorder (BAD) is generally considered to be an uncommon disorder in children and adolescents. A recent community survey of adolescents found a lifetime prevalence rate of approximately 1%. However, this figure encompassed a broad definition of mania, and the rate of classical mania was much lower, being only 0.1% (Lewinsohn *et al.* 1995b). When a subgroup of adolescents with MD were then followed into adulthood, less than 1% went on to develop mania (Lewinsohn *et al.* 2002), but figures far higher than this have been reported in clinical inpatient samples. In a 15-year follow-up study of young people hospitalized for depression, Goldberg *et al.* (2001) reported that 19% cases went on to develop mania, and 27% developed hypomania. Those with a psychotic depression or a family history of BAD where more at risk of switching to a bipolar illness.

A number of studies have reported an elevated risk for conduct disorder among children with mania. For example, Kovacs and Pollack (1995) found a 69% rate of conduct disorder in a referred sample of youths with mania. In a larger study, Biederman *et al.* (1999) reported that, of 186 children and adolescents with mania and of 192 with conduct disorder, 76 satisfied criteria for both conduct disorder and mania, representing 40% of youths with conduct disorder and 41% of youths with mania, respectively. These studies indicate that a high proportion of youths with conduct problems will also go on to develop manic symptoms. Further research is required to substantiate these findings, as it unlikely that rates this high are routinely seen in clinical practice. Nevertheless, BAD has been under-diagnosed in the past (AACAP 1997) and these findings suggest that it may be more prevalent than previously thought in clinical samples.

Diagnostic issues

Children and adolescents with mania frequently present with symptoms that are considered atypical (Bowring and Kovacs 1992), and irritability and belligerence are more common symptoms than euphoria. Thus, these presenting features can easily be misdiagnosed as purely conduct problems. Typical examples of reckless behaviour may include fighting, dangerous play, inappropriate sexualized activity, and school failure. Juvenile-onset mania may be particularly explosive and disorganized, resulting in more contact with the police (McGlashan 1988) for behaviours such as burglary, stealing and vandalism, as well as an increased likelihood of school suspensions (Kovacs and Pollack 1995).

Adolescents with mania frequently have complicated presentations including psychotic symptoms, labile moods with mixed manic and depressive symptoms, and severe deterioration in their behaviour (AACAP 1997). These varying presentations may have also contributed to the under-diagnosis of BAD in teenagers. For example, in the study by Lewinsohn *et al.* (1995b) only one of the 18 adolescents with BAD had been treated with lithium, although more than half had received some form of mental health treatment.

The diagnosis of mania in children and adolescents remains controversial, as there is much overlap between symptoms of mania and other childhood disorders. For example, the symptoms of overactivity and inattention are also cardinal symptoms of attention deficit hyperactivity disorder; flight of ideas and rapid speech may be seen in language disorders; and irritability is a symptom of oppositional defiant disorder, depression and anxiety. It has been suggested that there is a group of seriously emotionally disturbed children who meet the criteria of mania by virtue of their problems with irritability, emotional lability, increased energy and reckless behaviours. These symptoms often have a chronic and sometimes rapidly fluctuating course, which may represent the child's

baseline state rather than the classical episodic course usually seen in adults (AACAP 1997). This idea was substantiated in the epidemiological study by Lewinsohn *et al.* (1995b, 2002), who reported that a group of adolescents with subthreshold symptoms also exhibited high levels of impairment and comorbidity that were often comparable with that of subjects with BAD and MD. These findings provide some support for a bipolar spectrum and suggest that youngsters with subthreshold symptoms also need to be taken seriously. Therefore, BAD in children and adolescents may present with two different phenotypes: the classical phenotype which consists of clearly delineated episodes of mania, hypomania and depression, and a broader phenotype that encompasses more heterogeneity, and includes children who do not quite meet the criteria but are impaired by symptoms of mood instability (Nottelman *et al.* 2001). This latter group needs to be considered when assessing the complex clinical picture presented by youths with comorbid mood and behaviour problems.

Risk factors associated with developing bipolar I disorder, or mania, in adolescents and adults with MD include early-onset depression, depression with psychomotor retardation or psychosis, family history of bipolar disorder or heavy loading for mood disorders, and pharmacologically induced mania. In addition, risk factors for converting to the milder bipolar II disorder (MD and hypomania) in depressed adults include early-onset depression, atypical depression, mood lability, comorbid substance abuse, and high rates of psychosocial problems (Birhamer *et al.* 1996). It is notable that many of these risk factors are often associated with depressive conduct disorder and thus the index of suspicion for manic or hypomanic symptoms needs to be high in this group.

Associated clinical features

Compared with adults, adolescents with BAD may have a more prolonged early course and be less responsive to treatment (McGlashan 1988; Strober *et al.* 1995). There is also evidence to suggest that the comorbid condition may be more severe than either disorder alone. Although Biederman *et al.* (1999) found that symptoms were qualitatively similar in the comorbid group compared to youths with mania or CD alone, they were more severe than the symptoms of those with only one disorder. Kovacs and Pollock (1995) also found that youngsters with comorbid CD and BAD had a somewhat worse clinical course than those with bipolar disorder alone, particularly with regard to school suspensions, and were likely to have had a pre-existing disruptive disorder. The comorbid group also had higher rates of paternal substance abuse and antisocial personality disorder, although there was more likely to be a history of maternal mania in the bipolar group. The rates of maternal history of depression was the same for both groups. A more recent longitudinal study of inpatients with psychotic BAD (Carlson *et al.* 2002) reported that additional childhood psychopathology predicted a poorer outcome at 2-year follow-up.

Some studies have reported that BAD is associated with an increased risk of suicide. For example, Brent *et al.* (1993) found that a bipolar mixed state was associated with completed suicide in adolescents and was the most significant psychiatric risk factor after MD. Lewinsohn *et al.* (1995b) reported that a greater proportion of bipolar subjects attempted suicide compared to subjects with MD, and subthreshold bipolar cases were likewise associated with an elevated risk for suicide attempts. Studies have not examined the risk of suicidality in comorbid mania and CD, although the Brent *et al.* (1993) study found that the risk of suicide was greater with CD alone than when comorbid with affective disorder, which also included a bipolar mixed state group.

With regard to other comorbidity, high rates of substance abuse have been found in some samples of youths with BAD which may affect treatment and course adversely (AACAP 1997). In addition, the above Brent *et al.* (1993) study showed that the combination of an affective disorder with substance abuse results in a significantly elevated risk of completed suicide.

Treatment

As with DCD, treatment needs to be multimodal, combining psychosocial interventions with medication. Early recognition of manic symptoms in youths with conduct problems is important, and adolescents with subthreshold symptoms also need to be identified for treatment as the level of impairment in these cases can be just as great. There should be a high index of suspicion for manic symptoms in all youths with CD, particularly if there has been a marked deterioration in functioning associated with either mood or psychotic symptoms.

With regard to pharmacological treatment, there has only been one double-blind, placebo-controlled trial for the treatment of child and adolescent mania (Geller and Luby 1997). This study of adolescents with bipolar disorder and substance abuse found that lithium was more effective than placebo. Other studies have found that lithium can also be effective in aggressive children with CD (e.g. Campbell *et al.* 1995), although Rifkin *et al.* (1997) were not able to replicate this finding in adolescents with CD. Therefore, there is some evidence to suggest that lithium may be useful for both manic and conduct symptoms. However, lithium is not a drug that should be given to either chaotic families or those who are not able to keep regular appointments for the monitoring of lithium levels and renal and thyroid function. As it is likely that adolescents with comorbid CD will come from chaotic backgrounds, a careful evaluation of the risks of prescribing lithium is necessary. In particular, lithium is toxic in overdose so an assessment of suicide risk in mandatory, as well

as the ability of parents to provide a safe environment, particularly as the comorbid condition is associated with paternal substance abuse and antisocial personality disorder. It is also possible that a parent has a bipolar illness which has not been recognized.

Uncontrolled studies have suggested that anticonvulsants such as carbamazepine and valproate may be useful as mood stabilizers in the treatment of adolescents (Himmelhoch and Garfinkel 1986; West *et al.* 1994). Benzodiazepines may be useful adjuncts to antimanic agents for patients with acute mania, but their long-term use should be discouraged, given the lack of supporting research in children and adolescents, and potential dependency problems. Again there has been no research to examine the efficacy of neuroleptics in this age group, but they have been shown to be useful in adults for the treatment of acute mania. There is little evidence in adults that neuroleptics by themselves should be used for maintenance treatment (APA 1994). Careful monitoring is necessary because of their side-effect profile, and, in addition, the combination of lithium and neuroleptics has been associated with an increased risk of extrapyramidal side-effects and neurotoxicity (Alessi *et al.* 1994). Atypical antipsychotic agents such as clozapine may also have mood-stabilizing effects (APA 1994). Stimulants have been reported to both worsen (Koehler-Troy *et al.* 1986) and improve (Max *et al.* 1995) bipolar symptoms, so they should be used with caution. Antidepressants may induce mania and/or rapid cycling in bipolar patients, so these should be used only as adjuncts to antimanic therapy for persistent depressive symptoms.

Treatment with a mood stabilizer needs to be long-term as the relapse rate is high in early-onset bipolar disorder. Strober *et al.* (1990) reported a 90% relapse rate in adolescents who were non-compliant with their lithium treatment. However, as discussed earlier, long-term maintenance medication may be difficult to achieve in these chaotic adolescents, and also there are significant side effects associated with long-term use, such as thyroid and renal dysfunction.

As with DCD, psychosocial interventions are necessary as part of an integrated multimodal treatment approach. Particular issues to consider in this comorbid group of adolescents are the extent of school problems, and family history of psychiatric disorder, especially paternal substance abuse. Any comorbid substance abuse should be addressed as this will interfere with treatment and also substantially increase the risk of suicide.

In summary, adolescents who present with conduct problems and mood instability may be at risk of developing BAD, particularly if there is a history of severe depression and/or a family history of BAD. Subthreshold cases need to be taken seriously as these are likely to be significantly impaired. There is also evidence to suggest that the comorbid group of adolescents may have a more severe form of BAD than those without CD, so early treatment and intervention is warranted. However, treatment may be more difficult in these individuals, and a thorough assessment of risks and benefits is required before commencing lithium to ensure there will be compliance with monitoring and safe usage.

CONCLUSIONS AND FUTURE DIRECTIONS

Affective disorder is a common problem in the forensic adolescent population, and is associated with a high degree of morbidity. There are implications for service provision at various stages, namely in terms of prevention, early intervention, and treatment. As there is some evidence to suggest that CD tends to precede depression, early intervention with conduct-disordered youngsters may have a preventive role in the development of depression. The best established risk factors for depressive disorder in young people are earlier depressive symptoms and a family history of depression, and there is evidence that targeted interventions with these youths is helpful in reducing symptoms and preventing depressive disorder (Harrington 2002). In addition, children with early-onset CD are at a particularly high risk of developing depression and have a poorer prognosis.

Early detection and intervention is important as there is evidence to suggest that adolescents with comorbid conduct and affective disorder may be at risk of a worse outcome, compared with each single disorder alone. Subthreshold cases of BAD have been shown to have equally poor outcomes, so these also need to be detected and treated. However, young people with psychiatric disorders have a low rate of service utilization (Fergusson and Lynskey 1995), although they are more likely to access services if they have an externalizing disorder (Fergusson and Lynskey 1995), or comorbidity (Lewinsohn et al. 1995a). Therefore, adolescents coming into contact with the juvenile justice system who have an affective disorder may not have had any contact with clinical services, and thus the index of suspicion for detecting such a disorder needs to be high in this population. Clinicians must be aware of the fact that CD will often precede affective disorder and thus the depressive symptoms may be masked by conduct symptoms. In addition this group of young people is difficult to engage, and treatment of affective symptoms is more challenging if there are comorbid conduct symptoms. Treatment will also need to be maintained for over a long period if it is to be effective and also prevent relapse. Of particular importance is the risk of deliberate self-harm which is very high in this comorbid group and needs to be frequently assessed.

Therefore the assessment and treatment of adolescents with comorbid affective and conduct disorder is challenging and intensive, but if this group of young people is left undetected and untreated, they are likely to suffer a high level of continuing morbidity and impairment, which has implications for future costs to health services.

Research in the area of comorbidity has only recently begun to develop, so many questions remain unanswered. Longitudinal studies are needed which can examine developmental issues, the correlates of comorbid affective and conduct disorder, its course and long-term outcomes. Epidemiological studies need to include comorbid conditions as these are often excluded. Likewise, clinical studies need to examine affective disorder which is comorbid with CD, particularly with regard to treatment outcomes. Further research can inform causal mechanisms which can then be used to address prevention and early intervention. Finally, research findings can assist with the complex issue of classification, which has implications for the treatment of comorbid affective and conduct disorder.

APPENDIX: CASE STUDIES

Vignette 1: Shared and correlated risk factors

Clare was a 15-year-old girl who was admitted to a paediatric ward following an overdose of 100 paracetamol tablets. On mental state examination she was severely depressed with biological symptoms and clear suicidal intent. The overdose was precipitated by an argument with her single mother regarding her mother's continuing drug habit. Following the argument, Clare's mother disappeared for several days and was subsequently admitted to a psychiatric ward after attempting to throw herself off a bridge. She had numerous admissions in the past for depression and drug misuse. Clare then went to stay with her older sister who blamed her for their mother's admission to hospital. This resulted in Clare taking the overdose which she had been planning for some time.

In the past, Clare had been seen in the child psychiatry department at the age of eight for behaviour problems. It was noted then that Clare's mother was hostile and critical of Clare and there were some concerns regarding possible neglect. However, her mother failed to attend appointments and there was insufficient evidence to place Clare on the child protection register at the time. There were frequent moves throughout Clare's childhood so she rarely had the opportunity to make friendships and she missed a great deal of schooling. In addition, she was suspended on numerous occasions for aggressive behaviour and cannabis use. She had also been cautioned by the police for theft and being drunk and disorderly. Clare never had contact with her father and there was no extended family.

Initially it proved very difficult to engage Clare and she was keen to leave the hospital as soon as possible. However, in view of her marked depressive symptoms, ongoing suicidal intent and lack of social support, it was not safe to discharge her. Eventually Clare agreed to a continuing admission in an adolescent unit. She was commenced on antidepressant medication and gradually began to build up a trusting relationship with staff on the unit. Attempts were made to invite Clare's mother for joint therapeutic sessions. Unfortunately she only attended one session during which she was very critical of Clare. Although this session greatly distressed Clare, she was able to make good progress with individual work as she was motivated and psychologically insightful.

After discharge Clare went into foster care although she tried to maintain an ongoing relationship with her mother. Unfortunately, each contact with her mother resulted in a further relapse of her depressive symptoms, although these episodes were not severe. Further management involved helping Clare separate from her mother, supporting her in a future move from foster care to her own flat, and encouraging her to continue with antidepressant medication.

This vignette illustrates a case where a variety of shared and correlated risk factors for depression and conduct disorder have accumulated to substantially increase the risk for both these disorders. Child rejection and neglect, along with poor social support and socio-economic disadvantage are all examples of shared risk factors. In addition, a parental history of depression results in a genetic risk for depression in a child, but this is also an environmentally mediated risk for conduct disorder; in other words, these are correlated risk factors for both disorders.

Vignette 2: Conduct disorder creates an increased risk for depression

A 13-year-old boy called Paul presented in the child psychiatry clinic with a recent deterioration in behaviour. He had a long history of conduct problems and had been seen previously in the clinic. Parents had made some limited progress at home in the past with behavioural strategies, but Paul was eventually excluded from school and now attended a residential school during the week for children with behavioural difficulties. He struggled academically and recently his work had deteriorated even further. Paul had found it hard to make new friends in his new school and had lost contact with friends in his previous school. He had become more withdrawn and irritable. At weekends Paul was spending all his time with a group of delinquent older boys and becoming involved with drug and alcohol abuse and petty crime. He used to enjoy football but was unable to play any more as a result of a serious leg injury following a road traffic accident in a stolen car. Parents were now totally exasperated with him and blamed Paul for all his current difficulties.

At interview Paul was hostile initially and did not wish to be seen on his own. However, during the family interview he became more engaged and revealed that he was currently being bullied at school. Paul had found the move to his new school very difficult, particularly as he was no longer able to participate in football which was one of the few things he used to do well. Paul had been unable to tell his parents his concerns as his relationship with them had broken down. He only had one confiding relationship which had been his previous key-worker at school. Unfortunately this person had left the post several months earlier and, owing to staff shortages, a new key-worker had not yet been allocated. This particular event appeared to be the main trigger for the deterioration in his behaviour. On mental state examination Paul showed signs of a moderate depressive illness which had been masked by his difficult behaviour.

Management consisted of liaison with school and further family meetings. School were made aware of the bullying and quickly allocated a key-worker with whom Paul already had begun to establish a relationship. Parents also improved their communication with school. During family meetings efforts were made to improve the parent's understanding of Paul's depression and how this had affected his behaviour. This resulted in a less blaming attitude towards Paul. The importance of regular structured activities at weekends was also discussed. This would limit the amount of time Paul had to spend with the older boys; avoid the possibility of Paul spending time on his own and ruminating over his depressive thoughts, and also encourage parents to spend time with him in order to improve their relationship. Despite his initial hostility, Paul became involved in the family sessions, particularly when his parent's attitude began to shift from one of blame to one of acceptance of his current difficulties. His behaviour began to improve, he became less irritable and withdrawn and began to develop new friendships at school.

This vignette demonstrates how a long history of conduct problems resulted in a trajectory of difficulties which accumulated to increase the risk of depression. In this case the symptoms of depression were masked by well-established behaviour problems and thus went unrecognized by parents and school. Instead, the overt symptoms of depression such as his irritability and social withdrawal were attributed to misbehaviour. Thus the opportunity to discuss the child's worries was missed, and his feelings of isolation and low mood were intensified.

REFERENCES

AACAP (American Academy of Child and Adolescent Psychiatry) 1997: Practice parameters for the assessment and treatment of children and adolescents with bipolar disorder. *Journal of the American Academy of Child and Adolescent Psychiatry* **36**: 138–57.

AACAP (American Academy of Child and Adolescent Psychiatry) 1998: Practice parameters for the assessment and treatment of children and adolescents with depressive disorders.

Journal of the American Academy of Child and Adolescent Psychiatry **37**(10 suppl.): 63S–83S.

Achenbach, T.M., Howell, C.T., Quay, H.C. *et al.* 1991: *National Survey of Problems and Competencies among 4- to 16-year-olds*. Monographs of the Society for Research in Child Development 56 (serial no. 225).

Alessi, N., Naylor, M.W., Ghaziuddin, M. *et al.* 1994: Update on lithium carbonate therapy in children and adolescents. *Journal of the American Academy of Child and Adolescent Psychiatry* **33**: 291–304.

Anderson, J.C., Williams, S., McGee, R. *et al.* 1987: DSM-III disorders in preadolescent children: prevalence in a large sample from the general population. *Archives of General Psychiatry* **44**: 69–76.

Angold, A., Messer, S.C., Stangl, D. *et al.* 1998: Perceived parental burden and service use for child and adolescent psychiatric disorders. *American Journal of Public Health* **88**: 75–80.

Angold, A., Costello, E.J. and Erkanli, E. 1999: Comorbidity. *Journal of Child Psychology and Psychiatry* **40**: 57–87.

APA (American Psychiatric Association) 1994: Practice guideline for the treatment of patients with bipolar disorder. *American Journal of Psychiatry* **151**(suppl.): 1–36.

Asarnow, J.R., Tompson, M., Burney, E. *et al.* 1994: Family-expressed emotion, childhood-onset depression, and childhood-onset schizophrenia spectrum disorders: is expressed emotion a nonspecific correlate of child psychopathology or a specific risk factor for depression? *Journal of Abnormal Child Psychology* **22**(2): 129–46.

Barrett, M.L., Berney, T.P., Bhate, S. *et al.* 1991: Diagnosing childhood depression: who should be interviewed – parent or child? The Newcastle Child Depression Project. *British Journal of Psychiatry* **159**(suppl. 11): 22–7.

Beardslee, W.R., Keller, M.B., Seifer, R. *et al.* 1996: Prediction of adolescent affective disorder: effects of prior parental affective disorders and child psychopathology. *Journal of the American Academy of Child and Adolescent Psychiatry* **35**: 279–88.

Biederman, J., Faraone, S., Mick, E. *et al.* 1995: Psychiatric comorbidity among referred juveniles with major depression: fact or artifact? *Journal of the American Academy of Child and Adolescent Psychiatry* **34**: 579–90.

Biederman, J., Faraone, S.V., Chu, M.P. *et al.* 1999: Further evidence of a bidirectional overlap between mania and conduct disorder in children. *Journal of the American Academy of Child and Adolescent Psychiatry* **38**: 468–76.

Birmaher, B., Ryan, N.D., Williamson, D.E. *et al.* 1996: Childhood and adolescent depression: a review of the past 10 years – II. *Journal of the American Academy of Child and Adolescent Psychiatry* **35**: 1575–83.

Borst, S.R., Noam, G.G. and Bartok, J.A. 1991: Adolescent suicidality: a clinical-developmental approach. *Journal of the American Academy of Child and Adolescent Psychiatry* **30**: 796–803.

Bowring, M.A. and Kovacs, M. 1992: Difficulties in diagnosing manic disorders among children and adolescents. *Journal of the American Academy of Child and Adolescent Psychiatry* **31**: 611–14.

Boyle, M.H. and Offord, D.R. 1991: Psychiatric disorder and substance use in adolescence. *Canadian Journal of Psychiatry* **36**: 699–705.

Brent, D.A., Perper, J.A., Moritz, G. *et al.* 1993: Psychiatric risk factors for adolescent suicide: a case–control study. *Journal of the American Academy of Child and Adolescent Psychiatry* **32**: 521–9.

Brent, D.A., Holder, D., Kolko, D. *et al.* 1997: A clinical psychotherapy trial for adolescent depression comparing cognitive, family, and supportive treatments. *Archives of General Psychiatry* **54**: 877–85.

Brent, D.A. 2001: The art of treating treatment resistant depression. In Villani, S. (ed.), *Scientific Proceedings of the 48th Annual Meeting of the American Academy of Child and Adolescent Psychiatry* (pp. 9). Washington: American Academy of Child and Adolescent Psychiatry.

Brown, G.W., Harris, T.O. and Eales, M.J. 1996: Social factors and comorbidity of depressive and anxiety disorders. *British Journal of Psychiatry* **168**(suppl. 30): 50–7.

Cadoret, R.J., Troughton, E., Merchant, L.M. *et al.* 1990: Early life psychosocial events and adult affective symptoms. In Robins, L.N. and Rutter, M. (eds), *Straight and Devious Pathways from Childhood to Adulthood*. Cambridge: Cambridge University Press, 300–13.

Campbell, M., Adams, P.B., Small, A.M. *et al.* 1995: Lithium in hospitalised aggressive children with conduct disorder: a double-blind and placebo-controlled study. *Journal of the American Academy of Child and Adolescent Psychiatry* **34**: 445–53.

Capaldi, D.M. 1992: Co-occurrence of conduct problems and depressive symptoms in early adolescent boys: II. A 2-year follow-up at grade 8. *Development and Psychopathy* **4**: 125–44.

Carlson, G.A. and Cantwell, D.P. 1980: Unmasking masked depression in children and adolescents. *American Journal of Psychiatry* **137**: 445–9.

Caron, C. and Rutter, M. 1991: Comorbidity in child psychopathology: concepts, issues and research strategies. *Journal of Child Psychology and Psychiatry* **32**: 1063–80.

Chiles, J.A., Miller, M.L. and Cox, G.B. 1980: Depression in an adolescent delinquent population. *Archives of General Psychiatry* **37**: 1179–84.

Cloniger, C.R., Sigvardsson, S., Bohman, M. *et al.* 1982: Predisposition to petty criminality in Swedish adoptees: II. Cross-sectional analysis of gene–environment interaction. *Archives of General Psychiatry* **39**: 1242–53.

Cohen, P., Brook, J.S., Cohen, J. *et al.* 1990: Common and uncommon pathways to adolescent psychopathology and problem behaviour. In Robins, L. and Rutter, M. (eds), *Straight and Devious Pathways from Childhood to Adulthood*. Cambridge: Cambridge University Press.

Dischion, T.J., McCord, J. and Poulin, F. 1999: When interventions harm: peer groups and problem behaviour. *American Psychologist* **54**: 755–64.

Emslie, G.J., Rush, A.J., Weinberg, W.A. *et al.* 1997: A double-blind randomised, placebo-controlled trial of fluoxetine in children and adolescents with depression. *Archives of General Psychiatry* **54**: 1031–7.

Emslie, G.J., Heiligenstein, J.H., Wagner, K.D. *et al.* 2002: Fluoxetine for acute treatment of depression in children and adolescents: a placebo-controlled, randomized clinical trial. *Journal of the American Academy of Child and Adolescent Psychiatry* **41**: 1205–15.

Feehan, M., McGee, R. and Williams, S.M. 1993: Mental health disorders from age 15 to age 18 years. *Journal of the American Academy of Child and Adolescent Psychiatry* **32**: 1118–26.

Feehan, M., McGee, R., NadaRaja, S. *et al.* 1994: DSM-IIIR disorders in New Zealand 18-year-olds. *Australian and New Zealand Journal of Psychiatry* **28**: 87–99.

Ferdinand, R.F. and Verhulst, F.C. 1995: Psychopathology from adolescence into young adulthood: an 8-year follow-up study. *American Journal of Psychiatry* **152**: 1586–94.

Fergusson, D.M. and Lynskey, M.T. 1995: Childhood circumstances, adolescent adjustment, and suicide attempts in a New Zealand birth cohort. *Journal of the American Academy of Child and Adolescent Psychiatry* **34**: 612–22.

Fergusson, D.M., Lynskey, M.T. and Horwood, L.J. 1996a: Origins of comorbidity between conduct and affective disorders. *Journal of the American Academy of Child and Adolescent Psychiatry* **35**: 451–60.

Fergusson, D.M., Lynskey, M.T. and Horwood, L.J. 1996b: Childhood sexual abuse and psychiatric disorder in young adulthood: I. Prevalence of sexual abuse and factors associated with sexual abuse. *Journal of the American Academy of Child and Adolescent Psychiatry* **35**: 1355–64.

Fleming, J.E., Boyle, M.H. and Offord, D.R. 1993: The outcome of adolescent depression in the Ontario Child Health Study follow-up. *Journal of the American Academy of Child and Adolescent Psychiatry* **32**: 28–33.

Flisher, A.J. 1999: Annotation: mood disorder in suicidal children and adolescents: recent developments. *Journal of Child Psychology and Psychiatry* **40**: 315–24.

Fombonne, E., Wostear, G., Cooper, V., Harrington, R. and Rutter, M. 2001a: The Maudsley long-term follow-up of child and adolescent depression. 2. Suicidality, criminality and social dysfunction in adulthood. *British Journal of Psychiatry* **179**: 218–23.

Fombonne, E., Wostear, G., Cooper, V., Harrington, R. and Rutter, M. 2001b: The Maudsley long-term follow-up of child and adolescent depression. 1. Psychiatric outcomes in adulthood. *British Journal of Psychiatry* **179**: 210–17.

Geller, B. and Luby, J. 1997: Child and adolescent bipolar disorder: a review of the past 10 years. *Journal of the American Academy of Child and Adolescent Psychiatry* **36**: 1168–76.

Goldberg, J.F., Harrow, M., Leon, A.C. *et al.* 2001: Risk for bipolar illness in patients initially hospitalized for unipolar depression. *American Journal of Psychiatry* **158**: 1265–1270.

Goodyer, I.M., Herbert, J., Secher, S.M. *et al.* 1997a: Short-term outcome of major depression: I. Comorbidity and severity at presentation as predictors of persistent disorder. *Journal of the American Academy of Child and Adolescent Psychiatry* **36**: 179–87.

Goodyer, I.M., Herbert, J., Tamplin, A. *et al.* 1997b: Short-term outcome of major depression: II. Life events, family dysfunction, and friendship difficulties as predictors of persistent disorder. *Journal of the American Academy of Child and Adolescent Psychiatry* **36**: 474–80.

Gould, M.S., King, R., Greenwald, S. *et al.* 1998: Psychopathology associated with suicidal ideation and attempts among children and adolescents. *Journal of the American Academy of Child and Adolescent Psychiatry* **37**: 915–23.

Graham, P. and Rutter, M. 1973: Psychiatric disorders in the young adolescent: a follow-up study. *Proceedings of the Royal Society of Medicine* **6**: 1226–9.

Groholt, B., Ekeberg, O, Wichstrom, L. *et al.* 1998: Suicide among children and younger and older adolescents in Norway: a comparative study. *Journal of the American Academy of Child and Adolescent Psychiatry* **37**: 473–81.

Hammen, C., Rudolph, K., Weisz, J. *et al.* 1999: The context of depression in clinic-referred youth. *Journal of the American Academy of Child and Adolescent Psychiatry* **38**: 64–71.

Harrington, R. 2002: Affective disorders. In Rutter, M. and Taylor, E. (eds), *Child and Adolescent Psychiatry: Modern Approaches*. 4th edition. Oxford: Blackwell Science, 463–85.

Harrington, R. 1994b: Comorbidity between childhood depression and conduct disorder: preliminary findings from a longitudinal and family genetic study. In Poustka, F. (ed.), *Basic Approaches to Genetic and Molecularbiological Developmental Psychiatry*. Berlin: Quintessenz, 123–7.

Harrington, R., Fudge, H., Rutter, M. *et al.* 1991: Adult outcomes of childhood and adolescent depression: II. Links with antisocial disorders. *Journal of the American Academy of Child and Adolescent Psychiatry* **30**: 434–9.

Harrington, R., Bredenkamp, D., Groothues, C. *et al.* 1994: Adult outcomes of childhood and adolescent depression: III. Links with suicidal behaviours. *Journal of Child Psychology and Psychiatry* **35**: 1309–19.

Harrington, R., Rutter, M. and Fombonne, E. 1996: Developmental pathways in depression: multiple meanings, antecedents and endpoints. *Development and Psychopathy* **8**: 601–16.

Harrington, R., Whittaker, J. and Shoebridge, P. 1998: Psychological treatment of depression in children and adolescents: a review of treatment research. *British Journal of Psychiatry* **173**: 291–8.

Hazell, P., O'Connell, D., Heathcote, D. *et al.* 1995: Efficacy of tricyclic drugs in treating child and adolescent depression: a meta-analysis. *British Medical Journal* **310**: 897–901.

Henggeler, S.W. 1999: Multisystemic therapy: an overview of clinical procedures, outcomes, and policy implications. *Child Psychology and Psychiatry Review* **4**: 2–10.

Himmelhoch, J.M. and Garfinkel, M.E. 1986: Mixed mania: diagnosis and treatment. *Psychopharmacology Bulletin* **22**: 613–20.

Hughes, C., Preskorn, S., Weller, E. *et al.* 1990: The effect of concomitant disorder in childhood depression on predicting treatment response. *Psychopharmacology Bulletin* **26**: 235–8.

Jasper, A., Smith, C. and Bailey, S. 1998: One hundred girls in care referred to an adolescent forensic mental health service. *Journal of Adolescence* **21**: 555–68.

Kashani, J.H., Beck, N.C., Hoeper, E.W. *et al.* 1987: Psychiatric disorders in a community sample of adolescents. *American Journal of Psychiatry* **144**: 584–9.

Kazdin, A.E. 2001: Treatment of conduct disorders. In Hill, J. and Maughan, B. (eds), *Conduct Disorders in Childhood and Adolescence*. Cambridge: Cambridge University Press, 408–48.

Keller, M.B., Ryan, N.D., Strober, M. *et al.* 2001: Efficacy of paroxetine in the treatment of adolescent major depression: a randomized, controlled trial. *Journal of the American Academy of Child and Adolescent Psychiatry* **40**: 762–72.

Kempton, T., van Hasselt, V.B., Bukstein, O.G. *et al.* 1994: Cognitive distortions and psychiatric diagnosis in dually diagnosed adolescents. *Journal of the American Academy of Child and Adolescent Psychiatry* **33**: 217–22.

King, C.A., Ghaziuddin, N., McGovern, L. *et al.* 1996: Predictors of comorbid alcohol and substance abuse in depressed adolescents. *Journal of the American Academy of Child and Adolescent Psychiatry* **35**: 743–51.

Koehler-Troy, C., Strober, M. and Malenbaum, R. 1986: Methylphenidate-induced mania in a prepubertal child. *Journal of Clinical Psychiatry* **47**: 566–7.

Kolvin, F.J., Miller, J.W., Fleeting, M. *et al.* 1988: Social and parenting factors affecting criminal offence rates: findings from the Newcastle thousand family study 1947–1980. *British Journal of Psychiatry* **152**: 80–90.

Kovacs, M. 1992: *Children's Depression Inventory (CDI) Manual.* North Tonawanda, NY: Multi-Health Systems.

Kovacs, M. 1996: Presentation and course of major depressive disorder during childhood and later years of the life span. *Journal of the American Academy of Child and Adolescent Psychiatry* **35**: 705–15.

Kovacs, M. and Devlin, B. 1998: Internalizing disorders in childhood. *Journal of Child Psychology and Psychiatry* **39**: 47–63.

Kovacs. M. and Pollock, M. 1995: Bipolar disorder and comorbid conduct disorder in childhood and adolescence. *Journal of the American Academy of Child and Adolescent Psychiatry* **34**: 715–23.

Kovacs, M., Paulauskas, S., Gatsonis, C. *et al.* 1988: Depressive disorders in childhood: III. A longitudinal study of comorbidity with and risk for conduct disorders. *Journal of Affective Disorders* **15**: 205–17.

Kovacs, M., Goldston, D. and Gatsonis, C. 1993: Suicidal behaviours and childhood-onset depressive disorders: a longitudinal investigation. *Journal of the American Academy of Child and Adolescent Psychiatry* **32**: 8–20.

Kovacs, M., Kroll, R.S.M. and Voti, L. 1994: Early-onset psychopathology and the risk for teenage pregnancy among clinically referred girls. *Journal of the American Academy of Child and Adolescent Psychiatry* **33**: 106–13.

Kovacs, M., Devlin, B., Pollock, M. *et al.* 1997a: A controlled family history study of childhood-onset depressive disorder. *Archives of General Psychiatry* **54**: 613–23.

Kovacs, M., Obrosky, S., Gatsonis, C. *et al.* 1997b: First-episode major depressive and dysthymic disorder in childhood: clinical and sociodemographic factors in recovery. *Journal of the American Academy of Child and Adolescent Psychiatry* **36**: 777–84.

Kroll, L., Harrington, R. and Jayson, D. 1996: Pilot study of continuation cognitive–behavioural therapy for major depression in adolescent psychiatric patients. *Journal of the American Academy of Child and Adolescent Psychiatry* **35**: 1156–61.

Lahey, B.B., Waldman, I.D. and McBurnett, K. 1999: Annotation: the development of antisocial behaviour: and integrative causal model. *Journal of Child Psychology and Psychiatry* **40**: 669–82.

Ledingham, J.E. and Schwartzman, A.E. 1984: A 3-year follow-up study of aggressive and withdrawn behaviour in childhood: preliminary findings. *Journal of Abnormal Child Psychology* **12**: 157–68.

Lewinsohn, P.M., Rohde, P. and Seeley, J.R. 1995a: Adolescent psychopathology: III. The clinical consequences of comorbidity. *Journal of the American Academy of Child and Adolescent Psychiatry* **34**: 510–19.

Lewinsohn, P.M., Klein, D.N. and Seeley, J.R. 1995b: Bipolar disorders in a community sample of older adolescents: prevalence, phenomenology, comorbidity, and course. *Journal of the American Academy of Child and Adolescent Psychiatry* **34**: 454–63.

Lewinsohn, P.M., Seeley, J.R., Buckley, J.R. *et al.* 2002: Bipolar disorder in adolescence and young adulthood. *Child and Adolescent Psychiatric Clinics of North America* **11**: 461–76.

Marmorstein, N.R. and Iacono, W.G. 2001: An investigation of female adolescent twins with major depression and conduct disorder. *Journal of the American Academy of Child and Adolescent Psychiatry* **40**: 299–306.

Marriage, K., Fine, S., Moretti, M. *et al.* 1986: Relationship between depression and conduct disorder in children and adolescents. *Journal of the American Academy of Child and Adolescent Psychiatry* **25**: 687–91.

Marton, P., Churchard, M., Kutcher, S. *et al.* 1991: Diagnostic utility of the Beck Depression Inventory with adolescent psychiatric outpatients and inpatients. *Canadian Journal of Psychiatry* **36**: 428–31.

Maughan, B. and McCarthy, G. 1997: Childhood adversities and psychosocial disorders. *British Medical Bulletin* **53**: 156–69.

Max, J.E., Richards, L. and Hamdan-Allen, G. 1995: Case study: antimanic effectiveness of dextroamphetamine in a brain-injured adolescent. *Journal of the American Academy of Child and Adolescent Psychiatry* **34**: 472–6.

McGee, R., Feehan, M., Williams, S. *et al.* 1990: DSM-III disorders in a large sample of adolescents. *Journal of the American Academy of Child and Adolescent Psychiatry* **29**: 611–19.

McGlashan, T.H. 1988: Adolescent versus adult onset of mania. *American Journal of Psychiatry* **145**: 221–3.

Meller, W.H. and Borchardt, C.M. 1996: Comorbidity of major depression and conduct disorder. *Journal of Affective Disorders* **39**: 123–6.

Mufson, L., Weissman, M.M., Moreau, D. and Garfinkel, R. 1999: Efficacy of interpersonal therapy for depressed adolescents. *Archives of General Psychiatry* **56**: 573–79.

Nottelmann, E.D. and Jensen, P.S. 1995: Comorbidity of disorders in children and adolescents: developmental perspectives. In Ollendick, T.H. and Prinz, R.J. (eds), *Advances in Clinical Child Psychology*, Vol. 17. New York: Plenum Press, 109–55.

Nottelmann, E. *et al.* 2001: National Institute of Mental Health Research Roundtable on Prepubertal Bipolar Disorder. *Journal of the American Academy of Child and Adolescent Psychiatry* **40**: 871–78.

O'Connor, T.G., Neiderhiser, J.M., Reiss, D. *et al.* 1998: Genetic contributions to continuity, change, and co-occurrence of antisocial and depressive symptoms in adolescence. *Journal of Child Psychology and Psychiatry* **39**: 323–36.

Orvaschel, H., Lewinsohn, P.M. and Seeley, J.R. 1995: Continuity of psychopathology in a community sample of adolescents. *Journal of the American Academy of Child and Adolescent Psychiatry* **34**: 1525–35.

Os, J.V., Jones, P., Lewis, G. *et al.* 1997: Developmental precursors of affective illness in a general population birth. *Archives of General Psychiatry* **54**: 625–31.

Post, R.M., Weiss, S.R.B., Leverich, G.S. *et al.* 1996: Developmental psychobiology of cyclic affective illness: implications for early therapeutic intervention. *Development and Psychopathy* **8**: 273–305.

Puig-Antich, J. 1982: Major depression and conduct disorder in prepuberty. *Journal of the American Academy of Child Psychiatry* **21**: 118–28.

Puig-Antich, J., Goetz, D., Davies, M. *et al.* 1989: A controlled family history study of prepubertal major depressive disorder. *Archives of General Psychiatry* **46**: 406–18.

Randall, J., Hengeller, S.C., Pickrel, S.G. *et al.* 1999: Psychiatric comorbidity and the 16-month trajectory of substance-abusing and substance-dependent juvenile offenders. *Journal of the American Academy of Child and Adolescent Psychiatry* **38**: 1118–24.

Reiss, D., Hetherington, M., Plomin, R. *et al.* 1995: Genetic questions for environmental studies: differential parenting and psychopathology in adolescence. *Archives of General Psychiatry* **52**: 925–36.

Renaud, J., Brent, D.A., Birmaher, B. *et al.* 1999: Suicide in adolescents with disruptive disorders. *Journal of the American Academy of Child and Adolescent Psychiatry* **38**: 846–51.

Renouf, A.G., Kovacs, M. and Mukerji, P. 1997: Relationship of depressive, conduct, and comorbid disorders and social functioning in childhood. *Journal of the American Academy of Child and Adolescent Psychiatry* **36**: 998–1004.

Rifkin, A., Karajgi, B., Dicker, R. *et al.* 1997: Lithium treatment of conduct disorder in adolescents. *American Journal of Psychiatry* **154**: 554–5.

Riggs, P.D., Baker, S., Mikulich, S.K. *et al.* 1995: Depression in substance-dependent delinquents. *Journal of the American Academy of Child and Adolescent Psychiatry* **34**: 764–71.

Riley, A.W., Ensminger, M.E., Green, B. *et al.* 1998: Social role functioning by adolescents with psychiatric disorders. *Journal of the American Academy of Child and Adolescent Psychiatry* **37**: 620–8.

Robins, L.N. 1986: The consequences of conduct disorder in girls. In Olweus, D., Block, J. and Radke-Yarrow, M. (eds), *Development of Antisocial and Prosocial Behaviour.* New York: Academic Press, 385–414.

Robins, L.N. and Price, R.K. 1991: Adult disorders predicted by childhood conduct problems: results from the NIMH Epidemiologic Catchment Area project. *Psychiatry: Journal for the Study of Interpersonal Processes* **54**: 116–32.

Rohde, P., Lewinsohn, P.M. and Seeley, J.R. 1991: Comorbidity of unipolar depression: II. Comorbidity with other mental disorders in adolescents and adults. *Journal of Abnormal Psychology* **100**(2): 214–22.

Rohde, P., Lewinsohn, P.M. and Seeley, J.R. 1994: Are adolescents changed by an episode of major depression? *Journal of the American Academy of Child and Adolescent Psychiatry* **33**: 1289–98.

Rossello, J. and Bernal, G. 1999: The efficacy of cognitive-behavioural and interpersonal treatments for depression in Puerto Rican adolescents. *Journal of Consulting and Clinical Psychology* **67**: 734–45.

Rowe, J.B., Sullivan, P.F., Mulder, R.T. *et al.* 1996: The effect of a history of conduct disorder in adult major depression. *Journal of Affective Disorders* **37**: 51–63.

Rutter, M. 1997: Comorbidity: concepts, claims and choices. *Criminal Behavior and Mental Health* **7**: 265–85.

Rutter, M. and Graham, P. 1966: Psychiatric disorder in 10- and 11-year-old children. *Proceedings of the Royal Society of Medicine* **59**: 382–7.

Rutter, M., Harrington, R., Quinton, D. *et al.* 1994: Adult outcomes of conduct disorder in childhood: implications for concepts and definitions of patterns of psychopathology. In Ketterlinus, R.D. and Lamb, M. (eds), *Adolescent Problem Behaviours: Issues and Research.* Hillsdale, NJ: Lawrence Erlbaum, 57–80.

Sanders, M.R., Dadds, M.R., Johnston, B.M. *et al.* 1992: Childhood depression and conduct disorder: I. Behavioural, affective, and cognitive aspects of family problem-solving interactions. *Journal of Abnormal Psychology* **101**: 495–504.

Sandford, M., Szatmari, P., Spinner, M. *et al.* 1995: Predicting the one-year course of adolescent major depression. *Journal of the American Academy of Child and Adolescent Psychiatry* **34**: 1618–28.

Shaffer, D., Gould, M., Fisher, P. *et al.* 1996: Psychiatric diagnosis in child and adolescent suicide. *Archives of General Psychiatry* **53**: 339–48.

Simic, M. and Fombonne, E. 2001: Depressive conduct disorder: symptom patterns and correlates in referred children and adolescents. *Journal of Affective Disorders* **62**: 175–85.

Steinhausen, H.-C. and Reitzle, M. 1996: The validity of mixed disorders of conduct and emotions in children and adolescents: a research note. *Journal of Child Psychology and Psychiatry* **37**: 339–43.

Strober, M., Morrell, W., Lampert, C. *et al.* 1990: Relapse following discontinuation of lithium maintenance therapy in adolescents with bipolar I illness: a naturalistic study. *American Journal of Psychiatry* **147**: 457–61.

Strober, M., Schmidt-Lackner, S. and Freeman, R. 1995: Recovery and relapse in adolescents with bipolar affective illness: a five-year naturalistic, prospective follow-up. *Journal of the American Academy of Child and Adolescent Psychiatry* **34**: 724–31.

Verhulst, F.C. and Ende, van der J. 1993: 'Comorbidity' in an epidemiological sample: a longitudinal perspective. *Journal of Child Psychology and Psychiatry* **34**: 767–83.

Warner, V., Weissman, M., Fendrich, M. *et al.* 1992: The course of major depression in the offspring of depressed parents. *Archives of General Psychiatry* **49**: 795–801.

West, S.A., Keck, P.E., McElroy, S.L. *et al.* 1994: Open trial of valproate in the treatment of adolescent mania. *Journal of Adolescent Psychopharmacology* **4**: 263–7.

Williamson, D.E., Ryan, N.D., Birmaher, B. *et al.* 1995: A case–control family history study of depression in adolescents. *Journal of the American Academy of Child and Adolescent Psychiatry* **34**: 1596–607.

Wood, A.J., Harrington, R.C. and Moore, A. 1996: Controlled trial of a brief cognitive-behavioural intervention in adolescent patients with depressive disorders. *Journal of Child Psychology and Psychiatry* **37**: 737–46.

Zoccolillo, M. 1992: Co-occurrence of conduct disorder and its adult outcomes with depressive and anxiety disorders: a review. *Journal of the American Academy of Child and Adolescent Psychiatry* **31**: 547–56.

Zoccolillo, M. and Rogers, K. 1991: Characteristics and outcome of hospitalized adolescent girls with conduct disorder. *Journal of the American Academy of Child and Adolescent Psychiatry* **30**: 973–81.

11

Learning disability, autism and offending behaviour

GREGORY O'BRIEN AND GILLIAN BELL

INTRODUCTION

The adolescent with learning disability or autism faces the same myriad challenges and tasks as do all young people, but does not share in the general intellectual and social capacities required for resolution of these complex matters. Without the ability to understand, communicate and consider their situation, antisocial and disturbed behaviour is common in young people with these disabilities. In this chapter we consider the factors which predispose adolescents with learning disability and autism to offending, and the extent to which offending behaviour in these groups has a distinct profile. We suggest some pointers towards the basis of a coherent service response. It is emphasized that the same issues which are relevant to the offending behaviour of adolescents in general, as reviewed elsewhere in this volume, apply to some extent to adolescents with learning disability and autism.

In line with UK policy, the term 'learning disability' is used throughout this chapter, being synonymous with the internationally employed expression 'mental retardation' (WHO 1992). In line with conventional classification, mild learning disability corresponds to an IQ of 50–69; moderate to an IQ of 35–49; severe to an IQ of 20–34; and profound to an IQ below 20.

THE ADOLESCENT OFFENDER WITH LEARNING DISABILITY

In this section, the adolescent offender with learning disability is considered according to:

- the general issue of offending among all people with learning disability
- the role of the severity of learning disability in offending behaviour among adolescents
- the relevance of the cause/aetiology of learning disability to the offending behaviour
- the impact of the nature of an individual's learning disability/cognitive profile on offending
- the importance of super-added psychiatric disorder among learning disabled adolescents
- the role of life experience and personal history in the offending behaviour of these young people.

Offending and learning disability

GENERAL ISSUES

Most studies of offending among people with learning disability have concentrated on adults, or have not considered adolescents separately. If we first consider all people with learning disability, certain themes are identifiable.

Firstly, there is no clear evidence of any definite overall excess of offending behaviour – although most studies have reported marginally higher rates than among non-intellectually disabled populations (MacEachron 1979). However, there is longstanding interest in the offending profile of people with learning disabilities, and whether this shows any differences from that in the general population. Two types of offending behaviour have long been believed to be more prevalent among people with learning disability: sexual deviance and arson (Holland 1997). As yet, these claims have not stood up to scrutiny. Study of both offence types has suggested that the apparent over-representation of people with learning disabilities among those convicted may be more a reflection of criminal apprehension and the conviction process, rather than a result of any true excess of offending (Bradford 1982; Swanson and Garwick 1990). On the other hand, it is the case that some patterns of offending, most notably property crime such as planned theft and associated activity, require intellectual capacities which are lacking among young people with learning disabilities. This effect is more relevant to the situation of more severely intellectually disabled people, while it has long been reported that individuals with milder degrees of learning delay have similar offending propensities to those of low-to-normal intelligence (MacEachron 1979; Day 1988).

Regarding outcome and legal process, there is long-standing evidence that having some degree of learning disability renders the individual more liable to conviction. Through greater suggestibility and other social and linguistic deficits, people with learning disabilities are particularly prone to a pattern of acquiescence in the face of interrogation and questioning (Gudjonsson *et al.* 1995). These findings have been reported among adults with learning disabilities: the effect may be even more marked among young people. Furthermore, on consideration of issues such as peer pressure and group criminal activity through similar traits of suggestibility and social acquiescence, it has long been held that young people with learning disability may be particularly prone to becoming involved in crime by the instigation and influence of others (Holland 1997).

A number of interrelated factors might predispose adolescents with learning disability to high rates of offending behaviour and to recorded or processed offending. One major issue to consider is whether having a learning disability *per se* renders the adolescent more prone to offending behaviour. As a basic tenet, this theory has long been supported in certain quarters. Indeed such thinking was enshrined in the Mental Deficiency Act of 1913. It is more appropriate that contemporary thinking should take a more sophisticated view, and consider which influences are relevant to the occurrence and nature of offending in young people with learning disability.

SEVERITY OF THE LEARNING DISABILITY

One approach is to consider to what extent there is any evidence of an association between the severity of learning disability and the occurrence of offending behaviour. Putting it simply, if learning disability among adolescents operated as an independent determinant or predictor of offending, then borderline and mild learning disability would be associated with some excess of offending, while more severe learning disability would be associated with higher rates. Here, it is notable that having a degree of intellectual disability that does not comprise learning disability – in other words being of low-to-normal or borderline intelligence – has been identified as one of a number of risk factors in children which predispose to subsequent delinquency and offending (Farrington 1994; Fergusson and Horwood 1995). This observation suggests that the very fact of being learning disabled may of itself be a risk factor to offending. However, the same studies which have considered this subject have stressed that other factors operate, most notably social influences. It is also important to consider the impact of the most severe degrees of learning disability, for it is evident that many profoundly learning-disabled individuals are incapable of offending behaviour, lacking the capacity for independent social behaviour (O'Brien 1998). Clearly, there is no evidence of any simple association or direct correlation between the severity of learning disability and the occurrence of offending.

CAUSE OF THE LEARNING DISABILITY

One issue, which was until recently overlooked in some quarters, is the role of the cause of the individual's learning disability in behaviour. For, where a biological type – or cause – of learning disability carries a predisposition towards a given pattern of behaviour, then this can be crucial in understanding the offending behaviour of the adolescent with learning disability. For example, aggressive propensities have long been reported as a feature of *the behavioural phenotype* of certain causal syndromes of learning disability. One of the best known claims in this connection was for the XYY genotype. However, the history of this claim – which was originally based on spurious links found in a selected sample – is a salutory reminder of the need for caution in proposing simple or inevitable gene – behaviour links (O'Brien and Yule 1995). More recently there have been reports of increased aggression in respect of a few rather more rare genetic conditions, including notably Sotos and Smith–Magenis syndromes (see the chapter appendix). As with XYY, immense care must be taken both in the investigation and the interpretation of any such putative behavioural phenotypes, not least in relation to issues of labelling and personal responsibility for behaviour.

Less controversially, and more clearly, the *site* of learning disability – in terms of *focal brain damage* – may be an important predisposing factor to aggression and related offending behaviour. Where the cause of the learning disability is brain damage from head injury in childhood, aggression in adolescence and early adult life is a common problem (O'Brien 1999). Also, aggression is commonly seen where brain damage is progressive. For example, in clinical practice a period of aggressive propensities may be seen over the course of neurodegenerative disorders as brain damage progresses, such as in tuberous sclerosis (see the appendix). However, here it is the nature, site and disinhibiting effect of the central neurodegeneration that is implicated, rather than there being evidence of aggressive traits as part of the behavioural phenotype of tuberous sclerosis.

NATURE OF THE LEARNING DISABILITY

The offending behaviour of the adolescent with learning disability can be better understood when the *nature* of the individual's learning disability is given careful consideration, in addition to the overall severity and cause of the learning disability, as above. Attention to the severity of learning disability is concerned with the role of general intelligence in offending, while study of the influence of the cause of the learning disability on offending points towards the role of biological influences on behaviour.

However, people with learning disability commonly do not have 'flat' or uniformly suppressed cognitive profiles; specific deficits in one or more domains of cognitive functioning are often present, well beyond that expected for the given level of severity of intellectual disability. This phenomenon – the cognitive or neuropsychological profile of the learning disabled adolescent – is the nature of the learning disability, according to this approach. In clinical practice, psychometric testing will determine whether an individual with a certain overall level of learning disability possesses a specific deficit in some area of intellectual or cognitive functioning. Where a deficit is identified which is well in excess of that to be expected for a given developmental or intellectual level, this facilitates understanding any predisposition towards offending behaviour.

Communication deficits are of particular importance in this connection. The learning-disabled adolescent who has a general impairment of the capacity for everyday communication, most commonly described in terms of a significantly lower verbal than performance score on IQ testing, is at risk. More detailed psycholinguistic assessment may further clarify the nature of such deficits. In particular, the young person with more severe expressive language disability may be at even greater risk (Fraser and Rao 1991).

Psychiatric disorder and learning disability

As we consider the impact of intervening variables on the occurrence of offending among adolescents with learning disability, psychiatric disorder proves to be of key importance. There are several reasons for this. Firstly, psychiatric disorder is very common among adolescents with learning disability. One major epidemiological Swedish survey of 16- to 19-year olds with learning disability found rates as high as 64% in moderately to severely learning-disabled young people (IQ < 50), and 57% in the mildly learning-disabled (IQ 51–70) (Gillberg *et al.* 1986). Similarly, a recent community-based UK survey carried out in Cambridgeshire, UK, of 18- to 22-year-olds with

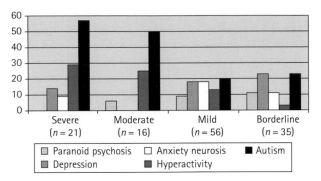

Figure 11.1 *Psychiatric diagnoses by severity of learning disability in a community study of 18- to 22-year-olds (O'Brien 1998).*

a history of child learning disability found a prevalence of 68% (O'Brien 1998). This phenomenon, of the prevalence rate of psychopathology 'peaking' in adolescence among people with learning disability, is well recognized (Corbett 1977). Such a high rate of psychiatric disorder has an obvious impact on rates of antisocial and offending behaviour.

Regarding the *nature of psychopathology* – the psychiatric disorders which constitute this major excess – the single most common disorder is autism. Given the extent and social impact of this disorder, and the suggestion that the young person with learning disability who also has autism may be at particularly high risk of offending behaviour (Baron-Cohen 1990), the second part of this chapter is devoted to consideration of autism and offending.

Apart from autism, the other common psychiatric disorders which constitute the high rate of psychopathology among these young people notably include attention-deficit disorder with hyperactivity (ADDH) and paranoid psychosis. The latter group includes those affected by schizophrenia or manic–depressive psychosis, and those individuals who suffer from a psychotic illness which cannot easily be classified, this being a common occurrence in young people with learning disability (WHO 1992).

A recent UK community-based survey of 18- to 22-year-olds with learning disability yielded the rates of these disorders shown in Figure 11.1 (O'Brien 1998). The figure shows the distribution of psychiatric diagnoses among young people with a history of child learning disability of varying severity, from borderline (IQ 70–79), to mild (IQ 50–69), through moderate (IQ 35–49) to severe (IQ under 35). In twelve cases, more than one disorder was diagnosed. The marginally higher rates of autism and hyperactivity among the borderline cases was due to attribution bias. Given the propensity for disruptive, antisocial and offending behaviour which is seen in these disorders, these high prevalences are of considerable relevance to consideration of the offending behaviour of young people with learning disability.

In summary:

- Psychiatric disorder is common among adolescents with learning disability.
- Autistic spectrum disorder is the most frequent diagnosis, followed by attention-deficit disorder with hyperactivity.
- Both autism and hyperactivity are increasingly more common in more severely learning disabled individuals.
- Paranoid psychosis is more common than among the non-intellectually disabled population, and is more often non-specific or poorly-differentiated in type.
- Psychiatric disorder of this extent and nature has major implications for both understanding and management of learning-disabled adolescent offenders.

Personal history

Any exploration of background, underlying or predisposing factors relevant to the development of offending in young people with learning disability would be incomplete without consideration of personal history and life experience. For example, aggression may have been learnt through the experience of being a victim of aggression, or may be some other reflection of an abusive or otherwise adverse early life experience. Indeed, it is now accepted that children and adolescents with learning disabilities, particularly those with more severe disabilities who are dependent on the care of others, may be more at risk of sexual and other physical abuse (O'Brien 1996; Holland 1997). Also, what seems at first sight to be a trait of serious and goal-directed aggression may reflect some longstanding aspect of individual development, where previous aggressive acts were in some sense 'rewarded', and therefore have continued, or even worsened. Such a set of circumstances commonly presents in the learning disabled adolescent who has, virtually by a process of trial and error, learned that aggression can serve to remove him/herself from some undesirable situation. A common scenario therefore emerges wherein the adolescent with learning disability finds some situation difficult or threatening, consequently employs disruptive or other aggressive behaviour to avoid the distress of the situation, and in doing so learns that aggression can help to control difficult situations. In such circumstances, aggression can easily become a way of life.

Other important life-experience influences lie in role-modelling within violent families and subcultures, and deficiencies of limit-setting and promotion of appropriate behaviour over development, as in all young offenders. For young people with learning disability, these influences may have even greater impact than usual. In many cases, however, it is not possible to identify the mechanisms of specific early-life adverse experience, and how these have predisposed to offending. More often, general indicators of adverse early-life experience are identified, such as early

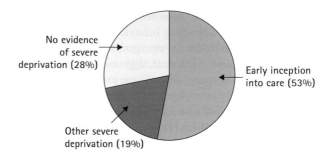

Figure 11.2 *Indicators of early-life severe deprivation in 53 mentally impaired adolescent and young adult inpatients.*

inception into care (usually due to deficient or otherwise inappropriate parenting) and severe emotional deprivation. For example, in a recent clinical study of 53 adolescents and young adults admitted to a medium secure unit for mentally impaired offenders, one of the present authors found that 28 had been received into care early in life, while 10 had been subject to other types of severe deprivation, as illustrated in Figure 11.2.

THE ADOLESCENT OFFENDER WITH AUTISM

General issues

The original clinical descriptions of autism and Asperger syndrome included reports of odd and bizarre antisocial behaviours, alongside the accounts of the core clinical features (Asperger 1944). As the literature has grown so has our awareness that there is an increasing catalogue of offending behaviour by autists, which is most remarkable in its bizarre quality. All four young people in Asperger's original paper on autistic psychopathy had conduct problems. This may be due in part to the population from which he drew his observations: at the time Asperger was working in the field of remedial pedagogy. Others, however, have echoed the nature of their behaviour, in their contributions to the literature.

Thus, in Lorna Wing's review paper on the clinical features of Asperger syndrome (1981) she notes 'a small minority have a history of rather bizarre antisocial acts, perhaps because of their lack of empathy'. This observation, coupled by Wolff and Chick's (1980) comments on Asperger's original sample, led Mawson *et al.* (1985) to comment even further on antisocial behaviours in individuals with autism. These writers suggested that violence, aggression and offending may be of clinical import in the presentation of Asperger syndrome. This has spawned a number of single-case studies of offending behaviour in subjects with Asperger syndrome.

There is increasing anecdotal evidence that aggression and violence may occur as part of the clinical presentation of autism and Asperger syndrome, but no systematic studies in the literature have as yet investigated the nature of

behaviour. Another approach was put forward by Lorenz (1960), who purported that aggression is a drive common to most animals and humans, and that aggression has a role in both animal and human society. It is not surprising, then, that autists who have difficulty understanding social rules and interaction show abnormal aggressive behaviours. Overall, it does seem that one crucial element in understanding the mechanisms at play in the aggressive behaviour of any one individual affected by autistic spectrum disorder lies in endeavouring to appreciate the singular cognitive set and view of the world in question, perhaps most usefully, after the fashion of Howlin, as above.

Conclusion and pointers to diagnosis

In common with all commentators on this field, we propose that autistic spectrum disorder is an important and under-diagnosed entity. All evidence indicates that the correct identification of autism or Asperger syndrome yields crucial insights into the understanding of offending behaviour, most especially among adolescents with learning disability. The authors suggest that a diagnosis of autistic spectrum disorder especially should be routinely considered (even if it is rapidly discounted) where an offence or assault is characterized by:

- bizarre nature
- a degree or nature of aggression which is 'unaccountable'
- a repeated and very stereotypic pattern of offending.

APPENDIX: DEFINITIONS

Smith–Magenis syndrome
This rare condition, with incidence probably around 1 in 50,000 live births, has a variable physical phenotype, with most notably a 'cupid's bow' shape to the upper lip, broad face and nasal bridge, flat mid-face and a deep hoarse voice. The severity of learning disability is variable, from mild to severe, most cases lying in the moderate band (IQ 35–49). The behavioural phenotype is florid and dramatic, with self-injury which typically includes head-banging, wrist and hand biting, and even pulling out finger and toe nails. In the context of this generally disruptive pattern, aggression towards others is much more common than in others of a similar degree of intellectual disability (Greenberg *et al.* 1991).

Sotos syndrome
This is a sporadic, non-familial condition, and is sometimes called *cerebral gigantism*. The prevalence is unknown, because the features are so variable in expression. Individuals typically present with large body size, accelerated growth, advanced bone age, and a characteristic facial appearance with high forehead, prominent jaw, premature eruption of teeth and sparseness of hair,

in addition to other eye and nasal features. The main behavioural problems are of aggressive behaviour and emotional immaturity. These assume even greater importance, given the large stature and appearance of sufferers of the syndrome.

Tuberous sclerosis
Tuberous sclerosis is not uncommon, with a prevalence of approximately 1 in 7000. The condition has a classic triad of epilepsy, learning disability and certain skin problems – notably the so-called 'adenoma sebaceum' rash. The severity of learning disability of the condition varies enormously, according to the brain involvement of blood vessel malformations, which are essentially the same as those which appear on the face. As these are progressive, so is deterioration in intelligence. The most prominent psychological findings are of generally disturbed, distractable and disinhibited behaviour, often amounting to an autistic/hyperactive constellation which may worsen in late adolescence and early adulthood (Hunt and Dennis 1987).

REFERENCES

Asperger, H. 1944: Die autischen Psychopathen im Kindesalter. *Archives für Psychiatrie und Nervenkrankheiten* **117**: 76–136.

Baron-Cohen, S. 1990: An assessment of violence in a young man with Asperger's syndrome. *Journal of Child Psychology and Psychiatry and Allied Disciplines* **29**: 351–60.

Bradford, J. 1982: Arson: a clinical study. *Canadian Journal of Psychiatry* **27**: 188–92.

Corbett, J. 1977: Studies of mental retardation. In Graham, P.J. (ed.), *Epidemiological Approaches in Child Psychiatry*. London: Academic Press.

Day, K.A. 1988: A hospital-based treatment programme for mentally handicapped offenders. *British Journal of Psychiatry* **153**: 635–44.

Dollard, J., Doob, L., Miller, N., Howrer, O.H. and Sears, R.R. 1939: *Frustration and Aggression*. Yale University Press.

Farrington, D. 1994: The development of offending and antisocial behaviour from childhood: key findings from the Cambridge Study in Delinquent Development. *Journal of Child Psychology and Psychiatry and Allied Disciplines* **36**: 929–64.

Fergusson, D.M. and Horwood, L.J. 1995: Early disruptive behaviour, IQ, and later achievement and delinquent behaviour. *Journal of Abnormal Child Psychology* **23**: 183–99.

Fraser, W.I. and Murti Rao, J. 1991: Recent studies of mentally handicapped young people's behaviour. *Journal of Child Psychology and Psychiatry* **32**: 79–108.

Gillberg, C., Persson, E., Grufman, M. and Themner, U. 1986: Psychiatric disorders in mildly and severely retarded urban children and adolescents: epidemiological aspects. *British Journal of Psychiatry* **149**: 68–74.

Greenberg, F., Guzzetta, V., Montes de Oca-Luna, R. *et al.* 1991: Molecular analysis of the Smith–Magenis syndrome: a possible contiguous gene associated with del(17)(p11.2p11.2) in nine patients. *American Journal of Medical Genetics* **24**: 393–414.

Gudjonsson, G.H., Clare, I.C.H. and Rutter, S. 1995: *Persons at Risk during Interview in Police Custody: Identification of*

Vulnerabilities. Royal Commission on Criminal Justice, Research Study 12. London: HMSO.

Holland, A. 1997: Forensic psychiatry and learning disability. In Russell, O. (ed.), *Seminars in the Psychiatry of Learning Disabilities.* London: Gaskell, 259–73.

Howlin, P. 1997: *Autism: Preparing for Adulthood.* London: Routledge.

Hunt, A. and Dennis 1987: Psychiatric disorder among children with tuberous sclerosis. *Developmental Medicine and Child Neurology* **29**: 190–8.

Kanner, L. 1943: Autistic disturbances of affective contact. *Nervous Child* **2**: 217–50.

Lorenz, K. 1960: *On Aggression.* London: Methuen.

Lyall, I., Holland, A. and Collins, S. 1995: Offending by adults with learning disabilities and the attitudes of staff to offending behaviour: implications for service development. *Journal of Intellectual Disability Research* **39**: 501–8.

McArdle, P., O'Brien, G. and Kolvin, I. 1995: Hyperactivity: prevalence and relationship with conduct disorder. *Journal of Child Psychology and Psychiatry* **36**: 279–304.

MacCulloch, M.J., Snowden, P.R., Wood, P.J.W. and Mills, H.E. 1983: Sadistic fantasy, sadistic behaviour and offending. *British Journal of Psychiatry* **143**: 20–9.

MacEachron, A.E. 1979: Mentally retarded offenders: prevalence and characteristics. *American Journal of Mental Deficiency* **84**: 165–76.

Mawson, D., Grounds, A. and Tantam, D. 1985: Violence and Asperger's syndrome: a case study. *British Journal of Psychiatry* **147**: 566–9.

O'Brien, G. 1996: The psychiatric management of adult autism. *Advances in Psychiatric Treatment* **2**: 173–7.

O'Brien, G. 1998: *The Adult Outcome of Child Learning Disability.* MD thesis, University of Aberdeen.

O'Brien, G. 1999: Traumatic brain damage. In Gillberg, C. and O'Brien, G. (eds), *Developmental Disability and Behaviour.* London: MacKeith Press.

O'Brien, G. and Yule, W. (eds) 1995: *Behavioural Phenotypes.* London: MacKeith Press.

Ramirez, J.M. 1985: The nature of aggression in animals. In Ramirez, J.M. and Brain, P.F. (eds), *Aggression: Functions and Causes.* Seville: Publicaciones de la Universidad de Savilla, 15–35.

Scragg, P. and Shah, A. 1994: Prevalence of Asperger's syndrome in a secure hospital. *British Journal of Psychiatry* **16**: 679–82.

Swanson, C.K. and Garwick, G.B. 1990: Treatment for low functioning sex offenders: group therapy and inter-agency co-ordination. *Mental Retardation* **28**: 155–61.

Tantam, D. 1988: Lifelong eccentricity and social isolation: I. Psychiatric, social, and forensic aspects. *British Journal of Psychiatry* **153**: 777–82.

WHO (World Health Organization) 1992: *The ICD-10 Classification of Mental and Behavioural Disorders.* Geneva: WHO.

Wing, L. 1981: Asperger's syndrome: a clinical account. *Psychological Medicine* **11**: 115–29.

Wolff, S. and Chick, J. 1980: Schizoid personality in childhood: a controlled follow-up study. *Psychological Medicine* **10**: 85–100.

12

Schizophrenia

ANTHONY JAMES

INTRODUCTION

Schizophrenia is a major mental disorder with an onset in late adolescence and early adulthood. DSM-IV (APA 1994) diagnostic criteria include the presence of psychotic symptoms (delusions and/or hallucinations) and social dysfunction for a period of at least six months. Early-onset schizophrenia (EOS; onset between the ages 13 and 18 years), although a relatively rare disorder, is associated with a proportion of offending and violent crime. A birth-cohort study (Arseneault *et al.* 2000c) suggests that schizophrenia spectrum disorders account for 10% of the total violent crimes committed by youths up to the age of 21.

Schizophrenia occurring in childhood and adolescence was described by Kraepelin (1919[1899]) and Bleuler (1951[1911]). It is a relatively rare disorder in the age range 16–19, with a crude annual incidence of 0.6 (confidence interval 0.2–1.5) per 10,000 population for schizophrenia type F20.0 (Brewin *et al.* 1997). The peak onset for males is slightly earlier than that for females, with 49% of males and 28% of females developing schizophrenia before age 19 (Loranger 1984). The phenomenology is similar to that in adult-onset cases, with 81% reporting delusions, 68% auditory hallucinations, and 73% thought disorder (Cawthron *et al.* 1994).

DIAGNOSIS

Schizophrenia is characterized by a fundamental 'distortion of thinking and perception, and by inappropriate affect or blunted affect. Clear consciousness and intellectual function are usually maintained' (WHO 1992). The essential features of schizophrenia are the psychotic symptoms:

1 thought echo, thought insertion or withdrawal, and thought broadcasting
2 delusions of control, influence or passivity
3 hallucinatory voices giving a running commentary on the patient's behaviour, or discussing the patient amongst themselves
4 persistent delusions which are culturally inappropriate, bizarre or impossible
5 persistent hallucinations with half-formed, non-affective delusions
6 thought disorder with resultant incoherent speech or irrelevant speech and neologisms
7 catatonic behaviour
8 negative symptoms of apathy, paucity of speech, social withdrawal, etc.
9 a significant and consistent change in personal behaviour: loss of interest, aimlessness, etc.

For a diagnosis under ICD-10 there must be one clear or two less clear-cut symptoms from 1–4, and at least two symptoms from 5–8. The symptoms must be present for one month or more. The DSM-IV criteria specify six months' duration of symptoms, and is therefore a more restrictive or narrower diagnostic system.

In early-onset schizophrenia, subgrouping is not overly helpful or, indeed, researched. Amongst first presentations a disorganized subgroup is most common (mean age of onset 16.7 years; standard deviation (SD): 2.5 years), followed by an undifferentiated type (23.5 years;

SD: 5.5 years), with paranoid type occurring later (29.9 years; SD: 9.9 years) (Beratis *et al.* 1994). A useful distinction is the positive (active delusions, hallucinations, thought disorder) versus negative (apathy, poverty of thinking, speech) symptom profile.

There are standardized instruments to aid diagnosis (e.g. K–SADS: Kiddie's Schedule of Affective Disorders and Schizophrenia; Chambers *et al.* 1985).

AETIOLOGY AND PATHOGENESIS

Aetiology

GENETIC FACTORS

The aetiology of adolescent or early-onset schizophrenia is multifactorial. Evidence from family, twin and adoption studies indicates that the genetic component to the liability to schizophrenia is about 75% (McGuffin *et al.* 1994). Pooled twin-data estimates of the mean concordance rate within monzygotic pairs (MZ) of 46% and within dizygotic pairs (DZ) of 14% suggest an inheritance pattern, across the age range, compatible with an oligogenetic disorder (Risch 1990) – that is, transmission by a few but not many genes. An increased genetic loading for early-onset cases is supported by the findings of an increased morbidity risk in relatives of males aged under 17 (Pulver *et al.* 1990) and of females under 21 (Sham *et al.* 1994). Genetic mechanisms are important in neuronal development and interconnectivity of neurones (Jones and Murray 1991; Vicete and Kennedy 1997) and possibly the development of cerebral asymmetry, which is reduced in schizophrenia (Crow *et al.* 1989); all of which suggest a genetic basis for prenatal developmental lesions. There is a suggestion that early-onset schizophrenia may be a more severe form of the disorder or perhaps phenotypically different from adult-onset cases, with D_3 receptor heterogeneity (Maziade *et al.* 1997).

An argument for the operation of environmental factors in the aetiology of schizophrenia comes from the findings that the monozygotic concordance rates for schizophrenia are less than unity. Structural modelling of family and twin data also indicates substantial environmental effects (Rutter *et al.* 1999). CT and MRI studies of monozygotic twins discordant for schizophrenia have shown ventricular enlargement and reduction in volume of the temporal lobes in the affected twin compared to his/her unaffected twin (Reveley *et al.* 1984; Suddath *et al.* 1990). While this does not prove the role of environmental factors, it is suggestive, because monozygotic twins share all their genes.

ENVIRONMENTAL FACTORS

Environmental factors implicated in the genesis of schizophrenia include an excess of pregnancy and obstetric complications (Geddes and Lawrie 1995; Cannon *et al.* 2002a),

which, it is estimated, doubles the lifetime risk to 2%. Gillberg *et al.* (1986) found an excess of perinatal events in teenage psychotics. Some controversy remains over the finding, from several studies, of an excess of winter births and exposure to maternal influenza between the fifth and seventh month of gestation (Sham *et al.* 1992). Crow and Done (1992), using direct maternal reports, found no such excess.

In the adolescent age range, the family environment is crucial. The importance of abnormal family communication ('communication deviance') and affective style was demonstrated in a 15-year prospective study of families of non-psychotic adolescent clinic attenders (Goldstein 1987). A combination of negative affective style and deviant communication was shown to have predictive power for the development of schizophrenia and schizophreniform illnesses. Further findings from the Finnish Adoptive Family Study of Schizophrenia, involving 58 adoptees at high genetic risk – children of mothers with schizophrenia – versus 96 comparison adoptees suggest a model of gene–environment interaction: those with high genetic loading who experience deviant communication are much more likely to develop schizophrenia (Wahlberg *et al.* 1997).

There are psychosocial risk factors operative at the societal level which include race or cultural factors. There is, for instance, a six times higher rate of schizophrenia in Afro-Caribbean second-generation people aged 16–25 (Harrison *et al.* 1988). Social isolation in ethic minorities also appears an important factor in the development of schizophrenia (Boydell *et al.* 2001).

PRODROME

The prodromal phase of non-psychotic behavioural disturbance (NPBD) occurs in about half of early-onset schizophrenia (55%) and can last between one and seven years (Maziade *et al.* 1996a). NPBDs include internalizing behaviours (obsessive–compulsive disorder, avoidant personality, anxiety states) and externalizing behaviours (attention-deficit disorder, conduct disorder).

Acute presentations are more common in adolescence, but an insidious onset with predominantly negative symptoms – affective blunting, apathy, etc. – occurs, and heralds a poor prognosis (Maziade *et al.* 1996a; Hollis 2000).

Pathogenesis

In early-onset schizophrenia there is accumulating evidence of neurodevelopmental abnormalities (Murray *et al.* 1992; Weinberger 1987) resulting in abnormal brain structures such as ventricular enlargement, smaller brain size (Frazier *et al.* 1996) and loss of normal brain asymmetry (Crow *et al.* 1989). Schizophrenic subjects are reported as having higher rates of obstetric complications, and low birthweight (Foerster *et al.* 1991). They also show deviance in social and intellectual development.

Pre-schizophrenic boys are more hostile and anxious by the age of 7 years, while pre-schizophrenic girls demonstrate higher rates of withdrawal and under-reaction by age 11 (Done *et al.* 1994). Academic impairments – language and reading difficulties – are evident at age 7, and by age 16 years pre-schizophrenic children are rated as more clumsy with a history of poor coordination, delayed continence and poor vision. Perhaps surprisingly, in a longitudinal population study in Finland (Cannon *et al.* 2002b), those with a diagnosis of schizophrenia who went on to offend had higher birthweights, larger head circumferences and attentional problems at school, but not more birth complications.

Neuropharmacological models implicate the mono-amines dopamine and serotonin and the excitatory amino acid glutamate. Following the introduction of chlorpromazine as an antipsychotic, a dopaminergic hypothesis was formulated with suggested dopamine over-activity affecting the D_2 receptor. The success of atypical antipsychotics such as clozapine, with differing binding affinities including the D_4 receptor and 5-HT_{2AC} receptors in the medial prefrontal cortex, necessitated a more complex view. One integrative model has been proposed with glutamate, an excitatory neurotransmitter, GABA (gamma amino butyric acid) and dopamine interacting in a cortico-temporal-limbic circuit, with the thalamus acting as a sensory filter to the cortex. A model of dopamine supersensitivity is supported by the finding that prolonged heavy use of cannabis, particularly from an early age, is associated with the development of psychosis (Arseneault *et al.* 2002a).

A biological basis for the violent behaviour in schizophrenia is suggested by the genetic findings of an association of increased violence with the A2 allele variant of the tyrosine hydroxylase gene (Wei and Hemmings 1998) and homozygous catechol-O-methyltransferase (COMT) genes (Jones *et al.* 2001). Violent schizophrenic subjects have been found on MRI to have smaller hippocampi bilaterally, and greater right-to-left asymmetry of the amygdala volumes (van Amelsvoort *et al.* 1998). Early results from a study of seven repetitively violent adult schizophrenics and seven matched controls, using functional magnetic resonance spectroscopy (^{1}HMRS), indicate possible loss of neuronal integrity in the frontal lobes of the schizophrenic subjects, with reduced N-acetylasparate (a marker for neuronal density) and reduced creatine (a measure of cellular metabolic turnover). The reduction in these metabolites correlated with the number of violent episodes per month (Robertson *et al.* 1998).

SCHIZOPHRENIA AND OFFENDING BEHAVIOUR

General issues

Data on forensic aspects of early-onset schizophrenia are limited, so some reliance is put upon studies of adult-onset schizophrenia. There are clearly problems with this: adolescence represents a unique developmental phase with issues of increasing autonomy and independence and changes in relation to family, peers, school and occupation. However, there are clear clinical similarities between early-onset and adult forms of the schizophrenia illness with similar phenomenology, stability of diagnosis from adolescence to adulthood (Maziade *et al.* 1996a; Hollis 2000), and similar structural brain abnormalities (Nicolson *et al.* 1999).

Where possible, attempts have been made to extract findings relating to late adolescence and early adulthood from epidemiological surveys such as the Camberwell study (Wessely *et al.* 1994) and WHO studies (Volavka *et al.* 1997). Some caution is necessary as there are differences between early- and late-onset schizophrenia subjects who are also violent offenders (Tengström *et al.* 2001). The early-onset group is more often characterized by histories of parental substance abuse, early school failure, conduct disorder and later antisocial personality functioning. The early-onset group appear generally more deviant, committing more crimes including violent crimes, and displaying greater rates of substance abuse.

There are problems is assessing the strength of association between EOS and criminal behaviour, not least of which is the rarity of the disorder and the diagnostic difficulties in the early or prodromal phase of the illness. Once psychotic symptoms develop, the youth who has committed a crime, with the exception of serious crimes such as rape, arson and murder, is often diverted from the criminal justice system by referral to the mental health services, making official crime figures unrepresentative.

As mentioned earlier, the prodromal phase of non-psychotic behavioural disturbances occurs in just over half of cases and can last on average six years. About half of these are externalizing behaviours – conduct disorder and attention-deficit disorder. As shown in the seminal studies of Farrington and West, of non-mentally ill boys, these behaviours, in conjunction with poverty, school failure, adverse parenting, and so on, represent risk factors for later offending behaviour. The importance of this lies in the finding that one of the strongest predictors of offending behaviour during a schizophrenic illness is pre-illness offending (Wessely and Taylor 1991).

Violent episodes are most likely to occur in the month prior to admission (Johnstone *et al.* 1986; Humphreys *et al.* 1992). In the Northwick Park study, violence was noted in a third of 253 first-onset cases (Johnstone *et al.* 1986). The WHO study of severe mental disorders in developed and developing countries revealed that, amongst the 1017 patients with schizophrenia presenting with psychotic symptoms, 112 out of 194 assaults coincided with the onset of the illness, contrasting with 13 before and 69 after the onset (Volavka *et al.* 1997). Violence was more likely with an acute onset of schizophrenia. Systematic under-reporting may account for the finding that few of these episodes of ward-based violence are recorded in official crime statistics.

Relationship between offending and schizophrenia

The relationship is complex. Data from the Camberwell study (Wessely *et al.* 1994) suggest, overall, that schizophrenia is not associated with an increased rate of criminality; however, this is not true for violent or serious crimes, where the rate for males with schizophrenia is three times that of the matched population (95% CI: 1.8–5.5). The risk factors for a criminal conviction include: being male, coming from an ethnic minority grouping (particularly Afro-Caribbean), poor social and work adjustment, misusing drugs and alcohol, earlier age of onset, and lower social class. These factors are interactive, schizophrenia being the weakest predictor. In a prospective 26-year follow-up study of a total birth cohort in Northern Finland (*n* = 12,058), the rate of any criminal behaviour amongst those with schizophrenia compared to normal healthy males was raised (odds ratio (OR): 3.0; 95% CI: 0.9–12.3), with an even greater risk of recidivism (more than two crimes) amongst schizophrenic males (OR: 9.5; 95% CI: 2.2–30) (Räsänen *et al.* 1998). However, the rate was significantly greater for violent offences, especially with coexistent alcohol abuse (OR: 25; 95% CI: 6.1–97.5), clearly pointing to the importance of comorbid alcohol and substance abuse as risk factors for violent crime. Overall, 7% (11/165) of violent male offenders were psychotic (Tiihonen *et al.* 1997).

Schizophrenia constitutes a specific risk for acquiring a criminal record. The likelihood of a male with schizophrenia getting a criminal record by the age of 30 is about 28% – very similar to that for normal males from an inner city (Farrington 1981). However, patients with schizophrenia continue to acquire criminal records after the age of 40, with lifetime rates for males of 52% versus 32% for controls, and for females 16% versus 9% (Wesseley *et al.* 1994). A Swedish study using centralized police records (Lindqvist and Allebeck 1990) revealed comparable results, with a crime rate amongst younger males with schizophrenia similar to that of the general population. Interestingly, amongst females with schizophrenia the rate was twice that of the normal female population. Overall, the level of violence was four times higher amongst those with schizophrenia; however, most offences were of minor severity.

Assaultative behaviour is associated with hearing voices, manic excitement and going on a spending spree (Volavka *et al.* 1997). Amongst adult psychotic prisoners, 20% are driven to offend by their symptoms; and alarmingly, 8% of those charged with homicide have schizophrenia – a high rate indeed (Taylor 1985).

The rate of violent or assaultative behaviour and criminality amongst first-presentation early-onset DSM-III-R schizophrenia can be judged from the Oxford Early Psychosis study (James *et al.* 1999). This prospective five-year study with psychiatric controls (Table 12.1) showed

Table 12.1 *Early-onset schizophrenia compared with psychiatric controls*

	Schizophrenia (*n* = 30)	Controls (*n* = 20)
Mean age in years (SD)	16.9 (1.2)	16.1 (1.9)
Student's *t*-test	–	0.83
		($p = 0.48$)
Sex		
males	20	12
females	10	8
χ^2- test		0.23
		(d.f. = 1, $p = 0.63$)
Social class		
I	1	1
II	5	9
III	14	9
IV	9	1
V	1	1
χ^2-test	–	7.92
		(d.f. = 4, $p = 0.09$)

that the rate of offending behaviour was low (13% versus 15%; Fisher exact test $p = 1.00$), although violent or assaultative behaviour was slightly more common, albeit not significantly, in the schizophrenic group (30% versus 10%; Fisher exact test $p = 0.16$).

Violent behaviour was confined to the month prior to admission and the period of initial hospitalization and, as in adult studies, even though severe, did not result in criminal proceedings. The violent episodes were in response to delusional, paranoid beliefs or hallucinatory experiences. Whilst the criminal behaviour amongst the psychiatric controls was mundane (traffic and drug offences), that amongst the schizophrenic group was either serious (arson, stabbing, threatening behaviour with a shotgun) or bizarre (being arrested for stealing £1 and causing a public nuisance by sitting cross-legged on a telephone kiosk). All were the direct result of delusional experiences. After assessment, two were treated in open units, one in a medium-secure unit and one in Broadmoor under s41 of the Mental Health Act 1983. Two made good symptomatic recoveries; one remained symptomatic and socially impaired but no longer dangerous; and one, who had a pre-existing schizoid personality, remained dangerous with fantasies of stabbing and rape. Although interesting and representative of a catchment area of 2.5 million in rural mid-England, the Oxford study is limited by the greater social affluence generally of this population, which contrasts with the deprivation of large inner cities, where the rates of criminality and psychiatric disorder are raised.

Data from the National Confidential Inquiry into Homicides for the 18-month study period 1996/97 indicate that there were 100 youth homicides (youths aged 20 and under) of whom four had schizophrenia (Shaw *et al.* 1999; Appleby, personal communication 1999). This low rate accords with the rate of admissions for mental illness to the special hospitals between 1972 and 1996, where the average for males was 2.4 per year and 0.9 per year for females for those aged less than 18 years (Taylor, personal communication 1997). The majority of those suffering from mental illness had schizophrenia and had been admitted for dangerous and/or violent behaviour. In contrast, a birth-cohort study in Dunedin (Arseneault *et al.* 2000c) up to the age of 21 years, representing 94% of the total city population ($n = 941$), found those with schizophrenia spectrum disorders were 2.5 times (95% CI: 1.1–5.7) more likely than controls to be involved in violent crimes and they accounted for 10% of the total violent crimes committed. A paranoid cognitive personality style was particularly likely to be associated with violence. Importantly, youths with schizophrenia spectrum disorders were more likely than those with substance abuse to victimize co-residents (Arseneault *et al.* 2002b).

There are no reasons to assume those with schizophrenia are more or less likely to be influenced by those factors known to be associated with a higher youth crime rate. There appears, however, to be a pathoplastic effect of culture: in developing countries the rate of assaultative behaviour amongst those with schizophrenia is three times (95% CI: 2.26–3.95) that in developed countries (Volavka *et al.* 1997).

DIFFERENTIAL DIAGNOSIS

The diagnosis of schizophrenia is often complex, requiring detailed phenomenological enquiry and longitudinal observation. In late childhood and early adolescence the differentiation of psychotic phenomenon from non-psychotic, idiosyncratic thinking associated with developmental delays, exposure to traumatic events and overactive imagination, poses problems. Differentiating the odd child with developmental and personality difficulties from the insidious, premorbid state found in schizophrenia is usually difficult, but the presence of active hallucinations and delusions is diagnostic of the latter. Likewise, distinguishing between the speech and language problems of children with pervasive developmental delays and formal thought disorder is often problematic, but loosening of associations and incoherence point toward a diagnosis of psychosis.

Mood disorders
Bipolar disorder with psychotic symptoms is misdiagnosed as schizophrenia in up to 50% of cases (Werry *et al.* 1991). Longitudinal observation and the presence of a positive family history of affective illness helps differentiate

these disorders, although there is a raised rate of depression in relatives of probands with schizophrenia.

Organic disorders
All adolescents presenting with a psychotic illness should receive a thorough medical examination including blood tests, urine analysis and an MRI scan. The range of organic pathologies to be screened include:

- delirium
- central nervous system lesions – seizure disorders, brain tumours, congenital malformations, head injury
- neurodegenerative disorders – Huntington's chorea, lipid storage disorder
- metabolic disorders – Wilson's disease, endocrinopathies
- infections – meningitis, encephalitis, human immunodeficiency virus-related syndromes
- toxic encephalopathies – corticosteroids, illegal drugs (cannabis, amphetamines, LSD, cocaine, ecstasy, etc.).

The rate of illegal drug usage amongst first presentations of schizophrenia is high – up to 50% in some studies. In order to distinguish a drug-induced psychosis a period of verified detoxification is necessary.

Pervasive developmental disorders
Asperger syndrome and autism pose particular differential diagnostic problems, especially as psychotic episodes can occur in both conditions. Although there are often developmental delays in cases of schizophrenia, including language, in autism and Asperger syndrome there is a lifelong history of aberrant social relatedness and characteristic speech abnormalities. The absence or transient nature of positive psychotic symptoms and the absence of a normal period of development help distinguish the conditions.

Personality disorders and dissociative states
Adolescents with severe conduct disorder may report psychotic-like symptoms, particularly auditory hallucinations. However, not all such experiences are part of a psychotic process (Garralda 1984), and the lack of thought disorder and delusions helps distinguish this presentation from schizophrenia. Psychotic-like symptoms are seen in dissociative states that follow histories of severe abuse. Likewise, borderline personality disorders can be difficult to differentiate. The transient nature of the psychotic experiences in this disorder and the lack of delusions and thought disorder combined with the chaotic, demanding and dependent social relationships contrast with the schizoid, socially isolated and awkward relationships of the pre-schizophrenic adolescent.

Obsessive–compulsive disorder
Severe obsessive–compulsive symptoms, such as intrusive thoughts or fears of contamination, without the patient being able to recognize these ideas as his or her own, can lead to diagnostic difficulty.

ASSESSMENT

The forensic assessment of schizophrenia can be divided into two interrelated parts: clinical assessment and risk assessment.

Clinical assessment

The assessment of schizophrenia can be a complex task, broadly consisting of three areas.

History

Whenever possible, an independent account of the early history should be sought. In particular, a developmental history of early language problems or disorder is important, as there is a link between these and later schizophrenia. The clinician should be alerted to the quality of peer relationships, interests and academic achievements, all of which may be adversely affected. Acute presentations occur in about half of cases; in the others there is an insidious onset with gradual withdrawal and isolation, loss of interest in activities – even those previously enjoyed – and a decline in sociability. The crucial factor is a change in personality functioning.

Examination of mental state

Rigorous attention to seeking the presence or otherwise of the psychotic symptoms, listed above, is an absolute necessity. This requires patience, time and an empathic, enquiring attitude; the patient may be suspicious, frightened of his or her experiences or worried about sanity. Semi-structured interviews such as K-SADS (Kiddie's Schedule for Affective Disorders and Schizophrenia; Chambers et al. 1985) are useful.

Observation

If the patient is severely ill, at risk of self-harm or being violent or behaviourally disturbed, admission to hospital is indicated. Clear accounts of the patient's behaviour are extremely useful. It should be possible to judge the patient's:

- response to abnormal experiences and his/her ability to resist these
- sociability and the potential to form relationships
- interaction with family and other significant figures
- level of general functioning
- likely response to treatment.

Risk assessment

The risk assessment should be specific and address the following.

Historic risk behaviours
- When?
- In what situation?

- With whom or to whom were these behaviours directed?
- Precipitating, aggravating and ameliorating factors?
- What was the associated mental state?
- Usage of illicit drugs or alcohol?

Past behaviour is one of the best or strongest predictors of future behaviour.

Current risk behaviours
Have there been changes in:

- external circumstances or situation?
- mental state?
- usage of illicit drugs or alcohol?
- social support network, including psychiatric and social services?

Mental state examination
This should cover:

- *subjective feelings of tension* or 'explosiveness' – ideas or feelings of violence
- persecutory ideation – especially delusions, paying particular attention to whether those currently around the patient are incorporated into the delusional system
- *passivity phenomena* – note the important association of 'threat/control–override' symptoms with violence (Link and Stueve 1994)
- *hallucinations* – their nature and quality, whether the source is benevolent or malevolent; also the omnipotence of the source (e.g. what are the consequences of not complying with any commands, why comply with some and not others?)
- *depression* – for example 'I wish I was dead, there's nothing to live for, I might as well kill her and myself too.'
- *jealousy of morbid intensity* – nature and detail, and importantly who is targeted
- *insight* – not only into any psychiatric disorder but also previous violent or aggressive behaviour (insight, however, may have poor predictive value for future violent episodes: Yen et al. (2002)).

Discussion
The risk assessment is not an all-or-nothing event; rather it should be an ongoing process, which needs to be incorporated into the day-to-day management of the patient.

Several broad statements can be made about the risk of violent or dangerous behaviour in those who are mentally disordered (Reed 1997):

- The great majority of those who are mentally ill present no increased risk to others.
- The best predictors of future offending among mentally disordered people are the same as for the whole population: previous offending, criminality within the family, poor parenting, etc.
- People suffering from severe mental illness such as schizophrenia may present an increased risk to others when they have active symptoms.

- People suffering from severe mental illness who have active symptoms and also abuse drugs or alcohol present a seriously increased risk to others.

Even with the use of risk assessments, the prediction of the dangerousness by mental health workers overall is very inexact. For adults with psychosis, detailed enquiry about delusions – strength of conviction, belief acquisition, maintenance factors, affect, preoccupation, systematization and insight – may be important (Buchanan 1997). Preliminary evidence suggests that those more likely to act on a delusion do the following: identify evidence, especially in the last week, to support their delusional beliefs; seek evidence to confirm their beliefs; feel frightened as a result of delusional beliefs; and have more insight (Buchanan 1997). In adolescents, however, one retrospective study has shown that violent behaviour is more closely related to a history of emotional and physical abuse (Clare et al. 2000).

TREATMENT

General issues

The treatment of schizophrenia can be divided broadly into two parts: specific treatment of the psychotic symptomatology, and general treatment of the psychological, social and educational needs of the adolescent (AACAP 2001).

Early intervention is important (Birchwood et al. 1997). Several studies such as the Northwick Park study (Johnstone et al. 1986) have demonstrated that the time to treat, often over one year with adults, is adversely associated with increased complications of severe behavioural disturbance and family difficulties, and a three-times greater likelihood of subsequent relapse. Some have suggested (e.g. Wyatt 1995) that untreated psychosis may be toxic, although recent MRI studies (Hoff et al. 2000) and neuropsychological studies (Barnes et al. 2000) have not supported this view.

Specific treatment

PHARMACOLOGICAL INTERVENTIONS

The only specific treatment for schizophrenia, demonstrated in over 100 double-blind trials, is neuroleptic medication (Davis et al. 1987). The evidence for effectiveness in adolescence is less strong and there is a suggestion that the non-response rate is higher (Campbell and Spencer 1988).

Recent practice and research suggests that the atypical neuroleptics are effective in the treatment of schizophrenia. Risperidone, an atypical antipsychotic, with potent properties to inhibit serotonin (5-HT$_{2A}$) and dopamine receptors, may be more effective than convential neuroleptics (Peuskens et al. 1995); however, although encouraging, the evidence in early-onset schizophrenia is more limited (Armenteros et al. 1997). Other novel antipsychotics are available including olanzapine, amisulpiride and quetiapine, which appear at least as effective as conventional neuroleptics. Clozapine is the most effective of all of the neuroleptics with reports of 67% significant improvement and 21% partial improvement in a group of 57 'predominantly' adult schizophrenic subjects (Blanz and Schmidt 1993). Clozapine was more effective than haloperidol in a sample of 21 individuals with childhood-onset schizophrenia, but there was a high rate of agranulocytosis and seizures in this younger group (Kumra et al. 1996). Because of the risk of agranulocytosis, estimated at 1%, weekly blood test monitoring is necessary. This medication is therefore reserved for cases of resistant schizophrenia where trials of two types of neuroleptics have failed to produce a response. Clozapine may offer particular benefit in a forensic population as it is suggested that it reduces aggression because of its central serotonergic effects (Meltzer 1992). There is evidence of improvement in cognitive functioning with atypicals such as quetiapine (Herold et al. 2002). Patients on atypical neuroleptics – risperidone, olanzapine, quetiapine, amisulpiride and clozapine – also appear to experience fewer side-effects, particularly tardive dyskinesia, but many do gain significant weight (Barnes and McPhillips 1999). Overall, patients on these medications may have a higher quality of life (Franz et al. 1997).

For severely disturbed patients, oral or intramuscular benzodiazepines are used to achieve sedation (McAllister-Williams 2001). Experience with the intramuscular forms of the newer atypical neuroleptics is as yet limited, but there are considerable side-effects with the older neuroleptics. In older adolescents, who have had previous exposure to neuroleptics, Acuphase (zuclopenthixol acetate), a depot medication, offers the advantage of single dosage with effects lasting for 72 hours. Depot medication is also useful where there are concerns about longer-term compliance, especially prior to discharge to the community.

PSYCHOLOGICAL INTERVENTIONS

In addition to medication, psychological approaches are necessary. A package of interventions over a six-month to two-year period, or longer, is beneficial, provided they are tailored to the patient, and not applied too intensively or ambitiously, but rather steadily, in a stable framework of supportive care (McGlashan 1988).

The individual

Cognitive–behavioural therapy, directed at helping the patient to gain some control over the hallucinatory experiences and challenge the delusions, is a very useful adjunct in those patients who are able to cooperate (Drake and Lewis 1997). This form of treatment can also be delivered by qualified psychiatric nurses with adequate supervision (Turkington *et al.* 2002).

The family

A psycho-educational approach with the family is essential and has been shown, in combination with other interventions such as long-term drug prophylaxis, to reduce relapse rates by up to 50% (Falloon and Brooker 1992). The aim is to educate the family about the illness and to reduce high levels of expressed emotion – particularly in critical and over-involved relationships (Falloon 1992).

It is important for the patient and family to be fully aware of the diagnosis and its implications so that they can cooperate with plans for social re-integration. There is evidence of considerable stress amongst carers, so that provision of support from either statutory or voluntary agencies is helpful.

Alerting the patient and family to the symptoms of possible relapse is useful, and should allow them to access help from the primary-care level via the general practitioner and community psychiatric nurse or hospital services.

Social functioning

Active rehabilitation is a necessary part of treatment. Evidence from long-term follow-up studies suggests that the major deterioration occurs within the first five years of the illness; this period, therefore, represents the most 'vulnerable period', and, perhaps, the most amenable time for psychosocial interventions (Birchwood 1992). A range of interventions is necessary and supported in the National Institute for Clinical Excellence guidelines (NICE 2002).

Skills for daily living

There are problems resulting from the illness, including negative symptoms of anergia, lack of volition, poverty of thought, and so on, which are difficult to treat and interfere greatly with rehabilitation. Pharmacological treatments are to a degree helpful (the novel neuroleptics risperidone and olanzapine do improve negative symptoms), but active, operant behavioural treatment programmes with social reinforcers may be required.

Rehabilitation to school/college or vocational training

There may be a real or apparent intellectual decline making it necessary to assess the individual's capacity for further education or vocational training. Active rehabilitation is a cornerstone to treatment and may help prevent relapse.

MANAGEMENT

It is a fundamental principle that the patient should be treated in the least restrictive setting appropriate to that person's needs. This judgement depends, therefore, on the risk assessment. It may be appropriate to treat the patient at home with attendance as a day patient, provided the home situation is safe and compliance with medication can be ensured. Inpatient treatment allows the opportunity for an in-depth assessment of the psychopathology and response to treatment. For those who refuse treatment, the latter may need to be through an order under s2 or s3 of the Mental Health Act 1983, or as directed by Hospital Orders 37 or 38 of the Act. Should the patient continue to present violent or dangerous behaviour, especially with the risk of absconding, secure care should be considered.

DISCHARGE

Patients over the age of 16 years and all those detained under ss 3, 37 or 38 of the Mental Health Act 1983, should be included under the Care Programme Approach (CPA; DoH 1990). Although this system has been criticized (Burns 1997), it does require:

- an assessment of need, including an assessment of risk
- an agreed package of care
- a nominated key-worker
- regular reviews and monitoring.

The most crucial aspect is maintaining contact with the patient. It is also essential to share relevant information with the family, carers, general practitioner and social services. Where there has been a history of violence, information should be included in the discharge summary on the assessment of ongoing risk, including, where possible, defining future circumstances likely to pose risks. However, a risk assessment is not enough; it must be accompanied by a risk management plan with reviews (Reed 1997). Clearly, this is an ongoing process.

A 'supervised discharge' under s25 of the Mental Health (Patients in the Community) Act 1995 allows continued compulsory treatment outside hospital. It may be necessary to ensure that an involuntary patient continues to receive medication after discharge, usually in depot form. This section of the Act applies only to those over 16 years of age.

OUTCOME

There is no systematic cure for schizophrenia. A small percentage (10–17%: Cawthron *et al.* 1994; Werry *et al.* 1991; Hollis 2000) appear to recover after the first episode, while the majority continue to experience symptoms, some disintegration of the personality and social handicap.

The extremely poor outcome of early-onset schizophrenia is predicted by premorbid functioning (Werry *et al.* 1991; Maziade *et al.* 1996b) and the severity of the positive and negative symptoms during the acute phase (Maziade *et al.* 1996b; Hollis 2000). Interestingly, the presence of non-psychotic behaviour disturbances or premorbid developmental problems are not related to severity of outcome. There is some consensus in the literature that the major deterioration occurs within the first few years of the onset, with a levelling off or plateauing thereafter (Bleuler 1978). Two broad patterns are seen: a relapsing course and a continuous illness.

The suicide rate, up to 15% in one study (Werry *et al.* 1991), is greatest within the first six years (Westermeyer *et al.* 1991) and is often associated with a depressive illness and feelings of hopelessness surrounding the illness itself. Continued social support and active treatment may mitigate against this. In particular, there is evidence that the atypical antipsychotics olanzapine and respiridone have antidepressant effects and clozapine reduces the suicide rate (Meltzer 1995).

Direct intervention aimed at supporting families with psycho-education and reduction of high expressed emotion, in conjunction with continuing medication, offers the best treatment package available and reduces the relapse rate substantially (Falloon and Brooker 1992).

A Dutch study (Linszen *et al.* 1998) found the effect of early intervention, in young patients (mean age 20) with first and second episodes of schizophrenia and related disorders, to be substantial, with a relapse rate of 15% during the intensive phase. Subsequently, the relapse rate rose to 64% at 17–55 months, with a deterioration in psychosocial functioning. Robust predictors of relapse were high expressed emotion and heavy cannabis use. The authors suggest continuation of the intensive intervention package for a minimum period of five years.

Overall, the picture is of continuing vulnerability. Treatment plans must allow for this and provision needs to made for longer-term coordinated care. This should involve links with social services, education, voluntary organizations and housing as appropriate. A recent systematic review has shown that, for adults, community mental health team management is superior to standard care (Simmonds *et al.* 2001), indicating that community and domiciliary delivery of care is important.

CONCLUSIONS AND FUTURE DIRECTIONS

RESEARCH

It is important to know the prevalence and development of offending behaviour in those suffering from, or at risk of, schizophrenia, in order to target interventions more accurately. This is a difficult task given the relative rarity of the disorder, and it requires collaboration between research centres. The first requirement is an accurately defined incidence and prevalence study on a defined population of DSM-IV or ICD-10 diagnosed early-onset schizophrenia. Prospective population studies would give greater understanding of the patterns of development and mechanisms of offending, and those factors specifically associated with persistence and remission of the violence and dangerous behaviour.

Despite some recent advances, there is a continuing need for further research into effective treatments, both pharmacological and psychological. The era of neuro-imaging will hopefully allow delineation of those brain structures and systems associated with violence, which may point to targeted pharmacological interventions, whilst further work on the applicability of cognitive–behavioural therapy aimed at challenging psychotic symptoms, improving insight and compliance is awaited.

POLICIES

In the UK there is a need for the development of forensic services on a regional basis with links to the now nationally commissioned, for England and Wales, inpatient medium-secure facilities for adolescents in Newcastle, Salford and Birmingham. At a local level, the development of protocols for risk assessment for this age group, and treatment guidelines, would help district child and adolescent psychiatrists manage these cases, in the first instance, more effective and safely.

A Research and Development Initiative by the National Health Service in the area of forensic adolescent psychiatry would be welcomed. Although research is expensive, it needs to be remembered that in 2002 it cost more than £250,000 per year to treat an adolescent in secure facilities, and any treatment which reduces the length of time in secure accommodation may pay dividends. An evidence-based approach, using numbers needed to secure, may aid planning in this area.

This group of disturbed and disturbing adolescents poses considerable problems in management. Alongside the systematic application of research-based risk assessments of dangerousness, the development of a measure of the 'burden of care' for the family and professionals is needed to help plan service delivery on a more rational basis.

REFERENCES

AACAP (American Academy of Child and Adolescent Psychiatry) 2001: Practice parameters for the assessment and treatment of children and adolescents with schizophrenia. *Journal of the American Academy of Child and Adolescent Psychiatry* **40**(suppl. 7): 4–23S.

APA (American Psychiatric Association) 1994: *Diagnostic and Statistical Manual of Mental Disorders*, 4th edn (DSM-IV). Washington, DC: APA.

Armenteros, J.L., Whitaker, A.H., Welikson, M., Stedge, D. and Gorman, J. 1997: Risperidone in adolescents with schizophrenia: an open pilot study. *Journal of the American Academy of Child and Adolescent Psychiatry* **36**: 694–700.

Arseneault, L., Cannon, M., Poulton, R. *et al.* 2002a: Cannabis use in adolescence and risk for adult psychosis: longitudinal prospective study. *British Medical Journal* **325**: 1212–13.

Arseneault, L., Moffit, T.E., Capsi, A. and Taylor, P.J. 2002b: The targets of violence committed by young offenders with alcohol dependence, marijuana dependence and schizophrenia-spectrum disorders: findings from a birth cohort. *Criminal Behaviour and Mental Health* **12**: 155–68.

Arseneault, L., Moffit, T.E., Capsi, A., Taylor, P.J. and Silva, P.A. 2000c: Mental disorders in a total birth cohort: results from the Dunedin study. *Archives of General Psychiatry* **57**: 979–86.

Barnes, T.R., Hutton, S.B., Chapman, M.J. *et al.* 2000: West London first-episode study of schizophrenia: clinical correlates of duration of untreated psychosis. *British Journal of Psychiatry* **177**: 207–11.

Beratis, S., Gabriel, J. and Hoidas, S. 1994: Age of onset in subtypes of schizophrenic disorders. *Schizophrenia Bulletin* **20**: 287–96.

Birchwood, M. 1992: Integrating psychosocial interventions in schizophrenia: critical periods and service structures. *Schizophrenia Monitor* **2**(3): 1–4.

Birchwood, M., McGregory, P. and Jackson, H. 1997: Early intervention in schizophrenia. *British Journal of Psychiatry* **171**: 2–5.

Blanz, B. and Schmidt, S. 1993: Clozapine for schizophrenia (letter). *Journal of the American Academy of Child and Adolescent Psychiatry* **32**: 323–4.

Bleuler, E. 1950[1911]: *Dementia Praecox or the Group of Schizophrenias* (trans. J. Zinkin). New York: International Universities.

Bleuler, M. 1978: *The Schizophrenic Disorders: Long Term Patient and Family Studies* (trans. C Clements). New Haven, CT: Yale University Press.

Boydell, J., van Os, J., McKenzie, K. *et al.* 2001: Incidence of schizophrenia in ethnic minorities in London: ecological study into interactions with environment. *British Medical Journal* **323**: 1336–8.

Brewin, J., Cantwell, R., Dalkin, T. *et al.* 1997: Incidence of schizophrenia in Nottingham. *British Journal of Psychiatry* **171**: 140–4.

Buchanan, A. 1997: The investigation of acting on delusions as a tool for risk assessment in the mentally disordered. *British Journal of Psychiatry* **170**(suppl. 32): 12–16.

Burns, T. 1997: Case management, care management and care programming. *British Journal of Psychiatry* **170**: 393–5.

Burns, T.E. and McPhillips, M.A. 1999: Critical analysis and comparison of the side-effect and safety profiles of the new antipsychotics. *British Journal of Psychiatry* **174**: 34–43.

Campbell, M. and Spencer, E.K. 1988: Psychopharmacology in child and adolescent psychiatry. *Journal of the American Academy of Child and Adolescent Psychiatry* **139**: 758–62.

Cannon, M.C., Jones, P.R. and Murray, R. 2002a: Obstetric complications and schizophrenia: historical and meta-analytical review. *American Journal of Psychiatry* **159**: 1080–92.

Cannon, M.C., Huttunen, M.G., Tanskanen, A.J. *et al.* 2002b: Perinatal and childhood risk factors for later criminality and violence in schizophrenia. *British Journal of Psychiatry* **180**: 496–501.

Cawthron, P., James, A., Dell, J. and Seagroat, V. 1994: Adolescent onset psychosis: a clinical and outcome study. *Journal of Child Psychology and Psychiatry* **35**: 1321–32.

Chambers, W., Puig-Antich, J., Hirsh, M. *et al.* 1985: The assessment of affective disorders in children and adolescents by semi-structured interview: test–retest reliability of the K–SADS-P. *Archives of General Psychiatry* **42**: 696–702.

Clare, P., Bailey, S. and Clark, A. 2000: Relationship between psychotic disorders in adolescence and criminally violent behaviour. *British Journal of Psychiatry* **177**: 275–9.

Crow, T.J., Ball, J., Bloom, S.R. *et al.* 1989: Schizophrenia as an anomaly of development of cerebral asymmetry: a post mortem study and a proposal concerning the genetic basis of the disease. *Archives of General Psychiatry* **46**: 1145–50.

Crow, T.J. and Done, D.J. 1992: Prenatal exposure to influenza does not cause schizophrenia. *British Journal of Psychiatry* **161**: 390–3.

Davis, J.M., Comarty, J.E. and Janicak, P.G. 1987: The psychological effects of antipsychotic drugs. In Stefanis, C.N. and Rabavilas, A.D. (eds), *Schizophrenia: Recent Biosocial Developments*. New York: Human Science Press, 165–81.

DoH (Department of Health) 1990: *The Care Programme Approach for People with a Mental Illness Referred to the Specialist Psychiatric Service*. Hc(90) 23/LASSL(90)II. London: DoH.

Done, D.J., Crow, T.J., Johnstone, E.C. and Sacker, A. 1994: Childhood antecedents of schizophrenia and affective illness: social adjustments ages 7 and 11. *British Medical Journal* **309**: 699–703.

Drake, R.J. and Lewis, S.W. 1997: Cognitive behavioural therapy in schizophrenia. *Schizophrenia Monitor* **7**: 1–3.

Farrington, D. 1981: The prevalence of convictions. *British Journal of Criminology* **21**: 173–5.

Falloon, I.R. 1992: Psychotherapy for schizophrenic disorders: a review. *British Journal of Hospital Medicine* **48**: 164–70.

Falloon, I.R. and Brooker, C. 1992: A critical re-evaluation of social and family interventions in schizophrenia. *Schizophrenia Monitor* **2**(4): 1–4.

Franz, M., Lis, S., Pluddeman, K. and Gallhoper, B. 1997: Conventional versus atypical neuroleptics: subjective quality of life in schizophrenic patients. *British Journal of Psychiatry* **170**: 422–5.

Foerster, A., Lewis, S.W., Owen, M.J. and Murray, R.M. 1991: Low birth weight and a family history of schizophrenia predict poor premorbid functioning in psychosis. *Schizophrenia Research* **5**: 13–20.

Frazier, J.A., Giedd, J.N., Hamburger, S.D. *et al.* 1996: Brain anatomic magnetic resonance imaging in childhood onset schizophrenia. *Archives of General Psychiatry* **53**: 617–24.

Garralda, M.E. 1994: Hallucinations in children and adolescents with conduct and emotional disorders: I. The clinical phenomena. *Psychological Medicine* **14**: 589–96.

Geddes, J.R. and Lawrie, S.M. 1995: Obstetric complications and schizophrenia. *British Journal of Psychiatry* **167**: 786–93.

Gillberg, C., Wahlstrom, J., Forsman, A., Hellgren, I. and Gillberg, I.C. 1986: Teenage psychoses: epidemiology, classification and reduced optimality in the pre-, peri-, and neonatal periodes. *Journal of Child Psychology and Psychiatry* **27**: 87–98.

Goldstein, M. 1987: The ULCA High Risk Project. *Schizophrenia Bulletin* **13**: 505–14.

Harrison, G., Owens, D., Holton, T., Neilson, D. and Boot, D.A. 1988: A prospective study of severe mental disorder in Afro-Caribbean patients. *Psychological Medicine* **18**: 643–7.

Herold, R., Simnon, T., Tényi, T. and Trixler, M. 2002: Cognitive functioning and subjective well-being in schizophrenia after six-month quetiapine treatment. *Journal of the European College of Neuropsychopharmacology* **12**(suppl. 3): 267.

Hoff, A.L., Sakuma, M., Razi, K. *et al.* 2000: Lack of association between duration of untreated illness and severity of cognitive and structural brain deficits at the first episode of schizophrenia. *American Journal of Psychiatry* **157**: 1824–8.

Hollis, C. 2000: Adult outcomes of child- and adolescent-onset schizophrenia: diagnostic stability and predictive validity. *American Journal of Psychiatry* **157**: 1652–9.

Humphreys, M., Johnstone, E.C., MacMillan, J.F. *et al.* 1992: Dangerous behaviour preceding first admission for schizophrenia. *British Journal of Psychiatry* **161**: 501–5.

James, A.C., Crow, T.J., Renowden, S. *et al.* 1999: Is the course of brain development in schizophrenia delayed? Evidence from onsets in adolescence. *Schizophrenia Research* **40**: 1–10.

Johnstone, E.C., Crow, T., Johnson, A. *et al.* 1986: The Northwick Park study of first episode of schizophrenia: I. Presentation of the illness and problems relating to admission. *British Journal of Psychiatry* **148**: 115–20.

Jones, G., Zammit, S., Norton, N., Hamshere, M.L., Jones, S.J., Milham, C., Sanders, R.D., McCarthy, G.M., Jones, L.A., Cardno, A.G., Gray, M., Murphy, K.C. and Owen, M.J. 2001: Aggressive behaviour in patients with schizophrenia is associated with catechol-*O*-methyltransferase genotype. *British Journal of Psychiatry* **179**: 351–5.

Jones, P. and Murray, R.M. 1991: The genetics of schizophrenia is the genetics of neurodevelopment. *British Journal of Psychiatry* **158**: 615–23.

Kraepelin, E. 1919[1899]: *Dementia Praecox and Paraphrenia* (trans. R. Barclay). Edinburgh: S. Livingstone.

Kumra,, S., Frazier, J.A., Jacobsen, L.K. *et al.* 1996: Childhood-onset schizophrenia: a double-blind clozapine–haloperidol comparison. *Archives of General Psychiatry* **53**: 1090–7.

Loranger, A.W. 1984: Sex difference in the onset of schizophrenia. *Archives of General Psychiatry* **41**: 157–61.

Lindqvist, F. and Allebeck, P. 1990: Schizophrenia and crime: a follow-up of 644 schizophrenics in Stockhom. *British Journal of Psychiatry* **157**: 345–50.

Linszen, D.H., Dingemans, P.M. and Lentor, M.A. 1998: Early intervention and the course of schizophrenia. *Schizophrenia Research* **29**: 159.

Maziade, M., Bouchard, S., Gingras, N. *et al.* 1996a: Long term stability of diagnosis and symptom dimensions in a systematic sample of patients with onset of schizophrenia in childhood and early adolescence: I. Nosology sex and age of onset. *British Journal of Psychiatry* **169**: 361–70.

Maziade, M., Bouchard, S., Gingras, N. *et al.* 1996b: Long term stability of diagnosis and symptom dimensions in a systematic sample of patients with onset of schizophrenia in childhood and early adolescence: II. Positive/negative distinction and childhood predictors of adult outcome. *British Journal of Psychiatry* **169**: 371–8.

Maziade, M., Martinez, M., Rodrigue, B. *et al.* 1997: Childhood/early adolescence-onset and adult-onset schizophrenia: heterogeneity at the D_3 receptor. *British Journal of Psychiatry* **170**: 27–30.

McAllister-Williams, R.H. and Ferrier, I.N. 2001: Rapid tranquillisation: time for reappraisal of options for parental therapy. *British Journal of Psychiatry* **179**: 485–9.

McGlashan, T.H. 1988: A selective review of recent North American long-term follow-up studies of schizophrenia. *Schizophrenia Bulletin* **16**: 515–42.

McGuffin, P., Anderson, P., Owen, M. and Farmer, A. 1994: The strength of the genetic effect: is there room for an environmental influence on the aetiology of schizophrenia? *British Journal of Psychiatry* **164**: 593–9.

Meltzer, H.Y. 1992: Treatment of the neuroleptic nonresponsive schizophrenic patient. *Schizophrenia Bulletin* **18**: 515–41.

Murray, R., O'Challaghan, E., Castle, D. and Lewis, S. 1992: A neurodevelopmental approach to schizophrenia. *Schizophrenia Bulletin* **18**: 319–34.

NICE (National Institute for Clinical Excellence) 2002: *Schizophrenia: Core Interventions in the Treatment and Management of Schizophrenia in Primary and Secondary Care.* London: NICE.

Nicolson, R. and Rapoport, J.L. 1999: Childhood-onset schizophrenia: rare but worth studying. *Biological Psychiatry* **46**(10): 18–28.

Peuskens, J. *et al.* 1995: Risperidone in the treatment of patients with chronic schizophrenia: a multinational, multicentre, double-blind, parallel-group study of risperidone vs halopreidol. *British Journal of Psychiatry* **166**: 712–26.

Pulver, A.E., Brown, C.H., Wolyniee, P. and McGrath, J. 1990: Schizophrenia: age at onset, gender and familial risk. *Acta Psychiatrica Scandanvica* **82**: 344–51.

Räsänen, P., Tiihonen, J., Isohanni, M. *et al.* 1998: Schizophrenia, alcohol abuse and violent behaviour. *Schizophrenia Research* **29**: 22.

Reed, J. 1997: Risk assessment and clinical risk management: the lessons from recent inquiries. *British Journal of Psychiatry* **170**(suppl. 32): 4–7.

Reveley, A.M., Reveley, M.A. and Murray, R.M. 1984: Cerebral ventricular enlargement in non-genetic schizophrenia: a controlled twin study. *British Journal of Psychiatry* **144**: 89–93.

Risch, N. 1990: Linkage studies for genetically complex traits: 1. Multilocus models. *American Journal of Human Genetics* **46**: 242–53.

Roberstson, D., Critchley, H., Daly, E. *et al.* 1998: The neurobiology of severe and repetitive violence: a ^{1}HMRS study of frontal lobe. *Schizophrenia Research* **29**: 100.

Rutter, M., Silberg, J., O'Connor, T. and Simonoff, E. 1999: Genetics and child psychiatry: II. Empirical findings. *Journal of Child Psychology and Psychiatry* **40**: 19–56.

Sham, P., O'Challaghan, E., Takei, N. *et al.* 1992: Schizophrenic births following influenza epidemics: 1939–60. *British Journal of Psychiatry* **160**: 461–6.

Sham, P.C., Jones, P.B., Russell, A. *et al.* 1994: Age of onset, sex and familiar psychiatric morbidity in schizophrenia: Camberwell Collaborative Psychosis Study. *British Journal of Psychiatry* **165**: 466–73.

Shaw, J., Appleby, L., Amos, T. *et al.* 1999: Mental disorder and clinical care in people convicted of homicide: national clinical survey. *British Medical Journal* **318**: 1225–6.

Simmonds, S., Coid, J., Joseph, P. and Marriott, S. 2001: Community mental health team management in severe mental illness: a systematic review. *British Journal of Psychiatry* **178**: 497–502.

Suddath, R.L., Christison, G.W., Torrey, E.F. and Casanova, M.L. 1990: Anatomical abnormalities in the brains of monozygotic twins discordant for schizophrenia. *New England Journal of Medicine* **322**: 789–94.

Taylor, P.J. 1985: Motives for offending amongst violent and psychotic men. *British Journal of Psychiatry* **147**: 491–8.

Tengström, A., Hodgins, S. and Kullgren, G. 2001: Men with schizophrenia who behave violently: the usefulness of an early- versus late-start offender typology. *Schizophrenia Bulletin* **27**: 205–18.

Tiihonen, J., Isohanni, M., Rasanen, P., Koiranen, M. and Moring, J. 1997: Specific major mental disorders and criminality: a 26-year prospective study of the 1966 northern Finland birth cohort. *American Journal of Psychiatry* **154**(6): 840–5.

van Almsvoort, T., Critchley, H., Roberstson, D. *et al.* 1998: Violence and psychosis: an MRI and MRS study of medial temporal lobe asymmetry in violent people with and without a psychotic illness. *Schizophrenia Research* **29**: 73.

Vicente, A.M. and Kennedy, J.L. 1997: The genetics of neurodevelopment and schizophrenia. In Keshavan, M. and Murray, R. (eds), *Neurodevelopment and Adult Psychopathology*. Cambridge: Cambridge University Press, 31–56.

Volavka, J., Laska, E., Baker, S., Meisner, M. Krivelevich, I. 1997: History of violent behaviour and schizophrenia in different cultures. *British Journal of Psychiatry* **171**: 9–14.

Walsh, E., Buchanan, A. and Fahy, T. 2001: Violence and schizophrenia: examinig the evidence. *British Journal of Psychiatry* **180**: 490–5.

Wahlberg, K.-E., Wynne, L.C., Oja, H. *et al.* 1997: Gene–environment interaction in vulnerability to schizophrenia: findings from the Finnish Adoptive Family Study of Schizophrenia. *American Journal of Psychiatry* **154**: 355–62.

Wei, J. and Hemmings, G.P. 1998: Are behavioural syndromes of schizophrenia associated with allelic variations of the tyrosine hydroxylase gene? *Schizophrenia Research* **29**: 129.

Weinberger, D.R. 1987: Implications of normal brain development for the pathogenesis of schizophrenia. *Archives of General Psychiatry* **44**: 660–9.

Werry, J., McClellanm, J. and Chard, L. 1991: Childhood and adolescent schizophrenia bipolar and schizoaffective disorder: a clinical outcome study. *Journal of the American Academy of Child and Adolescent Psychiatry* **30**: 457–65.

Wesseley, S. and Taylor, P. 1991: Madness and crime: criminology or psychiatry? *Criminal Behaviour and Mental Health* **1**: 193–228.

Wesseley, S., Castle, D., Douglas, A. *et al.* 1994: The criminal careers of incident cases of schizophrenia. *Psychological Medicine* **24**: 483–502.

Westermeyer, J.F., Harrow, M. and Marengo, J.T. 1991: Risk for suicide in schizophrenia and other psychotic and non psychotic disorders. *Journal of Nervous and Mental Disease* **179**: 259–66.

WHO (World Health Organization) 1992: *Mental Disorders. Glossary and Guide to their Classification in Accordance with the Tenth Revision of the International Classification of Diseases (ICD-10)*. Geneva: WHO.

Wyatt, R.J. 1995: Early intervention in schizophrenia: can the course of illness be altered? *Schizophrenia Bulletin* **22**: 353–71.

Yen, C.F., Yeh, M.L., Chen, C.S. and Chung, H.H. 2002: Predictive value of insight for suicide, violence, hospitalization, and social adjustment for outpatients with schizophrenia: a prospective study. *Comprehensive Psychiatry* **43**: 443–7.

13

Substance misuse

IAN H. DUFTON AND RUTH E. MARSHALL

INTRODUCTION

The use of illicit drugs among young people has increased relentlessly over the last 25 years (Miller and Plant 1996; Balding 1996, 1997; Wright *et al.* 1995), though provisional findings of the most recent survey by Balding (1998) may represent for the first time a clear downturn in illicit drug use in young people. The nature of this use spans a broad spectrum, from experimental to dependence. The larger the number of young people who experiment with drug and alcohol use, the greater number will go on to develop problems, either within adolescence or in later adult life. Of these a significant proportion will be involved in criminal activity and have contact with the Courts.

The link between substance abuse and criminal activity has long been established, but the relationship is complex, not directly causal, and influenced by situational factors, individual vulnerabilities, personality characteristics, social, educational and family background.

There is a growing awareness of the presence of misuse (as opposed to use) in the adolescent population, and identification by psychiatry and other disciplines working with young people of more adult-like problems such as dependence.

Many commentators remark that substance use is an integral part of adolescence and the adolescent's natural exploration and search for identity. It is difficult to gauge what factors are specific to developing a drug problem at this stage in an individual's development, but it is clear that the presence of drug and alcohol misuse plays a synergistic role in the gestation and expression of a wide spectrum of other adolescent psychiatric diagnoses.

DEFINITIONS AND DESCRIPTION

General issues

Definitions of substance use vary. This is to some extent explained by attempts to avoid the pejorative descriptive terms that have attached themselves to substance abuse (e.g. junkie, addict, alcoholic) while at the same time aiming to include the ever-increasing circles of damage a drug problem can cause. Substance use is common in young people and cannot be considered abnormal in itself. The variety of use extends from one-off experimental use, through to dependence, including experimentation, recreational use, polydrug use, and varying methods of use (inhalation, ingestion, intravenous, subcutaneous).

The Advisory Council on Misuse of Drugs used the term 'problem drug taker' which was defined as 'any person who experiences social, psychological, physical or legal problems related to the intoxication and/or regular excessive consumption and/or [is] dependent as a consequence of … use of drugs or other chemical substances' (1982). This was clinically useful in separating drug-taking from being a problem *per se*.

The World Health Organization's *Documents on Nomenclature and Classification* (1981) further conceptualized substance misuse problems in the following way:

1 *Unsanctioned use* – use of a drug not approved by society, or by a group within that society.
2 *Hazardous use* – use of a drug that will probably lead to harmful consequences for the user, either dysfunction or harm.

3 *Dysfunctional use* – use of a drug that leads to impaired psychological functioning (e.g. loss of job or marital problems).
4 *Harmful use* – use of a drug that is known to have caused tissue damage or mental illness in a person (one type of harmful use is that which leads to dependence).

This succeeded in drawing a distinction between different levels and patterns of drug use and better encapsulated the variety of using behaviour.

In 1987 the Royal College of Psychiatrists defined drug misuse as any taking of a drug which harms or threatens to harm the physical or mental health or social well-being of an individual, of other individuals, or of society at large, or which is illegal. While this definition emphasized the potential risks of drug misuse, it served only to recount the previous views and added little new.

The ICD-10 classification of mental and behavioural disorders and DSM-IV both adopt similar broad approaches, in order to highlight the consumption, absence or presence of dependence and adverse physical, mental, and social consequences. Within each of these there are individual differences. The main criteria are described below. ICD-10 and to a lesser extent DSM-IV are heavily influenced by Edwards and Gross (1976).

The ICD-10 classification

ICD-10 has conceptualized substance misuse problems in the following way.

F10–F19: MENTAL AND BEHAVIOURAL DISORDERS DUE TO PSYCHOACTIVE SUBSTANCE USE

1 *Harmful use* (F1x.1) – a pattern of psychoactive substance use that is causing damage to health. The damage may be physical (e.g. in cases of hepatitis from the self-administration of injected drugs) or mental (e.g. episodes of depressive disorder secondary to heavy consumption of alcohol). Acute intoxication or hangover is not in itself sufficient, and harmful use is not to be diagnosed if dependence syndrome is present.
2 *Dependence syndrome* (F1x.2) – a cluster of physiological, behavioural and cognitive phenomena in which the use of a substance takes on a much higher priority for a given individual than other behaviours that once had greater value. A definitive diagnosis requires three or more of the following to have been present together at some time during the previous year:

- a strong desire or sense of compulsion to take the substance
- difficulties in controlling substance-taking behaviour in terms of its onset, termination, or levels of use
- a physiological withdrawal state when substance use has ceased or been reduced, as evidenced by: the characteristic withdrawal syndrome for the

substance; or use of the same (or closely related) substance with the intention of relieving or avoiding withdrawal symptoms
- evidence of tolerance, such that increased doses of the psychoactive substance are required in order to achieve effects originally produced by lower doses
- progressive neglect of alternative pleasures or interests because of psychoactive substance use, increased amount of time necessary to obtain or to take or to recover from its effects
- persisting with the substance despite clear evidence of overtly harmful consequences, such as harm to the liver through excessive drinking, depressive mood states consequent to periods of heavy substance use, or drug-related impairment of cognitive functioning: efforts should be made to determine that the user was actually, or could be expected to be, aware of the nature and extent of the harm.

Narrowing of the personal repertoire of patterns of psychoactive substance use has also been described as a characteristic feature.

The DSM-IV classification

DSM-IV conceptualizes substance misuse problems in the following way, providing a broader definition in comparison to ICD-10. DSM-IV considers two groups: the substance-use disorders (substance dependence and substance abuse) and the substance-induced disorders (substance withdrawal, substance intoxication, etc.).

SUBSTANCE DEPENDENCE

This is a maladaptive pattern of substance use, leading to clinically significant impairment or distress, as manifested by three (or more) of the following, occurring at any time in the same 12-month period:

- There is tolerance, as defined by either of the following: (a) a need for markedly increased amounts of the substance to achieve intoxication or desired effect, or (b) markedly diminished effect with continued use of the same amount of the substance.
- There is withdrawal as manifested by either of the following: (a) the characteristic withdrawal syndrome for the substance, or (b) the same (or closely related) substance is taken to relieve or avoid withdrawal symptoms.
- The substance is often taken in larger amounts or over a longer period than was intended.
- There is a persistent desire or unsuccessful attempts to cut down or control substance use.
- A great deal of time is spent in activities necessary to obtain the substance (e.g. visiting multiple doctors or driving long distances), use the substance (e.g. chain-smoking), or recover from its effects.

- Important social, occupational or recreational activities are given up or reduced because of the substance use.
- The substance use is continued despite knowledge of having a persistent or recurrent physical or physiological problem that is likely to have been caused or exacerbated by the substance (e.g. current cocaine use despite the recognition of cocaine-induced depression, or continued drinking despite recognition that an ulcer was made worse by alcohol consumption).

SUBSTANCE ABUSE

This is a maladaptive pattern of substance use leading to clinically significant impairment or distress, as manifested by one (or more) of the following, occurring within a 12-month period. The symptoms should have never met the foregoing criteria for substance dependence for the relevant class of substance.

- There is recurrent substance use resulting in a failure to fulfill major role obligations at work, school or home (e.g. repeated absences or poor work performance related to substance use; substance-related absences, suspensions, or expulsions from school; neglect of children or household).
- There is recurrent substance use in situations in which it is physically hazardous (e.g. driving an automobile or operating a machine when impaired by substance use).
- There are recurrent substance-related legal problems (e.g. arrests for substance-related disorderly conduct).
- There is continued substance use despite having persistent or recurrent social or interpersonal problems caused or exacerbated by the effects of the substance (e.g. arguments with spouse about consequences of intoxication, physical fights).

The elements of dependence

Dependence is often simplistically divided into 'psychological' and 'physical/chemical'. The former covers compulsion and craving to use the particular substance, while the latter relates to physiological withdrawal symptoms that require the consumption of the particular substance for relief. However, psychological factors have been implicated in the development of withdrawal symptoms and there is evidence of a neuropharmacological substrate for craving.

While the similarities of the two systems of classification are apparent, Cottler et al. (1991) found that when comparing DSM-IIIR and ICD-10, 11% of individuals were included as having a substance use disorder by one classification and not the other. It is likely a similar response would be elicited from DSM-IV.

Definition remains a controversial area and it must be emphasized that there is an absence of research establishing either the validity or reliability of these diagnostic entities as they may apply to children and adolescents.

Harrison et al. (1998), in a study that incorporated the DSM-IV substance-use disorder criteria into the Minnesota Student Survey, concluded that their epidemiological study did not support the abuse/dependence diagnostic framework. They commented that the abuse/dependence distinction was developed on the basis of data and observations from limited populations: adults, individuals in clinic settings, and individuals with alcohol use disorders and therefore not applicable to children and adolescents. They suggest that a diagnostic framework based on a continuum of problem severity would be more useful.

The DSM-IV substance-use disorder diagnoses probably define a heterogeneous population and communicate insufficient information in terms of natural history and treatment response (Bukstein and Kaminer 1993). Similarly ICD-10 suffers from this failing when applied to the adolescent population. Clearly it is important to recognize the frequent differences between adult and adolescent substance misuse.

The Health Advisory Service (1996), in its thematic review of substance misuse services for children and young people, conceptualized the area into the terms use and misuse. Broadly, 'use' was defined as experimental or recreational use of drugs or alcohol, on the grounds that experimentation alone cannot and should not be seen as indicative of personal disorder. 'Misuse' was defined as use that is harmful, dependent use or the use of substances as part of a wider spectrum of problematic or harmful behaviour. The review stressed the importance of clarity with respect to the meaning of terms used to describe drug and alcohol problems in this group in order to avoid confusion about the presence and severity of problems, the need for and the availability of services, the need to allocate resources appropriately, the effectiveness of interventions, and the balance between prevention, education and direct intervention.

PREVALENCE AND TRENDS OF DRUG USE

Prevalence

Knowledge of the extent and nature of drug use among young people is limited owing to the paucity of research and statistical data. Attempting to ascertain the extent of substance use and misuse is beset with difficulties, and studies to date suffer from a number of problems which include small numbers, varying response rates, whether surveys are of national or local populations, reliance on self-report which may under- or over-estimate use, non-contact and school studies that may be unrepresentative owing to their failure to include non-attendees. Determining the 'true' prevalence is therefore difficult, but in the information available there are consistent trends.

Adolescent substance use appears to have increased with time, both in the UK and North America. While illicit drug use among children and young teenagers remains rare, all types of substance experimentation have increased in the 15- and 16-year-old age group, with four out of ten having used an illegal drug and 1–2% having tried heroin or cocaine. This is equivalent to 15,000 teenager users nationally (Reid 1996). Around 16% of 11- to 14-year-olds in the Health Education Authority's 1995/96 Drug Realities survey reported ever taking drugs or misusing solvents. This sharply rises, as in the Balding (1997) survey, for the older school children to around 40% for 14- to 16-year-olds. The 1992 British Crime Survey (which included those individuals aged 12 and upwards) indicated that one child in thirty in the 12- and 13-year-olds reported ever having used cannabis. This figure increased to between one in ten and one in seven for the 14- and 15-year-olds, and to one in three and one in two for the 16- to 19-year-olds (Mott and Mirrlees-Black 1993; Ramsay and Partridge 1999).

The 1997 Balding survey questioned regular use of drugs. The survey revealed that up to the age of 13 years, between 1% and 2% use drugs regularly, with nearly 2% of 11- and 12-year-olds using within the last year, and 1% in the last month. This begins to rise steeply from the age of 13 years. The survey shows that roughly 7% of 13- and 14-year-olds had used a drug in the last month, rising to 13% for 14- and 15-year-olds and 20% for 15- and 16-year-olds.

The availability and supply of illicit drugs as well as local socio-demographic factors clearly influence the prevalence rates. This is confirmed by local surveys in the UK that provide a different picture of the prevalence of drug use among young people. Latest figures, for example, from the North of England reveal a high incidence of drug use among its young population (Parker et al. 1995; Aldridge et al. 1999). Reports suggest that roughly 40% of 16-year-olds have used a drug, with one in five (19.5%) and nearly one in three (31.5%) of these age groups having used a drug in the last month. A number of school-based cohort surveys conducted in the north of England reported a lifetime drug use prevalence of 56% in their respondents aged 15–16 years. On the face of it, school children in the north of England are almost twice as likely to be using a drug (within the last month) than in the rest of the England and Wales.

Specific drugs used

Cannabis is universally shown, by local and national surveys, to be the most widely used illicit drug in the UK; for example, 50% of Aldridge et al.'s 15- and 16-year-olds reported having used it at least once, as did 43.6% (males) and 38% (females) of Miller et al.'s (1996) 15- and 16-year-olds.

Amphetamine appears to be the next most popular substance; 18% of 16- to 19-year-olds in the 1998 British Crime Survey sample reported using it at least once.

Lifetime prevalence rates for LSD tend to be around 10% in national surveys, but closer to 25% in some local surveys.

The prevalence of ecstasy use varies from 5% in some studies (Parker et al. 1995) to 4–12% in other samples (Leitner et al. 1993).

Use of cocaine and opiates among the young is much rarer. Experience of using cocaine was reported by 6% of 16- to 29-year-olds in the 1998 British Crime Survey, while use of heroin was reported by just 1%. However, Aldridge et al. (1999) found a 3% lifetime prevalence rate for heroin among 15- and 16-year-olds in their northern study. Needless to say, estimates of prevalence within shorter time periods – say the last year or last month – are significantly lower across the board.

Trends

The available evidence suggests that drug use among the young has been increasing steadily over the past decade (but see Ramsay and Spiller 1997). A review by the Institute for the Study of Drug Dependence (ISSD 1997), taking a rather conservative stance, nevertheless concluded that between one-fifth and one-quarter of young people will have tried some form of illicit drug by age 15 or 16. Although in the main this will be cannabis, as many as one in ten young people are estimated to have used an amphetamine, LSD or ecstasy. The ISSD concludes, however, that regular use of these drugs is still confined to a minority, with perhaps only 1–2% of young people involved in such behaviour.

While variations are reported in North America, there has been a sharp resurgence in adolescent substance use in the early 1990s and rates for several drugs are higher than at any time in the 1980s (Weinberg et al. 1998). The research evidence from the USA is summarized in Table 13.1.

Drug use in the forensic adolescent population

PREVALENCE

There is little evidence referring to the prevalence of drug use among young offenders. Howard and Zibert (1990) focused on 293 young offenders and found that polydrug patterns were typical of the group, with a majority of the sample reporting having used substances from more than seven different groups of drugs. A study by Inciardi and Pottieger (1991) found that the entire sample were regular drug users (defined as using drugs on at least three or more occasions per week in the previous 90 days). Hagell

Table 13.1 *Prevalence of substance-abuse disorders among adolescents, based on recent general population studies*

Source	Notes	Sample and age	Substance and criterion	Estimated rate (%)
Warren *et al.* (1995)	National comorbidity survey, DSM-III-R Criteria: household interview by trained lay person	15–24 year olds (*n* = 1765)	Any drug, dependence, past 12 months	3.3 M: 4.5 F: 2.1
Cohen *et al.* (1993)	DISC-1 DSM-III-R Criteria: child and parent data combined using 'or' rule, household interview by trained lay person	10–20 year olds (*n* = 766) New York State, longitudinal sample	Alcohol abuse, point prevalence, age 14–16	3.5 M: 4.1 F: 3.1
			Marijuana abuse, point prevalence, age 14–16	1.4 M: 1.2 F: 1.5
			'Other drug', abuse, point prevalence, age 14–16	0.6 M: 0.4 F: 0.9
Lewishon *et al.* (1993)	Modified K-SADS with DSM-III-R Criteria: interviews in standard research setting by clinically trained personnel	Oregon students in grades 9–12 (*n* = 1710)	Alcohol abuse or dependence, point prevalence	1.0 M: 0.9 F: 1.1
			Any drug abuse or dependence, point prevalence	1.8 M: 2.1 F: 1.6
			Marijuana abuse or dependence, point prevalence	1.7 M: 2.1 F: 1.4
			'Hard drugs' abuse or dependence, point prevalence	0.4 M: 0.5 F: 0.3

Note: Studies may include additional substances, substance abuse criteria, reference periods, age groups, etc. DISC-1, Diagnostic Interview Schedule for Children version 1; K-SADS, Schedule for Affective Disorders and Schizophrenia for School-Age Children. Reproduced from Weinberg *et al.* 1998: *Journal of the American Academy of Child and Adolescent Psychiatry* **37**: 255.

and Newburn's (1994) study of persistent young offenders aged 10–16 found that both alcohol and drug use were widespread within the sample. The use of alcohol in the sample appeared to be heavier and more frequent than that typical of representative samples despite the lifetime prevalence of having tried alcohol (96%) remaining similar to that obtained from representative community-based samples of young people.

In the Audit Commission's study, *Misspent Youth* (1996), interviews were conducted with 103 young offenders on supervision orders. Of these, approximately 65% had used cannabis, 25% an amphetamine, over 20% ecstasy, just under 20% LSD, over 10% cocaine, and approximately 6% heroin. Of a larger group of 600 young offenders included in the Audit Commission study, 15% were judged by their youth justice worker to have a problem with either drugs or alcohol. Significantly, the more persistent the offending the greater likelihood that the offender would be judged to have a problem.

A UK study of 50 young offenders on probation for a wide range of offences (Williamson *et al.* 1996) found that almost all reported lifetime experience of at least one illicit substance; 82% had used cannabis in the month prior to interview, and 48% had used other drugs in the same period, including a large proportion that had used crack cocaine (38%), heroin (24%) or methadone (14%).

Collinson (1994, 1996) found in a sample of 80 young male offenders in custody 'drug use figured centrally and excessively in the lives of 59% of the sample' with a reported lifetime prevalence of LSD at 54%, of an amphetamine 48%, of ecstasy 43%, of heroin and crack/cocaine 20%.

From even this limited evidence the suggestion is that rates of drug use appear higher among young offenders compared with the general population of young people, and that young offenders may be particularly at risk of developing problematic use.

PATTERNS OF USE

Boys are more likely to have used illicit drugs, smoked cannabis and used LSD, whereas girls are more likely to have used tranquillizers, cigarettes and pills with alcohol. Higher levels of illicit use have been shown to be associated with poor school performance. Sex differences have been noted for the progression to illicit drug use. In males, progression to illicit cannabis use was dependent on prior alcohol use, whereas for females either cigarette or alcohol use was a sufficient condition (Miller *et al.* 1996).

A number of general trends have been noted. These include the increased use of a wide range of drugs in the younger age group, the narrowing of the gender gap, the emergence of polydrug use as the norm, and a decrease in the age of initiation into substance use. Substance use and misuse occurs across all socio-economic backgrounds, though there is some suggestion that opiate misuse is more frequent in young people from deprived backgrounds (HAS 1996). With the integration into youth culture, magazines, language and fashion and the growth of the 'pick-n-mix scene', drug use now is synonymous with youth identity, and portrayed as a normative experience and legitimate pathway towards autonomy.

ASSOCIATION BETWEEN CRIME AND DRUG MISUSE

While it has come to be accepted that substance misuse, in particular opioid use, is associated with both drug- and non-drug-related crime, explanations of that association vary. The paucity of research makes the role of adolescent substance misuse difficult to ascertain.

In the adult literature, proposed explanations of the association between substance misuse and crime include a simple causal relationship (Norco 1987), whereby during periods of heavy substance misuse, users commit more crimes to finance their expensive habits. This explanation perhaps gains weight when considering the adolescent population who have limited non-criminal means to fund their drug use.

A second proposed explanation of the association is that the two co-occur. Simply put, those people who become criminals are likely to become drug abusers.

Parker *et al.* (1986, 1987) found evidence for a relationship between opioid use and crime in a study of adult opioid users in the Wirral, Merseyside. A rapid rise in crime, especially burglary, was mirrored in the Wirral by a rapid rise in the number of heroin users and neither rise occurred elsewhere at the same time. Drug users in general and opioid users in particular were extremely over-represented in a sample of known offenders. In this sample there were more drug- and opioid-using burglars. Thirty-five per cent of the registered opioid users did not have a criminal record prior to their opioid use.

Interpretation of results such as these is difficult. Convictions are a poor estimation of criminal activity, arrest may not be a random process, and drug users and opioid users may stand a greater chance of being arrested, notification is not a random process and a drug user in crisis is more likely to be known to the police or seek treatment. When British users have been compared to controls they appear to be more criminal than those controls (Neville *et al.* 1988).

In contradiction to the causal view that the need for the misused substance drives the criminal activity, Johnson *et al.* (1985) in a study of opioid users in New York found that many opioid users have methods of obtaining opiates without paying for them which precluded the need for crime. The determinant of daily use was not dependence but often the availability of funds, the suggestion being that rather than stealing to fund their heroin use they adjusted their daily intake according to the funds available. The availability of funds may depend on the success of their criminal activities. Many opioid users obtained their funds through drug dealing rather than through non-drug crime.

Hammersley *et al.* (1989), in an attempt to address the questions whether drug use causes crime or vice versa, studied 151 adult Scottish prisoners and non-prisoners. They concluded that, in general, higher-level drug users committed more crimes than lower-level drug users. Heavy opioid use was associated with increased criminality and higher-level drug users tended to be polydrug users and have a wider criminal experience. Theft could be explained by two main variables, criminal experience and polydrug use. More frequent violence and delinquency was associated with having more social support and polydrug use. Fraud was related only to alcohol use. Drug dealing was explained by the frequency of opioid use, polydrug use, lack of social support, use of alcohol, and criminal experience.

Hammersley *et al.* (1990) studied the drug use and crime of 210 teenage licit and illicit drug users. While there were many similarities with the study in adults, the adolescent population differed in two important respects. Firstly, in the adolescent population, violence, vandalism and fraud were associated with drug use. Secondly, theft was not explained uniquely by drug use but co-occurred. Friends' behaviour and prior criminal history were both important determinants of crime.

AETIOLOGY OF SUBSTANCE MISUSE

Substance misuse is a heterogeneous phenomenon, encompassing a variety of drugs, patterns and aetiologies. Most recent research concentrates on risk and protective factors and incorporates them into a number of aetiological pathways.

Many of the risk factors for adolescent drug misuse also predict other adolescent behavioural problems (Hawkins *et al.* 1985). There is no convincing evidence that relates which risk factors are of greatest importance in the aetiology of substance abuse, nor is it clear what factors govern the early initiation into drug use and what factors influence the progression from recreational and experimental use to dependence. Clinically it is clear that some individuals appear to progress rapidly to dependence while for others there is a persistent progression from initiation, to moderate, then heavy, and finally dependent use.

Societal and cultural risk factors

Societal norms have shifted. Mixed messages about use are provided by the mass media. Children and pre-adolescents are particularly susceptible to media promotion of substance use, which may influence the initial use of such gateway substances as tobacco. Media reports of drug taking by youth subcultures and drug associations such as acid-house and rave have had an impact on drug policy at both local and national level. Forsyth *et al.* (1997) have shown a relationship between adolescent drug use and musical preference, stressing the cultural affiliation. It now appears normality for youth and drug use to be synonymous, and polydrug use has been accepted as the predominant recreational practice.

When examining the social and cultural risk factors, substance availability, perceived low risk, acceptance of drug use, extreme economic deprivation, low socioeconomic status, high crime, high population density, lack of community support structures and neighbourhood disorganization repeatedly arise as the main environmental variables.

Genetic influences

Family studies have consistently shown that alcoholism occurs more frequently among the relatives of alcoholics than among the relatives of non-alcoholics (Cotton 1979). Adoption studies have also shown consistent evidence for genetic inheritance (Cadoret *et al.* 1978, 1985, 1987, 1995; Goodwin *et al.* 1973, 1974, 1977; Bohman 1978). They show an excess of alcoholism in the biological rather than the adoptive relatives of problem drinkers. The extent of the genetic effect varies. For instance, Goodwin *et al.* showed a four-fold increase in the incidence of alcoholism among male adoptees adopted away from their alcoholic parents soon after birth; these effects have been demonstrated in both males and females. Despite the flaws in methodology, on balance they provide a strong case for genetic influence in the transmission of alcoholism. Twin studies in this area have been less conclusive.

Cadoret *et al.* (1995) proposed two models for the pathway from parental alcohol misuse to substance use in their biological offspring:

- alcoholism in biological parents predicts substance-use disorder in offspring
- biological parent demonstrating antisocial personality disorder, in the offspring increased rates of aggression, conduct disorder, antisocial personality disorder leading into substance use disorder.

Twin and adoption studies have also pointed to a probable contribution of constitutional factors to the risk for substance-use disorders (Dinwiddie and Cloniger 1991). High-risk individuals may be less sensitive to the effects of alcohol in terms of subjective intoxication (Shuckit 1984, 1985) or may display differences in static ataxia (body sway) or in the latency of P3 component of evoked potentials (Porjosz and Beigleiter 1990; Hill *et al.* 1987).

There is also the possibility of constitutional differences in the way individuals with substance-use disorders obtain different levels of reinforcement from their substances of choice, as described by Khantzian (1985).

No single gene appears to be involved. Blum *et al.* (1990) revealed an association between alcoholism and the A1 allele of the dopamine D_2 receptor gene, while Smith *et al.* (1992) showed a putative association of dopamine DR D_2 allele with polyagent abuse that may suggest vulnerability to substance-abuse disorders.

Individual and interpersonal influences

Temperamental features also influence risk. For example, sensation-seeking and difficulties which affect regulation may interact with environmental responses in children with behavioural and mood difficulties. This in turn can provoke a harsher parenting response and a subsequent gravitation towards deviant peer groups (Pandina *et al.* 1992). Blackson *et al.* (1994) established that difficult affective temperament (characterized by negative mood, mood lability, and social withdrawal) was associated with increased risk of substance abuse.

Substance-abuse risk factors and predictors are equivalent across race and sex groups (Gottfredson *et al.* 1996).

High-risk children have cognitive disorders of behavioural self-regulation – difficulties with planning, attention, abstract thinking and reasoning, foresight, judgement, self-monitoring, and motor control. These often lead to aggression, a frequently identified feature of children at risk of adolescent substance-use disorder (Giancola *et al.* 1996). There is also a possible association with learning and language difficulties.

Family influences

The family exerts a powerful influence upon the developing adolescent. Research confirms that factors within the family modify the individual adolescent's vulnerability and response to substance abuse.

Parental drug abuse and permissive attitudes to drug use are of particular importance in determining a young person's use of drugs. Parental tolerance and their approval of drinking have been shown to be predictors of adolescent drug and alcohol misuse (HAS 1996).

Assortative mating by drug-abusing parents is both common and a great risk for substance abuse in the offspring (Merikangas *et al.* 1992).

All of these may lead to a family environment where there is early exposure to alcohol and drugs. Fergusson *et al.* (1994) have shown that children who were introduced to alcohol before the age of 6 years are more than twice as likely to report frequent, heavy or problem drinking at the age of 15 than are children who were not exposed to alcohol before the age of 13. Robins *et al.* (1985), among others, have shown that beginning drug use before the age of 15 years predicted an increased risk of drug-related disorders, particularly of a severe type.

Non-standard family structures (e.g. single-parent homes in which a parent has died or left the home because of separation or divorce) are associated with early adolescent drinking. It has been suggested by Isohanni *et al.* (1994) that these situations push the adolescent towards premature autonomy, and that increases the risk of alcohol or drug use both as a sign of, and a mechanism to cope with, autonomy.

This could also be mediated through poor and inconsistent family management practices or they themselves could exert an independent effect. These include poor monitoring and unclear expectations of behaviour, few rewards and approval, and excessively harsh or inconsistent punishment for unwanted behaviour. It would be prudent to bear in mind that Stice *et al.* (1993) demonstrated that extremely high as well as low levels of parental control were associated with illicit substance use in adolescents.

Peer influences

It has long been held that peer influence and pressure is important in the development and maintenance of substance abuse. Factors believed to increase the risk are peer substance use, peer attitudes (i.e. accepting, permissive, favourable) about substance use, and the increased orientation of youth to their peers (Kandel *et al.* 1978). More recently commentators have suggested that the view of the role of peer pressure is misleading and that the terms 'peer preference' and 'assortment' are more appropriate (Coggans *et al.* 1994). Some have shown that peer influence is less significant a predictor of either substance use or abuse than previously thought, and that prior correlations are the result of adolescent users selecting a using peer group and then editing their drug history in the context of that peer group to explain their own drug use (Ianotti *et al.* 1996; Glantz and Pickens 1992; Bauman and Ennett 1994).

Comorbidity

There is acknowledgement of the high prevalence of co-occurring addictive and mental disorders in adult populations. Among adults with a primary diagnosis of mental disorder, the National Institute of Mental Health's Epidemiological Catchment Area (ECA) study revealed comorbidity rates of 28% for substance-abuse disorders. This co-occurrence impacted on the course and prognosis of both disorders (Reiger *et al.* 1990).

Singer and Song (1992) found a 40% rate of substance-use disorders comorbid with psychiatric disorders among 319 adolescents admitted consecutively over a two-year period to an adolescent psychiatric unit.

Many studies have demonstrated an association between substance abuse and conduct problems (Bukstein *et al.* 1989; Robins *et al.* 1990; Miln *et al.* 1991). The levels of conduct disorder detected comorbid with substance-abuse disorders varied from 54% to 91% (Stowell *et al.* 1992; Miln *et al.* 1991; Bukstein *et al.* 1992).

Substance use in the absence of conduct disorder is rare and findings are similar for both males and females (Robins *et al.* 1990). It has also been found that as the number of adolescent conduct problems increases, the age of first significant substance use decreases. The relationship between conduct problems and substance abuse appears to hold only for those whose substance use began in adolescence. There does not appear to be a relationship between conduct problems in adolescence and substance abuse in those whose use began in adulthood.

In males, conduct problems and depressive symptoms (the latter being more important for predicting later substance use) at age 11 years predicted later cannabis, glue and polydrug use. In females, depressive and conduct symptoms (most important predictor) at age 15 predicted substance use (Henry *et al.* 1993).

However, when behavioural diagnoses are excluded, there are still significantly high rates of psychiatric comorbidity. Miln *et al.* (1991) found that, when evaluating 111 juvenile offenders, following exclusion of all conduct and oppositional disorder diagnoses, 39% of substance abusers versus 14% of non-substance abusers demonstrated comorbid psychiatric diagnoses. These included depression, anxiety and eating disorders.

Alcohol and drug abuse were associated with major depressive disorder in a large sample of American college students aged 16–19, using the diagnostic interview schedule (Deykin *et al.* 1987). Kashani *et al.* (1985) found that 16% of adolescent substance users attending a drop-in counselling centre suffered from double depression (dysthymic disorder with superimposed major depression).

Deas-Nesmith *et al.* (1998) found that 33% of adolescents admitted to an acute inpatient psychiatric unit had a diagnosis of substance abuse or dependence. These adolescents were admitted for psychiatric reasons other than substance-use disorders and outpatient clinicians had not identified the presence of a substance-use disorder prior to admission. The diagnoses included affective disorders (74%), anxiety disorders (21%) and disruptive disorders (61%), and there were no significant differences between the substance- and non-substance-using groups in the frequency of specific psychiatric disorders.

Studies where the K–SADS was administered to adolescents within inpatient units for the treatment of substance-abuse disorders, comorbid mood disorders showed a prevalence between 31% and 61%, anxiety disorders approximately 45%, and depressive conduct disorder 14%. Burke *et al.* (1988, 1994) analysed data from the Epidemiological Catchment Area study and determined that there was an association between early-onset mood and anxiety disorder and an earlier peak in the onset of substance abuse.

The correlation with attention-deficit hyperactivity disorder (ADHD) is unclear. Studies have suggested a link between cocaine dependence and childhood attention-deficit disorder (ADD; Cocores *et al.* 1987). ADD residual type has been reported in abusers of cocaine (Gavin *et al.* 1985; Khantsian 1983; Weiss *et al.* 1985). Eyre *et al.* (1982) reported attention-deficit disorder to be a childhood antecedent to substance misuse in a treatment sample of drug abusers. Weiss *et al.* (1985) found that the prevalence of attention-deficit disorder in adult psychiatric inpatients was 4.7% of cocaine users and 0.7% of opioid and depressant users. Rounsaville *et al.* (1991) found that, in 298 cocaine abusers, 34.9% had had childhood ADD. In comparison, a lower rate of childhood ADD (22%) was found in opiate addicts presenting for treatment.

Comings (1994) and Cook *et al.* (1995) have suggested that the genes for ADHD play an important role in drug abuse/dependence. The dopamine D_2 receptor gene (DRD2) appears to be one of these, since variants at this locus are significantly increased in frequency in ADHD and drug abuse.

There are those who suggest that the statistical relationship appears to be largely due to the association of each with conduct disorder (e.g. Kaminer 1992).

There is some suggestion that sub-populations of ADHD, namely those that persist into adulthood, have a stronger association.

In considering the association with personality disorder, possible associations with the development of antisocial personality disorder and borderline personality disorder have been identified (Grilo *et al.* 1997).

EXPLANATORY MODELS

Various models have been put forward to explain the development of substance-abuse disorders. They include:

PROBLEM–BEHAVIOUR THEORY

Jessor and Jessor (1977) viewed behaviours such as substance use and premature sexual initiation as having a particular function, namely to offset social and psychological deficits and achieve personal goals. Adolescents with fewer social skills, lack of effective coping strategies in their repertoire, little belief in self-efficacy, and difficulties in coping with interpersonal situations are at greater risk of substance abuse.

DISTURBED PERSONALITY–PERSPECTIVE THEORY

Khantzian (1985) viewed substance misuse as a function of a person's personality structure and dynamics, as a result of the person's efforts to cope with stresses, anxiety and depression, and difficulties in personal relationships.

FOUR STAGES IN THE SEQUENCE OF DRUG INITIATION AND USE

Kandel (1975) proposed the concept of gateway substances leading from one stage of substance use to another. Beer and wine tend to be the first substances used, followed by tobacco and spirits, then marijuana and finally other illegal substances. Simply put, Kandel proposed that the use of 'hard' drugs was preceded by the use of 'soft' drugs.

SOCIO–CULTURAL MODEL

This model (Bachman *et al.* 1984) focuses on environmental factors as those that are important in the acquisition of drug-use patterns of behaviour. These include drug availability, selling pressures, peer pressure, and material and cultural social deprivation.

THREE POTENTIAL EXPLANATORY MODELS FOR THE RELATIONSHIP BETWEEN DRUG ABUSE AND PSYCHIATRIC DISORDER (Brook *et al.* 1998)

First model
Psychiatric disorders lead to the use of drugs by the following mechanisms:

- Psychiatric disorders produce difficulties in parental monitoring and in the parent–child attachment relationship, or in peer relationships, which then facilitate substance use.
- Adverse parental factors may be risk factors for both substance use and psychiatric disorder.
- Drug use is one way for adolescents to cope with intrapersonal distress, and legal and illegal drug use may reduce dysphoric mood at least temporarily.

Second model
- Drug abuse and psychiatric disorders share the same aetiological factors – for example, predisposing biological or genetic, psychosocial, and sociocultural factors.

Third model
- Drug use leads directly to certain psychiatric disorders, owing to the psychopharmacological or toxic effects of the drugs on the functioning of the brain.

While these models develop different themes and emphasis, in the absence of a single definitive model to explain the development of substance-abuse disorders and the likelihood that no single theory would explain the genesis of all substance-abuse disorders, they provide useful frameworks from which to inform a clinician's thinking in this arena.

ASSESSMENT OF A SUBSTANCE-ABUSING ADOLESCENT

Firstly it is important to recognize that only a small proportion of those with problematic drug and/or alcohol use will ever present for assessment and treatment. Often they present at a fairly advanced stage of the problem and when associated problems have emerged, for example legal difficulties. In the case of young people, they are infrequently the initiators of the referral, the driving force often being a parent or other carer. Conversely, sometimes there is collusion of the parents in denial (conscious or unconscious) of their child's substance misuse. Both of these scenarios present problems in making the initial assessment.

Often problems go undetected for long periods. This can be partly understood by recognizing that adolescence is a time of great change in a young person, making fluctuations due to substance abuse difficult to see. Defences are developing to provide barriers to questions by concerned adults. This can lead to helplessness and frustration in the adults and a gradual withdrawal from the adolescent's life along with an abdication of control.

It is essential to understand who initiated the referral, and why, at the first appointment. Assessment is dependent on engaging the young person and respecting his or her view of the situation, even if this view is that there is no need for assessment and there is no problem. However, colluding with the young person's denial of the problem is not helpful and it is important to let your view be known. If the young person is not willing to be compliant with the assessment process, then it is sometimes worth stressing that you would rather hear his or her account of the situation than hear only from the carer who has brought the young person for consultation. Equally it is important to see the adolescent alone for the first part of the assessment unless there are strong reasons for doing otherwise. This allows him or her to feel treated as an individual and may increase the accuracy of the responses to your questions.

After the initial interview with the young person, an opportunity to speak with the carer should be sought. The carer's view of the problem may be very different, so part of the assessment is to attempt to understand the differences. It is useful to use this as an opportunity to educate the carer, if appropriate, as to the particular substance problem, its implications, and the signs of intoxication to look out for. During this part of the assessment it is not useful to discuss exactly what the young person has told you about the problem, especially if the carer is unaware of some of the details. There are exceptions to this if the young person appears to be putting himself or herself at risk and steps need to be taken to reduce the risk. If this is the case then it is best to discuss this with the young person during the time alone.

Assessment should always be seen as an ongoing process and not completed after the first consultation. The initial meeting aims to engage the patient and the carer(s) and to establish some of the background and the details of the problem. A fundamental goal of assessment is to ascertain whether a problem of using one or more psychoactive substances exists, and if so does this amount to abuse or dependence according to the diagnostic criteria. After seeing the young person and then the carer(s), some time will need to be put aside to discuss what course of action is to be taken and when the next consultation will be.

Many young people with substance-misuse problems have coexisting psychiatric conditions (Bukstein et al. 1989). Knowledge of these disorders is essential for the treatment and management of the substance-misuse problem. Enquiries about psychiatric symptomatology should include whether the symptoms were present before the start of substance use, and how the use affected the symptoms. Did they occur only after use had begun? Are they exacerbated by use or relieved? A family history of psychiatric illness should be sought. Ideally the young person should be observed in a period of abstinence before a diagnosis is made concerning the symptoms, as the possibility of a substance-induced disorder cannot be excluded.

Assessment of the risk factors of substance misuse should be part of the overall assessment. These include individual, peer, family and community risk factors, parental substance misuse, and parental attitudes to illicit drugs. The level of attachment between parents and the young person, and the level of supervision and control of the young person, are all important questions to be asked.

Physical investigations, including urine and serum toxicology, can be helpful in confirming substance use if they are positive, but they do not confirm substance dependence. Negative results, however, do not necessarily exclude the possibility of substance use. Different substances are present in the urine for differing amounts of time. Stimulants and cocaine are detectable in the urine for 1–2 days, as are heroin and other opiates, but cannabis can be detected for over one month, particularly when use has been chronic.

For each substance being used, enquiry should cover the pattern of use including quantity and frequency. As this is likely to be variable, it can be helpful to limit the enquiry to a particular period of time, for example the past 30 days. The context of use includes when use takes place and where, if there are any antecedents, what the consequences are, who is there at the time and whether they are using drugs too, what mood the young person is in both before and after use, the expectancies of use, and what actions are taken afterwards. In determining the extent of the problem, control of use is a particularly important area in determining whether the use fits the diagnostic criteria for dependence. This includes the young person's view of the substance use as a problem, attempts to stop or to limit use, whether withdrawals are experienced after stopping use. When these occur, has the young person experienced craving for the substance? What lengths does the person go to in order to get more of the substance or the funds to buy more?

Typically problems exist for the substance-using adolescent in one or more areas of life. Enquiry should be directed to the different areas to determine which if any are being affected. These areas include psychiatric and behaviour problems, home and family life, school or work functioning, social and peer group relationships, and leisure and recreational activities.

Questions regarding high-risk behaviour – including sexual activities – need to be asked owing to the risks of HIV, other sexually transmitted diseases, and unwanted pregnancies. High-risk sexual behaviour is more common in adolescents who abuse substances (DiClemente and Ponton 1993).

TREATMENTS

General issues

Although the main goal is abstinence, sometimes the interim goal of harm reduction is a more realistic one. This includes a reduction in the use along with an improvement in functioning in at least one area of the young person's life, and a reduction in any risk-taking behaviours. Other treatment goals relate to coexisting psychiatric and behavioural problems, family functioning, peer relationships, social functioning and school or work performance.

The following characteristics of treatment have been identified as associated with improved rates of abstinence and lower relapse rates (Fleisch 1991; Beschner and Friedman 1985). Treatment needs to be intensive and of sufficient duration to achieve changes in both attitude and behaviour towards substance use. It should be comprehensive in order to cover as many areas of the adolescent's life where problems exist. Family involvement should be encouraged wherever possible. Attendance at self-help groups should be encouraged. Treatment should be sensitive to cultural and socio-economic issues of the adolescents and should be linked in with the local community and system of care. Aftercare should be an integral part of treatment to reinforce the changes that have been achieved. Most young people grow out of heavy drinking and offending (McMurran 1991). The question is: should we intervene at all as it is both costly and ineffective?

Treatment services for young people should be different from those aimed at other ages. They need to encompass an adolescent's particular developmental needs and should be peer-orientated. Particular attention has to be paid to the occurrence of comorbid psychiatric disorder, which affects up to two-thirds of adolescents who misuse substances (Kazdin 1995).

Facilities need to cover a range of settings. Inpatient beds will be necessary for those with more serious problems, including those likely to experience withdrawal symptoms and those with a serious psychiatric disorder. Adolescents who have experienced recurrent failure with less intensive treatments may benefit from an inpatient admission. Residential treatment provides an option that is less intensive than inpatient treatment but usually lasts longer. This is also a useful next step from hospital treatment. Day-hospital treatment offers the regular supervision of an inpatient stay for those who do not need 24-hour monitoring. Outpatient treatment provides an option for those who do not need any more intensive input; this is usually reserved for highly motivated, well-supported adolescents with less complex presentations. Outpatient treatment is usually problem-focused because of the limited time available. Community treatment and self-help groups can be used as adjuncts to outpatient treatment or as a follow-on to more intensive treatments.

Treatment modalities

Little is written about the success or failure of any particular treatment in relation to adolescents. It has been suggested that no one treatment approach appears notably superior, but that some treatment is better than no treatment (Hawkins et al. 1991).

PSYCHOSOCIAL TREATMENTS

Cognitive–behavioural therapy
Cognitive distortions and negative internalized self-statements are commonly reported by substance-misusing adolescents (Van Hasselt 1993). Addressing negative thinking patterns can help these problems and reduce substance use and associated behaviours. Relapse prevention is a well-used strategy in the treatment of substance misuse and relies on a cognitive behavioural approach. It helps the young person identify triggers to use and to develop strategies for dealing with these to decrease the risk of relapse.

Behavioural therapy
Techniques of operant conditioning can be useful with rewards and punishments dependent on behaviour. These are often used as part of a treatment programme. Aversion techniques are rarely thought to be appropriate.

Psychodynamic and interpersonal therapies
These therapies are appropriate for adolescents assessed as having specific difficulties that may benefit from this approach, particularly depression and anxiety. Adolescents with a past history of abuse may also benefit, but as with this treatment mode in any age, candidates must be carefully assessed. Adolescents with conduct disorders tend to be unsuitable for this approach (Woody et al. 1985).

Family therapy

Involvement of the family when treating an adolescent is very important. Addressing parental views on substance misuse as well as educating the family on drug issues are some of the uses. Helping the parents to understand the treatment plans helps them to maintain effective boundaries to behaviour with the adolescent. Another aim is to improve communication between family members.

PHARMACOTHERAPIES

Pharmacotherapy is useful for detoxification, the treatment of withdrawal symptoms, and as an adjunct to continued abstinence. It also has an important role in the treatment of comorbid psychiatric disorders. The treatment of withdrawal syndromes should be managed as for adults and the drugs available are the same.

Treatment of dependence with substitutions such as methadone should be carefully considered; unless there are exceptional circumstances, they are a short-term measure aimed at harm reduction before detoxification. The risk of fostering a dependence to methadone should be a disincentive to its use. Methadone can be important in the control of substance use if the adolescent is using opiates. It can aid in the reduction of disturbance of other areas of the young person's life, and can help to stabilize opiate use prior to detoxification. The other area of benefit is its use in the substitution of oral methadone for intravenous opiates.

Detoxification with reducing doses of methadone either as an inpatient or as an outpatient is a well-documented method of withdrawal. Another method is the use of opioid antagonists, either naltrexone or naloxone. The use of these drugs allows detoxification to be quicker than with the traditional methadone reduction, an advantage in retaining adolescents in treatment and avoiding prolonged hospital admissions.

Treatment of comorbid psychiatric conditions with medication should be avoided until the young person has been assessed drug-free. This is not always possible and then a judgement has to be made on the likely aetiology, whether the symptoms reported are likely to respond to medication. Persistence of symptoms over weeks, symptoms predating substance use, a significant family history, past treatment failures, and past successes of medication suggest that prompt pharmacotherapy may be appropriate.

Other modalities

Behavioural self-control training can effectively encourage moderate drinking. This includes the use of self-help manuals, peer interventions (by training adolescents to be educators and counsellors), and simulated bar settings (Swadi and Zeitlin 1988).

As adolescent drinking is the norm, abstinence-based programmes may be unrealistic. It may dissuade youngsters from entering treatment programmes. If asked, most opt to cut down drinking rather than abstaining. However, abstinence may be a goal for some young people, again emphasizing the need to assess each young person individually.

REFERENCES

Advisory Council on the Misuse of Drugs 1982: *Treatment and Rehabilitation Report.* London: Department of Health and Social Security.

Aldridge, J., Parker, H. and Measham, F. 1999: *Drug Trying and Drug Use Across Adolescence: a Longitudinal Study of Young People's Drug Taking in Two Regions of Northern England.* Drugs Prevention Advisory Service Paper 1. London: DPAS.

APA (American Psychiatric Association) 1994: *DSM-IV Diagnostic and Statistical Manual of Mental Disorders,* 4th edn. Washington, DC: APA.

Audit Commission 1996: *Misspent Youth: Young People and Crime.* London: Audit Commission.

Bachman, J.G., O'Malley, P.M. and Johnson, E.D. 1984: Drug use among young adults: the impact of role status and social environment. *Journal of Personality and Social Psychology* **47**: 629–45.

Balding, J. 1996: *Young People and Illegal Drugs 1989–1995: Facts and Predictions.* Exeter: Schools Health Education Unit, University of Exeter.

Balding, J. 1997: *Young People and Illegal Drugs in 1996.* Exeter: Schools Health Education Unit, University of Exeter.

Bauman, K.E. and Ennett, S.T. 1994: Peer influence on adolescent drug use. *American Journal of Psychology* **49**: 820–2.

Beschner, G.M. and Friedman, A.S. 1985: Treatment of adolescent drug abusers. *International Journal of the Addictions* **20**: 97–9.

Blackson, T. 1994: Temperament: a salient correlate of risk factors for alcohol and drug abuse. *Drug and Alcohol Dependence* **36**: 205–14.

Blackson, T., Tarter, R., Martin, C. and Moss, H. 1994: Temperament mediates the effects of family history of substance abuse and externalizing and internalizing child behaviour. *American Journal of Addictions* **3**: 58–66.

Blum, K., Noble, E.P. and Sheridan, P.J. 1990: Allelic association of human dopamine D_2 receptor gene in alcoholism. *Journal of the American Medical Association* **263**: 2055–60.

Bohman, M. 1978: Some genetic aspects of alcoholism and criminality. *Archives of General Psychiatry* **35**: 269–76.

Brook, J.S., Cohen, P. and Brook, D.W. 1998: Longitudinal study of co-occurring psychiatric disorders and substance use. *Journal of the American Academy of Child and Adolescent Psychiatry* **37**: 322–30.

Bukstein, O.G. and Kaminer, Y. 1993: The nosology of adolescent substance abuse. *American Journal of Addictions* **3**: 1–13.

Bukstein, O.G., Brent, D.A. and Kaminer, Y. 1989: Comorbidity of substance abuse and other psychiatric disorders in adolescents. *American Journal of Psychiatry* **146**: 1131–41.

Bukstein, O.G., Glancy, L.J. and Kaminer, Y. 1992: Patterns of affective comorbidity in a clinical population of dually diagnosed adolescent substance abusers. *Journal of the American Academy of Child and Adolescent Psychiatry* **31**: 1041–5.

Rousanville, B.J., Anton, S.F., Caroll, K. *et al.* 1991: Psychiatric disgnoses of treatment seeking cocaine abusers. *Archives of General Psychiatry* **48**: 43–51.

Shuckit, M.A. 1984: Subjective responses to alcohol in sons of alcoholics and control subjects. *Archives of General Psychiatry* **41**: 879–84.

Shuckit, M.A. 1985: Studies of populations at high risk for alcoholism. *Psychiatric Developments* **3**: 31–63.

Singer, M. and Song, L. 1992: Short-term follow-up of dual diagnosed adolescent psychiatric inpatients. *Substance Abuse* **13**: 63–70.

Smith, S.S., O'Hara, B.F. and Perisco, A.M. 1992: Genetic vulnerability to drug abuse. The D_2 dopamine receptor Taz 1 B1 restriction fragment length polymorphism appears more frequently in drug abusers. *Archives of General Psychiatry* **49**: 723.

Stice, E., Barrera, M. and Chassain, L. 1993: Relation of parental support and control to adolescent's externalizing symptomatology and substance use: a longitudinal examination of curvilinear effects. *Journal of Abnormal Child Psychology* **21**: 609–29.

Stowell, R.J.A. and Estroff, T.W. 1992: Psychiatric disorders in substance abusing adolescent inpatients: a pilot study. *Journal of the American Academy of Child and Adolescent Psychiatry* **31**: 1036–40.

Swadi, H. and Zeitlin, H. 1988: Peer influence and adolescent substance abuse: promising side. *British Journal of Addiction* **83**: 153–7.

Van Hasselt, V.B., Null, J.A., Kempton, T. and Bukstein, O.G. 1993: Social skills and depression in adolescent substance abusers. *Addictive Behaviours* **18**: 9–18.

Warren, L.A., Kessler, R.C., Hughes, M. *et al.* 1995: Prevalence and correlates of drug use and dependence in the United States. *Archives of General Psychiatry* **52**: 219–29.

Weinberg, N.Z., Rahdert, E., Colliver, J.D. and Glantz, M.D. 1998: Adolescent substance abuse: a review of the past 10 years. *Journal of the American Academy of Child and Adolescent Psychiatry* **37**: 252–61.

Weiss, G., Hectman, L., Milroy, T. *et al.* 1985: Psychiatric status of hyperactives as adults: a controlled prospective 15 year follow-up of 63 hyperactive children. *Journal of the American Academy of Child Psychiatry* **24**: 211–20.

Weiss, R.D., Mirin, S.M., Griffin, M.L. *et al.* 1988: Psychopathology in cocaine abusers. *Journal of Nervous and Mental Disease* **176**: 719–25.

Williamson, S., Griffiths, P., Noble, A. *et al.* 1996: *Patterns of Drug Use amongst a Sample of Young Offenders.* Report to Bexley and Greenwich Drug Action Team and Greenwich Safer Cities, April.

Woody, R.H. and Springer, J.R. 1985: A holistic health model for family therapy. *Family Therapy Collections* **13**: 36–45.

PART 4

Offending behaviours and victims as perpetrators

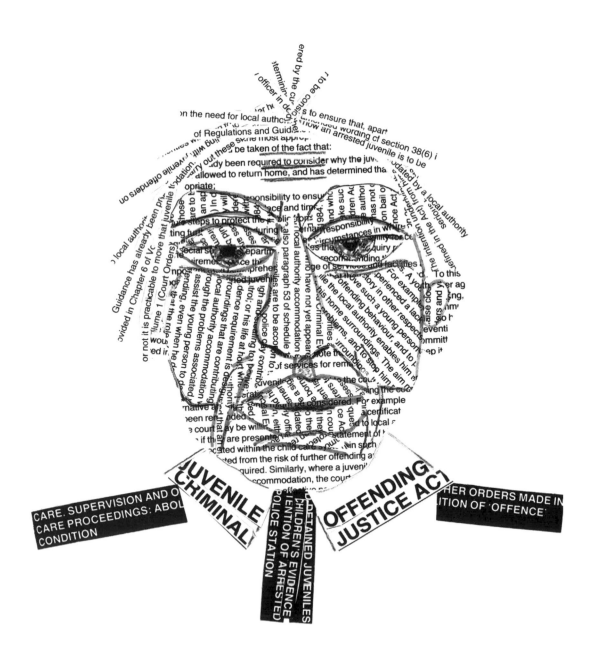

pathology of mixed relationships. These findings may have implications for the excess of referrals of mixed-race children by social services to Child and Adolescent Mental Health Services (CAMHS).

EDUCATION AND EMPLOYMENT

Research on exclusion from school (Osler 1997) quotes the Department of Education and Employment figures (1994/95). Black Caribbean pupils account for only 1.1% of the school population but form 7.3% of those permanently excluded. Of the total of school exclusions, 83% are from secondary schools, and of all those excluded 83% are male.

Using examination performance as an indicator, black and Pakistani/Bangladeshi pupils perform less well than white or Indian pupils. Gender differences are similar across ethnic groups, girls doing better in every cultural group.

While the great majority of 16- to 18-year-olds in England are in some form of education or training, 25% of the total in this age group are deemed not to be in any of these activities. Unemployment rates show large differences between the white population and minority ethnic groups, at all age levels, but these differences are most striking for the 18- to 24-year-olds.

TEENAGE PREGNANCIES

In the 1970s, teenage pregnancy rates in countries such as Germany, France and Italy were very similar to those in the UK. Birth rates for girls aged 5–19 have since fallen in other European counties, whilst in Britain they have remained much the same for 30 years. A possible reason may be the low level of contraceptive use in Britain (50%) at first sexual intercourse.

CONSTRUCTS OF RACE, ETHNICITY AND CULTURE

The words 'race', 'ethnicity' and 'culture' are often used interchangeably.

- *Race* is a person's biological inheritance.
- *Ethnicity* is the way a person thinks about that biological inheritance.
- *Culture* is the social network within which conversations about race and ethnicity evolve.

These constructs reflect beliefs about other cultural groups as well as beliefs within cultural groups. All three constructs are likely to be important in determining the use of services. While a person's race will evoke beliefs and prejudices of a potential referrer, primarily with respect to skin colour, ethnicity will reflect self-perceptions and self-beliefs. Culture will in fact reflect the referrer's beliefs and partly culturally specific beliefs about child-rearing, child development and mental health. This may subsume both the elements of the referrer's professional and personal culture.

The categories of ethnic groups used in officially collected data frequently compound these three constructs, and the growing number of culturally mixed unions constantly challenge traditionally ascribed categories (Hodes et al. 1998). The cultural attributes used to define different ethnic groups are often associated with a range of economic and political factors that are influential in affecting rates of child mental health disorders. Bird (1996) states that:

> 'Culture generates another source of contextual variability. Customs, religious beliefs, or attitudes all affect, not only what is perceived as the possible causation of symptomatology, but also the interpretation of behaviour, the meaning ascribed to it and the information actually reported.'

REFERRAL FOR BEHAVIOURAL PROBLEMS

In an early paper, Rutter et al. (1974) compared the rates of behavioural deviance and psychiatric disorders in a sample of 10-year-old West Indian children with those in non-immigrant children, both at school and at home. The data from parents of both sets of children displayed much the same rate of psychiatric disorder. However, the rate of deviance, as reported by teachers, in children from West Indian families was approximately double that for children from non-immigrant families. They suggested a number of reasons for these differences, including reading retardation, higher rates of pupil turnover and racial discrimination.

Epidemiological studies of pre-school children have shown no difference in the prevalence of behavioural and emotional disturbance in Asian and white English children when compared to indigenous English children (Hackett et al. 1991). Retrospective casenote studies of older children have found lower rates of conduct disorder in children of Punjabi Moslem families and higher rates of adjustment disorder, when compared with Caucasian children (Roberts and Cawthorpe 1995). A similar study of second-generation Afro-Caribbean children found an over-representation of children with psychotic disorders and autism (Goodman and Richards 1999).

Few studies have concentrated on the young people's perception of their own ethnic identity. Daryanani et al. (2001) investigated possible associations between ethnic background of referred children and non-attendance, referrer type, problem type, age and gender. The sample consisted of 769 children offered outpatient appointments. Ethnic background influenced the source of referral. Over-referrals against expectation were:

- white children referred more by GPs
- black and South Asian children referred more by specialist doctors
- black children referred more by education services
- mixed-race children referred more by social services.

However, there was neither a significant difference in ethnic background between attendees and non-attendees, nor were gender, age or problem types related to ethnic group. Daryanani *et al.* stress that clinicians should be aware that referral routes may appropriately, or inappropriately, be different for different ethnic groups and that differences found may be due to genuine variation in morbidity, thus leading to presentation to different referrers.

THE MENTAL HEALTH OF YOUNG PEOPLE

Meltzer (2000), in a study of 10,000 11- to 15-year-olds from England, Wales and Scotland, demonstrated higher rates of psychiatric disorder in black young people and very much lower rates among Indian adolescents. The most serious psychiatric disorders, in particular psychosis, can start in adolescence, and are associated with a deterioration in social functioning. Such illness is set in the social context, so the relevance and impact of ethnic variation is of great importance. It is therefore of concern to note that there have been few studies of early-onset psychosis in adolescents from ethnic-minority backgrounds, and more particularly into service responses and service use. In the USA, most ongoing studies are conducted in certain areas where the confounding factors of social adversity, poverty and deprivation play an important part in the origins, epidemiology and prognosis of psychiatric disorders. The interplay of ethnic groups' socio-economic status and family composition has to be carefully disentangled to establish the relative weighting that can or should be attributed to ethnic origin.

For practitioners, the issues remain the same: early detection of psychosis, and equitable service provision for young people from diverse ethnic backgrounds. This means greater user involvement, to ensure that child mental health services are fully utilized by families and children from ethnic-minority groups, and that service delivery has not only knowledge of ethnic issues but develops skilled mental health professionals that can engage in trusting relationships with empowered users.

YOUTH CRIME AND INSTITUTIONAL RACISM

One of the most controversial issues, and one that is difficult to disentangle in relation to youth crime, is ethnic minority backgrounds. This applies across Europe where different ethnic minority backgrounds are seen to be presenting with higher levels of offending (Doreleijers *et al.* 2000). In the UK it is often cited that Afro-Caribbean young men have greater involvement in offending behaviour than do young men from other ethnic groups. Simple statistics cannot satisfactorily address the complex issues that underlie such bald figures and statements (Smith 1995).

In Britain, the crime rate among Afro-Caribbeans is perceived as being substantially higher than among white youths. However, self-report data (2nd Sweep Youth Lifestyle Survey) among adolescents and young adults aged 12 though to 30 reveals higher rates of offending among white young men, with slightly higher rates among black young women. This raises the key issues of processing of offence behaviour and contact between youth, the police and the subtext of poverty and deprivation.

Violence is rated as one of the biggest public health problems facing black youth in the USA, and considerable investment has been made in researching the subject – with mixed results. UK media reports suggest that similar violence is increasing in inner city areas and may come to resemble the USA problem. This places us back in the dilemma surrounding all statistics on offending, whether looking at arrest, caution sentences or self-reported criminal activity.

Despite over-representation of black young people in institutions where persons are admitted involuntarily (e.g. care, young-offender institutions and prison) and in criminal statistics, there are few studies looking at offending and psychopathology in young black people. We already know that black people are over-represented in those who are excluded from school, and those who are excluded are at great risk of early entry into the criminal justice system.

Exploratory studies in the secure care system could and should seek out current and developing perspectives of young people and draw on insights from theories which might be relevant (e.g. attachment theory). These studies should examine issues of lifestyle choices, self-esteem, environmental adversity (racism), mastery over the environment, coping vulnerabilities, family and community dynamics, lifetime psychopathology, social/community/religious themes, peer support and influences, and cognitions.

In the *adult* literature, social division and difference can be seen as a factor in:

- the failure of primary-care filters to identify ethnic-minority people with psychological morbidity, to manage their presenting problems and retain them within primary care, with apparent failures of secondary-care filters and processing into tertiary services
- the absence of a dialogue between ethnic-minority service users and current psychiatric/medical services
- the over-representation of ethnic minorities in those receiving coercive interventions – compulsory admission, seclusion, control and restraint, medication, depot neuroleptic medication and polypharmacy, restriction orders, placement in locked wards and secure environments.

To black patients, *diagnosis* is a serious issue, shaping as it does the subsequent relationships between the black user and services, perceptions of treatment given, justification of coercion, patronizing users, and a culture of low expectation. Perceptions which can appear to be held by services, including side-effects of treatments being tolerated by clinicians and disliked and feared by others. It is helpful both in training and in assessment of complex cases to interchange the cultural background of the person and observe whether this makes a difference to the decision-making process.

In a helpful review, 'Racism in psychiatry: paradigm lost, paradigm regained', Bhugra and Bhui (1999a) describe racism and psychiatry as having been linked in the public imagination, largely because psychiatry is seen as an instrument of social control, and racism as a different form of oppression which permeates society at large. Racism in psychiatry is often believed to be the mediating factor in cases of 'psychiatric' misdiagnosis and 'mismanagement'. Misdiagnosis can include both under- and over-diagnosis. Bhugra and Bhui argue that institutional and individual racism are as a result of three levels or approaches: individual, intragroup and intergroup. The experiences a patient brings to the clinical encounter have to be seen in a historical and macro-economic as well as a social context. They conclude that the emphasis on biological race needs to be shifted on to a qualitative aspect of an individual's functioning, and the therapeutic encounter must take broader factors into account.

ISSUES OF DIAGNOSIS AND TREATMENT

Personality disorder

In any adolescent forensic population, concern is heightened if the prognosis is predicted to be antisocial personality disorder. The prevalence of personality disorder in community and forensic populations of ethnic minorities is unknown, with the exception of the recent ONS prison study (Singleton et al. 1998). Personality-disorder prevalence studies should use a combination of categorical and dimensional approaches in describing personality; they should not confine themselves to antisocial personality but include the whole range of personality disorders, subsuming a whole population and all cultures.

Schizophrenia

Most research on ethnic minorities has centred on the diagnosis of schizophrenia and explanation of black experiences in terms of the presence and the consequences of schizophrenia. The UK literature on psychopathology in ethnic minorities, particularly in persons of African heritage, is notable for the absence of diagnoses of personality disorder, neurotic disorder or affective disorder. Most research and commentary on black issues emanates from the USA.

Black forensic psychiatry is usually used to refer to people of African heritage (Afro-Caribbean, Afro-American

and African). Other ethnic minorities in the UK do not appear to be represented in forensic mental health settings in the same proportion relative to their numbers in the general population. The issue of validity of research instruments in cross-cultural studies has to take into account issues of linguistic equivalence, conceptual equivalence norm, equivalence and scale. Particular attention needs to be given to diagnostic systems which have a heavy reliance on Schneider's first-rank systems.

As in the child and adolescent literature, most studies which include ethnic-minority subjects are hampered by small samples. Examples of studies with large ethnic-minority samples are the Home Office's Youth Life Styles studies 1993 (second sweep 2000) and the Policy Studies Institute's survey of psychiatric morbidity (Nazroo 1997). As a starting point, therefore, debiasing of clinical judgement needs to be a much more prominent feature of clinical practice, and any research which may inform such practice. Factors like family organization, dynamics and support, individual identity, ability of family and individual to make choices, poverty and poor housing, all need to be added into future studies to help understand why single young black men are so vulnerable to adverse pathways into hospitals and the criminal justice system.

The existence of schizophrenia is deduced on the basis of clinical diagnostic practice, which varies within and across cultures, societies and economic systems. Diagnostic formulation may also emphasize as pathological those symptoms/phenomena that are prominent in non-schizophrenic psychoses and in culturally sanctioned states of distress.

In identifying the difficulties arising from the research literature in American studies and the UK findings, Bhugra and Bhui (2001) conclude that there is little doubt from the literature that rates of schizophrenia among Afro-Caribbeans in the UK are much higher than for whites (Carpenter and Brockington 1980; Harrison et al. 1997); findings for other ethnic groups are equivocal. Some of this can be explained by poor housing, high rates of unemployment and social isolation. Bhugra and Bhui suggest that an interactional model needs to be evaluated by empirical study of a number of factors, both environmental and psychological. Suggested hypotheses for high rates are: genetic factors, pregnancy and birth complications, social factors (social inequality, economic factors, discrimination), racism, harassment, racial life events, and population density.

Bhugra and Bhui suggest the following practice points in assessing a case of schizophrenia:

- Take a careful study.
- Understand delusional phenomena in a cultural context.
- Understand hallucinatory experience in a cultural context.
- Check though the disorder in the primary language.
- Ascertain abnormal mood states.

- Ascertain passivity phenomena.
- Carry out physical and neurological investigations.
- Check third-party information, including cultural identity.

Medication and other treatments

ISSUES FREQUENTLY RAISED BY BLACK PEOPLE

- Are there valid objective measures of disturbed or aggressive behaviour?
- Is the medication prescribed appropriate, given the issues of diagnosis and possible use of medication to control disturbed or aggressive behaviour, as opposed to the symptoms of the disorder under treatment? (Similar searches of objectivity are required in studies of seclusion, control and restraint.)
- The nature and use of medication in the first few hours, days and early weeks of treatment is crucial, when many changes are likely to be made to medication used and when most adverse events take place. There is the issue of polypharmacy and the need to monitor and examine for its scientific basis and for its prevalence.
- The outcomes of interventions in a psychiatric setting for black people are poor (Thornicroft *et al.* 1999). A number of questions can be asked. For example, are the observations the result of a poor assessment of presenting problems and thus targeting of inappropriate interventions for presenting problems?
- Is there a failure to recognize and treat problems related to substance abuse, which may in turn impact on the frequency of adverse contact with criminal justice agencies?
- Insight/compliance are recurring themes in the interface between black patients and services. Most studies of insight ignore the user's perspective or explanatory models. Compliance with treatment is an important issue to be addressed in attempts to reduce suicide and homicide (Appleby 2000). Callan *et al.* (1998) propose that where the patient's and the clinician's explanatory models merge, compliance is likely to be higher.
- What attempts are made to incorporate the patient's perspective in treatment plans, ensuring in particular that black people are offered psychological treatments such as cognitive-behavioural therapy and psychotherapy?

ETHNICITY AND PSYCHOPHARMACOLOGY

In a view of ethnic and cultural factors in psychopharmacology, Bhugra and Bhui (1999b) noted that 'ethnicity' is a social construction often invested with greater stability, permanence and biological importance than is justified. Definitions of ethnicity can be based at a social level at an individual identity level, or as is usual in medical practice at a level which recognizes a combination of social, cultural and phenotypic similarities rather than genotypic differences. It is the association of phenotypic similarities with pharmacogenic variations in drug metabolism that render ethnic-pharmacogenic variations of clinical importance.

The therapeutic effect of pharmacologically active drugs is determined by pharmokinetic and pharmacological processes. The recent recognition of a pharmacogenetic variation according to ethnic groups can lead to significant genetically determined modifications of metabolizing enzymes (the pharmokinetic handling of the drug by the body). This, in turn, leads to differing therapeutic levels and half-lives, and so to variable profiles of therapeutic and adverse effects.

Most of the data available on ethnicity and psychopharmacology come from the USA where the emphasis has been on the study of neuroleptics. Cross-racial differences in doses of neuroleptics which produce side-effects have been studied extensively in Asian–Americans (Bhugra and Bhui 1999b). Racial differences in red blood cell sodium and lithium levels are well recognized (Westermeyer 1989). For instance lithium has proved effective at lower levels among Japanese patients.

A wide variability in drug prescriptions and type of drugs across different cultures has been observed. Beliefs and attitudes on the part of both patient and clinician will determine what drugs are prescribed. For example, Afro-Caribbeans may be given higher doses of neuroleptics and be given depot injections, because a stereotype has arisen about Afro-Caribbeans being less compliant with medication. There is slow progress on cross cultural research on biological diversity and factors which affect metabolism of drugs. The use of clinical practice guidelines is escalating, but these originate from the existing evidence base, most of which has not included ethnic-minority patients. Compliance with medication depends upon a number of factors, such as side-effects experienced, and the person's model of illness and beliefs in healthcare. Divergence in the beliefs between patients and clinicians, and communication difficulties, have been regarded as the major reasons for such ethnic differences in compliance (Lin *et al.* 1995).

PRESCRIBING PRACTICE

Ethnic and cultural considerations are important in prescribing practice, and clinicians have to be aware of safety and efficacy effects of medications. In addition, these differences highlight the interaction between biological and cultural factors which may provide a clue to the pharmacological effects.

In the planning of pharmacological treatments for minority ethnic groups, Bhugra and Bhui (1999b) suggest the following:

- Prior to prescribing, check the person's diet and religious taboos about the diet. Also check the person's smoking habit, and alcohol and drug ingestion.

- When prescribing, start at as low a dose as possible, to have a low threshold for identifying side-effects. Adjust dosages regularly if required, and provide information to the patient.
- After prescribing, monitor side-effects, check compliance, and check environmental/dietary factors.

All the above is even more critical when prescribing to young people from ethnic-minority groups.

Issues in risk assessment

With a black or ethnic-minority patient, is the risk posed by the patient over-estimated, resulting in him or her receiving treatment in higher levels of security and for longer periods than is warranted? Although a number of checklists and formal assessment schedules have been developed to attempt to gauge the risk posed by an individual patient, most multi-disciplinary teams do not use these as routine but instead generally arrive at a decision through a multi-disciplinary team (Ford and Farrington 1999).

Risk assessments have not always been validated for ethnic-minority people, who often comprise an unfeasibly small proportion of the population. Also, an emphasis on historical factors renders these assessments static and unresponsive to changes in the patient. It could be argued that these facts increase the scores attained by ethnic-minority patients in relation to the general population; for example, ethnic-minority patients have a younger age at first conviction, are more likely to receive custodial sentences, and tend to receive longer sentences for more serious convictions. They are also more likely to be unemployed. All of these factors will increase the score of 'dangerousness' that will be relatively static and unaffected by any changes in the individual concerned.

There has been little examination of what ethnic-minority staff could and do bring to working with adolescent offenders from ethnic minority groups and the extent to which they are capable of influencing institutional processes. It could be that ethnic minority staff find the environment challenging. They may identify with the offenders and view themselves as advocates. Their presentations will undoubtedly be apparent to the offenders and may be viewed positively or negatively. There is therefore a need to examine what it is that staff from ethnic minorities bring to the adolescent forensic environment.

Bhugra and Bhui (1999a) stress that the impact of prejudice and racism is not static. The patient's set of assumptions, strategies and questions about behaviours meted out are crucial in making any interaction possible, therapeutic or otherwise. Interconnecting features are affected by various social, establishment and political systems. Both individual and social cognitions contribute to this interaction (Figure 14.1).

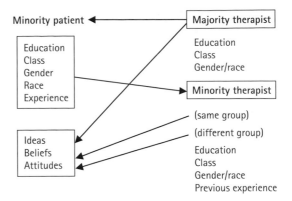

Figure 14.1 *The dynamic impact of prejudice and racism. (Reproduced from Bhugra and Bhui (1999a) with permission.)*

THEORY INTO PRACTICE: AN ADOLESCENT FORENSIC SERVICE

In the context of evolving knowledge about the safe and effective delivery of mental health care to all individuals, of whatever age, from ethnic-minority groups, the Adolescent Forensic Service in Salford undertook a pilot study of ethnic and non-ethnic admissions, and worked in partnership with the Greater Manchester African Caribbean Mental Health Project to develop a framework for delivery of a care programme attuned to the needs of young people from diverse cultural backgrounds.

The Salford adolescent forensic service

The adolescent forensic service in Salford is one of three NHS adolescent medium-secure inpatient units, accepting 12- to 18-year-olds with serious mental illness, early-onset psychosis who are deemed to be a high risk to others. In recent years, higher numbers of admissions have been of young people from diverse ethnic backgrounds, including increasing numbers of refugees. This has led the team to ensure the development of both the knowledge and skills to offer an ethnically and culturally attuned service. Given the diversity of culture, the approach has to be feasible and responsive.

As an example, in partnership with the African Caribbean Mental Health team in Manchester city centre, the service has strived to develop a team that can respond to the needs of, and indeed learn from the strengths of, diverse cultural and ethnic groups and families of the young people.

What follows is a practice framework for a unit working in partnership with African and Caribbean mental health services. Common issues arise from attempts to treat black young people within a predominantly white environment. Provision of culturally appropriate care to

Afro-Caribbean young people in a residential secure psychiatric unit is described for meeting the needs of young people from ethnic minority backgrounds.

The unit's environment

Provision of information

Information should be displayed in a prominent place and should include:

- a list of services for Afro-Caribbean people with mental health problems, including advocacy services
- a list of legal services, including access to black solicitors who specialize in mental health issues
- information about local community events, so that black young people can make a connection to the wider community.

The latter is particularly important, as this information is not normally available via the usual channels.

Pictures

The décor should as far as possible reflect the cultural origins of the young people being cared for. Pictures or photographs of black pioneers can be used as positive role models.

Library area

The library area should include books, magazines and newspapers for black people. These can be used as a resource for lessons, art and music sessions and for staff development around cultural awareness. They could then be used as the basis of discussion with all of the young people so as to inform their opinions about the experiences of black people in the UK.

Music

Music may be very important to young Afro-Caribbeans and is seen as a form of relaxation. Often the music is played very loudly, which may not be acceptable in a shared environment and can be seen as antisocial behaviour. It is considered normal to dance very closely with another person; although it may be considered inappropriate between young people, it is not usually seen as sexual in African and Caribbean cultures.

Approaches

AVOIDING INSTITUTIONAL RACISM

It is fair to say that sometimes in our professional or personal lives we are likely to be accused of colluding in institutional racism. As humans, we unwittingly behave in ways which are unacceptable to others, often through being dismissive of a specific need or situation. All staff need to consider:

- whether they see the young person's culture or race as a cause of the present problem

- whether they see the young person's culture as part of the solution to the present problem
- whether they can accept, acknowledge and understand the young person's culture
- whether cultural prejudice affects their relationships with the young people they are working with
- their ability to focus on feelings expressed in ways unfamiliar to their own culture
- how their own background may affect their own attitude to young black people.

ETHNIC MONITORING

Ethnic monitoring should be applied to issues where subjectivity could allow for racial discrimination to take place – for example, decisions about the number of escorts, how quickly young people are reintroduced back into the group after being managed separately, and whether risk assessments are routinely carried out.

LANGUAGE AND COMMUNICATION

Even where families speak English, this cannot necessarily be literally translated. Misunderstandings can occur within groups of people through regional differences. A common misunderstanding is to assume that because you hear a phrase used you have understood the meaning in terms of cultural references; for example nobody would literally translate 'having butterflies in my stomach'. Although this may appear to be common sense, taken to an extreme it can mean that workers could misunderstand fundamental aspects of a young person's family background as well as misinterpreting the attitudes of significant relatives.

Good communication could be considered to be the core of good service delivery. *Patois* is commonly used by Afro-Caribbeans. Some phrases have been appropriated into 'street talk' which is predominantly used by young people often in an attempt to alienate themselves from adults; therefore it is deliberately designed to be impenetrable and often words/phrases become defunct as soon as they become common knowledge. Although some street talk has its roots in *patois*, it should not be confused as one and the same. Young men may use *patois* to identify their cultural roots and links.

Cultural and family issues

For many black people, cultural identity plays an important part in their lives. Some issues for consideration are:

- whether the young person has the same culture as parents/brothers/sisters and how well they get on together
- those family members who live at home, and those who live in the neighbourhood/district/country

- the kind of contact the young person has with these family members, for example by personal/telephone contact, letters and cards
- the family members the young person sees as significant.

FAMILY ROLES

Often in black families the grandmother/aunt/sister/brother/uncle (extended family) can be seen as the most significant person in the young person's life. It is normal for the grandmother to bring up grandchildren, both because the mother can't cope, and to give her the opportunity to return to further education or to work.

It is also customary for the older brothers/sisters to take on caring responsibilities for the younger ones without this being seen as 'being taken advantage of'. If one or both parents are unwell the children would be expected to take on these caring responsibilities. Black children are shown from a very young age how to carry out basic tasks like cleaning, washing, cooking and shopping and are given these responsibilities. They are also able to address personal hygiene. The aim is to enable children to grow up as responsible, capable and independent human beings who are not reliant on others to do things for them.

CULTURAL NORMS

It is normal in the Afro-Caribbean culture to address an older person as aunt/uncle, as it is considered to be very rude to address an adult by their first name. This extends to adults themselves who would not feel comfortable addressing their elders on a first-name basis. Much cultural behaviour can be open to misinterpretation.

It is culturally normal for an Afro-Caribbean person to think aloud. This is used as a way of 'reasoning' or trying to put problems and situations in some context. It is useful for carers to check information with the young person or their family as to behaviour prior to illness, thus building on the creation of an atmosphere where questions can be asked from both sides without fear.

VISITING

Black families may not visit because of financial worries, the distance involved and the time this may necessitate off work. However, these may not be the only reasons why visiting does not take place.

Visits may not occur because relatives find it too upsetting and will therefore ask someone else to visit on their behalf. They often have anxieties about the situation and are worried that they may misunderstand or misinterpret the information. It is also quite normal for three or more members from one family to visit and attend meetings so as to offer emotional support to each other. They will also ask members/friends of the family who work in the caring profession to accompany them on visits and to attend meetings. This is because they feel that they will have a better understanding of the system. Possible solutions include:

- addressing issues concerning the sharing of information with significant relatives
- supplying copies of leaflets to all relatives
- exploring the possibility of holding regular briefing/training sessions with carers so as to address issues of high expressed emotion.

FOOD CHOICE

Food is significant within the black family. Children will be used to eating certain foods like chicken, rice and peas on a Sunday where it is traditional for all the family to gather at the family home. Meat and fish will be seasoned and left overnight before cooking, to enhance the flavour. All food including rice will be washed before use. Some young people check their plates and cutlery before using them; this reflects cultural norms around concerns about food hygiene.

Religions

People have ways in which their faith and worship defines them and which prescribe moral practices for everyday living. However, for most Afro-Caribbean people religion plays an important role. Even if the individual is not practising or attending a religious place for worship regularly, he or she will usually feel a spiritual connection. If the individual attends church, the overall church community will be very supportive often referring to each other as Brother Smith or Sister Brown as opposed to Mr Smith or Mrs Brown. There are a few specific denominations that are particularly relevant to African and Caribbean people.

Pentecostal/Church of God

People who are from the Pentecostal denomination believe that Jesus Christ is the Son of God and will worship by singing to the music of percussion, wind and brass instruments. A significant part of worship includes praying in an incoherent way (often referred to as 'speaking in tongues'). Oil is also used during worship to anoint sick people. This is viewed very much as a direct communication with God and should not therefore be interpreted as a symptom of psychosis. This is not to say that other symptoms of illness may not be present but merely to reinforce the notion that staff should clarify what is considered 'normal' behaviour for relatives, thereby ensuring that assumptions are not recorded as fact in people's notes.

It should be acknowledged that whilst the church community can be very supportive some individuals might find this level of support intrusive or overbearing. It is important to bear this in mind when working with young people who are 'in the church' as they will often have been brought up to abide by strict guidelines that may govern the way they feel can interact with other people.

The Rastafarian movement

The Rastafarian movement began in Jamaica in 1930. Its birth was inspired by Marcus Garvey. The Rastafarians ('Rastas') see Ethiopia as the Promised Land. Some members see their return to Ethiopia as a physical journey to Africa, while others acknowledge a cultural and spiritual unity with Africa and hope for social and political change. Within the Rastafarian culture there is a religious group identified as the Twelve Tribes of Israel, based on the biblical reference in the Old Testament (Genesis 49.33) to a lost tribe.

They have regular group meetings – 'reasoning sessions' – which provide a forum for people to air their views as well as to give social, cultural and religious support.

Rastas believe there is a living God incarnate in each individual and each can speak directly to God. They use the term 'I and I' instead of you and me and see their body as the temple of god and therefore try to guard against pollution, especially by chemicals.

They usually eat no salt, are vegetarian and eat natural (known as 'I-TAL') food. Pork is excluded from their diet, as are shellfish, alcohol and processed food. Milk is usually not drunk; fruit juice is consumed in large quantities. As with all religious groups there is a sliding scale as to the degree to which individuals choose to adhere to the above 'guidelines'.

One usual sign of Rastafarians is long hair plaited in locks ('dreadlocks'). Rastas wear their hair in locks as a symbol that represents their strength. It would, however, be wrong to assume that everyone who wears their hair in locks follows the Rastafarian religion. Hair is uncut, and hats or 'crowns' are worn with colours of red, green and gold, which are the colours of the Ethiopian flag. Each person is also assigned a colour depending on the tribe of origin; these may be referred to as the person's colours. Colours may also be worn on bracelets or other articles of clothing.

Smoking 'ganja' (cannabis) is used by some Rastas as a religious ritual. This is seen as a gift of God, which comes from the tree of life, and the act of smoking is a form of religious worship. This area of activity has been a source of much debate and conflict. Again, cannabis can also be consumed not as a religious ritual but as a social drug of choice. Meditation is also a significant part of this religion.

Seventh Day Adventists

Many African and Caribbean people belong to the Seventh Day Adventist church, or variations of it. This involves worshipping on Saturdays and keeping the Sabbath. They too will not eat pork and will avoid alcohol. Young people who belong to this religious group may not be used to taking part in social activities after dusk on Fridays and will be expected to study the Bible on Saturdays. Again there will be differences to the degree to which they conform to this. It is therefore important to clarify the extent of the young person's commitment to the faith as this may differ from that of their parents.

Personal characteristics

CLOTHING

Some Afro-Caribbeans dress in colourful clothing, which can be viewed as an expression of their personality. Good grooming is considered an essential part of the Afro-Caribbean culture. At times some people may wear articles of clothing that are not particularly well coordinated but are clean and well ironed. It is important to recognize that the majority of African and Caribbean young people will be used to the emphasis being placed on the wearing of clean 'pressed' clothes and would expect that staff would appreciate the care and attention that has gone into ensuring that they are well presented.

SKIN TONE

There is a great deal of variation in skin tone amongst black people who are not of mixed race. It is not uncommon to find several different members of the same family with different skin tone. This does not always mean that they have different parents but is a reflection of their racial heritage, which can often be traced back to Scottish, Irish, Spanish, Indian and Portuguese ancestors. This can be an issue for some black people as during the slave trade, which was less than 160 years ago, and more recently colonialism, lighter-skinned people were afforded certain privileges and were allowed access to positions that were closed to those with darker skin. Other black people often refer to lighter-skinned black people who are not mixed race as 'redskin'.

SKIN AND HAIR CARE

Black people need to pay special attention to their skin in the same way that white people do when they are exposed to the sun. Black people's skin becomes dry and patchy if not properly creamed. Most people 'cream' their skin more than once a day to ensure moisture is maintained and the skin is kept in good condition. The young people may tease other children if their skin is dry. Staff should ensure that cocoa butter or Vaseline is available for those young people whose relatives are not able to provide it, as without it their skin will become dry and start to crack.

Hair also needs attention; it usually needs to be 'greased' on a regular basis with hair oil and requires regular applications of conditioner to maintain its condition. Even if hair is braided it will still need to be washed and treated; hence the importance of being able to use the expertise and services of local Afro-Caribbean hairdressers.

Pulling the themes together

It has been recognized that the experiences of black young people prior to admission to the unit need to be taken seriously particularly in relation to narratives of persecutory or paranoid ideas. It is important to recognize that, although people can be paranoid as a symptom of illness, their experience as a black young person in Britain will be affected by the knowledge that institutional and direct racism is alive and well and could have directly affected their care. The case of the mudered black teenager Stephen Lawrence did much to reinforce black people's fear and concern. Indeed, the daily experiences of black life in Britain have been found to impact on mental health and need therefore to be handled with sensitivity. Here is a list of practice guidelines:

1 Create a unit that reflects the diversity of the multi-cultural environment that many of the young people will have come from.
2 Establish links with ACMHS Carers Group and other support available across the city for parents/relatives to aid facilitation of family support and as a national service to seek advice from as wide a field as necessary.
3 Establish links with youth workers experienced with working with black young people.
4 Establish a mentoring service so that each black young person in the unit can be assigned a mentor upon admission.
5 Evaluate the recruitment and selection process to make sure that qualified 'bank' staff are recruited and retained effectively within the unit.
6 Encourage staff to attend the Drop Ins at ACMHS so that they can become used to working in a black person's environment. This would also allow for workers to experience the feeling of being a minority within an environment, a valuable experience to draw on when working with black young people.
7 Consider placements for staff in black organisations so that they can experience first hand the provision of culturally appropriate care.
8 Make provision for black young people's spiritual needs to be assessed in a cultural context.
9 Revisit *all* policies and procedures, including risk assessment, in order to avoid institutional racism.
10 Conduct continuous monitoring and evaluation.

Moodley (2002) stresses that to build a culturally capable workforce it is necessary to have a broader-based knowledge of the constitution of psychiatry and psychiatric diagnoses and the cultures of psychiatry and psychology as we learn and teach them. An understanding of different notions of self and identity, including the manner in which they are constructed, is crucial. Different cultures have different rituals, rites of passage, taboos and idioms of distress. It is necessary to know about migration, acculturation, and international affairs such as regional wars or conflicts, which may have significant impact on local demographics and needs.

Moodley goes on to state that every psychiatrist needs to know how organizations function, how institutional racism operates, and how these may impact on access to services and pathways to care. Knowledge of local and national non-statutory organizations is essential, as is knowledge of evidence-based data on ethnic psychopharmacology and international therapies as applied to people of diverse backgrounds. Nowhere can this be more important than in adolescent forensic mental-health service delivery.

ASPECTS OF GENDER: LEARNING FROM THE ADULT LITERATURE

WOMEN AS INDIVIDUALS

Adult females suffer from a range of mental disorders similar to those that men may experience. However, there are some striking differences in the prevalence of specific disorders, and in their presentation and management. Some mental illnesses occur only in women. It seems that women patients may have a different experience of treatment, a consequence of differences in their needs and also of the way in which health professionals perceive those needs. These differences are embedded in the wider cultural milieu in which we live. There are particular issues for women patients in relation to childhood sexual abuse, rape and domestic violence. At present, tools to measure needs of individual patients are generally not gender-specific (Ramsay *et al.* 2001).

With specific disorders, there may be significant differences in the presentation and outcome for women and men. For example, in schizophrenia, men appear to have a more severe form of the illness, characterized by an early age of onset, poor premorbid adjustment, both atypical and negative symptoms and poor outcome, while in women the onset is later and a more affective component is apparent (Castle and Murray 1991; see also Chapter 12). Among patients with a dual diagnosis admitted for treatment, women seem to have more social contact problems and fewer legal difficulties but more problems with victimization and medical illness (Brunette and Drake 1997).

The Office of Population Censuses and Surveys' survey of 10,000 adults living in private households in the UK found that women were more likely than men to suffer from a neurotic health problem; men were three times more likely than women to suffer from alcohol dependence and twice as likely to suffer from a drug dependence problem (Meltzer *et al.* 1995). This gender difference is most marked for eating disorders; over 90% of patients with anorexia nervosa are female.

Women also experience specific times in relation to their life cycle when they are at increased risk of developing particular disorders and on occasions actions that bring them into contact with the police.

Two particular crimes of violence associated with females are those of infanticide and physical abuse of children. When women kill, it is often assumed that they are mentally disturbed. In particular, the mysterious workings of the female body have long been blamed for women running riot and becoming violent. The creation by the law of the offence of infanticide was an important stage in this tradition. The offence applies only to women who kill their children under the age of 12 months when the balance of their mind is disturbed as a result of childbirth or lactation. The offence reached the statute books in England in 1922, and was later modified in 1938 (Wilczynski 1997).

The infanticide provisions are underpinned by two contradictory assumptions. On the one hand, mothers are presumed to be naturally benign, tender and nurturing, and therefore incapable of harming their children unless mentally disturbed. On the other hand, there are fears that women's very biology makes them inclined towards murderous attacks on their children, and that this requires special provision within the criminal law. The uneasy balancing act between these twin assumptions is reflected in a number of unique features of the infanticide legislation which run counter to traditional criminal law principles. When offenders commit crimes, the law presumes they are sane until it is shown otherwise. Yet the infanticide provisions enshrine a virtual presumption that a certain class of offender is mentally disturbed. Further, it has to be shown only that the offender's imbalance of mind coincided with the criminal act, rather than having directly caused it. Of particular interest in adolescent females is the act of neonaticide (killing of an infant within 24 hours of birth) and undisclosed teenage pregnancy, which will be discussed later.

To a lesser extent than infanticide, the killing of family members is more characteristic of females than males. Homicides by females are three times as likely to be of a family member and less likely than in males to be of a stranger. Feminist sociological perspectives have suggested that there may be routes into crime for females which are much less characteristic of males. Examples include crimes that arise from a relationship with a violent male or through friends or partners who misuse drugs, and more limited evidence of serious crimes of violence related to severe depressive illness which is more common in females (Daly 1994).

WOMEN AND FAMILIES

Mothers who themselves have had poor experiences of parenting may be the least likely to receive practical help with childcare and social support to help them function in their new role (Pound and Abel 1996). Women threatened with having their children taken into care may distrust services and feel inhibited from seeking help. A significant proportion of women with a severe mental illness have children, but health professionals are only beginning to recognize the importance of these women's role as parents, regarding parenting as a social services problem rather than a health issue (Nicholson et al. 1993).

WOMEN AND ABUSE

There has been increasing awareness of the impact of violence against women, in particular the effects of childhood sexual abuse, domestic violence and rape.

Childhood sexual abuse

Women who have experienced childhood sexual abuse are more likely to suffer social, interpersonal and sexual difficulties in adult life. They seem to have particular problems with intimate relationships, owing to difficulties with trust and a perception of their partners as uncaring and over-controlling. Abuse may also correlate with an increased risk for a range of mental health problems (Mullen et al. 1994).

Domestic violence

A high proportion of women attending accident and emergency departments report a history of domestic violence, and in this group there is a high level of mental health problems. A history of childhood abuse increases a woman's risk of subsequent mental health problems, especially if she is also abused as an adult. In this double-abuse group, there may also be an increased risk of substance abuse (Roberts et al. 1998).

Rape

Victims of completed rape are at increased risk of suicide attempts and of having a depressive illness. In addition, perceptions of life threat and actual injury increase the risk of post-traumatic stress disorder (Mezey and Stanko 1996).

WOMEN FROM ETHNIC MINORITIES

Our understanding of mental health problems follows a western conceptualization of mental illness, and women from ethnic minorities may face additional barriers such as language difference in engaging with healthcare professionals. Factors such as this may partly explain the under-recognition of mental illness in these groups – for example, in Indian women in the UK (Jacob et al. 1998). Women from refugee groups are particularly likely to have experienced multiple losses and may be at risk of depression and post-traumatic stress disorder.

ADOLESCENT FEMALE OFFENDERS

Statistics

Official crime statistics of all countries have consistently demonstrated that the crime rate amongst young females is several times less than for young males (Heidensohn 1997).

Young women appear less likely to be recidivist or to commit very serious crimes; their offending careers tend to be shorter. It is, therefore, somewhat surprising that there has been relatively little interest shown in the research into female/male differences in antisocial behaviour in general, and violence in particular (Rutter *et al.* 1998).

Criminal statistics for England and Wales in 1998 show much the same level of offending for girls between the ages of 14 and 19, with still slightly higher levels at ages 14 and 15, indicating a peak age of offending of 15 years for females (Graham and Bowling 1995). Wikstrom (1990) reported a peak age of between 22 and 24 for young females in Sweden. All the evidence supports the conclusion that, compared with young males, young females commit fewer and different crimes and follow different offending careers. Although there has been evidence over the years that young females are treated differently by the criminal justice system (Morris 1987), this does not account for the overall difference in statistics with respect to young offenders; a real difference in behaviour exists. Known risk factors for delinquency do vary by sex, but this still does not offer a full explanation of gender differences in rates of juvenile crime and the associated evolution of severe antisocial behaviour and parallel acts of violence through childhood and into adolescence (Loeber and Hay 1994).

During the 1970s, young females tended to be treated more harshly than young males, being brought before the Courts for such non-criminal matters as being in moral danger or beyond control. Young females were more likely to be formally cautioned, to be brought to Court and placed in some form of institutional care for lesser offences. However, recent British statistics (Home Office 1997) indicate that young females tend now to be dealt with less harshly than their male counterparts. In 1994, 56% of females appearing in Court for the first time were given an absolute or conditional discharge, compared with 47% of male first offenders. In the case of individuals aged 21 years or more with at least ten convictions, 22% of males but only 13% of females were sentenced to immediate imprisonment. This differential processing of males and females should tend to lead to an increase in the sex ratio over time; in fact the opposite has taken place and the sex ratio has gradually but steadily diminished over the last 40 years. Crimes by females have been increasing at a faster rate than crimes by males. Consideration is now given to how gender, crime and violence are linked, how the small but significant rise in violent crimes carried out by adolescent females is understood, and the ways in which these issues are being addressed by the mental health services.

Assessment of young females

Psychiatric assessments (see Chapter 1), in general, place emphasis on the qualities of psychological and social functioning rather than on the criminogenic process. However, in adolescent forensic psychiatry there is a clear emphasis on the relationship between any mental disorder and offence specifics.

Given the transitional nature of adolescent influences on mental health and young females, assessment involves not only the consideration of the presence or absence of illness or disorder, but also an evaluation of the various components of development, which must encompass personality, social and moral development, including empathy and ability to form relationships. Physical and intellectual development will have a considerable bearing on psychological development. Any judgement about the presence or absence of psychiatric disorder has to take into account different presentations at different stages through development. The interplay between assessment, development and presence or absence of disorder is highlighted in the assessment of adjustment to a trauma, or a series of negative life events. Concepts of resilience and vulnerability are concerned with the factors that impinge on the ability to cope. Nowhere is this seen more vividly than in the lives of violent adolescent females whose critical early years have been characterized by a series of abusive experiences. Those coming to the attention of the adolescent forensic services have commonly started to (repetitively) self-harm and exercise control over their lives through an array of high-risk behaviours, such as firesetting and sustained repetitive, assaultative behaviour, the latter not infrequently against their residential carers.

Psychiatric disorders in adolescence fall into three main developmental categories: continuing childhood disorder; mental illness typical of adulthood; and disorders which, although not confined exclusively to adolescence, are characterized in the main by difficulties in surmounting this particular stage of development (see Chapter 1).

The acquisition of a personal identity remains the main developmental task for young females reared in supportive and caring environments; supplementary tasks are attainment and proficiency in the adult sexual role, the transition from being nurtured to being able to care for others, learning to work and be self-supporting, and leaving home. The early life experiences of adolescent females presenting with aggressive and violent behaviour render such tasks at times not only alien but frequently impossible to achieve. This situation, in turn, acts as a strong reinforcer for escalating maladaptive coping strategies to survive for the moment, while young women are unable to plan or think of the future.

In the field of forensic psychiatry, written communication between a range of disciplines, particularly in the medico-legal arena, is a key component. Thus, a common language of reliable and valid diagnoses is vital if safe practice is to be implemented. Both the World Health Organization's *International Classification of Disease* (ICD-10) and the *Diagnostic and Statistical Manual of the American Psychiatric Association* (DSM-IV) allows a multi-axial approach to classification, thus allowing different aspects of an adolescent's problems to be recorded separately without requiring an artificial judgement about the privacy of each. Both systems are for use across the whole lifespan and therefore increase the opportunity for safe transition, both meeting needs and managing risk as an adolescent female moves into adult services.

Assessment of a high-risk female adolescent with a possible mental health problem can be beset with many difficulties. Not least of these is the viewing of the adolescent solely as a target for complaint, the still prevalent attitude of stigma attached to mental illness adding to discrimination against this already negatively labelled group of young female offenders.

In reality, however, the greatest obstacle remains lack of confidence and previous negative experiences for young females who are trying to articulate their innermost thoughts and feelings to and with others. At the point of assessment by an adolescent forensic mental health team, there is often an already established pattern of poor relationships with the authority figures of parents, teachers, social workers and the police. Add to this the expectation from the judicial process of clear explanations for crimes, with accompanying exact diagnosis and prediction of future risk, and the process of assessment for both assessor and young female can appear a daunting one. In practice, assessment has to strike a balance between engagement, the need to elicit information, and formal mental state examination. There can be, and often is, conflict between these three, further compounded by whether the assessment is a stand-alone exercise for the purpose of a report to a Court, when the practice of least harm must be one of a set of competing priorities, or whether the assessment is but a prelude to long-term treatment for the young female facing the possibility of a life sentence for an act of extreme violence. In a world that demands increased sharing of information, and at times full disclosure of all information between professional agencies, in order to protect the public, this is further compounded and complicated by walking the difficult tightrope of the traditional patient–doctor confidentiality boundaries (Bailey and Harbour 1999).

PSYCHIATRIC DISORDERS AND VIOLENCE: A GENDER PERSPECTIVE

Oppositional defiant disorders (see Chapter 8), characterized by frequent severe temper tantrums for the child's developmental level, arguments with adults, defiance of rules and blaming others for mistakes, have similar rates in girls and boys. Children are often touchy, angry, resentful, spiteful and hold vindictive attitudes (Campbell 1995). Conduct disorders, however, were shown by an American twin study to occur in males up to four times more frequently than in young females (Simonoff *et al.* 1997). Conduct disorder is defined in terms of rather more serious behaviour including violence, fighting, cruelty and setting fires as well as by overtly delinquent acts such as stealing and burglary. It does, however, subsume lying and truanting. McGee *et al.* (1990) found that non-aggressive conduct disorders, mainly comprising truancy and the use of alcohol or cannabis, are more frequent in girls. However, Zoccolillo (1993) has argued cogently that the prevailing systems of psychiatric disorders are much more frequent in males, with a sex ratio of about four to one.

Antisocial personality disorders in adult life are some 5–6 times as frequent in males as in females (see Chapter 9). This condition is defined in terms of pervasive patterns of disregard for, and violation of the rights of, others that have been present from as early as mid-adolescence. The US epidemiological catchment area (ECA) showed a lifetime prevalence in males of 4.3% and in females of 0.07% (Robins and Regier 1991). Follow-up studies (Zocolillo *et al.* 1992) revealed that the ways in which pervasive social malfunction is shown varied by gender. Crime in adult life is a common feature in men but less common in women, who are more likely to show problems in interpersonal relationships. Information on young females is again scant.

The emphasis on the study and development of psychopathic personality in late adolescence has focused predominantly on males (Christian *et al.* 1997). There is an urgent need to explore the evolution of such personality types in young females. Key indicators include:

- *family features* – parental antisocial personality disorder; witnessing violence; abuse, neglect or rejection
- *personality features* – callous, unemotional, interpersonal style; evolution of violent and sadistic fantasy; people regarded as objects; morbid identity; paranoid ideation; hostile attribution
- *situational features* – history of repeated loss and rejection in relationships; threats to self-esteem; crescendos of hopelessness and helplessness; social disinhibition (group processes, substance misuse); changes in mental state over time.

Most of the literature on adult females who are violent consists of the study of women held in penal establishments or maximum security hospitals. The emphasis in the American literature is on borderline personality disorder, with pervasive instability of mood, difficulties in interpersonal relationships and self-image associated with marked impulsivity, huge fear of abandonment, identity disturbance and recurrent suicidal behaviour. These features are also highly characteristic of the young females in a study of the first 100 admissions to an adolescent forensic secure psychiatric unit (Bailey *et al.* 1994). Follow-up of these young women has shown that they fared badly in adult life, developing major psychotic illness, schizophrenia and high rates of successful suicide in their early twenties. Their histories and clinical presentation bear a strong resemblance to those adult females admitted to maximum-security hospitals, particularly those with histories of firesetting, violence and early histories of loss, trauma, sexual abuse and post-traumatic stress disorder.

Early onset of psychosis is, in itself, rare in both males and females. It can be associated with violent behaviour but the association is complex. Psychosis with onset in the teenage years has a tendency to go unrecognized, the psychotic behaviour being attributed to the very process of adolescence. The risk of violence, however, tends to lie less in the actual psychosis than in the previous history of antisocial behaviour and unsupportive rearing. Nevertheless, it remains important, in any overall assessment of young females by multi-professional agencies, to consider the possibility of early-onset psychosis. Literature in this field has been limited to date but there is emerging strong evidence that there is a prodromal phase of non-psychotic behavioural disturbance which can last between one and seven years in about half of early-onset cases of schizophrenia (Maziade *et al.* 1996). The importance to non-mental health practitioners lies in the nature of the non-psychotic behavioural disturbance which can include obsessive–compulsive disorder, avoidant personality, anxiety states, self-harm and, in particular, externalizing acts of violence.

Characteristically, the violent adolescent female will experience multiple periods of 'at-risk mental states', which are significantly affected by life events and family stress. In the lives of chaotic young females who repetitively self-harm, and are in unsupportive environments, it is important to look for any clear change in the baseline level of social functioning, even if the baseline itself is normally chaotic. At-risk mental states associated with violence include perceptual changes in ideas of reference, and paranoid delusions. Mental states in young females which should alert professionals to risk of imminent violence include subjective feelings of tension, ideas of violence, delusional systems that incorporate those currently close to the young female, persecutory delusions with fears of imminent attack, feelings of sustained anger and fear, passivity experiences, reduction of self-control, believing oneself to be controlled by others, and command hallucinations telling one what to do (see Chapter 12).

Protective factors in working with such young females are their capacity to respond to and comply with both social treatments and medical treatments, good social networks, valued home environments, and no interest in or knowledge of weapons of other means of violence. Especially important is not only good insight into their psychiatric illness but equally insight into any previous violent aggressive behaviour. A critical protective factor against violent acts is a fear of their own potential for violence, not only against others but turned against themselves. Such severe self-harm includes atypical cutting, of breasts and genitals, and attempts at self-immolation. The latter can, and does, result in serious risk to self when they discover the power of fire in removing their flashbacks of past abuse.

UNDERSTANDING GENDER DIFFERENCES

General issues

It can be argued that criminological research is either very male-orientated or gender-blind, in the sense that there is no consideration of whether or not crime in females may differ in its origin (Gelsthorpe 1997). In seeking to understand differential risk factors between girls and boys, it appears likely that the gender difference in hyperactivity plays a major role in the parallel difference between females and males and the life course of persistent antisocial behaviour (Taylor 1994; see also Chapter 8).

Biologically based gender differences in aggression are reasonably well documented. There is evidence from early in childhood that they apply across cultures (Quay 1993). High physiological reactivity seems to serve as a protective factor against antisocial and violent behaviour, and that could be implicated in the gender difference between females and males (Rubin *et al.* 1997; see also Chapter 6).

Rutter *et al.* (1998) suggest that adolescent females respond to stress and adversity in a different way to boys, though boys and girls seem equally vulnerable to the ill-effects associated with institutional care, as emphasized by the high rate of crime in women who had an institutional upbringing as children. They conclude that, over the course of the last 40 years, the male:female sex ratio of crime in the UK has fallen from about 11:1 to just below 4:1. This variation alone makes it implausible that biological difference is the only factor at work.

It is possible, however, that biological factors link with other factors predisposing to violence. Antisocial girls are much more likely than other girls to become teenage mothers. This may well expose such girls to a range of social difficulties and make it more likely that they will experience failure in parenting. As a consequence they may have a higher rate of interpersonal conflict, including violence with partners and children alike. On the other hand, their domestic commitments in late adolescence and early adult life may possibly make it more difficult for them to be part of a delinquent peer group and thus to engage in criminal activities, including violence outside the home (Maccoby 1998). However, there has been a noticeable and significant shift over the last 20 years, and between 1985 and 1994 female juvenile crime arrests more than doubled. It is unlikely that a change in women's social representations of aggression, or the shift in views and expectations that accompanied the women's rights and feminist movement, could be seen as responsible for this phenomenon (Snyder and Sickmund 1995).

According to Coleman and Schofield (2001), in England and Wales approximately 15,000 adolescent girls are in care, either accommodated by the local authority or subject to a Court order. Offences of violence are the second most common crime committed by female offenders and, with no current specific provision for young female offenders under 17 within the prison system (see later), it is likely that the majority remain within social services provision and supervision. It is known that, of the adult female prison population, 30–50% have been in care compared with 2% of the general population (Quinton and Rutter 1998). Drug and alcohol misuse by females is reported to be influenced by different factors than for males (Bodinger-Deuriate 1991). In their seminal epidemiological study of adult female offenders in British prisons, Maden et al. (1994) revealed a higher proportion of psychiatric disturbance, personality disorder and substance misuse than in adult male prisoners. Research in the USA shows that adolescent female offenders have experienced more sexual abuse at a higher frequency than their male counterparts (Chesney-Lind 1987), with significant relationships between child abuse before the age of 11 and later delinquency. Widom and White (1997), in an important American prospective design cohort study, report that among abused and neglected children, females but not males are at a significantly higher risk for substance misuse, dependence diagnosis and arrest for violent crimes in adulthood. These females are also at greater risk for comorbidity, for substance abuse and violence arrest compared with controls.

The number of young female offenders under sentence in young offender institutions has risen from 110 in 1991 to 183 in 1995, and had reached 385 by September 2000; the number of young male offenders under sentence reached 8224 by September 2000. Although the sample of female offenders in the ONS study of the mental health of young offenders (Lader et al. 2000) was too small in most categories to draw any reliable conclusions, amongst sentenced young women the rate of neurotic disorder was 68% compared with 19% in the general population (see also Chapters 27 and 28).

The younger group of females, as with young males, have higher rates for re-offending than their male and female adult counterparts. Flood-Page et al. (2000), in a study of self-reported offending behaviour in 4000 teenagers and young adults, showed that 11% of females under age 30 reported involvement in crime compared with 26% of young men.

Thus, understanding both the changing trend of violent behaviour in girls and protective factors which still operate for girls should help inform preventive measures for both sexes. The link between childhood abuse and adult substance abuse and violent behaviour is emerging for women, but not yet for men. Substance misuse and drug dependency present a considerable problem for adult women in prison. Girls who engage in violent behaviour present a useful and vital study group in trying to understand the pathway from experiences in childhood to serious antisocial violent behaviour in adulthood.

Emerging research origins from adolescent forensic mental health services

The adolescent forensic service based at the Salford NHS Trust accepts nationwide referrals. The service consists of two components: a ten-bed medium-secure inpatient psychiatric unit; and a forensic adolescent consultation and treatment service providing an outreach component. The two services form part of a broad-based supraregional adolescent forensic service. Local referrals are from the areas of health, social services, education and the criminal justice system, but referrals beyond the catchment area are via health services only.

Girls constitute a constant fifth of all referrals to the service. Although they are in a minority, the number of girls referred is substantial enough to consider whether their health, social and educational needs differ from those of boys. Existing services for adolescent offenders have been developed from a knowledge base of studies on male adolescent offenders (Miller et al. 1995). Thus, little information has hitherto been available about girls with high-risk behaviours who come to the attention of the mental health services. More recently however, a series of studies conducted by the service has given some insight into violence, vulnerability and gender.

In a health needs survey of a sample of 192 young offenders appearing before a large city-centre youth Court, 19% had significant medical problems, 42% had a history of significant and damaging substance misuse, and 7% had psychiatric problems of a nature and degree that required immediate treatment and intervention (Dolan et al. 1999). Of the group requiring acute intervention, the majority were young females. Although they represented only a small proportion of the overall sample (9 out of 192 youngsters), they presented as being at most risk, in particular, risk to self. The most vulnerable group, with most psychosocial difficulties, these young females were most likely to be placed in custodial remand. It is difficult to establish whether, in these cases, the Courts were acting totally on the basis of the level of risk the young female presented to others, or in the benign belief that they were rescuing young girls at risk of sexual activity and substance misuse.

A study of 100 'looked after' girls referred to the adolescent forensic service over a six-year period has given further insight on adolescent females who presented to health services through a pathway from social service provision for children with difficult behaviour. Nearly half these females were already in a social services secure provision at the time of referral (Jasper *et al.* 1998). Specific findings included:

- Seventy-nine per cent had behavioural disturbances in more than one major area of functioning (violence, substance misuse, non-violent offending, deliberate self-harm), with nearly a quarter demonstrating disturbed behaviour in all four of these areas.
- The referrers identified only 54% of those who could be described as violent or aggressive as such; 68% of those who self-harmed were described as such by the referrers.
- Forty-seven per cent of those who were recognized as having behaved in a way which was against the law had been charged with an offence; 71% of those who had physically attacked someone had not been charged by the police.
- Seventy-one per cent had experienced at least one form of childhood abuse, the majority (56%) having been multiply abused.
- Many were not having their educational needs met, with 45.5% of those who should have been attending school not doing so, and only 11% of the group having ever been 'statemented' as having special educational needs.

The subgroup of 68 violent girls was not greatly different from those who did not harm others through violence. In particular, they did not contain a greater proportion of girls who had experienced childhood abuse. A significantly greater proportion of the violent girls appeared to misuse substances then in the non-violent group.

The subgroup of 71 girls who had experienced childhood abuse contained a significantly greater proportion of those who set fires and were destructive to objects. No specific associations were found between the type of abuse experienced and behaviour, other than for deliberate self-harm.

The subgroup of 76 girls who self-harmed contained a greater proportion of those who had experienced childhood sexual abuse and those who misused substances. It is worth noting that, for 35 of the girls who self-harmed, there was no evidence in the vast array of information available that they had been sexually abused; this is an important finding in view of the belief widely held amongst professionals working with young people that girls who harm themselves have been sexually abused. There appeared to be very little difference between those a Court had deemed to require secure accommodation and those who had not.

Focusing service responses towards violent females

Any national strategic framework offering treatment for young violent offenders must consider appropriate provision for young females which takes into account their special needs. A study of children in the criminal justice and secure care systems surveyed secure units, young offender institutions, social services, youth justice, probation, and child and adolescent forensic psychiatrists in England and Wales, with a number of important findings (Kurtz *et al.* 1998).

- There were overwhelmingly more boys than girls in secure units, both child and adolescent psychiatry and social services.
- Children's services considered twice as many boys as girls for secure placement.
- Forty-two per cent of social services' children's services had not placed a single girl during the year of the study.
- The ratio of boys to girls in the caseload of forensic psychiatrists was 7 to 1.
- Court reports were prepared for about ten times as many boys as girls.
- The most common problem, as presented for boys and girls, was violence.
- The need for secure placement was confirmed by child and adolescent psychiatrists in 82% of those referred to them, boys and girls equally.

How can the needs of high-risk girls be met in the predominantly male environment of secure care, with no young offender institutions for girls? The Crime and Disorder Act 1998, establishment of youth offending teams, and a government mandate via the National Youth Justice Board should, theoretically, ensure equality of service provision for dangerous girls, but the implementation and nature of developing services is yet to be established and then has to be evaluated.

Intensive community-based services for substance-misusing aggressive girls, especially those with past histories of abuse, need to develop along the lines of the Multisystemic Therapy programmes operating in South Carolina (Henggeler 1996). The juvenile justice system expects a long-term reduction in rates of offending. Young offenders, including violent girls, have a right to a full range of cost-effective interventions. It is suggested that service delivery for these girls should:

- fit the developmental needs of female adolescents
- include specific risk and need assessment schedules
- address pertinent factors across family, peer, school and residential contexts
- offer treatment specificity and integrity of treatment delivery
- increase the competence of families and carers in intensive community programmes, offering support 24 hours a day, seven days a week.

Within secure care provision, the research suggests that many girls in these settings, and those who have behaved in similar high-risk ways, have a range of mental health needs rather than presenting with a single problem. Some of these needs are related to their high-risk behaviour, others are not, but nevertheless require intervention. The clinical staff providing mental health services to these girls, therefore, need access to expertise in a range of skills, not all of which are the sole domain of the forensic specialist. Girls who behave violently and those in secure care cannot readily access services. Needs in the following areas should be specifically addressed:

1 Information should be provided on sexual/reproductive health; contraception; sexually transmitted diseases; problems concerning menstruation; relevant resources in the event of a pregnancy.
2 There should be post-abuse counselling, when the adolescent female is ready to engage in it, from an appropriate adult, taking the issue of the gender of the therapist into account.
3 There should be medical and psychiatric assessment, followed by appropriate treatment of parasuicidal behaviour, remembering that the distraction and attention provided by the emergency may be an important component in reinforcing the use of this behaviour as a coping strategy.
4 Different leisure interests developed by girls should be catered for in their placement.
5 Eating problems are far more common in girls than in boys and may need to be managed. Girls will want to eat different foods from boys and maintain their fitness through different forms of exercise.

In terms of long-term prevention and protective processes, resilience mechanisms need also to be developed in girls. These include:

- reducing sensitivity to risk
- understanding the impact of risk
- reducing negative and increasing positive chain reactions, thereby promoting the self-esteem and self-efficacy of females
- opening up positive opportunities and enabling violent females to process negative experiences in a positive manner
- acceptance rather than denial of violent behaviour.

Girls are a significant minority in the workload of a forensic child and adolescent mental health service. They have complex multiple needs which require both assessment on an individual basis and appropriate treatment planned on the basis of that assessment. In terms of violence, their thinking is much like that of violent boys. However, they need services to recognize and adapt to their differences from boys. Failure to meet their specific therapeutic and associated practical needs could well result in the perpetuation of cycles of abuse from one generation to the next.

THE DISADVANTAGE OF GENDER: MALE OFFENDERS

Learning from the adult literature

In adult men with severe mental illness, addictions and affective illnesses are greatly over-represented in forensic populations when compared with the general population, whether in Court diversion schemes, remand, or sentenced prison populations (Kennedy 2001). This means that substantial numbers of men are falling through the net of primary care and mental health services and failing to seek help voluntarily. The rising suicide rate among young men in inner cities at a time when suicide rates for other groups are falling (Drever and Bunting 1997) underlines the same apparent failure in early case finding and early intervention for adolescent males. This failure probably in part arises from a combination of lack of public awareness and stigma particularly among men, and for young men the lack of accessibility or acceptability of how services are offered.

Morbidities that continue to go unrecognized include 'atypical affective disorders', distorted grief reaction, rage attacks, attachment disorder, and disorders of habit and impulse related to addictions, including repetitive self-harm. Failure to address these early places young males at risk and adds to the frequency and nature of their subsequent offending histories.

Suicide and deliberate self-harm

In the UK as a whole, 571 young men between the ages of 15 and 24 successfully took their own lives in 1998. Rates show large regional variations. Young males in care and those within the criminal justice system, in particular those in custody, can reflect their distress in self-destructive behaviour.

Among children and adolescents, the only group to have shown an increase in the official suicide rate since 1970 has been males aged 15–19 years. This increase is still evident when one examines the changes in undetermined and accidental rates during 1970–1998 (McClure 2001). The suicide rate for young males continues to rise (Fombonne 1998). The male:female ratio of deaths from suicide in 15- to 19-year-olds is approximately 4:1, and the ratio for deliberate self-harm is approximately 1:6 (Cotgrave et al. 1995).

The most common form of DSH is cutting or scratching, but the most frequently recorded form of DSH in the UK is self-poisoning (the majority with a paracetamol overdose). The most common form of completed suicide for males in the UK is hanging, while in the USA guns are used in over 50% of adolescent suicides. Adolescents who self-harm are a heterogeneous group.

In assessing risk, Stanway and Cotgrave (2001) summarize the main characteristic features which predispose to completed suicide in adolescence:

- *Individual features of psychiatric disorder* – depression; psychosis; substance misuse; conduct disorder; isolation; low self-esteem; physical illness.
- *Family and environmental factors* – loss of parent in childhood; family dysfunction; abuse and neglect; family history of psychiatric illness or suicide.

Immediate precipitants to DSH and suicide overlap with predisposing characteristics. They include interpersonal conflicts with family and friends, loss through bereavement or break-up of relationships, external stressors, involvement in the criminal justice system, unemployment, abuse/neglect, and exposure to DSH or suicide. These features will interact with the adolescent's emotional state, feelings of hopelessness, anxiety and anger.

A study of community referrals of adolescent males to Salford's forensic service has shown them to have significant self-harm histories, but this was mentioned only in a minority of referrals (Ross *et al.* 2000). Deliberate self-harm was mentioned in only 22 of the referrals of the 50 cases in the self-harm group. There were no significant differences in the nature of the self-harm or the frequency of the self-harm between those cases in which it was identified as a problem and those in which it was not. Attempted hangings, cuttings, overdosing and jumping from heights occurred in both groups. The self-harming group were more likely to have a mother with psychopathology – either mental illness or personality difficulties. The self-harming group were more likely to have a history of abusing alcohol, cannabis or a number of substances. The self-harming group were more likely to be socially isolated or to have a mixed-gender peer group. High-risk behaviours (substance abuse and offending behaviours) were more common in the self-harm group. The non-self-harming group were significantly more likely not to abuse any substances.

These statistics may reflect an inherent bias in the referrers to the Salford adolescent forensic service. Self-harming behaviour may be seen as less important or urgent than externalizing behaviours such as aggression. A study from the same service of referred adolescent females found the opposite result (Jasper *et al.* 1998). Self-harming behaviour was highlighted and externalizing behaviours minimized or not mentioned. The self-harming group of adolescent males form a high-risk group within a population already at increased risk of psychopathology. Thus self-harm in the adolescent forensic male population is often seen as being of less importance than externalizing behaviours. Given the increased risk of suicide in this population this must change if the rates of completed suicide are to be addressed.

The findings of this and previous research emphasizes that substance abuse, maternal psychopathology, and poor relationships, both with peers and fathers, should alert professionals to a higher risk of self-harming behaviours. The risk of self-harming behaviour should be assessed in cases with these features and appropriate therapeutic interventions sought. It is unclear as to why having a mixed-gender peer group should be associated with an increased rate of self-harm, but one possible explanation is the cross-fertilization of self-harming behaviour from female peers.

Deliberate self-harm may be a serious attempt to die or to escape from unbearable feelings or situations. It can be a dramatic action to change things the individual feels powerless about – a communication that includes a cry for help but so often involves hostility and anger directed at self or others. The act can release feelings of inner tension, or may reflect low self-worth or be a means of self-punishment.

Management of the problem in an individual is strongly influenced by a good risk assessment. The first part of this must consist of giving due consideration in young males to both the underlying meaning of externalizing behaviours, but also taking due note of any history of DSH and the meaning of it for the young male, his current circumstances, his past experience and the presence of any current psychiatric disorder.

Following an episode of DSH, 10% will repeat within a year (Cotgrave *et al.* 1995). Estimates of those who go on to kill themselves vary, but at the extreme Otto (1972) found that 4% of girls and 11% of boys had killed themselves at five-year follow-up.

Current initiatives from the Youth Justice Board in England and Wales to increase the mental health input to Youth Offending Teams are to be welcomed. Stress is placed on the importance of appropriate mental health training to all professionals working in the criminal justice system, together with rigorous mental health screening of all young offenders to ensure an early recognition and safe response to deliberate self-harm.

REFERENCES

Ammerman, R.T. and Hersen, M. 1992: Current issues in the assessment of family violence. In Ammerman, R.T. and Hersen, M. (eds), *Assessment of Family Violence*, Vol. 1. New York: John Wiley, 3–11.

Appleby, L. 2000: Safer services: conclusions from the report of the National Confidential Inquiry. *Advances in Psychiatric Treatment* **6**: 5–15.

Bailey, S. and Harbour, A. 1999: The law and a child's consent to treatment (England and Wales). *Child Psychology and Psychiatry Review* **4**: 30–4.

Bailey, S., Thornton, L. and Weaver, A. 1994: First 100 admissions to an adolescent secure unit. *Journal of Adolescence* **17**: 207–20.

Banks, N. 1995: Children of black mixed parentage and their placement needs. *Adoption and Fostering* **19**: 19–24.

Barn, R., Sinclair, R. and Ferdinand, D. 1997: *Acting on Principle: an Examination of Race and Ethnicity in Social Services Provision for Children and Families.* London: British Agency for Adoption and Fostering.

Bhugra, D. and Bhui, K. 1999a: Racism in psychiatry: paradigm lost, paradigm regained. *International Review of Psychiatry* **11**: 125–243.

Bhugra, D. and Bhui, K. 1999b: Ethnic and cultural factors in psychopharmacology. *Advances in Psychiatric Treatment* **5**: 89–95.

Bhugra, D. and Bhui, K. 2001: African–Caribbean's and schizophrenia contributing factors. *Advances in Psychiatric Treatment* **7**: 283–93.

Bird, H.R. 1996: Epidemiology of childhood disorders in a cross-cultural context. *Journal of Child Psychology and Psychiatry* **37**: 35–49.

Bodinger-Deuriate, C. 1991: *Female Adolescents: What Prevention Programmes Need to Know.* The North West Report, update 9, September.

Brunette, M.F. and Drake, R.E. 1997: Gender differences in patients with schizophrenia and substance abuse. *Comprehensive Psychiatry* **38**: 109–16.

Callan, A. and Littlewood, R. 1998: Patient satisfaction: ethnic origin or explanatory model? *International Journal of Social Psychiatry* **44**: 1–11.

Campbell, S.B. 1995: Behaviour problems in pre-school children: a review of recent research. *Journal of Child Psychology and Psychiatry* **36**: 113–49.

Carpenter, L. and Brockington, I.F. 1980: A study of mental illness in Asians, West Indians and Africans living in Manchester. *British Journal of Psychiatry* **127**: 201–5.

Castle, D.J. and Murray, R.M. 1991: The neurodevelopmental basis of sex differences in schizophrenia. *Psychological Medicine* **21**: 565–75.

Chesney-Lind, M. 1987: Girls and violence: an explanation of the gender gap in serious delinquent behaviour. In Cromwell, D., Evans, I. and O'Donnell, R. (eds), *Childhood Aggression and Violence: Sources of Influence, Prevention and Control.* New York: Plenum Press, 207–29.

Christian, R.E., Frick, P.J., Hill, N.L., Tyler, L. and Frazer, D.R. 1997: Psychopathy and conduct problems in children: implications of subtyping children with conduct problems. *Journal of the American Academy of Child and Adolescent Psychiatry* **36**: 233–41.

Coleman, J. and Schofield, J. 2001: *Key Data on Adolescence.* Brighton: Trust for the Study of Adolescence, 1–16.

Coleman, J. and Schofield, J. 2003: *Key Data on Adolescence.* Trust for the Study of Adolescence. Brighton: TSA Publications.

Cotgrave, A.J., Zirinsky, L., Black, D. and Weston, D. 1995: Secondary prevention of attempted suicide in adolescence. *Journal of Adolescence* **18**: 569–77.

Daly, K. 1994: *Gender, Crime and Punishment.* New Haven, CT: Yale University Press.

Daryanani, R., Hindley, P., Evans, C., Fahy, P. and Turk, T. 2001: Ethnicity and use of a child and adolescent mental health service. *Child Psychology and Psychiatry Review* **6**(3): 127–32.

Dolan, M., Holloway, J., Bailey, S., Smith, C. 1999: Health status of juvenile offenders. A survey of young offenders appearing before the juvenile courts. *Journal of Adolescence* **22**: 137–44.

Doreleijers, T.A.H., Moser, F., Thys, P., Van Engeland, H., Beyaert, F.H.L. 2000: Forensic assessment of juvenile delinquents: prevalence of psychopathology and decision making at court in the Netherlands. *Journal of Adolescence* **23**: 263–75.

Drever, F. and Bunting, J. 1997: Patterns and trends in male mortality. In Drever, F. and Whitehead, M. (eds), *Health Inequalities.* London: HMSO.

Flood-Page, C., Campbell, S., Harrington, V. and Miller, J. 2000: Youth Crime: Findings from the 1998/99 Youth Lifestyles Survey, Home Office Research Study 209. Home Office: London.

Fombonne, E. 1998: Suicidal behaviours in vulnerable adolescents: time trends and their correlates. *British Journal of Psychiatry* **173**: 154–9.

Ford, K. and Farrington, A. 1999: Assessing dangerousness in a regional secure unit: decision making in the multi-disciplinary team. *Mental Health Care* **21**(6): 201–4.

Gelsthorpe, L. 1997: Feminism and criminology. In Maguire, M., Morgan, R. and Reiner, R. (eds), *The Oxford Handbook of Criminology,* 2nd edn. Oxford: Clarendon Press, 511–33.

Goodman, R. and Richards, H. 1999: Child and adolescent psychiatric presentations of second-generation Afro-Caribbeans in Britain. *British Journal of Psychiatry* **167**: 362–69.

Graham, J. and Bowling, B. 1995: *Young People and Crime.* Home Office Research Study 145. London: HMSO, 1.

Hackett, L., Hackett, R. and Taylor, D.C. 1991: Psychological disturbance and its associations in the children of the Gujarati community. *Journal of Child Psychology and Psychiatry* **32**: 851–6.

Harrison, G., Glazebrook, C. and Brewin, J. 1997: Increased evidence of psychotic disorders in migrants from the Caribbean in the UK. *Psychological Medicine* **27**: 299–307.

Heidensohn, F. 1997: Gender and crime. In Maguire, M., Morgan, R. and Reiner, R. (eds), *The Oxford Handbook of Criminology,* 2nd edn. Oxford: Oxford University Press, 761–98.

Henggeler, S.W. 1996: Multi-systemic therapy: an effective violence prevention approach for serious juvenile offenders. *Journal of Adolescence* **19**: 47–61.

Hodes, M., Creamer, J. and Woolley, J. 1998: Cultural meaning of ethnic categories. *Psychiatric Bulletin* **22**: 20–34.

Home Office 1997: *Criminal Statistics England: Aspects of Crime – Gender.* London: Home Office Research and Statistics Directorate.

Jacob, K.S., Bhugra, D. and Lloyd, K.R. 1998: Common mental disorders, explanatory models and consultation behaviour among Indian women living in the UK. *Journal of the Royal Society of Medicine* **91**: 66–71.

Jasper, A., Smith, C. and Bailey, S. 1998: One hundred girls in care referred to an adolescent forensic service. *Journal of Adolescence* **21**: 555–68.

Kennedy, H. 2001: Do men need special services? *Advances in Psychiatric Treatment* **7**: 93–101.

Kurtz, Z., Thornes, R. and Bailey, S. 1998: Children in the criminal justice and secure care systems: how their mental health needs are met. *Journal of Adolescence* **21**: 543–53.

Lader, D., Singleton, N. and Meltzer, H. 2000: *Psychiatric Morbidity Among Young Offenders in England and Wales.* London: Office for National Statistics.

15

Victims as perpetrators

CESAR LENGUA

INTRODUCTION

Most clinicians will accept that young sex offenders, bullies and young perpetrators of violence have often been themselves the subject of abuse. On occasion they have been the subject of specific abuses that they later perpetrate in a similar way. We live in a society that is attempting to cope with a constant increase in violence. Crimes against the person (for all ages) increased by about 73% in the period between 1981 and 1995 (Audit Commission 1996). We know that two out of five offenders are under the age of 21 years, but in fact the overall juvenile crime rate has decreased. However, the violent crime rate has increased in the 10- to 17-year-old group especially in girls (Home Office 1992). Our society has probably become less outraged by images of the perverse and at times celebrates discourses on expressions of 'art' which portray the abuse of children (Burchill 1997).

The notion that violence breeds violence is firmly routed in people's minds. The idea that abusing parents were themselves abused makes intuitive sense, and the histories of patients often supports this notion. We seek reasons to understand what is sometimes incomprehensible and often collude with patients in externalizing causes of antisocial behaviour. We conceptualize a sociology of 'badness' and often find external reasons for 'naughtiness' in children.

This chapter examines the evidence for the presumption that victims become victimizers. In the first instance, it reviews the literature on the consequences of sexual abuse and what is known of the characteristics of offenders in general. It also specifically notes the characteristics of those offenders who perpetrate serious abusive violence. This is an important group of offenders whom we might expect to have suffered high levels of abuse. As a group, they provide insight into possible aetiologies to understand the transition between being a victim and becoming a perpetrator. The evidence presented would be incomplete unless attention is paid to why some children who have suffered abuse (sexual, physical or emotional) do *not* in fact show apparent psychological or psychiatric disturbance. In consequence, some of the literature on resilience will also be reviewed.

The chapter goes on to present some of the hypothetical frameworks that have arisen out of the evidence. It will be noted that the hypothetical constructs that have been developed have an increasing level of complexity as more is understood about cycles of violence and the relationship between victim and victimizer.

Finally there is an evidence-based approach to clinical considerations. Some of the implications that arise from the research are discussed, and in particular the notion of prevention. Important issues relating to the assessment of children and adolescents who commit serious violence and who themselves have past histories of severe abuse are discussed. Treatment issues are discussed only in general terms since specific treatment interventions are dealt with in other chapters. However, an attempt is made to demonstrate the complexity of clinical considerations by way of a case vignette.

EVIDENCE SUPPORTING A LINK BETWEEN VICTIMS AND PERPETRATORS

The fact that some children were sexually abused by adults was not widely recognized until the late 1970s, and we have only recently come to accept that adolescents can also perpetrate sexual abuse.

In the UK the definition of what constitutes abuse in children is laid out within our legislative framework. The Children Act 1989 contains concepts like 'significant harm' to describe processes of emotional abuse, physical abuse and neglect. However, the definition of these concepts is subject to discrepancies not only in law but also in day-to-day clinical practice and research. Certainly even the definition of what constitutes sexual abuse varies considerably. Equally, in the literature, the terms 'violence' and 'aggression' are used interchangeably. Most people will agree that aggression is a much broader term, but definitions of violence invariably contain ill-defined adjectives like 'chronic', 'serious' or 'antisocial'. There are in consequence considerable problems in the recognition of abusive acts and establishing their prevalence in children.

If we were to restrict cases of sexual abuse to those involving physical contact between the abuser and a child under 16 years of age, the estimated international prevalence rates for people who have suffered sexual abuse range from 7% to 62% for women and 3% to 59% for men (Leventhal 1990; Mathews 1996). In the field of sexual offending, in the UK, about 30% of all sexual offences are committed by people under 21 (Home Office 1992). This figure is considered to be an under-estimate since it excludes children under 10, it does not include informal cautions, and offences are either under-reported or simply not discovered.

There is considerable research into the sequelae of abuse and in particular sexual abuse. Although it is reported that a third of survivors of sexual abuse suffer no long-term negative effects (Kendal-Thackett et al. 1993), two-thirds therefore experience traumatogenic consequences. It is also known that worse outcomes are associated with:

- parental abuse, as opposed to stranger or sibling abuse (Finkelhor 1979)
- penetrative sexual acts (Bagley and Ramsey 1986)
- use of violence during the abuse (Russell 1986)
- bizarre abuse, pseudo-religious rituals and repugnant acts (Briere 1988).

Symptoms of depression and low self-esteem, anxiety, sadness, school and behaviour problems and a sense of powerlessness are all associated with sexual abuse. Longer-term sequelae include depression, low self-esteem, increased risk of further victimization, eating disorders, functional bowel disease, chronic pelvic pain, attempts at suicide and self-injury, interpersonal difficulties, drug abuse and criminality. Within this spectrum of possible problems, the possibility of further abuse is also recognized (Finkelhor 1990; Beitchnan 1992). In Widom's (1989a) retrospective longitudinal study, early childhood victimization produced long-term consequences for delinquency, adult criminality and violent criminal behaviour. Specifically, physical abuse and neglect were found to further increase the likelihood of later violent offending.

We now consider what is known about the propensity to commit crime in general. This will aid later consideration of the specific issues of serious perpetration of aggression.

The known elevating factors to a propensity for crime include family criminality, large and poor broken families, low intelligence, school failure, and learning difficulties. 'Maltreatment' (physical, sexual, emotional abuse and neglect) of children increases their risk for both later alcohol and drug abuse (Dembo et al. 1992). However, involvement in crime itself increases the risk of further victimization (Lauritsen et al. 1991), because of the physical proximity to other offenders, exposure to other possible offenders, attractiveness to potential targets and the absence of a guardian (Miethe and Meir 1990; Sampson and Lauritsen 1990). The studies of serious abusers give a number of important demographic and psychological variables. Spitzer et al. (1991), describing sadistic personality disorder in the patients of forensic psychiatrists, found that 90% had childhood backgrounds of emotional abuse. Parental figures had been hostile, demeaning or neglecting. Seventy-six per cent had been physically abused. Fifty-two per cent had experienced losses (death or abandonment by parental figures) and 41% had been sexually abused. In other words a past history of abuse is highly correlated with sadistic violence.

It is evident that the background of violent offenders often includes a history of neglect and/or abuse. In a sub-population of young people detained under s53 of the Children and Young Person's Act 1933, Boswell (1997) found that about a third had suffered emotional abuse, another third had suffered sexual abuse, 40% had had physical abuse, and 15% had been the subject of organized or ritual abuse. Seventy-two per cent of the total sample have experienced one or a combination of the forms of abuse looked for. Furthermore, 57% of the sample had experienced significant loss. The research only points to associations and it implies no causality. Interestingly, childhood sexual abuse per se (compared to other types of child abuse and neglect), does not on its own increase an individual's risk for later delinquent or adult criminal behaviour (Widom and Ames 1994). Many victims of abuse are more likely to be arrested for prostitution as adults (Widom and Ames 1994; Lake 1993), affording females the control they did not have in their own abuse (Jehu 1991). This adds further evidence to Widom's own research indicating that physically abused children have the highest rate of arrest for violence (Widom 1989c).

In summary, and despite the definitional difficulties, the literature suggests that experiences of abuse have lifelong consequences for later criminal behaviours. Experiences of emotional abuse, neglect and loss are also strongly associated with later delinquency. The backgrounds of later serious offenders include significant histories of abuse and loss. In order to make a connection between these two observations we need a developmental understanding on pathways to deviance. First we shall look at the possible factors behind why some children who are abused do not in fact show psychiatric or psychological disturbance.

PROTECTIVE FACTORS: RESILIENCE TO A NEGATIVE OUTCOME

It is estimated that the percentage of child victims of sexual abuse who do not apparently suffer adverse consequences as a result of their experience falls somewhere in the region of 20–40% (Finkelhor 1990; Lynskey and Ferguson 1997). Certainly the overall view is that the nature of the relationship that young people have with their parents and peers is a contributing risk factor for later psychopathology. Given the above, therefore, it would seem that there is no direct relationship between abuse and offending behaviour (Falshaw *et al.* 1996), as it is evident that the majority of abused children do not develop psychiatric or psychological problems.

'Resilience' refers to factors (individual, familial and social) that prevent or diminish a negative outcome. They are sometimes referred to as *protective factors*. Widom (1989b) defines protective factors as those dispositional attributes, environmental conditions, biological predispositions and positive events that can act to mitigate early negative experiences. Another definition of protective factors is that they are at the opposite end on a scale to risk factors. However, a variable with a non-linear relationship to antisocial behaviour might be regarded as a protective factor but not a risk factor. For instance, intelligence may be linked to low risk of antisocial behaviour, but medium-to-low intelligence might make no difference to the risk. Alternatively, a protective factor can be defined as a variable that interacts with a risk factor to minimize its effects – for example, the use of violence during sexual abuse might lead to offending in single-parent families but not in reconstituted families. Family reconstitution would then be seen as a protective factor against the risk factor of violence during sexual abuse.

The factors associated with resilience remain on the whole hypothetical. However, when resilience is further operationalized (Spaccarelli and Kin 1995) as achieving (a) maintenance of social functioning and (b) absence of clinical levels of symptomatology, then we find that the measuring of post-abuse resilience requires individual and parental assessments, since a significant proportion of young people are able to maintain adequate social competence but still have high levels of depression, anxiety or aggressive symptomatology. In these cases, the support that parents can give is seen as a key factor in maintaining social competence, and in particular, school progress and peer relations (parameters of social functioning).

Predictors of resilience are inversely correlated to the level of abuse and stresses experienced as a result of abuse. The predictors are also positively correlated to the quality of the victim's relationship with their non-offending parents. Personal characteristics that have been put forward as factors of relevance in the resilience of children include (Mrazek and Mrazek 1987):

- rapid responsivity to danger
- precocious maturity
- dissociation of affect
- information-seeking behaviour
- formation and utilization of relationship survival
- positive projective anticipation
- decisive risk-taking
- the conviction of being loved
- idealization of an aggressor's competence
- cognitive restructuring of painful experiences
- altruism
- optimism and hope.

Other identified protective factors include:

- not being abused by parents or guardians
- having had an emotionally supportive relationship with a family member during childhood
- having a supportive spouse
- having positive school experiences in childhood
- having received therapy
- coming to terms with the abuse.

The identification of individual, family and social characteristics fostering resilience offers hope for preventing psychopathology in victims of abuse. It also may provide answers on how to stop the escalation of violence and prevent the possible later perpetration of serious violence.

HYPOTHETICAL AETIOLOGIES

General issues

What can probably be seen as a progression of victim to victimizer involves complex multi-systemic, multi-dimensional mechanisms. These are probably best understood in terms of emotional, cognitive, social and biological attributes each contributing to the development of abusive behaviour in victims. Feelings of vulnerability, identification with the aggressor and conditioning to sexual responsiveness have been commented on by Mezey *et al.* (1991). Although the authors make specific reference to child sexual abuse, the mechanisms they consider can very likely be generalized into other forms of abuse.

The notion that 'violence breeds violence' or that children that have been abused are likely to abuse their own children (Curtis 1963; Spinetta and Rigler 1972) was discounted in the late 1980s (Widom and Ames 1994; Murphy and Smith 1996). The rate of intergenerational transmission of abuse (abusive episodes repeated from one generation to the next) was estimated to be 25–35% (Kauffman and Zigler 1987). However, this only means that the path between being abused and becoming an abuser is neither direct nor inevitable.

The literature seems to suggest that it is important to consider experiences of neglect as distinct from those of abuse. The largest studies demonstrate higher rates of physical aggression in neglected children (McCord 1983). Abuse and neglect in children is associated with early aggressive or problematic behaviours. These children tend to be more aggressive in play and fantasy (George and Main 1979; Reidy 1977) and have deficits in emotional development and self concept (Kinard 1980).

The above studies are important given what is already known about the developmental pathways of aggression, conduct disorder and later adult personality disorder. We know for instance that the majority of youngsters' antisocial behaviour is 'normal': it is usually about protest and it is transient. When early in onset the risk for adult continuity increases, in particular for antisocial behaviour and affective disturbance. Most developmental psychopathologists will emphasize the importance of inherited characteristics, although these tend to be seen as dispositions to vulnerability. Considering the stability with time of the 'temperament' parameters, it is interesting that temperament, as defined by Chess and Thomas (1990), does not include assessments of aggression. It might very well be that the consistency of temperament is less cohesive and the concept of aggression might be much wider. Certainly the studies of Olweus (1988) demonstrate persistency of aggression from childhood to adulthood and serious violence tends to increase with age, especially in adolescence. An argument can be made for hypothesizing that early experiences of abuse require processes of emotional, cognitive, familial and social assimilations before a later manifestation into a victimizer role.

Loeber and Hay (1994) argued that the development pathways of aggression from pre-school age to young adulthood represents diverse youth groups:

- young people who desist from aggression
- young people where aggression is stable and continues at the same level
- youths who escalate in the severity of their aggression and make the transition into violence
- youths whose aggression stabilizes.

In 1997 their research led them to conclude that maladaptive aggression, in comparison to aggression in response

to unfavourable circumstances, is relatively insensitive to variations of settings. It is also likely that impulsive and unsocialized sensation-seeking behaviours underpin antisocial personality traits in adulthood (Loeber and Hay 1997). Certainly in children, an unemotional 'interpersonal style' when combined with conduct disorder designates a specific subgroup of antisocial children who correlate with adult conceptualizations of psychopathy (Christian et al. 1997; Forth et al. in press).

Specific theories

There are a number of theories to explain the link between the experience of abuse and becoming an abuser.

- *Intergenerational transmission of violence* (Curtis 1963; Spinetta and Rigler 1972). This theory is close to Bandura's (1973) social learning theory. In this, the normalization of aggression in families provides models of learning for children whereby aggression is seen as an appropriate means of goal realization.
- *Differential association–reinforcement* (Akers et al. 1979; Burgess and Akers 1966). This theory incorporates conditioning and modelling elements by bringing in the effects of peers and families.
- *Traumagenic dynamics* (Browne and Finkelhor 1985). This incorporates a psychodynamic and social learning model to deal with traumatic sexualization, betrayal, powerlessness and stigmatization. The importance of the model is that it highlights the traumatic effects of sexual abuse and places emphasis on the wider aspects of the relationship between the victim and its abuser, the type of abuse endured and the possible reactions to it. It has also been suggested that victims manipulate their own psychological mechanisms in order to overcome the controlling strategies of their perpetrators (Hartman and Burgess 1989).
- *Strain theory* (Cohen 1955). This presumes a loss of self-esteem and a drift into delinquency closely tied in with social class dissatisfaction.
- *Control theory* (Hirschi 1969). This proposes that poor parental supervision and harsh discipline disrupts parent–child bonding, leading to poor identification with the primary object, poor internal controls and eventual delinquency.
- *Psychoanalytic theory*. This emphasises the role of early parental internal representations. Psychoanalysis goes some way to explaining how the abuser also identifies with the victim and in the act of abuse is threatened by a re-experiencing of his or her own trauma (Woods 1997). The re-enactment of past abusive experiences has been seen as a sado-masochistic way of relating (Dillon-Weston 1997) or the 'erotic form of hatred' (Stoller 1975). The bond victims have with their abusers is based on identification with their aggressors, and victims convert their past passive

traumas into active events when perpetrating abusive acts (Glasser *et al.* 2001)

- *Biological theories* (Mednick and Volavka 1980). Most of the findings have no implications on causality of offending but do suggest disturbances on learning and socialization. Certainly it is known that psychic trauma has lasting effects on the neurological functioning of individuals and has lasting effects on brain function at emotional, cognitive, behavioural and physiological levels (Perry 1994). Furthermore, studies of memory and trauma are already beginning to locate 'explicit memories' (conscious past events intentionally recalled) to specific areas of the brain such as the medial temporal lobe systems (hippocampal formation) (Squire 1992a,b), and 'implicit memories' (not readily accessible past events seen as unintentional unconscious forms of retention) to areas such as the basal ganglia, amygdala and possibly motor, somatosensory and sensory cortices (Squire 1992a). The role of intrapsychic adaptation (suppression/repression, denial, fantasy and dissociation) and its effects on memory remain well within the remit of neuropsychology (Siegel 1997).
- *Criminal personality theory* (Yochelson and Samenow 1976, 1997). This emphasizes cognitive processes in the maintenance of criminal behaviour.
- *Trauma-learning* (Burgess *et al.* 1987). This refers to a process of re-victimization. The attempts of victims to come to terms with their experiences (sensory, perceptual and cognitive) are made difficult by finding themselves in situations of either further abuse or by perpetrating abusive acts.
- *Labelling theory* (Smith *et al.* 1980). This proposes that systems label the victims and the abusers, thereby serving to perpetuate their career paths. In fact there is nothing new in this view, and in the nineteenth century 'pauper' children and their criminal activities were seen as resulting from their social class. There was a predominant view that institutionalization crushed the spirit of children who, if treated like adult criminals, became later criminals themselves (Pearson 1975).
- *Dysfunctional response cycle* (Ryan 1989). In this model, feelings of helplessness, loss or betrayal by parents and the actual trauma of the abuse together is relived in situations reminiscent of the past abuse which may trigger 'the commission of abusive acts'. These experiences are influenced by the past child's experience of nurture. Victims and offenders have to deal with similar characteristics, which provides evidence for their similar 'core' pathologies. These characteristics are denial and minimization, guilt and accountability, power and control, anger and retaliation, fantasies and reinforcements, secrets, confidentiality and empathy.
- *Social-interactional theory* (Forehand *et al.* 1975; Patterson 1982; Snyder 1977; Wahler and Dumas 1984). This proposes that familial coerced behaviours are reinforced within families where children learn to do the same.

No single model produces a satisfactory answer to the essential question of why some victims become perpetrators. The models do, however, shed some on possible mechanisms for the transition. They also help us understand the individuals involved and to contextualize their often extreme experiences.

Integrative theories

Recently, a number of workers have attempted to integrate some of the hypotheses considered above. The importance of these models is that they allow for a more comprehensive and holistic approach to assessments and treatments which take account of a number of variable factors known to be of relevance to both onset and chronicity of disturbance in this group of patients.

The diathesis–stressor paradigm model

This model (Davison and Neale 1990) views normal behaviour as the outcome between personal vulnerability factors and external stressors. It provides a simple and yet comprehensively expandable way of looking at abnormal behaviour. Models of relevance to sexual abuse in adolescence have been developed taking into account (Hoghughi 1997):

- genetic and constitutional factors
- home atmosphere and child-rearing factors
- developmental milestones
- personality factors
- social, biological and developmental stages
- current life circumstances
- socio-demographic variables
- personal variables (cognition, perceptions and motivation)
- behavioural analysis.

The developmental model

Williams and New (1996) proposed that sexual abusive behaviour is the result of contextual and situational factors with contributions from ecological, individual, familial and social factors, sexual victimization and identified risk factors (i.e. exposure/witness to violence, discontinuity of care, rejection by peers, past victimization of the mother, etc.). These factors are considered over a time frame from childhood to adolescence.

The integrated perspective model

This has been proposed by Hawkes *et al.* (1997) for sex offenders. The model takes into account the theoretical perspectives but adds a developmental sphere that includes traumatic events, child development, sexual development, social development and parenting. The model graphically attempts to explain the genesis and the sustaining factors of relevance in sexual abusive behaviours across generations.

CLINICAL CONSIDERATIONS

There is a small but nevertheless significant group (estimates are at around 20%) of victims of sexual abuse who will become perpetrators of abuse during adolescence (Watkins and Bentovim 1992). This group of children and adolescents will be of concern to a wide range of agencies and will not solely present on the basis of mental health concerns. A number of external agencies have highlighted the importance of achieving a multi-agency approach based on supportive networks of identified plans and procedures that clarify roles and responsibilities; examples are Area Child Protection Committees (ACPCs) or the Youth Justice Board (YJB).

'Treatments' in the wide sense of the word (i.e. those interventions addressing psychological and emotional needs of children, rather than those implying specific therapies for disturbance) are on the whole recognized as being helpful. The important issues are what type of treatments work better, with which children, for which problems, and under what circumstances. It seems, nevertheless, that the overall aims of various treatments are to *interrupt* the experiences of abuse and address the consequences of abuse, whether this is perpetrated or suffered. The hypotheses that have been put forward to explain the victim/victimizer cycle to an extent lay out the conceptual framework needed. For example, a family-systems view will attempt change, through family interactions, beliefs and responses. A traumatogenic model will focus on the alleviation of past traumatic experiences. Most workers on the field will demonstrate flexibility in approaches towards informed eclectic models which work with patients rather than models of work that simply impose interventions.

The research on abuse-specific treatment programmes (Finkelhor and Berliner 1995) demonstrates that some symptoms are more resistant than others to change, and several studies have found that aggression and sexualized behaviour are not readily amenable to standard therapeutic interventions. This is an important issue because these characteristics are particularly common in perpetrators of abuse who have themselves been victims. It is unclear at this stage whether these difficulties arise because of specific factors in the victim/victimizer cycle or are part of therapist and/or therapy characteristics.

The planning of interventions needs to consider whether children will be physically and emotionally safe during the intervention process. It is often easy to recognize what children need; it is less straightforward to decide how and when to administer particular therapeutic modalities and interventions.

PREVENTION OF THE VICTIM/VICTIMIZER PROGRESSION

This author would argue that interventions require a focus on preventative strategies. These can be either in terms of reducing risk of re-offending, or in terms of contributing to wider inter-agency prevention, aimed at improving social opportunities and the quality of family life and reducing the predictive factors that give rise to abuse. These strategies, although impinging on mental health services, require multi-agency involvement and action by the criminal justice system and education and social welfare services. Tonry and Farrington (1995) distinguish four types of prevention:

- *criminal justice system prevention* – with an emphasis on deterrence, incapacitation and rehabilitation
- *situational prevention* – to reduce opportunities for antisocial behaviour
- *community prevention* – to change the social conditions and social institutions (i.e. community norms and organizations) that influence antisocial behaviour in communities
- *developmental prevention* – strategies aimed at inhibiting the development of antisocial behaviour in individuals.

Traditional public health definitions of prevention (NAS 1994) recognize three kinds of prevention:

- *primary prevention* – targeting whole communities and aiming to prevent problems before they become manifest
- *secondary prevention* – targeting children at risk (those who are already showing signs of problems)
- *tertiary prevention* – to reduce the risk of recurrence of disorder and reduce complications arising from it.

Hardiker (1991) also talks about tertiary prevention for complex multiple problems. At this level, prevention offers focused interventions with children to solve particular problems amongst a number of others. An example could be direct work on reducing use of amphetamines abuse in a polydrug abuser with a past history of abuse committing a wide range of offences. *Quaternary prevention* refers to work to reduce the impact of other interventions – an example could be work to minimize the impact of school exclusion in children.

There is a robust body of knowledge that recognizes the factors for onset of offending. These include low parental supervision, truancy and exclusion from school, having friends and/or siblings in trouble with the police, and poor family attachments (Graham and Bowling 1995). Preventative work with the aim of enabling victims not to become offenders should be part of a wider strategy which focuses on the prevention of abuse, neglect and the prevention of offending in general.

Universally targeted interventions could focus on factors relevant in the reduction of both onset of abuse and of offending. These interventions are essentially psycho-educational and might include (Bailey 1997):

- parental education about child abuse and neglect
- the education of children who might be in abusive or potentially abusive situations
- the education of children on the recognition of alcohol and drug abuse and dysfunctional lifestyles
- helping children to access services and professionals and increase community awareness on the role they have in helping children make prosocial choices.

The messages from preventative work are clear: it must involve families, nurseries, schools, employment training, positive leisure opportunities and improved facilities to tackle substance abuse (Audit Commission 1996). These strategies must also be effective in providing approaches to targeted groups and services, thus providing for the most needy. They must be cost-effective. Services must be easily available to individuals and the community they serve. They must be also be acceptable to users and be non-stigmatizing, listener-friendly and capable of empowering parents on existing skills. The services must be accessible in terms of distance and aware of cultural/ethnic characteristics as well as social/class considerations. Probably the services need to be accountable to parents and satisfy the right of children as consumers. They must also be jointly planned, funded and delivered by appropriate agencies (health, welfare, education, housing, etc.). Finally, services must not be static; they should follow a developmental model as children grow into adolescence. Government initiatives – such as the National Child Care strategy and the work of the Social Exclusion Unit – illustrate movement towards more integrated preventative strategies aimed at addressing social exclusion (factors which lead to families being unable to participate fully in society).

ASSESSMENT ISSUES

Given that the implementation and success of preventative strategies are essentially long-term, we need to return to consider some of the issues which victims who become perpetrators raise in clinical assessments.

In fact, the specific issues of assessment that arise in victims who go on to perpetrate abuse are the same as in other clinical assessments. They must include a comprehensive history-taking and information-gathering clinical effort. Cases are particularly difficult because of issues of denial and minimization. These are characteristics of both victims and offenders. The reasons for this range from shame to overwhelming distress if events are brought to consciousness. Young offenders often perceive Courts as unfriendly places where truth might lead to punishment. Engaging and relating to disturbed children

is an acquired skill; it requires a way of relating that is understandable to them and at the same time provides safety and emotional containment and at times physical containment (by means of security). There are no easy answers. Time is often needed particularly for those children with significant histories of abnormal and/or abusive early attachments.

Issues of confidentiality are as important to children as they are for adults. In children their right to confidentiality needs to be balanced with the 'duty to protect' and sometimes the 'duty to warn'. An honest approach on the remit we have as professionals and an explanation of what we can or cannot achieve serves to emphasize the importance of the contact professionals have with children, and dispels myths. This is particularly important for those children or adolescents who have magical thinking as part of their cognitive make-up.

The assessment is a process of study of the information gathered on personal developmental, social, educational, medical/psychiatric and family history of the child. Specific examinations of mental states investigate:

- phenomenology
- thoughts, feelings and perceptions in a developmental framework
- psychological mechanisms of defence
- the role of fantasy.

It is often necessary to make an assessment of a young person's mental state retrospectively to understand the reasons behind the abuse suffered or the abuse the individual has perpetrated. Until recently, Courts were particularly interested in whether children can discern right from wrong. Between the ages of 10 and 13, they were presumed to be incapable of forming criminal intent (*doli incapax*). Section 34 of the Crime and Disorder Act 1998 has now abolished this. Children who are now over the age of criminal responsibility (10 years in England) will be treated as any other juvenile when deciding whether or not prosecution is appropriate.

The purposes of assessment can be manifold. Psychiatric assessments should be seen as complementary to a number of other assessments that need to be carried out by other professionals and agencies. When properly coordinated, the sharing of information should prevent overwhelming the child with yet another face and another assessment. Psychiatric assessments have an emphasis on formulations and diagnostics because it determines our future intervention strategies. The diagnoses of mental disorder should form part of risk assessments and inform on the role mental disorder plays in worrying behaviours. Attempts also need to be made at establishing the link between mental disorder and the propensity some children have to re-enact the abuse they have suffered (by putting themselves in situations of risk) or establish the role mental disorder plays in the abuse they might perpetrate (children at risk to others).

TREATMENT APPROACHES

Approaches to treatment for specific mental disorders should consider whether or not other agencies are actively involved. This is particularly relevant within this group of patients who are more likely to become involved with other agencies because of their behaviour and/or their offending. They may already, sometimes with their families, be subject to a wide variety of other treatment programmes. Often, children are the subject of statutory orders which either supervises them and/or their families or legislation that restricts their liberties either as part of 'care' within the Children Act of 1989 or as part of punishment within the criminal justice system. Extreme behaviours and psychological disturbances, of course, may or may not form part of recognized psychiatric syndromes or diagnoses. Often, however, they are highly associated with mental disorder–aggression in the psychoses, self-injurious behaviour in conduct disorder, enuresis in hyperactivity disorder, etc.

Perpetrators with past histories of victimization present particular difficulties. They are a heterogeneous group that present with a wide variety of problems and diagnoses. It is often difficult to decide whether a child perpetrator with a history of abuse should be treated in the light of the victimization he or she has suffered, or in terms of the criminal behaviour displayed (Epps 1993). In non-medical settings this view can often be polarized. Furthermore, a society which focuses on the punishment of offenders may attach little importance to the effects past abuse has had on individuals and might decide to channel interventions on pragmatic approaches to extinguish criminal behaviour. Whether it achieves so by punishment or by focusing on here-and-now interventions to deter from further offending will be part of a political agenda hopefully informed by expert evidence. It is this author's view that the long-term consequences of abuse are serious enough to warrant exploration, examination and possible interventions particularly in those children where the trauma of abuse is serious but its psychological consequences are denied. Having established that some of the long-term consequences of abuse include adult criminal behaviour, it would make sense to provide interventions that deal with the effects of abuse as part of strategies to deal with offenders.

Interventions should aim to reduce the risk to self and others in the first instance. Only then can other interventions be made safely. It would, for instance be inappropriate to engage in psychodynamic psychotherapy to help resolve an early attachment disorder to a young person afflicted with thoughts of stabbing others, unless that young person is adequately contained in an environment that provides sufficient emotional understanding and nurture, or sometimes in a physically secure environment. It is sensible to reduce the risk a young person

places to himself or herself and/or others by manipulation of the external environment before attempting to manage the other problems that arise secondary to the rest of the individual's psychopathology.

CONCLUSIONS

The mechanisms that underlie the path of being a victim and becoming a perpetrator of serious violence are by no means straightforward and certainly not unequivocal. There are a number of interactive factors that require consideration. It seems, however, that the 'normal' set of events is actually not to develop observable psychopathology in the light of abuse.

For a proportion of young people where the path is all too evident, theoretical aetiological constructs must aim to take account of developmental perspectives. They should also take cognisance of the apparent individual differences in what is at the moment still a heterogeneously defined group of patients. In the meantime, assessment and treatment models must keep an open mind in the search for causes of psychopathology and extreme behaviours. Interventions must be assessed for their efficacy and their safety in the light of carefully planned, evidence-based risk assessments.

APPENDIX: CASE STUDY

Z was a 16-year-old English Afro-Caribbean adolescent serving a sentence under s53(2) of the Children and Young Persons Act 1933. She had been transferred from prison to secure accommodation because during her first year as a sentenced prisoner she talked about an earlier murder she had committed at the age of 12 but was never found out. She was provisionally transferred to the child-care secure system whilst investigations on her allegations were made.

She had a history of physical abuse and neglect from her mentally ill mother since birth. Her play in childhood made references to death and she ceremonially buried the pets she had killed. At the age of 9, and for about 3–4 years, she was the subject of multiple sexual abuse as she was the victim in a paedophile ring. She killed her first victim at the age of 12 by stabbing, and seriously wounded her second victim at the age of 14, also by stabbing. She had spent time in secure care from the age of 13 and had also spent time in psychiatric hospitals. She was affectionless, had disturbed sexual orientation, sexual excitement to violence, physical violence and a history of self-harm by cutting. She had diagnoses of conduct disorder (ICD-10) and sexual arousal disorder (Vizard et al. 1996). She was already serving a fixed sentence for her second stabbing and was expecting a life sentence for her recently discovered first offence. She made a full confession of her first murder to the police. The details of that confession were incorporated in her risk assessment which had identified the vulnerability of small, white attractive females, issues of jealousy, revenge and quick disinhibition into violence which was at times instrumental.

The management of her care during her time in security was geared towards the protection of others and herself. Attempts made at curbing her expressions of anger by cognitive challenges quickly met with intense suicidal and homicidal impulses to one of her key-workers. She was assigned one male and one female key-worker to guide her on medium-term wishes and offer support on what had been a catalogue of disasters throughout her life.

When she was approaching 17 years, it was deemed not appropriate to deal with her intrapsychic conflicts. Furthermore the provision of skills to control her anger led to serious risk to others, as she was unable to completely obliterate her past as effectively as she would have liked to. At the age of 17, after she was found guilty of her first offence, she was transferred back to prison.

The case is a pessimistic one. It is an example of the importance of assessing interventions and evaluating risks. Z required interventions to affectively deal with her past abuse experiences. They were prominent in her mind, manifested in her behaviours and had the characteristic intrusive nature associated with post-traumatic states. She also needed specific inputs to curb her physical violence. It was too traumatic for her to deal with her past abuse, and the level of containment she required to deal with her physical aggression had eventually incarcerated her. Very often patients can deal only with small doses of their previous trauma. The important strategy to bear in mind is that treatments be made readily available when patients are able to take them on board and retreat when it proves that the interventions might worsen the situation. The dictum should always be to minimize harm, to effectively protect and manage risk.

REFERENCES

Akers, R.L., Krohn, M.D., Lanza-Kaduce, L. and Radosevich, M. 1979: Social learning and deviant behaviour. A specific test of a general theory. *American Sociological Review* **44**: 636–55.

Audit Commission 1996: *Misspent Youth: Young People and Crime*. Audit Commission Publications.

Bagley, C. and Ramsay, R. 1986: Sexual abuse in childhood, psychological outcomes and implications for social worker practices. *Journal of Social Work on Human Sexuality* **4**: 33–47.

Bailey, S. 1997: Sadistic and violent acts in the young. *Child Psychology and Psychiatry Review* **2**(3): 92–102.

Bandura, A. 1977: *Social Learning Theory*. London: Prentice-Hall.

Beitchman, J.H., Zucker, K.J., Hood, J.E. *et al.* A review of the long term effects of child sexual abuse. *Child Abuse and Neglect* **16**: 101–18.

Boswell, G. 1997: The backgrounds of violent offenders: the present picture. In Varma, V. (ed.), *Violence in Children and Adolescents*. London: Jessica Kingsley Publishers.

Browne, A. and Finkelhor, D. 1985: The traumatic impact of sexual abuse: a conceptualization. *American Journal of Orthopsychiatry* **55**: 530–41.

Burchill, J. 1997: Death of innocence. *The Guardian*, 12 November.

Burgess, R.L. and Akers, R.L. 1966: A differential association-reinforcement theory of criminal behaviour. *Social Problems* **14**: 128–47.

Burgess, A.W., Hartman, C.R. and McCormack, A. 1987: Abused to abuser: antecedents of socially deviant behaviours. *American Journal of Psychiatry* **144**: 1431–6.

Briere, J. 1988: Long-term clinical correlates of childhood sexual victimisation. In Prentky, R. (ed.), *Human Sexual Aggression: Current Perspectives*. New York: New York Academy of Science, 327–34.

Chess, S. and Thomas, A. 1990: Continuities and discontinuities in temperament. In Robins, L. and Rutter, M. (eds), *Straight and Devious Pathways from Childhood to Adulthood*. Cambridge: Cambridge University Press.

Christian, R.E., Frick, P.J., Hill, N.L., Tyler, L. and Frazer, D.R. 1997: Psychopathy and conduct problems in children. *Journal of the American Academy of Child and Adolescent Psychiatry* **36**: 233–41.

Cohen, A.K. 1955: *Delinquent Boys: the Culture of the Gang*. New York: Free Press.

Curtis, G.C. 1963: Violence breeds violence – perhaps? *American Journal of Psychiatry* **120**: 386–7.

Davison, G.C. and Neale, J.M. 1990: *Abnormal Psychology*. New York: John Wiley.

Dembo, R., Williams, L., Wothke, W., Schmidler, J. and Brown, C.H. 1992: The role of family factors, physical abuse and sexual victimisation experiences in high risk youths' alcohol and other drug use and delinquency: a longitudinal model. *Violence and Victims* **7**: 245–66.

Dillon-Weston, M. 1997: From sadomasochism to shared sadness. In Welldon, E.V. and Van Velsen, C. (eds), *A Practical Guide to Forensic Psychotherapy*. London: Jessica Kingsley Publishers.

Epps, K. 1993: From victim to offender. Paper presented at the BPS Developmental Section Annual conference, University of Birmingham.

Falshaw, L., Browne, K.D. and Hollin, C.R. 1996: Victim to offender: a review. *Aggression and Violent Behaviour* **1**: 389–404.

Finkelhor, D. 1979: *Sexually Victimised Children*. New York: Free Press.

Finkelhor, D. 1990: Early and long term effects of child sexual abuse: an update. *Professional Psychology: Research and Practice* **21**: 325–30.

Finkelhor, D. and Berliner, L. 1995: The research on the treatment of sexually abused children: a review and recommendations. *Journal of the American Academy of Child and Adolescent Psychiatry* **34**: 1408–23.

Forehand, R., King, H.E., Peed, S. and Yoder, P. 1975: Mother–child interactions: comparison of a non-compliant clinic group and a non-clinic group. *Behaviour Research and Therapy* **13**: 79–85.

Forth, A.E., Kosson, D. and Hare, R.D. in press: *The Hare Psychopathy Checklist: Youth Version*. Toronto: Multi-Health Systems.

George, C. and Main, M. 1979: Social interactions of young abused children: approach, avoidance and aggression. *Child Development* **50**: 306–18.

Glasser, M., Kolvin, I., Campbell, A. *et al.* 2001: Cycle of child sexual abuse: links between being a victim and becoming a perpetrator. *British Journal of Psychiatry* **179**: 482–94.

Graham, J. and Bowling, B. 1995: *Young People and Crime*. London: HMSO.

Hardiker, P., Exton, K. and Barber, M. 1991: *Policies and Practice in Preventive Child Care*. Aldershot: Gower.

Hartman, C.R. and Burgess, A.W. 1989: Sexual abuse of children: causes and consequences. In Cichetti, D. and Carlson, V. (eds), *Child Maltreatment: Theory and Research on the Causes and Consequences of Child Abuse and Neglect*. Cambridge: Cambridge University Press.

Hawkes, C., Jenkins, J.A. and Vizard, E. 1997: Roots of sexual violence in children. In Varma, V. (ed.), *Violence in Children and Adolescents*. London: Jessica Kingsley Publishers.

Hirschi, T. 1969: *Causes of Delinquency*. Los Angeles: University of California Press.

Hoghughi, M. 1997: Sexual abuse by adolescents. In Hoghughi, M.S., Bhate, S.R. and Graham, F. (eds), *Working with Sexually Abusive Adolescents*. London: Sage.

Home Office 1992: *Criminal Statistics for England and Wales*. London: HMSO.

Jehu, D. 1991: Clinical work with adults who were sexually abused in childhood. In Hollin, C.R. and Howells, K. (eds), *Clinical Approaches to Sex Offenders and their Victims*. Chichester: John Wiley.

Kauffman, J. and Zeigler, D. 1987: Do abused children become abusive parents? *American Journal of Orthopsychiatry* **57**: 186–92.

Kendal-Thackett, K.A., Meyer Williams, L. and Finkelhor, D. 1993: Impact of sexual abuse of children: a review and synthesis of recent empirical findings. *Psychological Bulletin* **113**: 164–80.

Kinard, E.M. 1980: Emotional development in physically abused children. *American Journal of Orthopsychiatry* **50**: 686–96.

Lake, E.S. 1993: An exploration of the violent victim experiences of female offenders. *Violence and Victims* **8**: 41–51.

Lauritsen, J.L., Sampson, R.J. and Laub, J.H. 1991: The link between offending and victimisation among adolescents. *Criminology* **28**: 265–91.

Leventhal, J.M. 1990: Epidemiology of child sexual abuse. In Oates, R.K. (ed.), *Understanding and Managing Sexual Abuse*. London: Harcourt Brace Jovanovich.

Loeber, R. and Hay, D.F. 1994: Developmental approaches to aggression and conduct problems. In Rutter, M. and Hay, D. (eds), *Development Through Life: a Handbook for Clinicians*. New York: Blackwell Scientific.

Loeber, R. and Hay, D. 1997: Key issues in the development of aggression and violence from childhood to early adulthood. *Annual Review of Psychology* **48**: 371–410.

Lynskey, M.T. and Ferguson, D.M. 1997: Factors protecting against the development of adjustment difficulties in young adults exposed to childhood sexual abuse. *Child Abuse and Neglect* **12**: 1177–90.

McCord, J. 1983: A forty-year perspective on the effects of child abuse and neglect. *Child Abuse and Neglect* **7**: 265–70.

Mednick, S.A. and Volavka, J. 1980: Biology and crime. In Morris, N. and Tonry, M. (eds), *Crime and Justice: an Annual Review of Research*, Vol. 2. Chicago: University of Chicago Press.

Mathews, F. 1996: *The Invisible Boy: Revisioning the Victimization of Male Children and Teens*. Health Canada, National Clearinghouse on Family Violence.

Mezey, G.C., Vizard, E., Hawkes, C. *et al.* 1991: A community treatment program for convicted child sex offenders: a preliminary report. *Journal of Forensic Psychiatry* **2**: 12–25.

Miethe, T.D. and Meir, R.F. 1990: Opportunity, choice and criminal victimisation: a test of a theoretical model. *Journal of Research in Crime and Delinquency* **27**: 243–66.

Mrazek, P.J. and Mrazek, D.A. 1987: Resilience in child maltreatment victims: a conceptual exploration. *Child Abuse and Neglect* **11**: 357–66.

Murphy, W.D. and Smith, T.A. 1996: Sex offenders against children: empirical and clinical studies. In Briere, J., Berliner, L. and Buckley, A. (eds), *The APSAC Handbook on Child Maltreatment*. London: Sage.

NAS (National Academy of Sciences) 1994: *Reducing the Risk for Mental Disorders: Frontiers for Preventive Intervention*. New York: National Academy Press.

Olweus, D. 1988: Environmental and biological factors in the development of aggressive behaviour. In Bluckhuisen, W. and Mednick, S.A. (eds), *Explaining Criminal Behaviour: Interdisciplinary Approaches*. Leiden: E.J. Brill, 90–120.

Patterson, G.R. 1982: *A Social Learning Approach: 3. Coercive Family Process*. Castalia.

Pearson, G. 1975: *The Deviant Imagination: Psychiatry, Social Work and Social Change*. London: Macmillan.

Perry, B.D. 1994: Neurobiological sequelae of childhood trauma: PTSD in children. In Murburg, M.M. (ed.), *Post-traumatic Stress Disorder: Emerging Concepts*. Washington, DC: American Psychiatric Press, 233–55.

Reidy, T.J. 1977: The aggressive characteristics of abused and neglected children. *Journal of Clinical Psychology* **33**: 1140–5.

Russell, D.E.H. 1984: *Sexual Exploitation*. London: Sage.

Russell, D.E.H. 1986: *The Secret Trauma: Incest in the Lives of Girls and Women*. New York: Basic Books.

Ryan, G. 1989: Victim to victimizer. *Journal of Interpersonal Violence* **4**: 325–41.

Sampson, R.L. and Lauritsen, J.L. 1990: Dominant life styles, proximity to crime and the offender–victim link in personal violence. *Journal of Research in Crime and Delinquency* **27**: 110–39.

Siegel, D.J. 1997: Memory and trauma. In Black, D., Newman, M., Harris-Hendriks, J. and Mezey, G. (eds), *Psychological Trauma: a Developmental Approach*. Location: Gaskell.

Smith, C.P., Berkman, D.J. and Fraser, W.M. 1980: *Reports of the National Juvenile Justice Assessment Centers*. Washington, DC: American Justice Institute.

Snyder, J.J. 1977: Reinforcement analysis of interaction in problem and non-problem families. *Journal of Abnormal Psychology* **86**: 528–35.

Spaccarelli, S. and Kin, S. 1995: Resilience criteria and factors associated with resilience in sexually abused girls. *Child Abuse and Neglect* **19**: 1171–82.

Spinetta, J.J. and Rigler, D. 1972: The child abusing parent: a psychological review. *Psychological Bulletin* **77**: 296–304.

Spitzer, R.L., Feister, S., Gray, M. and Pfohl, B. 1991: Results of a survey of forensic psychiatrists on the validity of the sadistic personality disorder diagnosis. *American Journal of Psychiatry* **148**: 875–9.

Squire, L.R. 1992a: Declarative and non-declarative memory: multiple brain systems supporting learning and memory. *Journal of Cognitive Neuroscience* **4**: 232–43.

Squire, L.R. 1992b: Memory and the hippocampus: a synthesis from findings from rats, monkeys and humans. *Psychological Review* **99**: 195–231.

Stoller, R.J. 1975: *The Erotic Form of Hatred*. Location: Maresfield Library.

Tonry, M. and Farrington, D.P. 1995: Strategic approaches to crime prevention. In Tonry, M. and Farrington, D.P. (eds), *Building a Safer Society: Strategic Approaches to Crime Prevention*. Chicago: University of Chicago Press.

Vizard, E., Wynick, S., Hawkes, C., Woods, J. and Jenkins, J. 1996: Juvenile sexual offenders: assessment issues. *British Journal of Psychiatry* **168**: 259–62.

Wahler, R.G. and Dumas, J.E. 1984: Family factors in childhood psychopathology: toward a coercion neglect model. In Jacob, T. (ed.), *Family Interaction and Psychopathology*. New York: Plenum Press.

Watkins, B. and Bentovim, A. 1992: The sexual abuse of male children and adolescents: a review of current research. *Journal of Psychology and Psychiatry* **33**: 197–248.

Widom, C.S. 1989a: Does violence beget violence? A critical examination of the literature. *Psychological Bulletin* **106**(1): 3–28.

Widom, C.S. 1989b: The cycle of violence. *Science* **244**: 160–6.

Widom, C.S. 1989c: The intergenerational transmission of violence. In Weiner, N.A. and Wolfgang, M.E. (eds), *Pathways to Criminal Violence*. London: Sage.

Widom, C.S. and Ames, M.A. 1994: Criminal consequences of childhood sexual victimisation. *Child Abuse and Neglect* **18**: 303–18.

Williams, B. and New, M. 1996: Developmental perspective on adolescent boys who sexually abuse other children: *Child Psychology and Psychiatry Review* **1**(4): 122–9.

Woods, J. 1997: Breaking the cycle of abuse and abusing: individual psychotherapy for juvenile offenders. *Clinical Psychology and Psychiatry* **2**: 379–92.

Yochelson, S. and Samenow, S.E. 1976: *The Criminal Personality: 1. A Profile for Change*. Location: Aronson.

Yochelson, S. and Samenow, S.E. 1977: A new horizon for total change of the criminal. In *The Criminal Personality: 2. The Change Process*. Location: Aronson.

16

Violence

SUSAN BAILEY AND MAIREAD DOLAN

INTRODUCTION

Violent juvenile offenders, although few in number, are responsible for a disproportionate number of crimes (Wasserman and Miller 1998). There is much debate in the literature about definitions of violence and aggression. For example:

- violence denotes the 'forceful' infliction of physical injury (Blackburn 1993)
- aggression involves harmful, threatening or antagonistic behaviour (Berkowitz 1993).

Loeber and Hay (1994) described four groups of young people:

- those who desist from aggression
- those whose aggression is stable and continues at the same level
- those who escalate in the severity of their aggression and make the transition into violence
- a group who show a stable pattern of aggression.

Longitudinal studies are invaluable in mapping out the range of factors and processes that contribute to the development of aggressive behaviour and in showing how they are causally related (Farrington 1995). However, in attempting to work with any individual who has committed a violent act, the question to be answered is why *this* individual has behaved in *this* unique fashion on *this* occasion (Lipsey 1995). Figure 16.1 shows a framework for the assessment of violence.

This chapter first looks at violence from an ecological perspective, exploring violence in the context of the

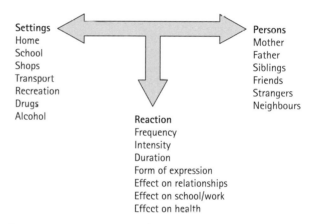

Figure 16.1 *Framework for the assessment of violence.*

community, the school and the home, to gain an understanding of grave acts of violence including juvenile homicide. The chapter concludes with a systematic approach to history-taking from the individual child or adolescent and their carers.

AN ECOLOGICAL PERSPECTIVE

Much of the work in this field has concentrated on the impact of violence on children who have experienced war and subsequently become refugees. *Minefields in their Hearts* (Apfel and Simon 1996) deals with the mental heath issues of children in war. UNICEF estimates that, whereas in 1900 the ratio of civilian to military casualties was about 1 to 9, it now stands at 8 to 1. Children constitute a significant proportion of these civilian casualties. Some countries – most often described in the USA but of increasing relevance to the UK – have chronic community violence in 'urban war zones', which affects the development of children (Kotlowitz 1991).

Garborino (2001) sets out an ecological framework to explain the processes and conditions that transform the 'developmental challenge' of violence into developmental harm in some children:

- an accumulation-of-risk model for understanding how and when children suffer the most adverse consequences of exposure to community violence and go beyond their limits of resilience
- the concept of 'social maps' as the product of childhood experiences
- the concept of trauma as a 'psychological wound'.

AN ACCUMULATION–OF–RISK MODEL

The idea is that risk accumulates whilst opportunity ameliorates. As negative (pathogenic) influences increase, the child may exceed his or her breaking point; consequently as a positive (salutogenic) influence increases, the probability of recovery and enhanced development increases.

The development model predicts that children and adolescents most at risk for negative consequences associated with community violence are those who already live in the context of accumulated risk – the socially marginal, those with fractured families and those with caregivers who have mental health problems or who are addicted to substances. In contrast, children who approach their community violence experience from a position of strength – with the salutogenic resources of social support, intact and functional families, and parents who model social competence – can accept better the developmental challenges posed by community violence and deal with them more positively in the long run (even if they show short-term disturbance). This model applies whether the experience is of actual war or 'urban war zones' (Garborino and Kostelny 1996).

SOCIAL MAPS

Garborino (1995) states that one of the most important features of child development is the child's emerging capacity to form and maintain 'social maps' – the cognitive competency of the child to be sure of how he is and has been, not just in the world where the child has been, but (given each child's moral and affective inclination) how the child views pathways to the future.

Pathways are crucial in mediating the experience of risk in later developmental outcomes (Rutter 1989). Young children have to contend with changes from two sources not so relevant to adults. Firstly there is their physical immaturity; and secondly they tend to believe in the reality of threats from what adults would describe as 'the fantasy' world. This increases their vulnerability to perceiving themselves in danger. Security is vitally important for a child's well-being.

For some children the level of their fright exceeds the actual dangers they face. For others, the fact of the matter is they are surrounded by violence – the world for them is a dangerous place, and they experience trauma.

TRAUMA AS A PSYCHOLOGICAL WOUND

Trauma arises when a child cannot give a meaning to dangerous experiences. The result is overwhelming negative emotion and cognition. Young children, in particular, have not developed fully functioning systems to modulate arousal and trauma can result in an inability to handle effectively the physiological responses of stress in situations of threat. The process required to 'understand' traumatic experiences can have pathogenic side-effects and the child may be forced into patterns of behaviour, thought and feelings that are themselves 'abnormal' compared with the un-traumatized healthy child.

Children and adolescents exposed to acute danger may develop symptoms of post-traumatic stress disorder (PTSD). These manifest themselves as sleep disturbance, day-dreaming, revelations of trauma in play, extreme startle responses, emotional numbing, and diminished expectations for the future. Trauma can also result in alterations in brain chemistry that can impair social and academic performance (Osofsky 1995; Pysnoos and Nader 1988). In some cases trauma may be seen as a significant aetiological factor for violent behaviour due to its adverse effects on psychological functioning, academic performance and normal parent–child relationships.

As difficult and damaging as acute trauma can be in the lives of children who in turn become violent, their neighbourhood and family experiences can also have a profound influence particularly if these environments are chronically traumatic. Garborino (1995) describes chronic traumatic danger as rewriting the child's story, redrawing the child's social map, and redirecting behaviour. Trauma represents an enormous challenge to any individual's understanding of the meaning and purpose of life. Children start life with a need and expectation for care, protection and love; when this need is absolutely violated, some children will seek out a negative universe on the grounds that anything is better than nothing. This can result in extreme acts of violence later in life (Douglas and O'Sharker 1995). It also importantly has implications for identity: when faced with the prospect of psychic annihilation, human beings will opt even for negative identities (Gilligan 1996).

COMMUNITY AND GANG VIOLENCE

General issues

Community violence and its consequences can make children prime candidates for involvement in social groups that augment or replace families and offer a sense of affiliation and security and perhaps a sense of revenge. In urban settings this can mean gangs.

The USA and inner-city areas of Britain have seen a proliferation in youth gangs. In the USA, an eleven-city survey of eighth-graders found that 9% were gang members and 17% had been at some time in their lives (Esbensen and Osgood 1997). Research indicates that the USA has seen several distinct periods of gang proliferation (Curry and Decker 1998). The gravest cause for concern in recent years has been the association with weapons of greater lethality (Block and Block 1993; Miller 1992) and drug trafficking (Miller 1992; Thornberry 1998).

The mean age of gang members tends to be 17 years (Curry and Decker 1998), but older individuals are found in cities with longer histories of gang-related activity (Spergel 1995). While gang membership is often viewed in terms of its degree of organization (Gordon 1994), three other types of gangs have been identified:

- organized/cooperative – strong leadership and a focus on illegal monetary gain
- territorial – belonging to a specific neighbourhood or turf
- scavenger – no strong leadership, but engaged in petty criminal activity.

Gang membership tends to be associated with lower social class and decaying urban areas, and ethnic-minority groups predominate (Miller 1974; Spergel 1995). In the USA, the ethnic-minority composition has changed dramatically since the 1800s with Irish and Italian gangs predominating in the nineteenth and twentieth centuries (Sante 1991) and Afro-Caribbean and Hispanic predominating in modern gangs (Spergel 1995). There is also some evidence of gang specialization in relation to ethnicity and offending behaviour. While Afro-American gangs are predominately involved in drug offences, Hispanic gangs tend to be associated in petty crime (Block et al. 1996; Spergel 1990). According to a most recent official US statistics, 10% of gang members are female (Miller 1992) but there is evidence of an increase in female gang membership; Esbenson and Osgood (1997) reported that approximately 38% of female eighth-graders claimed to be in a gang.

The extent of the problem

It is difficult to accurately ascertain the extent of the gang problem owing to varying definitions of what constitutes a gang. However, it is recognized that youth gangs are widespread and beginning to include non-urban areas. There are several factors that influence youth gang membership, including community, family, school, peer group and individual factors. Howell (1998) reported that low community integrity, poverty, parental absence/lack of supervision, academic under-achievement, peer influences

and drug use were significant predictors of gang membership, and similar findings were reported in a Seattle study (Hill et al. 1996; Kosterman et al. 1996). Findings from the latter study indicate that the greater the number of risk factors to which the individual is exposed, the greater the risk of joining a gang in adolescence. Children who experience seven or more risk factors at age 10–12 years are 13 times more likely to join a gang (Hill et al. 1996).

Miller (1992) provides a comprehensive review of the history of gang violence in the USA. In the 1970s, gang crime was more lethal because of the prevalence and sophistication of firearms.

Compared with non-gang adolescents, gang members commit serious and violent offences at significantly higher rates (Esbensen and Huizinga 1993; Bjerregaard and Smith 1993; Thornberry et al. 1995). The use of violence is a key characteristic to distinguishing gangs from other adolescent peer groups (Horowitz 1983; Sanders 1994). It serves to maintain organization within the gang, to control gang members (Decker and Van Winkle 1996). While there is a perception that gang violence is a significant threat to society, work by Block et al. (1996) indicates that, of 1000 gang-related homicides in Chicago between 1987 and 1994, 75% were between gangs, 11% were within gangs and 14% involved non-gang victims. Disputes were usually over turf, and the violent episodes occurred within a mile of the attacker's residence.

USE OF GUNS

Gangs are more likely to recruit adolescents who own firearms, and gang members are more likely than non-gang members to own a gun for protection (Bjerregaard and Lizotte 1995). The lethality of assault appears to have increased (Block and Block 1993) because of the proliferation of more sophisticated weapons. National trend data on gang homicides is scant, but Miller (1992) reported an increase in gang-related homicides since the 1980s particularly in cities like Chicago and Los Angeles. More recent studies indicate a doubling of gang-related homicides in Los Angeles county between 1987 and 1992 (Klein 1995). Decker and Van Winkle (1996) found that in St Louis the gang-member homicide rate was 1000 times higher than the overall US homicide rate.

Several factors appear to distinguish gang from non-gang homicides. In the former, homicides are more likely to occur in the street, involve strangers (drive-by shootings), and fluctuate from one racial or ethnic minority group to another at a given time point (Block and Christakos 1995).

REDUCING GUN VIOLENCE

Strategies for reducing gun violence include making them less available, and influencing how youths use them (Mercy and Rosenberg 1998). Recent research in the US has revealed ways to reduce gun ownership among teenagers, including identification and shutting down of suppliers (Kennedy 1998), and enlisting the help of adolescents to encourage their peers not to carry guns for their own protection (Chaiken 2000).

DRUG TRAFFICKING

While youth gangs appear to have increased their involvement in drug trafficking, the consensus in gang research is that the organizational structure of typical gangs is unsuited to drug trafficking business (Klein 1995; Spergel 1995). Studies indicate that the relationship between adolescent drug trafficking and violence is weak (Decker and Van Winkle 1996; Esbensen and Huizinga 1993). It appears that youth gang homicide erupts more from inter-gang conflict than from the drugs trade (Block and Block 1993) and that the majority of homicides are related to territorial disputes.

Solutions to the gang problem

There have been several initiatives in the USA to combat gang-related activities. The Gang Resistance Education and Training (GREAT) programme in students resulted in lower levels of gang affiliation and self-reported delinquent activities (Esbensen and Osgood 1997). The community-wide approach to gang prevention, intervention and suppression programme developed by Spergel *et al.* (1994) is a multi-agency programme to reduce gang activity; preliminary data from pilot projects indicate lower levels of serious gang violence, improved perception by residents on gang crime, and fewer arrests for serious gang crimes. In California, the Try Agency Resource Gang Enforcement Team (TARGET) identifies and tracks gang members to provide intelligence in the selection of appropriate gang members for interventions.

It seems that combined comprehensive programmes of prevention, social intervention and rehabilitation have some effect in reducing gang affiliation and gang violence. The Office of Juvenile Justice and Delinquency Prevention currently has a five-sided programme, which may shed more light on the most effective interventions.

SERIOUS AND VIOLENT JUVENILE OFFENDERS: A US PERSPECTIVE

The Office of Juvenile Justice and Delinquency Prevention (OJJDP) of the US Department of Justice convened a study group of 22 researchers to examine research on risk and protective factors in the development of serious and violent juvenile (SVJ) offending (Loeber and Farrington 1998). Their definition of serious and violent offences included homicide, rape, robbery, aggravated assault and kidnapping. The group found that the majority of SVJ offenders were male, their criminal careers began early and tended to escalate to serious violent offending through a variety of pathways, and they had multiple problems such as substance misuse and mental health difficulties. They described three pathways that can explain progression to SVJ offending (Loeber and Hay 1994):

- the Authority Conflict pathway
- the Covert pathway
- the Overt pathway.

The Authority Conflict pathway, which applies to boys under 12 years, is the earliest pathway. It begins with stubborn behaviour followed by defiance and finally authority avoidance, e.g. truancy. The Covert pathway starts with covert behaviours such as lying, followed by property damage and later more serious property crimes such as burglary. The Overt pathway has minor aggression as a first stage, physical fighting as the next stage and violence as a third stage (Kelley *et al.* 1997).

Serious and violent juvenile (SVJ) offenders tend to differ from non-SVJ offenders in a number of ways. The majority start offending earlier and continue offending longer than non-SVJ offenders. They have an earlier age of onset of non-delinquent behaviour problems. SVJ offending is more prevalent in Afro-American youth than among whites. SVJ offenders exhibit more aggression, dishonesty, property offences and conflict with authority in the transition from childhood to adolescence. Finally, SVJ offenders typically advance simultaneously in each problem behaviour area and progress to increasingly more serious forms of delinquency (Loeber and Farrington 1998).

The SVJ-offending study group also listed a number of predictors of SVJ offending:

- elementary school – persistent precocious behavioural problems
- age 6 to 11 – non-serious delinquent acts, aggression, substance misuse and family dysfunction
- age 12 to 14 – weak social ties, antisocial peers, poor school attitude and performance and the emergence of psychological conditions such as impulsivity
- adolescence to early adulthood – gang membership, drug dealing, unemployment and gun ownership.

Principles of effective delinquency prevention and early intervention

Approaches to prevention can be described as universal, selected or indicated (Wasserman and Miller 1998). Universal programmes apply to the community at large and target issues such as neighbourhood poverty. Selected programmes target high-risk children who may have exhibited some antisocial behaviour. Indicated programmes are for those with recorded delinquent behaviour. There are a number of key principles for effective delinquency prevention and early intervention (Loeber and Farrington 1998;

Bilchik 1998). These are listed below:

1 Address the highest priority problem areas and identify strengths.
2 Focus more strongly on populations exposed to a number of risk factors.
3 Address problem areas and identify strengths early and at appropriate developmental stages.
4 Address multiple risk factors.
5 Offer comprehensive interventions across many systems.
6 Build on a juvenile's strengths, rather than focus on deficiencies.
7 Deal with juveniles in the context of their relationship to and with others, rather than focus only on the individual.
8 Encourage co-operation among various community members.
9 Be aware of the nature and availability of the various community intervention programmes.

EFFECTIVE EARLY INTERVENTION PROGRAMMES

Loeber and Farrington (1998) and Wasserman and Miller (1998) have summarized what is known about effective early intervention programmes for serious violent juveniles. The programmes are separated into the contexts in which they are delivered and are listed under the following headings:

Parents
• Parent management training.
• Functional family therapy.
• Family preservation.

Children
• Home visiting for pregnant teenagers.
• Social competence training.
• Peer mediation and conflict resolution.
• Medication for neurological disorders and mental illness.

Schools
• Early intellectual environmental enrichment.
• School organization.

Community
• Comprehensive community mobilization.
• Situational crime prevention.
• Intensive police patrolling.
• Legal and policy change restricting availability of guns, drugs and alcohol
• Mandatory laws for firearms crime.

EFFECTIVE TREATMENT PROGRAMMES FOR VIOLENT DELIQUENTS

The OJJDP strategy for offenders promotes a graduated sanctions approach and builds on the *Comprehensive Strategy for Serious, Violent, and Chronic Juvenile Offenders* (Wilson and Howell 1993). The programme combines accountability and sanctions with increasingly intensive treatment and rehabilitation services. Sanctions are wide-ranging to fit the offence and include both interventions and secure correction components. The intervention component includes the use of immediate intervention and immediate sanctions, and the secure corrections component includes the use of community confinement and incarceration in training schools, camps and ranches. At each level the family must continue to be integral in treatment and rehabilitation. Aftercare must be a formal component of all treatment and rehabilitation efforts. The placement of the offender should be on a risk and needs assessment (Wasserman and Miller 1998).

VIOLENCE IN SCHOOLS: A UK PERSPECTIVE

Risk factors for violence in an educational setting

There are a number of factors in school environments that may contribute to violence among school children. These include academic failure due to bullying, exclusion or underling mental health and behavioural disorders such as attention-deficit hyperactivity disorder (ADHD).

Over the last decade of the twentieth century the majority of young people tended to remain in education until the age of 18. The pressure to acquire good qualifications, however, led some schools to exclude pupils who were under performing or disruptive. Between 1996 and 1997 there were 12,700 permanent exclusions in England, and these numbers continue to rise. Eighty-three per cent of these exclusions were from secondary schools and 12% from primary schools. Of all those excluded from school, 83% were male, a statistic which reflects the known preponderance of boys involved in both antisocial and challenging behaviour (Coleman 1999).

Bullying in school causes much concern to mental health professionals, and much thought has been given to devising methods of combating the problem. Smith and Sharp (1994) reported approximately 10% of young people being bullied at least once a term, but there were variations by age and gender. A study by Turtle et al. (1997) demonstrates that bullying has become a very serious problem, with 19% of boys and 17% of girls reporting being bullied during the current school term.

The onset of attention problems as described in ADHD occurs during the pre-school period, the time when aggression manifests itself in some children (Barkley 1990, 1997). Longitudinal studies show that children with attention problems exhibit increased levels of aggression in childhood, adolescence and adulthood. A major cluster of individual risk factors is starting to emerge which include hyperactivity, impulsivity, attention problems, clumsiness, daring or risk-taking and other elements of ADHD (Hagell and Shaw 1996). These factors are closely linked to childhood conduct disorder. Lynam (1996) has argued that children who had both hyperactivity/impulsivity/attention deficit and conduct problems were at risk of serious adult antisocial behaviour and personality disorder.

Maguine and Loeber (1996), in a meta-analysis, demonstrated that it is low intelligence and attentional problems rather than educational performance that predicts later delinquency. Maughan *et al.* (1996) followed poor and normal readers through adolescence and into early adulthood; reading-disabled boys showed high rates of inattentiveness in middle childhood. Increased risk of juvenile offending amongst the specific group has been linked to poor school attendance rather than reading difficulties *per se*.

Children who have frequent disagreements with peers do not make friends. Very aggressive children are rejected by their peers, a process that can start in the early school years. Aggressive children who are rejected show more diverse and severe conduct problems. Moreover, peer rejection promoted an association with antisocial peers; dyadic relationships are then formed that provide the focus for peer-diverted aggression. Victims often lack social skills and can be aggressive themselves. Repeatedly victimized young people are more likely to become aggressors as well. Aggressive young people may make alliances, bullying others which results in the emergence of aggressive peer groups and gangs where the individual's rate of violence usually increases. These groups may appear attractive to other previously non-aggressive young people, adding to the group late-onset aggressive adolescence.

The real costs of aggression and violence go far beyond the individual injury and physical suffering resulting from a violent act within a school setting. The fear and trauma in schools is having an impact on the entire school context and on all students in this context. They will influence teaching practices, children's readiness and capacity for learning, recruitment and retention of teachers and other school staff, the openness and accessibility of the school premises, students' rights to privacy, the nature of the physical building and the grounds, and overall the quality of the learning environment. The important question then is how safer schools can be created for children to be able to learn and to have an enriched education.

Youths living in areas characterized by a culture of violence in their homes and neighbourhoods often find it difficult to satisfy their needs for belonging, recognition and acceptance through non-violent outlets. School therefore has the potential to offer positive outlets. Failure by young people to achieve academic success, peer approval, personal independence, self-efficacy and satisfying interpersonal relationships within the school context may create stresses and conflicts that instead increase the likelihood

of aggressive and violent behaviour (Lowry *et al.* 1995). Thus it is important to bear in mind whilst violence in schools may reflect the violence that pervades the surrounding community, the school environment itself presents the potential for giving rise to violence. Most school-related violence is linked to competition for status amongst peers. The presence of gangs in schools increases the likelihood of victimization for non-gang members. An additional emerging peer-related concern is that of sexual assault, particularly within the context of dating.

Protective factors against violence: the 'social development model'

Catalana and Hawkins (1996) proposed a social development model to explain why prosocial and antisocial behaviours might emerge during the school going years. Between the ages of 6 and 18 – the period during which involvement in violent behaviour usually emerges and peaks – schools are a major social environment experienced by most children. Children who develop a commitment to succeed in school and have bonded with the school community are more successful academically than other children. They are also less likely to engage in serious crime, including violent behaviour. Academic success helps to protect against violent behaviour during adolescence.

The key features in the social development model are:

- social bonding and academic achievement
- promoting norms of non-violence
- teaching skills for living according to non-violent norms
- eliminating the presence or opportunity to obtain or use weapons.

Interventions include:

- use of management and instructional practices in classrooms and on playgrounds that promote the development of social bonding
- promotion of norms antithetical to violent behaviour
- teaching schools to resolve conflicts non-violently
- minimizing the availability of an acceptance of weapons, and more particularly their use
- efforts to change an entire school to make it more protective against violence or violent risk factors.

Interventions and solutions

In addressing the problem of violence in schools it is important to be able to take a life-course perspective and a developmental perspective. Interventions need to take into account the developmental stage of the child or youth. For example, dyadic parent–child training programmes may be effective with young children and early adolescents who are at risk of adopting violent coping strategies, but they are not appropriate and may even have negative effects if employed for older adolescents who at that stage of life seek independence from parents and look to peers for approval and status. Likewise, it may be tempting to teach primary school children how to deal with peer pressure for engaging in sex, violence or drugs before they have experienced the onset of puberty, but they have no understanding of the intense need for peer approval or badges of adult status and establishing one's sexual identity which emerge from the developmental stage of adolescence.

Applying a public health-based approach to reduction of violence in young people will address risks in the individual, the family, the school and the community. School-based interventions are those designed to alter school settings by (Hamburg 1998):

- changing teacher behaviour management strategies to prevent violent behaviour and encouraging student cooperation
- improving student motivation by enhancing reinforcement, improving communication between students, school staff and families, and enhancing monitoring of students to identify youths at risk of developing violent behaviour
- changing school organizational structures and atmosphere in order to increase student and parent involvement and to establish programmes to better meet students special needs.

Since Plato set out to train young people to find pleasure in actions which strengthen the bonds of human society rather than weaken them, the creation of social bonding has itself been a goal of education (Csikszentmihalyi and Larson 1980).

EARLY CHILDHOOD EDUCATION PROGRAMMES

There have been three major studies of early childhood education programmes supplemented with home visits and community support with follow-up of the children well into adolescence. Children who received these interventions did better academically in school and later had lower rates of violence and crime (Berreuta-Clement *et al.* 1984; Johnson and Walker 1987; Lally *et al.* 1988; see also Schweinhart *et al.* 1993).

- The Perry Pre-School Programme used the High/Scope cognitively orientated curriculum to foster social and intellectual developments in children aged 3–4 years from disadvantaged Afro-American children in a poor neighbourhood. At follow-up study to age 27, the experimental group had had only half as many arrests. They had significantly higher earnings. More of the women were married. They were likely to have graduated from high school and they had greater academic achievement.

- The Houston Parent/Child Development Center Programme featured home visitation services during the first years of a child's life followed by centre-based educational nursery school and parent effectiveness training.
- The Syracuse Family Development Research Programme included home visits, parental training, centre-based educational childcare and parent organization during the pre-school years for families in poverty.

Fast-track prevention programmes are the most recent effort targeted at high-risk school children. The interventions offered for 54 schools matched for size, poverty and ethnic composition consisted of a curriculum 'promoting alternative thinking strategies' (PATHS), parent groups, a child social-skills training group, parent–child sharing time, home visiting, child–peer groups, parenting groups, academic tutoring offered during school time, and community and home extra-curriculum enrichment programmes. In children at high risk of developing long-term antisocial behaviour, the initial findings of the fast-track preventive programme suggested improvement in some measures of social, emotional, behavioural and academic functioning.

Of more potential interest is part of the fast-track prevention programme that looks at classroom atmosphere and peer-reported behaviour problems. In this lies the subtlety of how we measure and regard improvement. The fast-track prevention programme improved behaviour according to peer reports and ratings of classroom atmosphere. However, teachers' reports did not show a difference in behaviour (McMahon 1999a,b).

Hunter and Chandler (1999) raise important issues about adolescent resilience, the value of not just quantitative but also qualitative research in evaluating impact on the individual. Using a triangulated research design, resilience was looked at in inner-city vocational high schools. The qualitative component to the study consisted of a free writing exercise. The adolescents' perceptions of resilience were based not on resilience as we would mean it, but rather on their sense of invincibility, sensibility, feelings, isolation of self from those who could hurt them, distrust of everyone around them, acting out, and being violent to be heard and seen. Resilience to them meant being a disconnected self-reliant self-protective individual with no one to depend on or trust but themselves. Thus being resilient for these high-risk adolescents was not having a healthy sense of self-worth or the ability to connect and trust others, but just surviving.

VIOLENCE IN THE FAMILY

Theoretical work in the 1970s provided a framework for understanding the multi-determined nature of abuse and neglect (Ammerman and Hersen 1992). Ecological models were posited to interact and converge to bring about family violence. This in turn led to an increased interest in clinical assessment and treatment. The epidemiological research of the 1980s documented widespread prevalence of child abuse, neglect, spouse battering, mistreatment of elders, and psychological abuse (Strauss *et al.* 1980; Strauss and Gelles 1988, 1990). This in turn fuelled the development and evaluation of interventions for both victims and perpetrators.

Predominant factors within families which contribute to longer-term aggressiveness and risk of violence are clearly established in child-rearing and parenting styles (Farrington 1995). Against a backdrop of multiple deprivation, three key clusters emerge. The first cluster is the presence of criminal parents and siblings with behavioural problems. In the second, day-to-day behaviour of primary caregivers is one of parental conflict, inconsistent supervision and physical and emotional neglect with little or no reinforcement of prosocial behaviours. The children learn that their own aversive behaviours stop unwanted intrusions by parents. Young people who assault others have lower rates of positive communication with their families. A third cluster of family factors linked with later violence in the child include: cruel authoritarian discipline, physical control, and shaming and emotional degradation of the child.

Where young people live in a culture of violence in their homes and neighbourhoods, school has the potential to offer positive outlets to satisfy needs for belonging and recognition and acceptance through non-violent means. Failure to achieve academic success, peer approval and the satisfaction of interpersonal relationships within school creates additional stresses and conflicts, with increased likelihood of aggression and violence linked to competition for status and status-related confrontations with peers (Laub and Lauristen 1998).

Domestic violence remains one of the most pervasive of all social problems affecting most of the population directly or indirectly (Blacklock 2001).

There is remarkably little known or documented about children who are violent to their parents. This is surprising given the level of knowledge and concern about antisocial and violent behaviour, committed by children within school or when out in the community. The subject of abused parents (with the exceptions of the elderly and the extreme act of parricide) can at best be seen as underresearched and at worst as a taboo subject associated with a sense of shame that parents cannot protect themselves against the violence of those with whose care and protection they are charged.

Strauss *et al.* (1980) estimated that 18% of children between the ages of 3 and 17 carried out one or more acts of violence towards parents. The victim was most often the mother, with range of severity from 10% of children hitting or striking a parent, 7% striking a parent with an object, 1% severely beating a parent, and 1% using a potentially lethal weapon. What therefore is known about children who are violent to parents?

Adolescents who have assaulted peers, siblings, teachers and strangers are at increased risk of having assaulted or threatened to inflict physical violence on their parents. Children who inflicted physical violence on parents were described by Harbin and Madden (1979) as more often economically dependent, male and aged between 13 and 24. Adolescents who are violent to parents appear to straddle socio-economic groupings. As such, family dynamics provide the greatest insight into the evolution of this particular form of violence in children. For example:

- Some parents convey inconsistent values about aggression.
- Although severe child abuse in this group is unusual, parents who use harsh child-rearing techniques are at increased risk of being victims of violence at the hands of their children.
- Role reversal between parent and child (parentification) takes place, to the extent that parental authority is given over to the child.

Parents will tend to deny the seriousness of acts of aggression and violence displayed against them. In the clinical situation when a child is referred for violent acts occurring in the community or school, parents will not always reveal the preceding or coexisting history of violence in the home.

Violent assaults against parents are most likely to occur in the context of parenting stress evolving out of parent–child disagreement. Failure to set consistent limits on unacceptable behaviour produces a dynamic in which the child experiences an evolving sense of empowerment, and indeed a sense of justification in dealing with increasingly failing attempts at parenting by both escalating frequency and severity of violent responses. The tyrannical child is then in turn rewarded and reinforced in his or her behaviour by parents giving in to this graded continuum of physical aggression. Authors have likened the evolution of parental inconsistency and loss of authority – which includes fear of the child – to the need to maintain the relationship through co-dependency, as seen in adult male-to-female domestic violence (Roth and Coles 1995). In domestic violence, violence and other abusive behaviours are used to control. The abusive behaviour is used to support the aggressor's sense of entitlement which allows an adult male to see his behaviour as reasonable given his partner's 'unreasonable' resistance to his expectation. This further fuels the process of partner-blaming (Blacklock 2001). Whatever other factors place a child at risk of being violent, this sense of entitlement, and experience of being in control, can lead to aggression and violence becoming the child's normal form of social transaction in the home, and then beyond.

JUVENILE HOMICIDE

The extent of the problem

In the UK and most industrialized countries outside the USA, juvenile homicide is very rare (Justice 1996). The low base rate inevitably makes it difficult to establish whether juvenile killers constitute a distinct group. In the USA, the rate of homicides by young people is some 15 times higher than in European countries (Snyder *et al.* 1996), and such a huge national difference in rate raises questions of comparability. Killing by children in the USA may occur more often in the course of acquisitive crime, and it probably reflects in part the much greater availability of guns. School-based killings by juveniles have reopened the debate, which is informed by a series of texts (Elliott *et al.* 1998; Kelleher 1998; Heide 1999).

In the USA, the surge of violence during the late 1980s and early 1990s included more than homicides. Between 1988 and 1991, the rate of juvenile arrests for non-lethal crimes (assault, robbery and rape) increased by 38% (Snyder and Sickmund 1995). The 'Monitoring the Future' study, involving a national sample of high school seniors, also found an 18% increase in the proportion of students reporting a serious assault on another person between 1984 and 1994 (Maguire and Pastore 1996). Although this increase was not particularly striking, fights that in earlier years resulted in black eyes and bloody noses now often involved death or serious injury as the number of youths carrying guns and other weapons has increased substantially (Elliott 1994).

In the 1990s, homicide became the second leading cause of death among adolescents in the USA, and the leading cause of death among Afro-American male adolescents (Snyder and Sickmund 1995). In the increase of the use of firearms, there were more seemingly 'random' violent events, and assaults on strangers without provocation (Fox 1996). Violence erupted in places previously though to be safe – trains, restaurants and schools. The result of this has been high levels of fear of violence experienced by both children and adults (Elliot 1994).

In her analysis of crime patterns in the USA over 13 years, Kathleen Heide revealed that homicides by juveniles rose every year from 1984 through to 1993, when the number of juveniles arrested (under 18 years of age), at 3284, was three times higher than the number arrested in 1984. This increase, although felt in urban, suburban and rural areas across the nation, was particularly noticeable in US cities: 8.3% of all homicide arrests in 1984 rose to 18.1% in 1994. In 1996, one in six homicide arrests in cities involved juveniles. From a public health perspective, the 50,000 deaths caused by violence across all age groups is much greater than the number caused by AIDS (30,000 per year) and greater than the number of deaths caused by drunk driving (18,000 per year).

The connection between race and juvenile homicide remains a controversial issue. From 1985 to 1994, homicide offending rates of white youths aged 14–17 doubled, from 7.0 to 15.6 per 100,000, but the rates for black youths tripled, from 44.3 to 139.6 per 100,000. Afro-Americans made up approximately 14% of the juvenile population in the USA.

Juvenile homicide offenders, like their adult counterparts, are far more likely to kill one victim than several. When two or more juveniles kill, the victim is more likely to be a stranger. During the last decade in the USA, gang membership has increased, and gangs have become increasingly responsible for a disproportionate amount of violence, related to the availability of firearms and the dynamics of gang violence (see earlier).

The perpetrators

Juvenile homicide remains an overwhelmingly male phenomenon. When girls kill, they are more likely than their male counterparts to kill people they know.

Although there is a paucity of systematic comparative studies of juvenile homicide, there are several reviews of what is known about the characteristics of young people who kill (Wilson 1973; Cornell *et al.* 1987; Goetting 1995; Cavadino and Allen 2000), a comparative study of adolescents convicted of homicide and those convicted of property offences (Toupin 1997), and one follow-up study of nine delinquents who subsequently killed (Lewis *et al.* 1985). In addition, there are a number of detailed studies of small groups (Myers *et al.* 1995; Bailey 1996; Bailey *et al.* 2001; Myers and Scott 1998).

Taking the evidence as a whole (Rutter *et al.* 1998), two conclusions seem reasonably well justified. Firstly, both the nature of the homicidal acts and the characteristics of the young people who commit the acts are heterogeneous. Secondly, the children who kill tend to have disturbed, often abusive family backgrounds and they also show a range of personal problems. Accordingly, in a great majority of cases it would seem appropriate to consider the homicides as a result of personal psychopathology and serious psychosocial adversities, rather than simple acts of serious wrongdoing or the consequences of 'innate evil'.

At present these considerations are poorly represented in the ways in which child killers are dealt with by the British judicial system. In a landmark judgement in December 1999, 'Children in criminal proceedings – the right to a fair trial – the cases of T and V' (V v UK, application number 248888/94, and T v UK, application number 2472/94), the European Court of Human Rights stated that Article 6, read as a whole, guarantees the right to a fair trial. In practice, the impact of his or her age, level of maturity and intellectual and emotional capacities should be considered, and steps taken to promote his or her ability to understand and participate effectively in the proceedings. This has major implications for psychiatrists and psychologists preparing pre-trial reports on all minors with regard to both training and a standardized systematic assessment process. This aspect of medico-legal work is already being addressed in the USA (Grisso and Schwartz 2000).

The causes

Following a spate of killings in schools in the USA, there has been discussion among professionals on both sides of the Atlantic on the extent to which juvenile homicide reflects the severe end of juvenile delinquent behaviour. It is apparent that there is much in common between juveniles who kill and other delinquents. However, there is one respect in which the two seem different, at least in the UK. Over the last 50 years there has been a massive increase in juvenile delinquency in most westernized industrialized countries (Rutter and Smith 1995), accompanied by similar (although less marked) rises in other psychosocial disorders in young people, such as drug and alcohol abuse, depression and suicide. The rate of juvenile homicide in the UK does not, though, appear to have risen to any appreciable extent (McNally 1995; Justice 1996). A proportion of these killings involved sexual assaults and/or extreme repeated violence (Bailey 1996). It may be inferred tentatively that in the UK killings by children or adolescents may be more likely to reflect serious personal psychopathology, although rarely illnesses such as schizophrenia, than is the case with most other serious crime committed by young people (Clare *et al.* 2000).

In *Lost Boys*, Garborino (1999) attempts to unravel the processes that lead to extreme aggression, citing genetic inheritance, parental upbringing and the 'increasing toxic nature of contemporary American society' as contributory factors. Adolescent males fall victim to an unfortunate synchronicity between 'the demons inhabiting their own internal world and the corrupting influences of modern American culture, vicarious violence, crude sexuality, shallow materialism, mean spirited competitiveness and spiritual emptiness'. For most, problems begin in early childhood, with boys describing abuse and/or abandonment; they gradually lose the capacity to feel emotions and externalization of the pain. This is echoed in the paranoid attributions noted by Myers and Scott (1998), and described in the evolution of violent and sadistic fantasy by Bailey (1997), and in the failure of home, school and community to respond to the clues presented by young males in the six months prior to the final indecent act. There is progression and combination in some young people from insecure attachment in infancy, early antisocial behaviour, adolescent rage, post-traumatic stress disorder to past trauma, and a sense of abandonment.

Any discussion of juvenile homicide has to explore not only the impact of gun availability in the USA, but also the influence of pervasive violence as portrayed through the media. In film and television violence, violent acts committed by not only the 'villains' but also the 'heroes' are often accompanied by no showing of remorse and no criticism of their acts. Increasing focus following a spate of teenage murderers in the USA has centred on the impact of violent video games (Anderson and Dill 2000). These games provide a forum for learning and practising aggressive solutions to conflict situations. The effect appears to be cognitive in the short term, primary aggressive thoughts in the long term leading to changes in everyday social interactions. Given the trend towards (1) greater realism and more graphic violence in video games, (2) their increasing popularity, (3) the game play becoming synonymous with the game character, (4) the active participation involved in video games, and (5) their addictive nature, close monitoring and new research are called for to clarify for society what risks are entailed – especially for disaffected, isolated, alienated young people who have failed in school and in normal peer interactions and who have neuropsychotic vulnerabilities.

Treatments

Following their arrest most adolescents – whether allowed to remain with the family, placed under the open or secure care of social services, or psychiatric secure care or remand to a Young Offender Institution – experience a progression of reactions and feelings akin to a grief reaction (Hambridge 1990). The majority initially dissociate themselves from the reality of their offence and situation, but gradually they start to grieve. This is usually first about their own loss of freedom, then their enforced separation from the family (however chaotic and abusive), and lastly about their victim. The current legal process itself often delays the onset of the last process.

Irrespective of the available treatment model, if any, provided by the care or custody institution, the parallel process of education, vocation, avocation, consistent role models and continued family contact are of critical importance (Bullock *et al.* 1994). This parallel process is best facilitated in a milieu characterized by warmth and harmony, with clear organization, practicality and high expectations (Harris *et al.* 1987), allowing for the establishment of positive staff–adolescent, staff–staff and adolescent–adolescent relations (Waplington 1994).

Psychopharmacological treatment should be retained for the management of a primary illness (e.g. epilepsy, psychosis), and in such cases there should be a clearly defined quantifiable means of assessing efficacy (Eichelman 1988). The clinician always needs to be alert to the possibility of an emerging mental illness, in particular depression, whilst the adolescent is serving a sentence (Stewart *et al.* 1990).

Hollin (1993) describes the emerging success of cognitive-behavioural therapy with serious delinquents, but stresses the importance of carefully targeted programmes.

The use of psychotherapy for the child or adolescent who has committed a homicidal act is an important adjunctive treatment and can play the central role in therapy. The capacity to form emotional attachments with others, thus potentially allowing the establishment of a working relationship with the clinician, is a common indication of treatability, together with the ability for self-examination and insight. Qualities such as frequent and severe aggression, low intelligence and a poor capacity for insight weigh against the reliance on psychotherapy as a primary means of treatment.

Burgess et al. (1990) described the use of drawing, painting and sculpture in accessing memory of the homicidal act, allowing further insights into the motivational dynamics of the act. This can enable the adolescent to face the more violent sadistic elements of the offence and his or her own previous abuse, particularly in those cases where the spoken word has become such a painful and destructive reminder of the pre-trial and trial process.

From the outset of treatment there has to be a clear understanding of the patient–therapist dyad, the boundaries of confidentiality, especially given the expectation that a forensic psychiatrist may well have to comment on the level of responsibility a child or adolescent can hold for the offence and give a prediction of future risk, particularly when the individual reaches the point when he or she becomes eligible for parole and supervised return to the community. This can lead to a testing of a trusting relationship between the adolescent and clinician.

Against the inevitable waxing and waning of outside pressures, the adolescent has to move safely through the process of disbelief, denial, loss, grief, anger/blame and possible post-traumatic stress syndrome arising either from the participation in the homicidal act directly, or observing the action of co-defendants, or arising from past personal abuse.

Addressing victim empathy, saying sorry, and re-attributing blame can lead to an expression of anger and distress within sessions, often sexualized in both form and content. When the emotion this engenders spills outside sessions it can lead to disruptive behaviour within the institution. This is difficult for both the adolescent and carers and can lead to both becoming rejecting and dismissive of the therapist. The therapist has to make constructive use of the parallel process of care, educational input and peer-group interactions to help the adolescent in a highly artificial environment to cope with psychosexual and personality development, and above all to enable the adolescent to attain safe autonomy.

The tools available to the therapist are first and foremost the empowerment from statutory agencies, placement, family and the individual to carry out the work, the baggage of history accompanying each adolescent, the depositions (police evidence regarding the offence)

and the therapist physically retracing the events prior to the homicidal act (the adolescent often having a distorted memory of time, size and geography). All have been used effectively in offence-specific work.

Each component has to be visited and revisited as and when the adolescent can cope with the relevant issues. At a later stage in therapy it is important that the adolescent understands the degree and level of public opinion arising from the offence (via newspaper and media coverage). As the adolescent approaches a return to the community, he or she needs to reach a safe resolution – which must include a mechanism for explaining the gap in his or her life to the outside world, and in particular to any future partner.

Focused cognitive-behavioural psychotherapy, combined with non-verbal therapies offered as part of the parallel process consistent limit-setting, education and vocational training, can aim for a sublimation of aggressive drives. This provides a context in which the adolescent can achieve safe autonomy and develop and sustain positive relationships with peers and family, both during the sentence and on release.

Heide (1999) and Kelleher (1998) both argue against the public perception of juvenile killers as a homogeneous group, characterized by threat, fear, loss of control, explosive rage, high levels of aggression, hostility, impulsivity and unpredictability. Both authors emphasize the fact that most convicted killers are eventually released back to the community. Heide argues that with sensitive interviewing and behavioural observations, it is possible to elucidate which and how factors act in concert, and the child's responses to each factor and the combination of factors. Of critical important is the clinician's ability to unravel sequences of input and output, parallel sequences in the process of killing, and the combination of thoughts, emotions and expectations, attitudes and other behaviours of the young person at the time. Heide concludes that clinical assessment is to help understand, not to stereotype or oversimplify. Echoed in similar long-term work with young killers in the UK (Bailey and Aulich 1997), Heide believes that these young people can change substantially, but they need considerable assistance, direction and treatment which can follow on only from a detailed initial evaluation, an acceptance that therapeutic gains come slowly, and a realization that work may have to be conducted against a background of changing legislation, policy and placement and sentence planning by the various government departments charged with responsibility for young offenders (Bailey et al. 2001).

A SEMI-STRUCTURED APPROACH TO HISTORY-TAKING

Assessment of violence in its various settings, degrees of severity and with the presence or absence of mental

Question asked of the child/adolescent	In home	In school	In the community
Has anyone ever thrown something at you?			
Have you thrown something at anyone else?			
Have you pushed, grabbed, shoved anyone?			
Have you slapped anyone?			
Have you tugged or pulled at anyone's hair?			
Have you bitten anyone?			
Have you punched anyone?			
Have you kicked anyone?			
Have you headbutted anyone?			
Have you kneed anyone?			
Have you ever put anybody in a headlock?			
Have you ever held on to anyone around their neck so that they might be starting to choke?			
Have you threatened anyone with a knife or any other object or weapon?			
Have you used a knife or other weapon?			
Have you done anything else that might be considered violent?			

Figure 16.2 *Suggested framework for a structured history interview.*

disorder, has to be approached systematically. As with adults, a graded series of questions to children and adolescents about their violence – starting with allowing them the opportunity to talk about violence done to them, whether at home, school or in the community – will enable the clinician to gain an informed understanding of why *this* child at *this* time is presenting with *this* particular violent act. Figure 16.2 shows an example.

The same structure can be used to take a history from parents or other carers, allowing them to gradually explore with the clinician the depth and extent of violence displayed towards them behind the closed doors of home.

CONCLUSION AND FUTURE DIRECTIONS

Risk assessment and management of violent children must be informed by those with expertise in understanding of young people's development. Child and adolescent mental health teams have an important role to play, a role that is likely to increase and will have particular importance when the young person has 'special needs' and/or recognized mental health problems. In order to fulfil this role safely, the practitioner needs to be equipped with

appropriate training and a framework within which to carry out assessments before advising on and being involved in treatment.

Health and human service administration at city, national and international levels should assess organizational versus disorganizational status in neighbourhoods prior to selecting and investing money, time and social capital in a particular intervention strategy (Bank and Dowled-Noursi 2001).

- There should be efforts to alter the 'legitimisation of aggression' among young people, to stimulate cognitive restructuring and behavioural reversal of non-violent responses to conflict, anger, frustration, injustice and threat. These efforts should start in early childhood.
- Early childhood educators need to be trained to recognize and respond to traumatic experiences in the lives of young children in their care.
- Prosocial adults and young members of the community can be mobilized to help draw the 'social maps' of children living in violent communities (Garborino 1995).
- The critical importance of 'moral' rehabilitation needs to be recognized. Trauma can and does distort values, and can draw vulnerable young people into groups that legitimize and reward their rage, fear and violence – an environment in which gangs can flourish and

community institutions deteriorate (Garborino and Bedard 1997).

- Finally, there should be a focus on issues of trust. Children in situations of conflict and distress are at risk of having a declining trust in prosocial adults, making the work of early intervention programmes more problematic.

REFERENCES

Anderson, C.A. and Dill, K.A. 2000: Video games and aggressive thoughts: feelings and behaviour in the laboratory and in life. *Journal of Personality and Social Psychology* **78**: 772–90.

Ammerman, R.T. and Hersen, M. 1992: Current issues in the assessment of family violence. In Ammerman, R.T. and Hersen, M. (eds), *Assessment of Family Violence*, Vol. 1. New York: John Wiley, 3–11.

Apfel, R. and Simon, B.C. (eds) 1996: *Minefields in their Hearts: the Mental Health of Children in War and Community Violence.* New Haven, CT: Yale University Press.

Bailey, S. 1996: Adolescents who murder. *Journal of Adolescence* **19**: 19–39.

Bailey, S. 1997: Sadistic and violent acts in young people. *Psychology and Psychiatry Review* **2**(3): 92–102.

Bailey, S. and Aulich, L. 1997: Understanding murderous young people. In Weldon, E.V. and Van Velsen, C. (eds), *A Practical Guide to Forensic Psychiatry.* London: Jessica Kingsley.

Bailey, S., Smith, C. and Dolan, M. 2001: The social background and nature of 'children' who perpetrate violent crimes: a UK perspective. *Journal of Community Psychology* **29**: 305–17.

Bank, L. and Dawud-Noursi, S. 2001: The impact of violence on children: home, community and national levels. *Journal of Community Psychology* **2**(3): 189–93.

Barkley, R.A. 1990: *Attention Deficit Hyperactivity Disorder: a Handbook for Diagnosis and Treatment.* New York: Guilford.

Barkley, R.A. 1997: *Defiant Children: a Clinician's Manual for Assessment and Parent Training*, 2nd edn. New York: Guilford.

Berkowitz, L. 1993: *Aggression: Its Causes, Consequences and Control.* New York: McGraw-Hill.

Berrueta-Clement, J.R., Schweinhart, L.J., Barnett, W.S., Epstein, A.S. and Weikart, D.P. 1984: *Changed Lives: the Effects of the Perry Preschool Programme on Youths Through Age 19.* Ypsilanti, MI: High/Scope Educational Research Foundation Press.

Bilchick, S. 1998: Serious and Violent Juvenile Offenders. Department of Justice, *Office of Justice Programs, Office of Juvenile Justice and Delinquency Prevention.* NCJ 170027. Washington, DC: US.

Bjerregaard, B. and Lizottte, A.J. 1995: Gun ownership and gang membership. *Journal of Criminal Law and Criminology* **86**: 37–58.

Bjerregaard, B. and Smith, C. 1993: Gender differences in gang participation, delinquency, and substance use. *Journal of Quantitative Criminology* **9**: 329–55.

Blackburn, R. 1993: *The Psychology of Criminal Conduct.* Chichester: John Wiley.

Blacklock, N. 2001: Domestic violence: working with perpetrators, the community and its institutions. *Advances in Psychiatric Treatment* **7**(1): 65–78.

Block, R. and Block, C.R. 1993: *Street Gang Crime in Chicago: Research in Brief.* Washington, DC: US Department of Justice, Office of Justice Programs, National Institute of Justice.

Block, C.R. and Christakos, A. 1995: *Major Trends in Chicago Homicide: 1965–1994.* Chicago, IL: Illinois Criminal Justice Information Authority.

Block, C.R., Christakos, A., Jacob, A. and Przybylski, R. 1996: *Street Gangs and Crime: Patterns and Trends in Chicago.* Chicago, IL: Illinois Criminal Justice Information Authority.

Bullock, R., Little, M. and Millham, S. 1994: *The Part Played by Carer, Individual Circumstance and Treatment Interventions in the Outcomes of Leavers from the Youth Treatment Centres.* Dartington: Dartington Social Research Unit.

Burgess, A.W., Hartman, C.R., Hawe, J., Shaw, E.R. and McFarland, G.C. 1990: Juvenile murderers: assessing memory thorough crime scene drawings. *Journal of Psychosocial Nursing* **28**: 26–34.

Catalana, R.F. and Hawkins, J.D. 1996: The social development model: a theory of antisocial behaviour. In Hawkins, J.D. (ed.), *Delinquency and Crime: Current Theories.* New York: Cambridge University Press, 149–97.

Cavadino, P. and Allen, R. 2000: Children who kill: trends, reasons and procedures. In Boswell, G. (ed.), *Violent Children and Adolescents: Asking the Question Why?* London: Whurr, 1–18.

Chaiken, M.R. 2000: Violent Neighborhoods Violent Kids. Juvenile Justice Bulletin. *Department of Justice, Office of Juvenile Justice and Delinquency Prevention.* NJC 178248. Washington, DC. US.

Clare, P., Bailey, S. and Clark, A. 2000: Relationship between psychotic disorders in adolescence and criminally violent behaviour. *British Journal of Psychiatry* **177**: 275–9.

Coleman, J., for the Trust for the Study of Adolescence 1999: *Key Data on Adolescence*, 2nd edn. Brighton: TSA Publishing, 15–23.

Cornell, D.G., Benedek, E.P. and Benedek, B.A. 1987: Juvenile homicide: prior adjustment and a proposed typology. *American Journal of Orthopsychiatry* **57**: 383–93.

Csikszentmihalyi and Larson 1980: Intrinsic rewards in school crime. In Baker, K. and Rubel, R.J. (eds), *Violence and Crime in the Schools.* Lexington, MA: Lexington Books, 181–92.

Curry, G.D. and Decker, S.H. 1998: *Confronting Gangs: Crime and Community.* Los Angeles, CA. Roxbury.

Decker, S.H. and Van Winkle, B. 1996: *Life in the Gang: Family, Friends and Violence.* New York, NY: Cambridge University Press.

Douglas, S.J. and O'Shaker, M. 1995: *Mindhunter.* New York: Schriber.

Eichelman, B. 1988: Toward a rational pharmacotherapy for aggressive and violent behaviour. *Hospital Community Psychiatry* **39**: 31–9.

Elliott, D.S. 1994: Youth violence: an overview congressional program. *Children and Violence* **9**(2): 15–20.

Elliot, D.S., Hamburg., B.A. and Williams, K.R. 1998: *Violence in American Schools.* Cambridge: Cambridge University Press.

Esbensen, F. and Huizinga, D. 1993: Gangs, drugs, and delinquency in a survey of urban youth. *Criminology* **31**: 565–89.

Esbensen, F. and Osgood, D.W. 1997: *National Evaluation of GREAT Research in Brief.* Washington, DC: US Department of Justice, Office of Justice Programs, National Institute of Justice.

Farrington, D.P. 1995: The development of offending and antisocial behaviour from childhood: key findings from the Cambridge Study in delinquent development. *Journal of Child Psychology and Psychiatry* **36**: 929–64.

Fox, J.A. 1996: *Trends in Juvenile Violence: Report to the US Attorney General on Current and Future Rates of Juvenile*

Offending. Washington, DC: US Department of Justice, Bureau of Justice Statistics.

Garborino, J. 1995: *Raising Children in a Socially Toxic Environment*. San Fransisco: Jossey–Bass.

Garborino, J. 1999: *Lost Boys: Why our Sons Turn Violent and How We Can Save Them*. New York: Free Press.

Garborino, J. 2001: An ecological perspective on the effects of violence on children. *Journal of Community Psychology* **29**: 361–78.

Garborino, J. and Bedard, C. 1997: *Making Sense of 'Senseless' Youth Violence: Preliminary Report*. New York: Cornell University.

Garborino, J. and Kostelny, K. 1996: The impact of political violence on the behavioural problems of Palestine children. *Child Development* **67**: 33–45.

Gilligan, J. 1996: *Violence*. New York: Pulman.

Goetting, A. 1995: *Homicide in Families and Other Special Populations*. New York: Springer Verlag.

Gordon, R.M. 1994: Incarcerating gang members in British Columbia: preliminary study. Unpublished study, Ministry of the Attorney General. Victoria, BC.

Grisso, T. and Schwartz, R.G. 2000: *Youth on Trial: a Developmental Perspective on Juvenile Justice*. Chicago, IL: University of Chicago Press, 1–6.

Hagell, A. and Shaw, C. 1996: *Opportunity and Disadvantage at Age 16*. London: Policy Studies Institute.

Hambridge, J.A. 1990: The grief process in those admitted to Regional Secure Units following homicide. *Journal of Forensic Sciences* **35**: 1149–54.

Hamburg, M.A. 1998: Youth violence is a public health concern. In Elliot, D.S., Hamburg, V.A. and Williams, K.R. (eds), *Violence in American Schools*, 2nd edn. Cambridge: Cambridge University Press, 31–54.

Harbin, H.T. and Madden, D.J. 1979: Battered parents: a new syndrome. *American Journal of Psychiatry* **136**: 1288–91.

Harris, D.P., Cote, J.E. and Vipona, E.M. 1987: Residential treatment of disturbed delinquents: description of a centre and identification of therapeutic factors. *Canadian Journal of Psychiatry* **32**: 579–83.

Heide, K.M. 1999: *Young Killers: the Challenge of Juvenile Homicide*. Thousand Oaks, CA: Sage.

Hill, K.G., Hawkins, J.D., Catalano, R.F. *ct al.* 1996: The longitudinal dynamics of gang membership and problem behaviour: a replication and extension of the Denver and Rochester gang studies in Seattle. Paper presented at the annual meeting of the American Socity of Criminology, Chicago, Illinois.

Hollin, C.R. 1993: Advances in psychological treatment of delinquent behaviour. *Criminal Behaviour and Mental Health* **3**: 142–57.

Horowitz, R. 1983: *Honor and the American Dream: Culture and Identity in a Chicano Community*. New Brunswick, NJ: Rutgers University Press.

Howell, J.C. 1998: Promising programs for youth gang violence prevention and intervention. In Loeber, R. and Farrington, D.P. (eds), *Serious and Violent Juvenile Offenders: Risk Factors and Successful Interventions*. Thousand Oaks, CA: Sage, 284–312.

Hunter, A.J. and Chandler, G.E. 1999: Adolescent resilience image. *Journal of Nursing Scholarship* **31**(3): 243–7.

Johnson, D.L. and Walker, T. 1987: Primary prevention of behavioural problems in Mexican/American children. *American Journal of Community Psychology* **15**: 375–85.

Justice 1996: *Children and Homicide: Appropriate Procedures for Juveniles in Murder and Manslaughter Cases*. London: Justice.

Kelleher, M.D. 1998: *When Good Kids Kill*. Westport, CT: Praeger.

Kelley, B.T., Loeber, R., Keenan, K. and DeLamatre, M. 1997: Developmental pathways in boys' disruptive and delinquent behavior. *Juvenile Justice Bulletin*, Department of Justice, Office of Justice Programs, Office of Juvenile Justice and Delinquency Prevention. NCJ 165692. Washington, DC.

Kennedy, D. 1988: Pulling levers: getting deterrence right. *National Institute of Justice Journal* **236**: 2–8.

Klein, M.W. 1995: *The American Street Gang*. New York: Oxford University Press.

Kosterman, R., Hawkins, J.D., Hill, K.G. *et al.* 1996: The developmental dynamics of gang initiation: when and why young people join gangs. Paper presented at the annual meeting of the American Society of Criminology, Chicago, IL.

Kotlowitz, 1991: *There Are No Children Here*. New York: Doubleday.

Laub, J.H. and Lauristen, J.L. 1998: The interdependence of school violence with neighbourhood and family conditions. In Elliot, D.S., Hamburg, B.A. and Williams, K.R. (eds), *Violence in American Schools*, 5th edn. Cambridge: Cambridge University Press, 127–55.

Lally, J.R., Mangione, P.L. and Honigh, A.S. 1988: *Long-Range Impact on an Early Intervention with Low-Income Children and their Families*. Syradise University Family Development Research Programme.

Lewis, D.O., Moy, E., Jackson, L.D. *et al.* 1985: Biopsychosocial characteristics of children who later murder: prospective study. *American Journal of Psychiatry* **142**: 1161–7.

Lipsey, M.W. 1995: What do we learn from treatment research studies on the effectiveness with juvenile delinquents? In McGuire, J. (ed.), *What Works: Reducing Offending*. Chichester: John Wiley.

Loeber, R. and Farrington, D.P. (eds) 1998: *Serious and Violent Juvenile Offencers: Risk Factors and Successful Interventions*. Thousand Oaks, CA: Sage.

Loeber, R. and Hay, D.F. 1994: Developmental approaches to aggression and conduct problems. In Rutter, M. and Hay, D. (eds), *Development Through Life: a Handbook for Clinicians*. Oxford: Blackwell Science.

Lowry, R., Sleet, D., Duncan, C. *et al.* 1995: Adolescents at risk for violence. *Educational Psychology Review* **7**: 7–39.

Lynam, D. 1996: Early identification of chronic offenders: who is the fledgling psychopath? *Psychologist Bulletin* **120**: 209–34.

Maguine, E. and Loeber, R. 1996: Academic performance and delinquency. In Tonry, M. and Morns, N. (eds), *Crime and Justice*. Chicago, IL: Chicago University Press.

Maguire, K. and Pastore, A.L. (eds) 1996: *Sourcebook of Criminal Justice Statistics 1995*. Washington, DC: US Department of Justice, Bureau of Justice Statistics, US Government Printing Office.

Maughan, B., Pickles, A., Hagell, A., Rutter, M. and Yule, W. 1996: Reading problems and antisocial behaviour: developmental trends in comorbidity. *Child Psychology and Psychiatry* **37**: 405–18.

McMahon, R.J. 1999a: Conduct Problems Prevention Research Group. Initial impact to the fast-track prevention trial for conduct problems: I. The high-risk sample. *Journal of Consulting and Clinical Psychology* **67**: 631–47.

McMahon, R.J. 1999b: Conduct Problems Prevention Research Group. Initial impact to the fast-track prevention trial for conduct problems: II. Classroom effects. *Journal of Consulting and Clinical Psychology* **67**: 648–47.

McNally, R.B. 1995: Homicidal youth in England and Wales 1982–1992: people and policy. *Psychology, Crime and Law* **1**: 333–42.

Mercy, J. and Rosenberg, M.L. 1988: Preventing firearm violence in and around schools. In Elliott, D.S., Hamburg, B.A. and Williams, K.R. (eds), *Violence in American Schools*. New York: Cambridge University Press.

Miller, W.B. 1974: American youth gangs: past and present. In Blumberg, A. (ed.), *Current Perspectives on Criminal Behaviour*. New York: Knopf, 410–20.

Miller, W.B. 1992: *Crime by Youth Gangs and Groups in the United States*. Washington, DC: US Department of Justice, Office of Justice Programs, Office of Juvenile Justice and Delinquency Prevention.

Myers, W.C. and Scott, K. 1998: Psychotic and conduct disorder symptoms in juvenile murderers. *Journal of Homicide Studies* **202**: 160–75.

Myers, W.C., Scott, K., Burgess, A.L. and Burgess, A.G. 1995: Psychopathology, biopsychosocial factors, crime statistics and classification of 25 homicidal youths. *Journal of the American Academy of Child and Adolescent Psychiatry* **34**: 1483–9.

Osofsky, J. 1995: The effects of exposure to violence on young children. *American Psychologist* **50**: 782–8.

Pynoos, R. and Nader, K. 1988: Psychological first aid and treatment approach to children exposed to community violence: research implications. *Journal of Traumatic Stress* **1**: 445–73.

Roth, D.L. and Coles, E.M. 1995: Battered women syndrome: a conceptual analysis of its status *vis à vis* DSM-IV mental disorders. *Medicine and Law* **14**: 641–58.

Rutter, M. 1989: Pathways from childhood to adult life. *Journal of Child Psychology and Psychiatry* **30**: 23–51.

Rutter, M. and Smith, D.J. 1995: *Psychosocial Disorders in Young People: Time Trends and their Causes*. Chichester: John Wiley.

Rutter, M., Giller, H. and Hagel, A. 1998: Varieties of antisocial behaviour. In *Antisocial Behaviour by Young People*. Cambridge: Cambridge University Press, 115–17.

Sanders, W. 1994: *Gangbangs and Drive-bys: Grounded Culture and Juvenile Gang Violence*. New York: Cambridge University Press.

Sante, L. 1991: *Low Life: Lure and Snares of Old New York*. New York: Vintage Books.

Schweinhart, L.J., Barnes, H.V. and Weikart, D.P. 1993: *Significant Benefits*. Ypsilanti, MI: High/Scope Educational Research Foundation Press.

Sheldrick, C. 1999: Assessment and management of risk in adolescents. *Journal of Child Psychology and Psychiatry* **40**: 507–18.

Smith, P. and Sharp, S. (eds) 1994: *School Bullying: Insights and Perspectives*. London: Routledge.

Snyder, H.N. and Sickmund, M. 1995: *Juvenile Offenders*. Washington, DC. National Institute of Justice.

Snyder, H.N., Sickmund, M. and Poe-Yamagata, E. 1996: *Juvenile Offenders and Victims: 1996 Update on Violence*.

Washington, DC: Office of Juvenile Justice and Delinquency Prevention.

Spergel, I.A. 1990: Youth gangs: continuity and change. In Tonry, M. and Morris, N. (eds), *Crime and Justice: a Review of Research*, Vol. 12. Chicago, IL: University of Chicago, 171–275.

Spergel, I.A. 1995: *The Youth Gang Problem*. New York: Oxford University Press.

Spergel, I.A., Chance, R., Ehransaft, R. *et al.* 1994: *Gang Supervision and Intervention: Community Models*. Washington, DC: US Department of Justice, Office of Justice Programs, Office of Juvenile Justice and Delinquency Prevention.

Stewart, J.T., Myers, W.C. and Burket, R.C. 1990: A review of the pharmacotherapy of aggression in children and adolescents. *Journal of the American Academy of Child and Adolescent Psychiatry* **29**: 269–77.

Strauss, M.A. and Gelles, R.J. 1988: How violent are American families? Estimates from the national family violence resurvey and other studies. In Hotaling, G.T., Finkelhor, D., Kirkpatrick, J.T. and Straus, M.A. (eds), *New Directions in Family Violence Research*. Newbury Park, CA: Sage, 14–36.

Strauss, M.A. and Gelles, R.J. 1990: *Physical Violence in American Families: Risk Factors and Adaptations to Violence in 8145 Families*. New Brunswick, NJ: Transaction.

Strauss, M.A., Gelles, R.J. and Steinmetz, S.K. 1980: *Behind Closed Doors: Violence in the American Family*. New York: Anchor/Doubleday.

Thornberry, T.P. 1998: Membership in youth gangs and involvement in serious and violent offending. In Loeber, R. and Farrington, D.P. (eds), *Serious and Violent Offenders: Risk Factors and Successful Interventions*. Thousand Oaks, CA: Sage, 147–66.

Thornberry, T.P., Huizinga, D. and Loeber, R. 1995: The prevention of serious delinquency and violence: implications from the program of research on the causes and correlates of delinquency. In Howell, J.C., Hawkins, J.D. and Wilson, J.J. (eds), *A Sourcebook: Serious, Violent and Chronic Juvenile Offenders*. Thousand Oakes, CA: Sage, 213–37.

Toupin, J. 1997: Adolescent murderers: validation of a typology and study of their recidivism. In Wilson, A.V. (ed.), *Homicide: the Victim/Offender Connection*. Cincinnati, OH: Aronson, 135–56.

Turtle, J., Jonesm A. and Hickman, M. 1997: *Young People and Health: the Health Behaviour of School-Aged Children*. London: Health Education Authority.

Waplington, D. 1994: Understanding adolescents: a key concept in constructing the regime for young offenders at HMP YOI Lancaster Farms. *Prison Service Journal*, no. 96.

Wasserman, G.A. and Miller, L.S. 1998: The prevention of serious and violent juvenile offending. In Loeber, R. and Farrington, D.P. (eds), *Serious and Violent Juvenile Offenders: Risk Factors and Successful Interventions*. Thousand Oaks, CA: Sage Publications.

Wilson, P. 1973: *Children Who Kill*. London: Michael Joseph.

Wilson, J.J. and Howell, J.C. 1993: *Comprehensive Strategy for Serious, Violent, and Chronic Juvenile Offenders*. Washington, DC: US Department of Justice, Office of Justice Programs, Office of Juvenile Justice and Delinquency Prevention.

17

Sexually abusive behaviour by children and adolescents

EILEEN VIZARD

INTRODUCTION

Adult sexual offenders against children are now acknowledged to exist both inside and outside of family systems and to pose a limited but recognizable threat to vulnerable children. Media coverage of sexually aggressive children and adolescents has brought awareness but not understanding of the problem, and recent changes in the law relating to young offenders highlights the need for professional assessment of risk (Soothill 1997; Vizard 1999). The concept of sexually aggressive and abusive children has been discussed in the light of research evidence that 30–50% of all sexual abuse of children is perpetrated by people under 21 years old (Vizard *et al.* 1995). The natural history of sexually abusive behaviour by children towards other children is still not fully understood, although work with adult and adolescent perpetrators of abuse suggests that at least some of these individuals have started patterns of abusive behaviour in puberty or earlier (Longo and Groth 1983).

A major problem in identifying this group of children has been the lack of definitional agreement about the nature of the problem in childhood. This, in turn, has led to confusion and ambivalence about naming the behaviour, and referring children and young people on for assessment and treatment services. Even when children and young people are identified as being sexual abusers, few sustained professional efforts are made to halt the escalation of this juvenile behaviour into adult offending patterns.

This chapter discusses definitional issues, the prevalence of sexual abusing behaviour in childhood and adolescence, classification, typologies and theories of adolescent abusers, the clinical features of sexual offences committed by adolescents against others, and assessment and treatment approaches including evidence-based treatment outcome. The need for a review of the classification systems in relation to children and adolescents who sexually abuse is emphasized. Recommendations on the management of these complex child protection cases is made, along with policy suggestions for the future direction of this work on a local and a national basis.

LITERATURE REVIEW

The search for definitions

Since the early 1990s in the UK (NCH 1992), and rather earlier in the USA (Davis and Leitenberg 1987), the existence of a group of sexually predatory adolescents has been recognized and attempts at defining the behaviour of these children have been made (Vizard *et al.* 1995; Calder 1997a). However, there is still reluctance to refer children and adolescents who sexually abuse for assessment and treatment. One reason for the reluctance to refer young sexualized children for assessment may relate to professionals' fear of 'labelling' sexually aggressive children and adolescents (Vizard *et al.* 1996; Araji 1997a).

In fact, Araji (1997a) notes that there are a range of labels used to describe children under 12 years of age, including:

- 'children who abuse' (Cunningham and MacFarlane 1996)
- 'children who molest' (Gil and Johnson 1993a)

- 'child perpetrators' (Cunningham and MacFarlane 1991)
- 'children with sexual behaviour problems' (Pithers *et al.* 1993)
- 'sexually aggressive children' (Cantwell 1995)
- 'children who sexually act with criminal intent' (Hindman 1994).

However, Cantwell notes that certain terms are not appropriate because they assume that the abusing child is a victim (e.g. 'abuse reactive' – Cunningham and MacFarlane (1991)). It is pointed out that 'molestation' (to meddle with or to annoy) does not necessarily have a sexual connotation and that the term 'offender' may not have relevance for sexually abusive children under 10 years old who cannot be charged with a criminal offence. Both Cantwell (1995) and Araji (1997a) agree that the term 'sexually aggressive children' is more appropriate for young sexual abusers.

In reviewing these definitional dilemmas, Calder (1997a) identified seven different terms for children's sexual behaviour as follows:

- 'child perpetrators' (Johnson and Berry 1989)
- 'sexually aggressive' (Elliott and Butler 1994; Cantwell 1995; Araji 1997a)
- 'sexualized children' (Gil 1993b)
- 'sexual' (Schwartz 1996)
- 'pseudomature' (Schwartz 1996)
- 'abuse-reactive' (Cunningham and MacFarlane 1991)
- 'children who sexually abuse other children' (Dey and Print 1992; NCH 1992).

Clinical experience suggests that controversy about nomenclature is much greater for the prepubertal than for the pubertal and adolescent child abuser. This may be because society and professionals still have great difficulty in accepting that normal prepubertal children have a developing sexuality and that this may be corrupted occasionally into the sexual abuse of other children.

The emergence of younger pubertal and prepubertal sexual abusers has meant that a developmental perspective is urgently needed in any definitional discussion (Bremer 1993; Vizard *et al.* 1995; Calder 1997a; Araji 1997a). This is because the coercive sexualized behaviour of a 6-year-old child, for instance, cannot be understood and defined in the same way as the coercive sexualized behaviour of a 16-year-old. It may not be at all clear that the 6-year-old knew what he or she was doing or understood the consequences of the particular behaviour, in contrast to the 16-year-old who would have a much clearer idea of the seriousness of the behaviour and the consequences for himself or herself, and perhaps for the victim.

The whole debate about defining 'abnormal' sexualized or sexually abusive behaviour in childhood is greatly hampered by the lack of information and research on 'normal' childhood sexuality, despite the fact that in 1971 Michael Rutter noted that 'psychosexual issues occupy a central place in child development' (p. 259). Reviews of the literature on 'normal' psychosexual development, behaviour and knowledge (Hanks 1997; Heiman 1998) and childhood sexuality identify role (professional status) and gender (Heiman 1998) factors as confounding issues for research in this area. Vizard *et al.* (1995) highlight the importance of culture and ethics in this research. 'Professional interpretations of sexualized interactions between children may vary between cultures and over time' (p. 733), and it is pointed out that there may be ethical reasons (not just professional recalcitrance) for the lack of research in this area of work:

> 'The paucity of observational or experimental data on childhood sexuality is being, in part, attributed to ethical considerations where the mere act of observing induced sexual responses in children could lay the experimenter open to charges of child abuse (Bancroft 1989)'. (Vizard *et al.* 1995, p. 733)

However, research with clinical samples does throw important light on the possible links between adverse childhood experiences such as abuse and the later development of perpetrating behaviours. For instance, the findings from Freidrich *et al.*'s (1991) analysis of the child sexual behaviour inventory shows that characteristics of the child's victimization were evident in the child's later sexualized behaviour, with the implication that sexual behaviour problems may discriminate between sexually abused and non-sexually abused children. Freidrich's group's norm-setting research (Freidrich *et al.* 1991, 1992) has allowed for the construction of further research studying 'developmentally expected and developmentally problematic sexual behaviors' in a clinical sample of 100 sexually abused boys and girls enrolled in two treatment programmes (Hall *et al.* 1998). This research highlighted five variables which were predictive of sexual behaviour problems among sexually abused children:

- sexual arousal
- sadism during the child's sexual abuse
- a history of physical abuse
- a history of emotional abuse
- who the child blamed for that abuse.

These findings from a clinical sample of sexual abuse victims with very familiar symptoms begin to bring into focus the myriad of potential risk factors present in the backgrounds of such victims. Other research from the Great Ormond Street Hospital team in the UK (Skuse *et al.* 1998), looking at risk factors for the development of sexually abusive behaviour in sexually victimized adolescent males, found that discontinuities of care, witnessing or experiencing violence in the home, rejection by parents and unusual psychiatric symptoms were more commonly found in the boys who perpetrated sexual abuse than in the control groups. A specialist outpatient service for young sexual abusers (Vizard 1988) has also identified clinical risk indicators described below. Watkins and Bentovim's (1992) review of research in relation to the sexual abuse of male children provides a model describing the risk factors likely to be associated with becoming an abuser, and includes details of victimization, age of child, impact of the abuse and diagnosis.

Helpful as these risk factors may be, Jones (1998) has remarked that 'as practitioners we also need to bear in mind that some children with these risk factors will not develop interpersonal sexual behaviour problems'. This point is underlined by Bentovim (1998) in discussing victims who become perpetrators, when it is stated: 'Despite the paucity of reliable evidence, it is clear that the majority of children who are sexually abused do not become abusers' (p. 101).

Given that it will be some time before definitive research is written up in relation to 'normal' and 'abnormal' sexuality in childhood, texts which offer guidance to parents and children (Johnson 1989; MacFarlane and Cunningham 1988) as well as academic papers for professionals (Hanks 1997; Bremer 1993) are to be welcomed. Hank's discussion of normal sexual behaviour in childhood, tabulated by age and developmental status, is helpful to clinicians working with sexualized young children where a key question is often 'Is this abuse or is it "normal" childhood experimentation?' The point is made by Hanks that normal childhood sexuality is also culturally determined, and that:

'The arguments for healthy sexual development are complicated and for every culture are enshrined in rules and attitudes which in essence protect children and lean towards a healthy sexual fulfillment and development from childhood into adulthood rather than towards perverse, cruel, punishing or deviant behaviour.' (Hanks 1997, p. 17)

The labelling versus identification debate appears to be counterproductive, however, in that needy and dangerous children are being deprived of help and their victims deprived of protection whilst professionals wrangle over nomenclature. It is clearly anomalous that there is no child or adolescent version of paedophilia in either ICD-10 or DSM-IV which would allow children and adolescents who fulfil criteria for this disorder to be identified earlier or to be seen as suffering from a compulsion which is beyond their control without professional help. It has been suggested (Vizard et al. 1996) that a descriptive term such as 'sexual arousal disorder of childhood and adolescence' could be an acceptable name for this behaviour in childhood; whilst Jones (1998) has argued that 'sexual behaviour problems' might also be an appropriate term, and Judith Becker (personal communication, 1998) has indicated that 'sexual behavior disorder' might be a useful concept to include in classification systems.

Whatever the eventual nomenclature devised, it will be important for it to be useful and intelligible to clinicians. Clinical operational criteria for sexual arousal disorder have been devised and piloted in a number of UK projects dealing with young sexual abusers. Early findings (Vizard 1998)

Table 17.1 *Indicators and prognoses*

High-risk indicators/poor prognosis
- Increasing frequency of abusing
- Increasing severity of abusing (e.g. from fondling to buggery)
- Increasing perversity of abusing (bondage, gagging, use of objects)
- Decrease in age of victim
- Indiscriminate choice of boys or girls
- Abduction of a child
- More than one other paraphilia of any type
- Comorbid for sexual sadism and zoophilia
- Very low IQ
- Specific learning difficulty (communication disorders)
- PTSD with arousal to memories of both own abusing and abused experiences
- *3–16 years*: conduct disorder; childhood onset; severe
- *17–21 years*: antisocial/dissocial personality disorder
- Serious own emotional abuse and bullying
- Reactive attachment disorder of childhood before age 5 years
- More than four changes of placement in care
- Poor GAF score (i.e. below DSM-IV 30)

Lower-risk indicators/good prognosis
- Stable pattern of masturbatory fantasies
- PTSD characterized by low/absent arousal towards own abuse flashbacks
- Only one (or no) other psychiatric disorders
- Absence of conduct disorder/personality disorder
- No other paraphilias
- Few placement breakdowns
- No contact with abusive family (if relevant)
- *3–10 years*: can understand that behaviour is seriously wrong
- *11–16 years*: can envisage a realistic future life without abusing
- Any real remorse
- Any real victim empathy

have provided a list of risk factors and predictor variables, similar to certain of those reported by Hall et al. (1998). The presumed links between high-risk indicators and poor prognosis are based on clinical assessment of 143 young sexual abusers and will be validated by a follow-up study. The high-risk indicators/poor prognosis and lower-risk indicators/good prognosis from clinical assessment are listed in Table 17.1.

It has been suggested (Vizard 1998) that a form of words should be inserted into the DSM-IV manual to acknowledge that children under 16 years of age *do* sexually abuse other children. A similar modification to ICD-10 will be necessary to ensure consistent practice and coding of any new category for research purposes. However, even if such a suggestion is taken on board within the psychiatric classification systems, this alone will not overcome all the problems of professional resistance to identification and referral described earlier; but it may help to bring to an end a rather pointless debate about whether and how to describe this client group.

Prevalence

Reviews of the literature on epidemiology (Leventhal 1998) and incidence and prevalence (Finklehor 1994; Becker 1994) suggest that it is still not possible to know accurately the exact incidence (new cases per population in one year) or prevalence (the proportion of a population who are 'cases') at any point in time (point prevalence) or over a period of time (period prevalence) of juvenile abusing behaviour. A review of 19 USA studies (Finklehor 1994) indicated that rates of sexual abuse of between 2% and 62% reported by women and of 3–16% reported by men were reasonable summary statistics. There are well-documented methodological reasons for this very wide range of prevalences (Vizard 1989; Leventhal 1998), but Becker (1994) draws three main conclusions about the specific epidemiology of male perpetrators from the literature:

1 Approximately one-quarter to one-third are reported to be juveniles.
2 Many perpetrators report own sexual abuse but estimates for victimization vary widely.
3 Many perpetrators have abused more than one child.

In a cross-sectional study of the prevalence of child sexual abuse among 1116 adolescents in Geneva, Halperin *et al.* (1996) found that 35% of the 201 abusers described in the study were adolescents under 18 years of age, and this is in line with the prevalence rates reported in most studies (Horne 1991; Davis and Leitenberg 1987; Kelly *et al.* 1991) and reviews (Vizard *et al.* 1995) – which have concluded that 30–50% of all child sexual abuse is perpetrated by people under 21. It must also be remembered that in specialist residential settings (Johnson and Aoki 1993; Boswell 1996) groups of young sexually abused and abusing children may be placed together, with resultant high rates of over sexualized, sexually aggressive and sexually abusive behaviour by children and adolescents occurring among the residents.

At present, there is no one statistic available to give an accurate level of the rates of sexually abusive behaviour by juveniles.

Rather, the literature provides a series of estimates based on reported cases and retrospective studies of various sorts which must be taken together to give an overall picture of these rates. Added to this is the fact that many juvenile offenders are not even cautioned, so known abusing behaviour does not enter into the official statistics. It has been estimated (Hoghugi 1997) that in the North East of England 'only 10–15% of all *known* sexually abusive and offending adolescents are officially dealt with or reported for further legal and professional intervention' (p. 6). If this estimate is correct, and clinical

experience suggests that it may be, then the recorded crime figures discussed below are clearly a serious underestimate of the extent of the problem.

Home Office Statistics (Home Office 1998a, p. 22) indicate that the number of 10- to 17-year-olds sentenced for indictable offences rose for the third successive year in 1996 following falls in most years from 1986 to 1993. Within this group, the number of males aged 10–13 years sentenced fell by 300 between 1995 and 1996. This overall rise in serious crime in the 10- to 17-year-olds is not, however, reflected in the recorded figures for sexual offending for that age group, in which the number of offenders found guilty or cautioned fell from 78.2 per 100,000 population in 1981 to 42.6 per 100,000 in 1996 (Home Office 1998a, p. 13). The reasons for this fall in recorded sexual crimes by juveniles is not clear, and on the face of it could represent a trend away from recognition of the seriousness of the problem. However, the drop in cautioning and sentencing of juvenile sex offenders is also reflected in the adult sex offender statistics over the same period and may therefore represent other difficulties, such as inadequate evidence from vulnerable victims of abuse within an adversarial setting.

It should also be remembered that juveniles under 10 years (the age of criminal responsibility in England) committing sexual offences against other children will not be identified in official statistics about offenders.

The number of sexual offences for which juveniles aged 10–17 years were cautioned or sentenced in 1996, for instance, stood at 1100 out of a total of 6400 sexual offences for offenders of all ages (Home Office 1998a, p. 11); that is, 17.2 % of all recorded sexual offences were committed by juveniles. Even earlier in a study undertaken in Liverpool in 1989/90, Horne *et al.* (1991) estimated that the percentage of perpetrators aged under 18 years sexually abusing children was 36% of the sample studied, and many other studies now confirm these retrospectively reported rates of juvenile sexual assault on other children (for a review, see Vizard *et al.* (1995)).

A one-year period prevalence study of juvenile sexual offending in Oxfordshire showed a prevalence of 1.5 per 1000 males aged 12–17 years (James and Neil 1996), indicating the high levels of sexually aggressive activity undertaken by this age group.

However, it has become apparent that ever-younger children, well below the age of criminal responsibility (10 years old in the UK) are now involved in abusing other children. In reviewing nine research studies describing the demographics of 652 sexually aggressive children under 12 years of age in the USA, Araji (1997b) notes that the age range across all studies was 4–12 years with an average age at intake of 6.7 years for the four studies where data were available. Even allowing for methodological problems in this meta-analysis of existing studies, it is clear from the literature that referral of prepubescent children for sexually abusive behaviour has been occurring in the USA for some time.

This is still not the case to any great extent in the UK, as noted earlier, and the average age of most referred young perpetrators of sexual abuse against other children still remains in the teens (Richardson *et al.* 1995: $n = 100$, age range 11–18, mean 15.0 years; Vizard *et al.* 1996: $n = 80$, age range 8–21, mean 14.7 years; Manocha and Mezey 1998: $n = 51$, age range 13.1–17.8, mean 15.4 years). It appears that the evidence base and clinical experience with sexually abusive juveniles and sexually aggressive children has not yet convinced referrers in the UK to send sexualized pre-pubertal children for assessment and treatment.

CLASSIFICATIONS, TYPOLOGIES AND THEORIES

As mentioned earlier, it is not considered acceptable to apply adult criteria for paedophilia in ICD-10 or in DSM-IV to the assessment of child and adolescent sexual abusers. Therefore an anomalous situation exists in that highly disturbed children with compulsive problems of sexual arousal and aggression towards other children cannot be mentioned or described in any current psychiatric classification system. Efforts are being made to change this situation, but inclusion of the concept of juvenile sexual abusing in DSM-IV and/or ICD-10 could only be a beginning of a process of clarification about the origins, natural history and treatment outcome for different types of young abusers. Research is clearly needed in this area of classification and this may now be possible given the increased amount of information available about the characteristics of the population.

Given the complexity involved in defining the problem of sexually abusive behaviour in childhood, and given the persisting lack of clarity about normal sexual development in childhood, the prospect of constructing a typology of young sexual abusers may seem rather remote. However, several interesting and informative attempts have been made to achieve this task based on extensive clinical experience with young abusers in specialist services.

The reasons for attempting a typology of sexually abusing juveniles are discussed by Calder (1997a) and primarily relate to the need to take on board developmental and cultural issues as well as the fact that this population is heterogeneous and comorbid for a range of disorders and problems. The typology employed by O'Brien and Bera (1992) and discussed by Calder (1997a, pp. 13–14) describes seven different categories of adolescent sexual abuser as follows:

- naive experimenter/abuser
- undersocialized child exploiter
- pseudo-socialized child exploiter
- sexual aggressive
- sexual compulsive

- disturbed impulsive
- group-influenced.

These terms are self-explanatory, but this typology appears to be more suitable for children aged 11–18 years and does not take account of earlier patterns of sexualized or aggressive behaviour.

Some understanding of the transition from 'normal' childhood sexual behaviours to more pathological patterns is described in the form of a continuum by Johnson and Feldmeth (1993), consisting of four groups of children:

- group 1 – normal sexual exploration
- group 2 – sexually reactive
- group 3 – extensive mutual sexual behaviours
- group 4 – children who molest.

A meta-analysis (Graves 1996) of demographic studies between 1973 and 1993 of the characteristics of young sex offenders identified three categories of juvenile sexual offenders with distinct psychosocial profiles. These abuser types were:

- the paedophilic offender
- the sexual-assault offender
- the mixed-offence offender.

Graves was able to identify the paedophilic offender as coming from lower to mid socio-economic group, molesting much younger, female children and having maladaptive backgrounds. The sexual-assault offender was also from a lower to mid socio-economic group, lone-parent dysfunctional family and assaulted female victims within a wider age range. The mixed-offence offender came from lower socio-economic backgrounds, with a neglectful and possibly drug-abusing mother. They committed a range of offences, including other paraphilias, started offending at an early age and were described as having the most severe psychological and social problems.

A clinician with extensive experience of working with pre- and post-pubertal sexual abusers of other children is Janis Bremer, and her typology or continuum appears to span the developmental spectrum from normal to highly abnormal behaviour across the full age range encountered in practice. Bremer's (1993) continuum of sexual behaviours is as follows:

- normative
- inappropriate
- hypersexualized
- orgasm-orientated
- aggressive.

Bremer makes the points that these categories are not mutually exclusive (p. 271), and that the continuum differentiates between types of sexual behaviour in order to assist clinicians in deciding what form of intervention, if any, should be made.

With regard to theories of sexual offending, it is important to note that many ideas about offence-related thinking and behaviour are rooted in work with adult sex offenders (Abel *et al.* 1987; Beck-Sander 1995; McGregor and Howells 1997; Mezey *et al.* 1991). There is no doubt that there has been much to learn from work with adults, but the wholesale transposition of theories from an adult population to a growing and developing child and adolescent population should be viewed with caution.

Certain principles of cognitive–behavioural work with adults, based on an addiction model of sexual offending (Salter 1988; Maletzky 1991; Craissati and McClurg 1997; McGregor 1997; Eldridge 1998) which has been fully validated, tried and tested on a range of incarcerated and community-based adult sex offenders, have obvious relevance for work with older adolescent abusers. However, although many of these cognitive–behavioural concepts are used increasingly in the construction of treatment programmes for child and adolescent sexual abusers (see below), it must be questioned whether the principle of a lifelong 'addiction' to sexually abusive behaviour is viable when discussing the sexually aggressive behaviour of younger children. In such young children, the natural developmental processes will usually push the child back towards a normative developmental trajectory when external corrupting influences are removed (e.g. the recovery of seriously abused children placed in safe alternative care). Set against this natural restorative drive, however, is the impact of puberty and hormonal changes which clinical experience suggests may exacerbate and reinforce existing deviant sexual fantasies and make treatment more difficult during and after puberty (Hawkes *et al.* 1996). Hawkes and associates suggested that puberty may act on a combination of existing neurobiological sequelae of childhood trauma (Perry 1994) in the brain of the young sexual abuser, coupled with fear conditioning (Le Doux 1994) to create a neurophysiological state of traumatic sexual arousal which is activated in the presence of certain external cues and stimuli to abuse. This suggestion does not in any way imply that perpetration of sexual abuse by a child or adolescent is an automated or reflex behaviour which is beyond the individual's control. Rather is raised the possibility of physiological mechanisms in childhood which may have a reinforcing effect upon existing behavioural sequelae of abuse. Hawkes *et al.* (1996) attempt to bring together these biological issues, external familial, cultural factors and psychodynamic factors to form an 'integrated perspectives model' (pp. 95–101) in which the whole concept of the child as a changing and developing organism is central.

Existing reviews of theoretical models in relation to adult sex offending list the usual range of theories brought to bear on this type of delinquent behaviour: situational theories; feminist analysis; psychoanalytic perspectives and behavioural theories; psychodynamic theories; biological theories; and empirical theories (Marshall 1990; Lanyon 1991). They discuss the origins of abusing in the light of these perspectives. Singularly lacking from these

reviews based on work with adults is any clear acknowledgement of relevant child developmental issues in the childhood of the adult abuser, including early sexual arousal to other children, although adverse childhood experiences and child abuse are mentioned. Unsurprisingly, child protection issues and the wider systemic context around the abuser are seldom mentioned in the adult literature, although attempts to work with 'victim empathy' and the effect of the abuse on the victim are a core part of most behavioural programmes with adults.

However, a research-based approach to thinking about adult sexual offending has recently described paedophilia 'both as a pathology and a form of criminality' in which distinct behavioural themes in relation to the offence have allowed the development of a more complex, multivariate model of offence behaviour in paedophilia (Canter *et al.* 1998). Interestingly in this study of 97 recorded incidents of child sexual abuse in Lancashire, the offenders' ages ranged from as young as 10 years to 61 years, with the highest proportion of incidents being in relation to offenders aged between 17 and 27 years (p. 539). It appears that a proportion of child and adolescent offenders were therefore the subjects of study by adult mental health services and criminal justice workers, but from this research it was not clear how many (if any) of these children and adolescents subsequently received help. This may illustrate how easy it has been for this group of children to slip through the net of specialist service delivery for their age group. It is important to recognize these origins in adult services of much current intervention with child and adolescent sexual abusers so that appropriate services can be designed for children rather than simply scaled down in some way from work with adults. Examples of child-orientated modifications of work with adults, such as relapse prevention (Gray and Pithers 1993), are given later in the section on treatments.

Even Araji and Finklehor's (1986) four factor model of sexual offending is based on 'individual psychological and sociocultural explanations' (p. 94) of sexual offending in adult paedophiles. It does not refer to work with abusive children and adolescents because at that time relatively little was known about these young abusers. However, Bentovim and Williams (1998) have taken the notion of 'traumagenic dynamics' further to describe pathways in which the traumatic sexualization of the child or adolescent can lead to later perpetrating behaviour in certain at-risk cases (Bentovim 1998, p. 102). Both Freidrich and Schwartz discuss the failure of some abused boys to process traumatic events and the resultant traumagenic 'dysregulation' (Freidrich 1995, p. 5) of emotions and behaviour which can present as 'compulsive sexual behaviour' (Schwartz 1995, p. 49), some of which may be sexually abusive behaviour.

Hoghughi and Richardson (1997) offer a review of theoretical approaches to work with juvenile sex offenders which spans the feminist, family systems, dynamic, psychological, developmental and learning theory approaches put together in a child protection context. An integrated systemic/cognitive/behaviourally orientated child protection perspective is described by Calder (1997a) and this approach has similarities to the integrated perspectives approach described by Hawkes *et al.* (1996). Earlier reviews in the UK (NCH 1992) of children who abuse other children strongly support the use of multiple integrated models to understand this complex problem, and the need to use a multi-factorial model has also been advocated by USA research (Araji *et al.* 1986).

CLINICAL FEATURES

Clinical experience with this group of children and adolescents shows that they have multiple, concurrent psychosocial and behavioural problems (Richardson *et al.* 1995; Vizard *et al.* 1995; Freidrich 1995; Cantwell 1995; Araji 1997b; Vizard 1988) amongst which sexually aggressive or abusive behaviour is simply one feature.

Some studies point to the existence of conduct disorder as an important factor in the backgrounds of adolescents who sexually abuse (Bagley 1992; Richardson *et al.* 1995; Vizard 1998) and comparison studies looking at differences between young sexual abusers and other categories of juvenile delinquents (Ford and Linney 1995; Hastings *et al.* 1997) have concluded that adolescent sex offenders and conduct-disordered adolescents had more similarities to each other than to the controls.

Histories of abuse

Reviews have looked in detail at the characteristics of juvenile sex offenders (Becker 1994, 1998; Vizard *et al.* 1995; Araji 1997b) and the issue of own history of child abuse has been comprehensively addressed. It is clear that the range of reported rates of own sexual, physical and emotional abuse in the childhoods of young sexual offenders varies very widely, from 17% to 70%. In a study of 143 young sexual abusers aged between 6 and 21 years (Vizard 1998), 64% of the assessed children had a confirmed history of own sexual abuse.

Much of the variation in the reported rates of sexual abuse in young sexual offenders in the literature appears to depend on who asked what questions (if any) about abuse histories and at which point in the life of the young person such clinical or research questions were asked. However, it is clear from all studies that there is a proportion of juvenile and adult sex offenders who have not been sexually abused. Reviews point to the relevance of a history of physical abuse within the juvenile sex-offender population ranging from 13% to 46%. Other studies have highlighted the role of a climate of violence and fear at home, and research has shown that witnessing or being involved in domestic violence may be one of several risk factors for becoming a sexual offender (Ford and Linney 1995; Skuse *et al.* 1998).

Why do children abuse?

Professionals and public alike naturally seek explanations about why this behaviour occurs in children and young people. Research and clinical experience confirms Araji and Finklehor's (1986) view that there is no single-factor theory (e.g. being sexually abused) which can explain the origins of sex offending in adult life. Rather Araji and Finklehor's view that a multi-factorial explanation should be sought appears to be correct in relation to younger sex offenders and sexually aggressive children.

It is also clear from the literature and from clinical experience that in these cases, most of whom are seriously abused and neglected children, comorbid for a range of psychiatric, emotional and behavioural problems, that a progression from early childhood sexually aggressive behaviour to adolescent sexually abusive behaviour is highly likely without professional intervention.

Girls who abuse

This chapter, and most other publications dealing with adolescents who sexually offend, assumes that the majority of such children are boys. This is borne out by statistics and reviews. However, it must be remembered that professional and public resistance to envisaging girls as sexual predators is high, that many sexually aggressive girls are currently described as victimized or abuse reactive and therefore do not get referred for sexually abusive behaviour, nor do they become entered on to official statistics very much at present. These low reported rates appear to relate to low awareness of the problem and resistance to the notion of girls as abusers, a situation that is best addressed through public education and professional training.

Fehrenbach and Monastersky (1988) found that, when 28 adolescent girls were referred as abusers, they had committed serious offences. Fifty-three per cent had been referred for rape and 46.4% for indecent liberties, against children who may be notably younger (mean age 5.2 years) than the average age of victims of boy abusers. Also, the history of own sexual victimization for girls was 53.3% in those referred for rape and 46.1% in those referred for indecent liberties, indicating that half the sample had been sexually abused. Hunter *et al.* (1993), in a study of female sexual offenders in a residential treatment programme, reported that all of these girls had been sexually abused and that nine out of ten had a diagnosis of post-traumatic stress disorder. However, the small sample size indicates the limited data currently available on female sex offenders and points clearly to a direction for future research.

Reviews of the sparse literature on female adolescent sexual abusers indicate that girls are more likely than boys to be known to the victim, that they use persuasion rather than force with victims, and that they may gain physical access to younger victims sooner, perhaps through baby-sitting activities – which are seen as innocuous with girls whereas a boy may be viewed with more caution by parents.

Learning-disabled abusers

In relation to learning-disabled adolescent sexual offenders against children, Tudiver and Griffin (1992) found that mentally retarded adolescent sex offenders were similar to normal-intelligence sex offenders in that they lacked social skills, had poor impulse control and little victim empathy. As far as prevalence of sexual offending by learning-disabled adolescent sex offenders is concerned, very few adequate data are available. A study by Murphy *et al.* (1983) indicated that 10–15% of the sex-offender population had learning difficulties defined by an IQ of less than 70. Clinical experience and reviews (Vizard *et al.* 1995) suggest that learning disability, academic under-achievement, poor literacy and developmental delays are commonly found among the adolescent sex-offender population, and that an important confounding factor in clarifying the exact rate of offending by the learning disabled is the difficulty in defining learning disability or mental handicap. However, in the population of 143 children and adolescents referred to the Young Abusers Project (Vizard 1998), 36% of these children had clinically diagnosed DSM-IV mild mental retardation, an IQ of 50–55 to approximately 70, and many of the remaining children and adolescents had serious academic and school-based problems even when their cognitive abilities were adequate.

A key issue yet to be resolved by research is the extent to which any correlation between learning disability and sexual offending may be mediated by trauma or related to early childhood abuse. The traumagenic origins of certain forms of mild and moderate mental retardation have been described by clinicians (Sinason 1992) working in the field of sexual abuse. However, it is more likely that a history of own sexual abuse would act together with other childhood adversities to produce mild mental retardation, which is in any event associated with higher rates of psychiatric disorder, and that a combination of these and other factors could lead to sexual offending as a presenting feature of serious conduct disorder. In other words, there is no evidence to suggest a simple link between mental retardation and juvenile sexual offending although there is a higher than might be expected rate of mental retardation in this population.

High-risk indicators

Research describing differences between abused, abusing and non-abusing boys (Skuse *et al.* 1998) has highlighted certain risk factors. These research results, literature reviews and clinical experience strongly support a case for the earliest possible intervention with sexualized and disturbed young boys in order to prevent a progression into abusing behaviour.

In summary, a typical presentation of a high-risk sexually abusive adolescent would be a (hypothetical) case as follows:

> The patient is a developmentally delayed, mild learning-disabled, abused and neglected boy with several placement changes in the past, few close friends, hobbies and interests centring on younger children, childhood-onset conduct disorder with evidence of sexual fantasies about younger children, and patterns of targeting, isolating and grooming victims becoming more evident with each known or suspected incident. Typically such a boy and his sexual proclivities are well known to agencies and this type of case is characterized by the 'fat file' syndrome where all the above features are meticulously recorded but little coherent multi-agency action is taken.

Sexual homicide and other offences

Most children and adolescents with sexually aggressive or abusive behaviour will hurt their victims through emotional blackmail and abuse, physical and sexual violence and betrayal of trust. A small minority of much more dangerous children does exist, who abduct, rape (Soothill 1997) and occasionally murder (Bailey 1996) other children. Early indicators of such behaviour are becoming apparent in clinical populations, and high-risk indicators with a poor prognosis seem to include sexual sadism, multiple paraphilias, post-traumatic stress disorder with arousal to own abuse experiences, and fantasies of child abduction.

Information about serious juvenile sexual offending such as homicide is not readily available from Home Office statistics. In a study of 20 adolescent murderers, 18 males and two females aged 11–18 years, Bailey (1996) found that over a third of the victims (of both sexes) had been sexually assaulted. A subsequent sample of 25 child and adolescent murderers 'displayed similar characteristics but were younger (some pre-pubertal), and the older group had more significant histories of drug abuse and more sadistic and sexual elements to the homicidal act'.

These findings are borne out by other work in the USA (Myers 1994) which looked at a small sample of 14 juvenile sexual homicides. There was a high prevalence of conduct disorder, sadistic fantasies, cruelty to animals and histories of childhood abuse in the backgrounds of these sexual killers.

Although sexual homicides by children and adolescents are rare, clinical experience strongly suggests the need for earlier assessment and identification of high-risk indicators for sadistic young sexual abusers who may go on to commit such crimes.

An association with other paraphilic offences has been reported (Vizard 1998) and links between the sexual abuse of children and the zoophilic abuse of animals has also been described (Duffield *et al.* 1998). In the latter cases admitted to the Young Abusers Project, seven male children aged 8–16 years were studied, with further information being available on seven more children who had a documented history of non-sexual cruelty to animals. The seven who had sexually abused other children as well as having performed a sexual act with an animal were seriously emotionally disturbed and aggressive, four out of the seven had learning difficulties, none was exclusively fixated on animals, and all showed rather indiscriminate object attachments. It was clear that the abuse of the animals had been as carefully planned and executed as the abuse of the child victims. All of this small sample were from deeply deprived and abusive home backgrounds, and the study concluded that zoophilia and cruelty to animals might well be under-reported in the literature because of embarrassment and reluctance by clinicians to take a full history. Other characteristics of the cases seen in the Young Abusers Project include sexual sadism (12%) and firesetting (21%), as well as zoophilia and cruelty to animals (20%).

In a larger sample of 143 young sexual abusers seen in the same service, Vizard (1998) found predominant diagnoses of conduct disorder, post-traumatic stress disorder, deliberate self-harm and high levels of own sexual abuse. The findings show that these children and young people are exceptionally disturbed, comorbid for more than one (and sometimes more than two) psychiatric disorders, and in need of specialist assessment and treatment. The traumagenic nature of their backgrounds suggests that the aggressive and deviant behaviour of young sexual abusers is rooted in seriously adverse early parenting experiences such as child abuse and multiple changes of placement, a finding highlighted elsewhere (Skuse *et al.* 1998).

More recently, even younger sexually aggressive children under 10 years old have been seen in the Young Abusers Project, and it may be relevant to a discussion about traumagenic origins of abusive behaviour to note that many of these younger children aged 6, 7 or 8 years fulfil criteria for reactive attachment disorder of childhood which links early childhood adverse and abusive attachment experiences with later maladjustment and relationship problems.

APPROACHES TO ASSESSMENT AND TREATMENT

Assessment

Most clinicians working with sexually aggressive younger children and sexually abusive older adolescents agree that a structured and carefully planned, multi-agency approach is most helpful (Becker 1990; O'Callaghan and Print 1994; Vizard 1996; Graham *et al.* 1997; Calder 1997b; Gray and Wallace 1992). Whether or not an outpatient or residential assessment is to be done, there is agreement that a focused approach is best. Specialist outpatient assessment of juvenile sexual offenders has been described as containing three stages (Vizard 1996):

1 Clarification and rapport building.
2 Mapping the abuse: the fantasies, strategies and behaviours.
3 The future: placement, treatment and personal change.

Within this semi-structured approach to interviewing, it is expected that the interviewers will take the lead in the assessment, that careful observations of the child or adolescent's verbal and non-verbal responses will be made, that a full mental state examination will be done on children and adolescents of all ages, and that child protection issues will be actively considered within a model of open confidentiality. Other clinical teams working with juvenile sexual abusers describe similar or more structured assessment protocols. Gray and Wallace's (1992) *Adolescent Sexual Offender Assessment Packet* starts with prescriptive and comprehensive lists of advice for interviewing high-risk youths. It comments at the outset: 'The following do's and don'ts are recommended when interviewing high-risk youth including antisocial clients, adolescent sexual offenders, aggressive and passive–aggressive clients, clients who frequently lie and exploit and juvenile firesetters' (p. 7). Some of the do's are the following:

- Do control the interview.
- Do state immediately and clearly the nature of the interview.
- Do keep the focus on the client and swiftly and repeatedly bring the client back to task.
- Do ask 'what' and 'how' questions, not 'why'.
- Do track your feelings during the interview (if you're feeling exploited, validate this through changing course).
- Do respect the client as a whole individual, capable of change.

Some of the don'ts are:

- Do not agree to keep secrets (obtain all necessary releases of information at the time of the initial interview).
- Do not relinquish interview control (do use control positively to reinforce the client when responsibility is taken for any personal behavior).
- Do not be diverted (do keep the focus firmly on the client, where you want it).
- Do not 'need' or 'want' something from the client (do care and detach).
- Do not isolate yourself (do seek colleague input and support, share concerns, ideas and feelings, attend trainings and network).

The general clinical experience in assessing clients with a problem of addiction such as sexual offending (whether adults or children) is that evasion, trivialization and denial of the seriousness of offending behaviour is the norm. Assessing such an individual therefore requires considerable forensic skills which are needed over and above the usual level of clinical interviewing skills expected in mental health work. This approach is one which may seem uncomfortable to professionals predominantly trained within a more client-centred, 'facilitating', psychotherapeutic or family-systems framework. Conversely, professionals trained in cognitive–behavioural work, parent training work or any type of Court-related forensic work may find this close-focused, therapist-controlled type of assessment much more straightforward. It may be particularly difficult for professionals who have been highly trained to work in a play-centred, 'facilitating' manner with child-abuse victims, to learn to practice in a different and much more strategic fashion with child and adolescent perpetrators. This skills deficit is often difficult for trained child-as-victim workers to accept since many child perpetrators are, of course, victimized themselves, look and behave just like other victims at times, and can inspire strong countertransference feelings of sympathy and sadness in experienced workers. It may, at times appear that such an assessment process is being 'cruel to be kind', but it has also been pointed out (Vizard 1996) that the child will not be helped by interviewer avoidance and that an acceptable language for unacceptable behaviour must be found by the interviewer so that everyone (including the child) can be clear about how to proceed.

For instance, even with quite young children who feel guilty about what they have done, interviewer qualities of focus and persistance are needed to ensure that the child is brought back to task and not allowed to drift off or to distract unduly into other topics. This does not prevent the interviewer from using age-appropriate methods to talk with young and learning-disabled child perpetrators. Drawing materials, small play therapy toys including human figures, wild and domestic animals and toy vehicles, etc., plus a set of anatomically correct dolls should always be provided on a low table in front of such young children during every assessment interview.

With older adolescents who may be more verbal than younger children, it should be made clear that they will be expected to contribute to the discussion, to put their own views across, to agree or disagree with the interviewer as necessary, and at all times to remember the serious nature of their problem which has brought them for help. It is often helpful to provide a flip chart and pens for children and adolescents of all ages.

Given the high levels of denial, prevarication and outright lies which can be expected from many sexual abuse perpetrators at all ages, it is essential that the interviewer be well versed and trained in questioning techniques (such as circular questioning) to avoid pointless arguments with the perpetrator, that the interviewer be constantly aware of his or her own feelings (countertransference) as the assessment proceeds, and that a very clear focus on the assessment issues is kept at all times. These requirements are not simple and the countertransference issues in work with child and adolescent perpetrators are considerable (Woods 1997; Vizard and Usiskin 1999). For these reasons, live supervision of the assessment work through earbugs/phone is strongly recommended. In this way, interviewer over- or under-reactions can be modified by advice from the supervising team, and any discrepancies in the story given by the perpetrator to the interviewer in the room can be picked up by the supervising team who will also be joined by the local referrer for most of the assessment interview.

Furthermore, it is clearly important that the wider systemic context and the local concerns which led to the case being referred are brought into the assessment interview in a concrete manner. This can be achieved by asking the referring professional to name the nature of the child perpetrator's problem at the outset of the meeting and to explain why help is being sought from the specialist team. It thus becomes clear to everyone, including the child or adolescent perpetrator, that the problem is serious, that outside help is needed, and that the referrer remains responsible for the case. These may seem mundane considerations but, in fact, it is commonplace for referrers and the abusing child or adolescent to believe that the case will be 'handed over' (indefinitely) to the specialist team to 'cure' the abusive behaviour. There are many advantages of recruiting the help of the local referrers and other colleagues into supporting the assessment process in this way, and these include the continued professional support for any further assessment, and support for subsequent treatment input (Vizard 1999).

It is of fundamental importance that the whole assessment process be undertaken in a full child-protection context (Home Office 1991). This means that the young sexual abuser is seen as a 'dual status' child who is both a perpetrator of abuse posing a risk to other children and liable to prosecution (if aged 10 years in England and Wales) as well as being a vulnerable child in need in terms of the Children Act 1989. A full multi-disciplinary and inter-agency approach (Home Office 1991; Vizard 1996) is required to implement a safe assessment and to ensure that appropriate subsequent intervention and help is made available. It follows, therefore, that there are serious professional and ethical problems facing solo practitioners who attempt to undertake one-off 'risk assessments' of such children and adolescents outside of a full multi-disciplinary, child-protection, systemic context.

Treatment: general issues

In recent years, greater awareness of the existence of juvenile perpetrators of sexual abuse has led to a proliferation of treatment programmes, noted by Becker (1998) to have increased from 20 in 1982 to more than 800 specialized programmes in 1993 in the USA. Nevertheless, the quality of work undertaken in many of the new programmes is as yet unclear. Treatment outcome studies suggest that there is rather little agreement about the key components of treatment (Vizard *et al.* 1995, p. 742). Nevertheless, it is encouraging that such therapeutic work is at last being undertaken in an attempt to break the cycle of sexual abuse.

Treatment of young sexual abusers may include work with the individual child through individual or group work, work with the family, and support from the professional network. In the UK it appears that, by the time a sexually aroused or sexually abusive adolescent arrives for treatment, he will almost certainly have been removed from his home context and placed in care with little realistic chance of rehabilitation. In contrast, referrals of younger sexually aggressive children aged under 10 years to the Young Abusers Project in the UK has shown that many of these children are still living with their own families or are very recently removed into foster care with the hope of rehabilitation home. In practice, this means that family work aimed at rehabilitation with an older adolescent sexual abuser aged 14 or 15 is less likely to be requested than family work with a young sexually aggressive child aged 8 or 9. Furthermore, the natural history of child and adolescent sexual arousal to other children also means that by age 15 years, say, it will be much more difficult for any form of treatment, including family work, to show convincing evidence of intrapsychic, attitudinal and behavioural change. This means is that the chances are rather low of an adolescent sexual abuser being returned home to live with younger siblings or with access to vulnerable children unless treatment can show convincing change in thinking, attitudes and behaviour. However, every case is different and there may be adolescent cases for whom treatment shows clear evidence of change and where a very carefully monitored return home is possible.

In reviewing family systemic approaches to work with young sexual offenders, Bentovim (1998) emphasizes the need for 'assessment of potential to engage in treatment' and recaps on the previously described categories (Elton 1988) of hopeful, doubtful or hopeless cases in relation to the prognosis for treatment. It is clear from this and other work that a very thorough assessment of treatability must precede any attempts at family therapy in child abuse cases, and particularly when the child or adolescent is a perpetrator.

When a decision to undertake family treatment has been made, Bentovim (1998) outlines the following stages in a possible treatment process:

- the crisis of disclosure
- family assessment
- therapeutic work in a protective context for the victim
- reconstruction and reunification of the family.

It is however, pointed out that the 'family' may not just be the biological family but may include the child's foster family or the network within a residential unit where these are the long-term placements for the child. Calder (1997b), Sirles *et al.* (1997) and Bentovim (1998) all emphasize the need to integrate any work with family or parent group work with other treatment interventions for the individual child so that a multi-pronged approach is always used.

With juvenile sexual abusers it is important to remember that the child as a whole person needs to be offered help and that treatment approaches which focus only on the issue of sexual abusing behaviour will not address the many other emotional developmental needs of this type of child. It is also essential that issues of ethnicity, culture and gender, of both the referred child and of the assessing team, are taken into account at the outset. The referral of a black or ethnic-minority child or adolescent sexual abuser to a predominantly white specialist team, for instance, may have the effect of making that child or young person feel even more stigmatized and unfairly treated than may already be the case, since many black and ethnic-minority children and adolescents suffer from racism regardless of their own behavioural problems. Hence, the issues of ethnicity, culture and gender need to be named and sensitively addressed by the specialist team when the case is referred, in the assessment interview with the child or young person, and in any reports subsequently produced. It does not follow, however, that in naming issues of ethnicity, culture or gender the child or young person is going to be treated differently from other young people, or that an easier or a harder line of questioning, for instance, will be pursued. Rather these issues are to be seen in the overall life context of the young person and need to inform any discussion of what sexually aggressive behaviour, for instance, might mean in his or her particular culture.

Given the high rates of co-morbidity reported for this population, it is clearly important that help be given for all other physical and mental health problems identified at the time of assessment. For instance, there is no point in starting a learning-disabled, hearing-impaired sex offender in challenging group work which will definitely stir up strong feelings, until the degrees of learning disability and hearing impairment have been fully assessed. Similarly, a diabetic child who is sexually aggressive and who controls adults and carers by manipulating his blood sugar levels will require psychological help for this behaviour, and the help may need to be undertaken concurrently with group or individual therapy for his sexual arousal. There are also children and adolescents with pre-existing medical problems such as asthma and eczema which assessment may suggest will be exacerbated by the stress of treatment; these issues should be fully explored with the child's carer and with the child before treatment begins.

A major issue to be resolved before any form of treatment is started is the child-protection context in which help will be given. It has been noted that all assessment and treatment of young sexual abusers needs to be undertaken in a full child-protection context, but this must remain in the forefront of thinking for the case manager and for the treatment team long after the child or young person has started in therapy. This is because new child-protection material may emerge at any time – on escorted trips to therapy, in the therapy session or in the care context between sessions. Quite often such material may not emerge for several months into therapy.

It must be established quite clearly that the sexually aggressive child or the sexually abusive adolescent cannot enter into group or individual therapy if he is known to be living at home with a potential victim, or if he is known to have access to vulnerable children. Pouring water into a bucket perforated with holes may be a reasonable metaphor here, where the bucket represents the leaky container of the child's mind and the water represents the wasted therapeutic effort. Another way of looking at this situation is to remember the role of masturbatory rehearsal of sexual fantasies about intended child victims of sexual abuse (Vizard *et al.* 1995) in relation to juveniles who sexually abuse. When a young sexual abuser is receiving psychotherapy which encourages him to stop entertaining deviant sexual fantasies about victims, then returns home to meet his intended victim or other vulnerable children, this situation is clearly going to give him several contradictory messages. These messages will be that (a) it must be all right to masturbate to sexual thoughts about children or there would not be children left in his home for him to see; (b) the therapy/therapist is powerless to stop him from continuing these thought processes; and (c) all adults are hypocrites and liars, like his own abuser, since they tell him one thing and then let him do another thing (have access to victims). In purely practical terms it is impossible for group or individual therapists to engage the mind of the young abuser in a process of change when the abuser's mind is still caught up in a reinforcing cycle of pleasurable sexual fantasy.

However, although it may be relatively straightforward to agree the removal of the more obviously dangerous adolescent sexual abuser from a home or care context with other vulnerable children, it is often much more difficult to agree appropriate arrangements for a much younger sexually aggressive child to receive treatment outside of a context where there are other children. It is in these cases that inter-professional disputes may begin about whether this is really sexual abuse, what it should be called if it is not abuse, and whether 'labelling' is damaging, etc. One negative result can be that the younger sexually aggressive child is relabelled as a sexual abuse victim and not as an aggressor, and the request for treatment of sexual arousal is quietly dropped whilst victim-focused services are approached instead. However, in better-managed cases (see below) a focus on sexual aggression is kept, child-protection measures are implemented, and treatment is set up within a care

plan which can envisage eventual rehabilitation home as one possibility. When local colleagues comment that even a temporary separation of young children from other children may seem harsh, this must be acknowledged but the question still remains: 'What is the course of action which is in the long-term best interests of this child and other children?' Furthermore, consideration must be given to the effect of this distorted message on the victim of abuse if his or her abuser is then allowed access whilst professionals continue to talk about keeping children safe. When such situations arise, at least two children (the victim and the abuser) lose trust in adults yet again.

It needs to be pointed out to anxious referrers of younger children that there is a surprisingly small time span, perhaps between the ages of 5 and 10 years, in which a truly primary preventative approach to sexual aggression and subsequent sexual offending can be taken. It should be emphasized that by the time most pubertal adolescent sexual abusers present for treatment services, they may have experienced up to five years of pleasurable masturbatory reinforcement of deviant sexual fantasies about children which they will be very unwilling to change, making the likelihood of safe rehabilitation of this group of children much less certain than for their junior, pre-pubertal counterparts.

The need for the therapist (group or individual) to establish clear rules with the referrer and the young person of 'open confidentiality' in relation to child protection matters has been described (Vizard and Usiskin 1999). Given that group and individual therapy are likely to stir up very strong feelings in the young sexual abuser, his carers and the treatment team, and given the constantly looming threat of the young person 'acting out' in therapy by re-offending, such openness in communication is not just desirable but is essential to ensure that more children are not abused. Interestingly, clinical experience of individual therapy with young sexual abusers (Woods 1997; Vizard and Usiskin 1999) confirms the paradox that more openness and directness with such secretive and evasive young people is perceived as containing and reassuring. This may be because it then seems as if the therapist has passed the first 'test' – not being a secretive, collusive and deceitful adult like previously abusive carers, and (see above) is not saying one thing and doing another.

Finally, a treatment context which provides regular support for the carers (Griffin *et al.* 1997) and consultation to the professional network is essential if the young person's treatment is to succeed.

Brief overview of some treatment programmes

The range of treatment approaches currently available in ten different programmes for young sexual abusers of other children is reviewed by Sirles *et al.* (1997), and a helpful summary of the programmes reviewed is laid out as a chart which includes the name of the program (SPARK, STEP, RSA, etc.), the ages served, the theories utilized and the treatment modalities offered. The review confirms that 'multiple theoretical approaches and treatment modalities have been found useful for intervening with sexually abusive or aggressive children' (p. 191), and that such complex, integrated interventions are preferable to a single-model approach.

It is striking that all ten programmes reviewed by Sirles and associates included a cognitive–behavioural component, whatever other modalities were also used. This reflects the predominance of the cognitive–behavioural approach in both assessment (Calder 1997b) and in treatment (Becker 1990; Bremer 1993; Richardson *et al.* 1997) which is linked to the same preference in work with adult offenders (Eldridge 1998). A key difference in cognitive–behavioural work with young sex offenders as opposed to their adult counterparts, however, is that virtually all the programmes offered are also rooted in systematic thinking and child-protection practice and there is, apparently, a flexibility and openness to other approaches.

It is not possible to advocate one treatment programme as preferable to another, but two approaches from the SPARK and STEP services will be mentioned, followed by a brief description of the treatment approaches used in the Young Abusers Project.

SPARK

In the SPARK programme, derived from earlier work by MacFarlane and Cunningham (1988), the treatment approach is based on theories derived from post-traumatic stress disorder, addiction theory and the sexual abuse cycle as well as other concepts from within the victim and offender field of work. Treating children between the ages of 4 and 13 years who have molested other children, the programme uses group therapy for children and parents groups as the primary treatment modalities. Group treatment goals are set out for each child in relation to the following topics: specific antecedents to sexual acting out for each child; social skills; self-esteem; internalized locus of control; feeling recognition; own victimization; decreasing impulsive behaviors; empathy development; gaining mastery over problematic behaviors; and identifying and using resources. The parent groups are held concurrently and focus on the same issues as the children's groups but also allow a forum for the parents to discuss their own victimization and parenting issues. In reviewing this programme, Sirles *et al.* (1997) note that its strengths are the inclusion of all the family members and the modification of the group treatment programme to the developmental stage of the child.

STEP

The STEP programme (Gray and Pithers 1993) is cognitive–behavioural but uses a modified relapse prevention approach which is adapted to the developmental needs of the much younger perpetrator who may also be a victim. Groups for children between the ages of 6 and 12 years are subdivided according to age and cognitive ability. Parent groups are also held, and both children and parents are in treatment for 32 weeks. The goals for the groups in the STEP programme are similar to those set by the SPARK programme, and there is an additional emphasis on learning adaptive skills and taking measures to prevent relapse.

YOUNG ABUSERS PROJECT

The group work programme in the Young Abusers Project is cognitive–behavioural and is set within a family and professional systems context, but it also draws on psychodynamics and trauma theory. At the outset of work with older adolescent sexual abusers in 1992, the Young Abusers Project provided a more discursive and dynamically orientated approach to group work in which cognitive–behavioural principles were increasingly used as the true addictive nature of the young people's problem became evident. Over the succeeding years the average age at referral fell from 17 years in 1992 to 14.7 years in 1996. However, the age range is 6 to 21 years, and many more children under 10 years old now attend for assessment and treatment. Furthermore, although 95% of the first 143 cases were male and only 5% female (by 1996), an increase in the number of girls referred to the Young Abusers Project has been noted, and several of these sexually aggressive girls have been pre-pubertal. These demographic changes have led to a substantial modification of the group treatment programme which has treated children as young as 11 years.

Initially, cognitive–behavioural groups were run with a highly structured closed-group format once per week for 30 weeks on an outpatient basis with a concurrent professional carer's group (Griffin *et al.* 1997). The work undertaken with the young people was along the lines of a 'quest' to find the hero inside themselves and to stop abusing. The programme sought to externalize a dialogue between the young persons' hero and his or her internal enemy (i.e. that aspect which wanted to abuse) through the use of role play, cognitive–behavioural excercises, reinforcement of positive attitudes, structured group discussion on certain topics, and homework supervised by carers. The treatment intervention was part of an agreed care plan for the young person in which therapy, education, healthcare and placement issues were all addressed. For several young people, concurrent individual psychotherapy (with a different therapist from those running the group) was also necessary. All young people in group work were seen for regular follow-up groups, and professional consultations were offered to the network supporting their care.

With time it became obvious in the Young Abusers Project that 30 sessions of therapy was far from adequate for this needy and dangerous client group and their carers. It was usually just becoming clear what the level of need of the young abuser really was when the 30-week programme drew to a close, and not all young people in group work are assessed as suitable for continuing in individual therapy. This is clearly one of the limitations of offering outpatient treatment services to young people whose extensive needs might be more intensively and more rapidly addressed in a residential setting. However, set against this limitation is the importance of keeping the young person within the community and in touch with existing friends and family so that rehabilitation home is more readily achieved.

Added to concerns about the shortness of the 30-week programme have been the constant requests to the Young Abusers Project for additional support and training of the carers, particularly the foster carers, with the clear feedback that parenting such sexually aroused and conduct-disordered children is an overwhelming task for which training and support is needed. The carers' feedback confirms that containment of young sexual abusers may be particularly stressful during treatment since the treatment process itself may stir up strong feelings which become enacted in the home context.

As a result, the project has revised the treatment programme to run for 45 weeks with concurrent sessions for the young people and for the carers lasting a full morning or afternoon. The overall model remains cognitive–behavioural within a systemic child-protection context. There is now a strongly educational component to the work with the carers, and regular reviews for each young person are built into the group programme.

As far as individual therapy with young abusers is concerned, cases seen in the Young Abusers Project have been described (Woods 1997). The themes emerging include 'sexualization of attachments, re-enactments of the abuse, and a constant testing of the boundaries of the therapeutic relationship' (p. 379). It is clear that individual therapy poses special challenges to the therapist, and that a flexible, child protection-orientated and (perhaps paradoxically) reality-based approach is required in order to access the inner worlds of these children. Vizard and Usiskin (1999) have described the professional framework within which such individual therapy is best conducted and have indicated the range of 'acting out' behaviours which may be seen in the young person, his or her carer and in the therapist. All of these 'acting out' behaviours may be damaging to the integrity of the treatment, and much of this is best addressed in case management meetings and in psychotherapy supervision of the individual's treatment. It is essential that only fully trained and supervised child psychotherapists undertake

this specialist individual therapy with young sexual offenders. This is because the level of perversity of the fantasy material presented, the intensity of the transference and countertransference issues, and the real possibility of physical and sexual threat to the therapist mean that these are particularly challenging cases requiring a careful approach and an appropriately supportive professional network (Vizard 1999).

Clinical experience (Vizard 1998) suggests that abusive children and young people assessed as having more lower-risk indicators are likely to do better in cognitive–behavioural group work and in individual therapy than the high-risk group who are often unable to tolerate the social and emotional constraints of a therapy setting.

In conclusion, in relation to the treatment of young sexual offenders, Bentovim summarizes some of the key requisites:

'There is no one narrow therapeutic approach which is appropriate for addressing the multiple, complex problems associated with adolescent perpetration of sexual abuse ... it has been argued that treatment must be multi-focused; involve the multiple agencies associated with child protection; and be grounded in a theoretical approach which is integrative and systemic.' (Bentovim 1998, p. 134)

Evidence–based treatment outcomes

Treatment outcome has been reviewed elsewhere (e.g. Becker et al. 1988; Vizard et al. 1995) and will not be discussed here in detail. However, it is clear that a major problem in measuring treatment outcome is the lack of consensus about what constitute relevant outcome goals and measures. As Sirles et al. (1997) remark:

'It is not sufficient to conduct practice based on the collective wisdom of experts, theoreticians or blind faith. Each case needs to be scrutinized for goal attainment as well as for areas that need further development or changes.'

At the time of writing, 12 young people had received individual weekly psychotherapy in the Young Abusers Project and all needed treatment for more than two years (with one young man in treatment for four years). Only one of these young people had re-offended (as far as is known), in line with most treatment outcome studies which show that treatment generally has a protective effect against recidivism, as does follow-up. Of the 16 young people who had received group therapy in the Young Abusers Project, three had re-offended, but on follow-up all remained offence-free. Whether or not individual psychotherapy alone can effect attitudinal change is doubtful, so it may be unwise to rely solely on any one form of therapy, particularly individual therapy.

In one study (Borduin et al. 1990), 16 adolescent sex offenders were randomly assigned to multi-systemic therapy (MST) for an average of 37 hours and to individual therapy (IT) for an average of 45 hours. The sexual-offence recidivism rate was significantly higher in the IT group. The authors point to the possible lack of a theoretical consensus amongst analytic practitioners resulting in a rather unfocused approach to the work, plus the lack of a supportive systemic context from which to deliver the IT as possible factors in its poor performance in this (admittedly very small) treatment outcome study.

Debelle *et al.* (1993), in reviewing intervention programmes for juvenile sex offenders, conclude that sexual recidivism in juvenile offenders is relatively low. However, this conclusion was based on a review of follow-up studies undertaken in the 1940s and 1950s, and Debelle and associates acknowledge that there may have been significant changes in both the client group and the therapy selection criteria since that time. However, they argue that the longer the follow-up period the greater the likelihood of re-offending. The issue missing from these research data is the extent to which the followed-up sex offender (adolescent or adult) continued to receive therapeutic or even supportive services from professionals. The strong clinical impression is that the young sex offender is very much *less* likely to try to re-offend if there is a watchful professional network in place to review his or her behaviour.

MANAGEMENT OF YOUNG SEXUAL ABUSERS

The management of young sexual abusers is within a full child-protection context (Home Office 1991) and involves close cooperation within the professional network dealing with the case. A case conference on the child as an abuser as well as the usual child-protection procedures for the victim(s) involved will usually be necessary.

Often child and adolescent abusers of other children have aroused extraordinarily strong feelings of revulsion in one or two members of the professional network, who may write a referral letter expressing the fear that the child will abduct or murder (a fear grounded in reality for some cases). Conversely, others in the professional network will be surprisingly relaxed about the patterns of emerging behaviour and appear to be under-reacting or denying the nature of the risks posed. The nature of work with abusers involves paradoxes such as strong feelings of empathy for the child as a victim which exist alongside equally strong feelings of revulsion aroused by the child's behaviour. These different feelings and reactions may combine in the minds of all professionals concerned (including specialists) to cause overt and covert conflicts about case management which can easily abort the referral and return the young abuser (unassessed and

untreated) to his home area. In a more hopeful end scenario, careful management of the referral process and awareness of these issues will result in positive recruitment of other professionals into the assessment and treatment process so that the young abuser is given appropriate services.

Management is also affected by professional perceptions and interpretations of what constitutes sexualized or abusive behaviour by children, and this in turn depends on the context in which the behaviour occurs. In a study of 158 children between the ages of 6 and 11 years in residential treatment centres, Johnson and Aoki (1993) noted that 155 out of 158 of these abused and neglected children regularly asked staff for hugs, and staff in turn had very mixed feelings about the ethics of whether and how to respond to these requests (which were often overtly or covertly sexualized). Furthermore, the mixed feelings about these sexualized children meant that staff recordings and observations of these behaviours were affected by their own countertransference feelings which needed to be addressed through regular team meetings and debriefing.

Professional anxiety about the sexually abusive behaviour appears to rise with the child's age until the point at which referral is made, with greatest professional resistance being seen in relation to referral of sexually aggressive younger children. However, it is often the case that by the time referral of an abusive, pubertal, large-stature young male is made to a specialist agency, the overwhelming focus will be upon his sexual problems and the need for risk assessment. At this point, professionals may have lost sight of the needs of the young person as a whole individual with many emotional, developmental and social problems. This presents management problems since child and adolescent sexual abusers require a holistic approach to assessment.

CONCLUSIONS AND FUTURE DIRECTIONS

Research

There are various reasons why one round figure for the rate of juvenile sexual offending is not available to quote with confidence.

Firstly, there has not been a government-funded incidence or prevalence study of the rates of sexual offending by young people which would allow an estimate of the national picture in the UK. Such a national study has not yet been done in the USA, although data are kept by the National Perpetrator Network on existing programmes in various USA states (National Task Force 1993). Clearly such studies do need to be undertaken as a matter of some urgency because the available data rely heavily on criminal, clinical and respondant populations and are therefore likely to be skewed towards the more serious end of the abusive spectrum, and to be missing the (presumed) majority of undisclosed and unprosecuted cases.

Secondly, and related to the above reason, funders do not seem to have accepted that the problem of sexual offending in childhood and adolescence is a major cause of psychopathology in later life in both victims and in the, soon to be adult, young sexual abuser. Juvenile sexual offending is still seen as a rather rare, esoteric sort of problem which does not merit serious research attention.

Thirdly, in the UK at least, juvenile sexual offending does not really 'belong' anywhere within the professional systems which look after children. Since the problem contains elements of child psychiatry, forensic psychiatry, psychology, criminology, sociology and psychotherapy, it might be thought that a multi-disciplinary approach would be highly appropriate. In practice, the problem falls between all the disciplines mentioned above and there is no sign of any one discipline taking the lead in developing this work. Such a situation means that coordinated research into incidence and prevalence is difficult to arrange and more difficult to fund.

Debelle *et al.* (1993, p. 83) make a strong case for the establishment of a multi-centre cohort study to be carried out at a national and possibly international level. However, even in 1993 they noted that the choice of suitable measures of short-term outcome was proving problematic. It is to be hoped that a more cooperative and effective approach to collaborative research with young sexual abusers can be created.

Whilst the serious nature of sexual offending cannot be doubted, it is also true that many children experiencing the same adverse family factors and child abuse as young abusers have experienced will *not* become abusers. There do seem to be resilience factors which allow some children to live through abusive experiences, although research data do not seem to be available to identify resilience-related issues clearly. In discussing the factors which might result in a positive outcome, Leventhal (1998) suggests that factors that might be examined include nurturing family characteristics, counselling at the time of disclosure, and intervening variables such as a supportive spouse. Further research into the resilience factors which may allow an abused young boy to turn away from sexually abusive behaviour towards a more normative sexual development is therefore urgently needed.

Research is also needed in the area of classification of the problem of sexual aggression and sexual arousal in children and adolescents so that a name can be given to a worrying problem. Such research may now be possible given the increased amount of information available about the characteristics of this population. The attempts to create clinical typologies described earlier in this chapter indicate the necessity to identify these children's needs in more detail and earlier in the developmental process.

Other areas in which research is urgently needed are the extent and nature of sexual offending by girls, and the true nature of any association between learning difficulties or mental retardation and sexual offending against children. There is a sense that political correctness is also a reason why girls (often traditionally thought of as disadvantaged or vulnerable anyway) are not encouraged to be seen as more calculating, predatory or able to commit offences independently without a male being present to push them into offending. Learning-disabled children and adolescents are often patronized with the same attitudes which assume that a lower IQ means that culpability is not possible and that sexual assaults, for instance, are somehow accidental rather than planned.

Policy

The abolition in the Crime and Disorder Act 1998 of the *doli incapax* supposition may have important implications for young sexual offenders. *Doli incapax* was a legally rebuttable supposition that a child between the ages of 10 and 14 years did not realize the seriousness of an alleged offence. If such a defence could be proven, a child defendant facing a sexual offence charge was unlikely to be prosecuted and might, therefore, have a more humane, 'welfare' response to the alleged behaviour. In the opinion of this author, however, the *doli incapax* provision itself was perverse and ultimately confusing since it seemed to pick out only one age group (10–14 years) whereas all adolescents from 10 to 18 years of age are developmentally immature and in need of special assessment and provision.

In the absence of *doli incapax*, concerns have been voiced about the civil liberties of such young and possibly developmentally delayed child defendants. Reports in the media of sexual assaults by young children, some of whom are below the British age of criminal responsibility (10 years), have raised questions about the true extent to which such young abusers can be held responsible for their actions.

The policy dilemma is how to balance the very important public safety issues raised by dangerous young sexual offenders against their undoubted welfare needs; in other words, how to deal with children and adolescents who are 'dual status'-delinquents under the Crime and Disorder Act, yet children under the Children Act. It seems unlikely that increased prosecutions alone will deal with the problem without a clear inter-agency care plan for the future development of each of these young sexual abusers. At the time of writing it is not clear how such an expensive and integrated approach to the care of these children will be funded.

Funding difficulties link to the persistent problems for local authorities and health trusts in agreeing priorities for mental health provision for adult and adolescent clients. The difficulties of the Young Abusers Project in persuading local authorities and trusts to refer for such specialist services (Vizard and Usiskin 1999) has had, on occasion, devastating consequences for the individual client or young person who is in great need of help. For instance, occasionally funding has been abruptly stopped when the local authority has interpreted the reduction in abusive behaviour by the client since starting therapy as an indication that therapy has worked and is obviously no longer needed. However, it is also true to say that the best managed cases with an agreed inter-agency care plan will seldom have such acute funding problems and joint funding is usually possible in cases where the professional network is able to work in a degree of harmony.

The major policy issue must be whether to heed the many messages from research and clinical practice with young sexual abusers over many years, and to put time, money and commitment into the prevention of this form of delinquency, rather than paying out for services for victims who need never have been created.

Acknowledgements

I would like to acknowledge with gratitude the assistance of Alex King, Colin Hawkes, Judith Usiskin, Claire Usiskin, Lesley French and Nicole Hickey in the preparation of this chapter. Thanks are very much due to my clinical colleagues in the Young Abusers Project for their constant support and encouragement to describe our extremely challenging work together. I am very grateful indeed to NSPCC for backing this project during difficult times. The assistance of the Home Office Crime and Criminal Justice Unit's Research, Development and Statistics Directorate was most helpful. However, any conclusions I may have drawn remain my responsibility alone.

Finally, I also wish to acknowledge the debt of gratitude which I owe to the young people who have attended the Young Abusers Project and from whom I have learnt so much about the long-lasting effects of abuse and trauma.

REFERENCES

Abel, G., Becker, J.V., Mittleman-Rathner, J., Rouleau, J. and Murphy, W. 1987: Self-reported sex crimes of 561 non-incarcerated paraphiliacs. *Journal of Interpersonal Violence* **2**(6): 3–25.

Araji, S.K. 1997a: Identifying, labelling and explaining children's sexually aggressive behaviors. In Sharon, K. Araji (ed.), *Sexually Aggressive Children: Coming to Understand Them*. London: Sage, 1–46.

Araji, S.K. 1997b: Sexually aggressive children: social demographics and psychological characteristics. In Sharon, K. Araji (ed.), *Sexually Aggressive Children: Coming to Understand Them*. London: Sage, 47–88.

Araji, S.K. and Finklehor, D. 1986: Abusers: a review of the research. In Finklehor, D. (ed.), *A Sourcebook on Child Sexual Abuse*. London: Sage, 89–118.

Bailey, S. 1996: Adolescents who murder. *Journal of Adolescence* **19**: 19–39.

Bancroft, J. 1989: *Human Sexuality and its Problems*. Edinburgh: Churchill Livingstone.

Beck-Sander, A. 1995: Childhood abuse in adult offenders: the role of control in perpetuating cycles of abuse. *Journal of Forensic Psychiatry* **6**: 486–98.

Becker, J.V. 1990: Treating adolescent sex offenders. *Professional Psychology: Research and Practice* **21**: 362–5.

Becker, J.V. 1994: Offenders: characteristics and treatment. *The Future of Children* **4**: 198–223.

Becker, J.V. 1998: The assessment of adolescent perpetrators of childhood sexual abuse. *Irish Journal of Psychology* **19**: 68–81.

Becker, J.V. and Coleman, E.M. 1988: Incest. In Hassalt, V.B., Morrison, R.L., Becker, J.V., Kaplan, M.S., and Kavoussi, R. (eds), Measuring the Effectiveness of Treatment for the Aggressive Adolescent Sexual Offender. *Annals of the New York Academy of Sciences* **528**: 215–22.

Bentovim, A. 1998: Family systemic approach to work with young sex offenders. *Irish Journal of Psychology* **19**: 119–35.

Bentovim, A. and Williams, B. 1998: Children and adolescents: victims who become perpetrators. *Advances in Psychiatric Treatment* **4**: 101–7.

Borduin, C.M., Henggeler, S.W., Blaske, D.M. and Stein, R. 1990: Multisystemic treatment of adolescent sex offenders. *International Journal of Offender Therapy and Comparative Criminology* **34**: 105–13.

Boswell, G. 1996: *Young and Dangerous: the Backgrounds and Careers of Section 53 Offenders*. Aldershot: Avebury.

Bremer, J.F. 1993: The treatment of children and adolescents with aberrant sexual behaviours. In Hobbs, C.J. and Wynne, J.M. (eds), *Baillière's Clinical Paediatrics. International Practice and Research: 1. Child Abuse*, 269–82.

Calder, M.C. 1997a: Defining the problem. In Martin, C. and Calder, M.C. (eds), *Juveniles and Children Who Sexually Abuse: a Guide to Risk Assessment*. UK: Russell House Publishing, 11–15.

Calder, M.C. 1997b: Assessing juveniles who sexually abuse: a framework. In Martin, C. and Calder, M.C. (eds), *Juveniles and Children Who Sexually Abuse: a Guide to Risk Assessment*. UK: Russell House Publishing, 50–98.

Canter, D., Hughes, D. and Kirby, S. 1998: Paedophilia: pathology, criminality or both? The development of a multivariate model of offence behaviour in child sexual abuse. *Journal of Forensic Psychiatry* **9**: 532–55.

Cantwell, H.B. 1995: Sexually aggressive children and societal responses. In Hunter, M. (ed.), *Child Survivors and Perpetrators of Sexual Abuse: Treatment Innovations*. London: Sage, 79–107.

Craissati, J. and McClurg, G. 1997: The Challenge Project: a treatment program evaluation for perpetrators of child sexual abuse. *Child Abuse and Neglect* **21**: 637–48.

Cunningham, C. and MacFarlane, L. 1991: *When Children Molest Children*. Orwell, VT: Safer Society Press.

Cunningham, C. and MacFarlane, L. 1996: *When Children Abuse: Group Treatment Strategies for Young Sexual Offenders*. Brandon, VT: Safer Society Press.

Davis, G. and Leitenberg, H. 1987: Adolescent sex offenders. *Psychological Bulletin* **101**: 417–27.

Debelle, G.D., Ward, M.R., Burnham, J.B., Jamieson, R. and Ginty, M. 1993: Evaluation of intervention programmes for juvenile sex offenders: questions and dilemmas. *Child Abuse Review* **2**: 75–87.

Dey, C. and Print, B. 1992: Young children who exhibit sexually abusive behaviour. In Bannister, A. (ed.), *From Hearing to*

Healing: Working with the Aftermath of Child Sexual Abuse. London: Longman, 105–29.

Duffield, G., Hassiotis, A. and Vizard, E. 1998: Zoophilia in young sexual abusers. *Journal of Forensic Psychiatry* **9**: 294–304.

Eldridge, H. 1998: *Therapist Guide for Maintaining Change: Relapse Prevention for Adult Male Perpetrators of Child Sexual Abuse.* London: Sage.

Elliott, C.E. and Butler, L. 1994: The Stop and Think Group: changing sexually aggressive behaviour in young children. *Journal of Sexual Aggression* **1**: 15–28.

Elton, A. 1988: Assessment of families for treatment. In Bentovim, A., Elton, A., Hildebrand, J., Tranter, M. and Vizard, E. (eds), *Child Sexual Abuse Within the Family: Assessment and Treatment.* London: John Wright, 153–81.

Fehrenbach, P.A. and Monastersky, C. 1988: Characteristics of female sexual offenders. *American Journal of Orthopsychiatry* **58**: 148–51.

Finklehor, D. 1994: Current information on the scope and nature of child sexual abuse. *The Future of Children* **4**: 31–53.

Ford, M.E. and Linney, A.J.A. 1995. Comparative analysis of juveniles sexual offenders, violent nonsexual offenders and status offenders. *Journal of Interpersonal Violence* **10**: 56–70.

Freidrich, W.N. 1995: Managing disorders of self regulation in sexually abused boys. In Hunter, M. (ed.), *Child Survivors and Perpetrators of Sexual Abuse.* London: Sage, 3–23.

Freidrich, W.N., Grambsch, P., Broughton, D., Kuiper, J. and Beilke, R.L. 1991: Normative sexual behavior in children. *Pediatrics* **88**: 456–64.

Freidrich, W.N., Grambsch, P., Damon, L. *et al.* 1992: Child sexual behavior inventory: normative and clinical comparisons. *Psychological Assessment* **4**: 303–11.

Gil, E. 1993a: Age-appropriate sex play versus problematic sexual behaviors. In Gil, E. and Johnson, T.C. (eds), *Sexualised Children: Assessment and Treatment of Sexualised Children and Children Who Molest.* Rockville, MD: Launch Press, 21–40.

Gil, E. 1993b: Sexualised children. In Gil, E. and Johnson, T.C. (eds), *Sexualised Children: Assessment and Treatment of Sexualised Children and Children Who Molest.* Rockville, MD: Launch Press, 91–99.

Graham, F., Richardson, G. and Bhate, S. 1997: Assessment. In Hoghughi, M. (ed.), *Working with Sexually Abusive Adolescents.* London: Sage, 52–91.

Graves, R.B., Openshaw, D.K., Ascione, F.R. and Erikson, S.L. 1996: Demographic and parental characteristics of youthful sexual offenders. *International Journal of Offender Therapy and Comparative Criminology* **40**: 300–17.

Gray, A.S. and Wallace, R. 1992: *Adolescent Sexual Offender Assessment Packet.* Orwell, VT: Safer Society Press.

Gray, A.S. and Pithers, W.D. 1993: Relapse prevention with sex offenders. In Barbaree, H.E., Marshall, W.L. and Hudson, S.M. (eds), *The Juvenile Sex Offender.* New York: Guilford, 289–319.

Griffin, S., Williams, M., Hawkes, C. and Vizard, E. 1997: The Professional Carers' Group: supporting group work for young sexual abusers. *Child Abuse and Neglect* **21**: 681–90.

Hall, D.K., Mathews, F. and Pearce, J. 1998: Factors associated with sexual behaviour problems in young sexually abused children *Child Abuse and Neglect* **22**: 1045–63.

Halperin, D.S., Bouvier, P., Jaffe, P.D. *et al.* 1996: Prevalence of child sexual abuse among adolescents in Geneva: results of a cross sectional survey. *British Medical Journal* **312**: 1326–9.

Hanks, H. 1997: 'Normal' psychosexual development, behaviour and knowledge. In Martin, C. and Calder, M.C. (eds), *Juveniles and*

Children Who Sexually Abuse: a Guide to Risk Assessment. UK: Russell House Publishing.

Hastings, T., Anderson, S.J. and Hemphill, P. 1997: Comparisons of daily stress, coping, problem behaviour and cognitive distortions in adolescent sexual offenders and conduct disordered youth. *Sexual Abuse: Journal of Research and Treatment* **9**: 29–42.

Hawkes, C., Jenkins, J. and Vizard, E. 1996: Roots of sexual violence in children and adolescents. In Varma, V. (ed.), *Violence in Children and Adolescents.* London: Jessica Kingsley, 84–102.

Heiman, M.L., Leiblum, S., Cohen Esquilin, S. and Melendez Pallitto, L. 1998: A comparative study of beliefs about 'normal' childhood sexual behaviors. *Child Abuse and Neglect* **22**: 289–304.

Hindman, J. 1994: *JCA – Juvenile Culpability Assessment,* 2nd edn. Ontario, OR: Alexandria.

Hoghugi, M. 1997: Sexual abuse by adolescents. In Hoghughi, M. (ed.), *Working With Sexually Abusive Adolescents.* London: Sage, 1–19.

Hoghughi, M. and Richardson, G. 1997: Theories of adolescent sexual abuse. In Hoghughi, M. (ed.), *Working With Sexually Abusive Adolescents.* London: Sage, 20–34.

Home Office, with Department of Health, Department of Education and Science, Welsh Office 1991: *Working Together under the Children Act 1989: a Guide to Arrangements for Inter-agency Cooperation for the Protection of Children from Abuse.* London: HMSO.

Home Office 1996a: *Criminal Statistics for England and Wales.* London: HMSO.

Home Office 1996b: The British Crime Survey 1990–94. In *Home Office Statistical Findings,* 1/96. London: HMSO.

Home Office 1998a: *Aspects of Crime: Young Offenders 1996.* Available from the Crime and Criminal Justice Unit, Research and Statistics Directorate, Home Office.

Home Office 1998b: *Aspects of Crime: Children as Victims 1996.* Available from the Crime and Criminal Justice Unit, Research and Statistics Directorate, Home Office.

Horne, L., Glasgow, D., Cox, A. and Calam, R. 1991: Sexual abuse of children by children. *Journal of Child Law* **3**: 147–51.

Hunter, J.A., Lexier, L.J., Goodwin, D.W., Browne, P.A. and Dennis, C. 1993: Psychosexual, attitudinal and developmental characteristics of juvenile female sexual perpetrators in a residential treatment setting. *Journal of Child and Family Studies* **2**: 317–26.

James, A.C. and Neil, P. 1996: Juvenile sexual offending: one-year period prevalence study within Oxfordshire. *Child Abuse and Neglect* **13**: 571–85.

Johnson, T.C. 1989: *Human Sexuality. Curriculum for Parents and Children in Troubled Families.* Available from Children's Institute International, Marshall Resource Library, Los Angeles, USA.

Johnson, T.C. and Aoki, W.T. 1993: Sexual behaviors of latency age children in residential treatment. In Braga, W. de C. and Schimmer, R. (eds), *Sexual Abuse and Residential Treatment.* London: Haworth Press, 1–22.

Johnson, T.C. and Berry, C. 1989: Children who molest: a treatment program. *Journal of Interpersonal Violence* **4**: 185–203.

Johnson, T.C. and Feldmeth, J.R. 1993: Sexual behaviours: a continuum. In Gil, E. and Johnson, T.C. (eds), *Sexualised Children: Assessment and Treatment of Sexualised Children and Children who Molest.* Rockville, MD: Launch Press, 41–52.

Jones, D. 1998: Sexual behaviour problems among sexually abused children (editorial). *Child Abuse and Neglect* **22**: 1043–4.

Kelly, L., Regan, L. and Burton, S. 1991: *An exploratory study of the prevalence of sexual abuse in a sample of 16–21 year olds.* Report for the ESRC Child Abuse Studies Unit. University of North London.

Lanyon, R. 1991: Theories of Sex Offending. In Hollin, C.R. and Howell, K. (eds), *Clinical Approaches to Sex Offenders and Their Victims.* John Wiley & Sons, 36–54.

Le Doux, J.E. 1994: Emotion, memory and the brain. *Scientific American*, June, 50–7.

Longo, R.E. and Groth, A.N. 1983: Juvenile sexual offences in the histories of adult rapists and child molesters. *Journal of Offender Therapy and Comparative Criminology* **27**: 150–5.

MacFarlane, K. and Cunningham, C. 1988: *Steps to Healthy Touching.* Mount Dora, FL: Kidsrights.

Maletzky, B.M. 1991: *Treating the Sexual Offender.* London: Sage.

Manocha, K.F. and Mezey, G. 1998: British adolescents who sexually abuse: a descriptive study. *Journal of Forensic Psychiatry* **9**: 588–608.

Marshall, W.L. and Barbaree, H.E. 1990: An integrated theory of the etiology and maintenance of sexual offending. In Marshall, W.L., Laws, D.R. and Barbaree, H.E. (eds), *Handbook of Sexual Assault: Issues, Theories and Treatment of the Offender.* New York: Plenum.

McGregor, G. and Howells, K. 1997: Addiction models of sexual offending. In Hodge, J.E., McMurran, M. and Hollin, C.R. (eds), *Addicted to Crime?* Chichester: John Wiley, 107–37.

Mezey, G., Vizard, E., Hawkes, C. and Austin, R. 1991: A community treatment programme for convicted child sex offenders: a preliminary report. *Journal of Forensic Psychiatry* **2**(1): 11–25.

Murphy, W.D., Coleman, E.M. and Abel, G.G. 1983: Human sexuality in the mentally retarded. In Matson, J.L. and Andrasik, F. (eds), *Treatment Issues and Innovations in Mental Retardation.* New York: Plenum Press, 581–643.

Myers, W.C. 1994: Sexual homicide by adolescents. *Journal of the American Academy of Child and Adolescent Psychiatry* **33**: 962–9.

National Task Force on Juvenile Sexual Offending 1993: Revised report. *Juvenile and Family Court Journal* **44**: 4.

NCH (National Children's Home) 1992: *Children Who Sexually Abuse Other Children.* London: NCH.

O'Brien, M. and Bera, W.H. 1992: The PHASE typology of adolescent sex offenders. Appendix C in Gray, A.S. and Wallace, R. (eds), *Adolescent Sexual Offender Packet.* Orwell, VT: Safer Society Press.

O'Callaghan, D. and Print, B. 1994: Adolescent sexual abusers. research, assessment and treatment. In Morrison, T., Erooga, M. and Beckett, R.C. (eds), *Sexual Offending Against Children: Assessment and Treatment of Male Abusers.* London: Routledge, 146–77.

Perry, B.D. 1994: Neurobiological sequelae of childhood trauma: PTSD in children. In Murray, M. (ed.), *Catecholamines in Post-traumatic Stress Disorder: Emerging Concepts.* Washington, DC: American Psychiatric Press.

Pithers, W., Gray, A.S., Cunningham, C. and Lane, S. 1993: *From Trauma to Understanding.* Brandon, VT: Safer Society Press.

Richardson, G., Graham, F., Bhate, S.R. and Kelly, T.P. 1995: A British sample of sexually abusive adolescents: abuser and abuse characteristics. *Criminal Behaviour and Mental Health* **5**: 187–208.

Richardson, G., Bhate, S. and Graham, F. 1997: Cognitive-based practice with sexually abusive adolescents. In Hoghughi, M. (ed.), *Working with Sexually Abusive Adolescents.* London: Sage, 128–43.

Rutter, M. 1971: Normal psychosexual development. *Journal of Child Psychology and Psychiatry* **11**: 259–83.

Salter, A. 1988: *Treating Child Sex Offenders and Victims: a Practical Guide.* London: Sage.

Schwartz, J.W. 1996: Assessing children's sexual behaviour in a protection context. Paper presented at the Eleventh ISPCAN Congress on Child Abuse and Neglect, Dublin, Ireland, 18–21 August.

Schwartz, M.E., Galperin, L.D. and Masters, W.H. 1995: Dissociation and treatment of compulsive reenactment of trauma. In Hunter, M. (ed.), *Adult Survivors of Sexual Abuse: Treatment Innovations.* London: Sage, 42–55.

Sinason, V. 1992: *Mental Handicap and the Human Condition: New Approaches from the Tavistock.* London: Free Association Books.

Sirles, E.A., Araji, S. and Bosek, R. 1997: Redirecting children's sexually abusive and sexually aggressive behaviours: programs and practices. In Sharon, K. Araji (ed.), *Sexually Aggressive Children: Coming to Understand Them.* London: Sage, 161–92.

Skuse, D., Bentovim, A., Hodges, J. *et al.* 1998: Risk factors for the development of sexually abusive behaviour in sexually victimized adolescent males: a cross-sectional study. *British Medical Journal* **317**: 175–9.

Soothill, K. 1997: Rapists under 14 years in the news. *The Howard Journal* **36**: 367–77.

Tudiver, J.G. and Griffin, J.D. 1992: Treating developmentally disabled adolescents who have committed sexual abuse. *Newsletter of the Sex Information and Education Council of Canada* **27**: 5–10.

Vizard, E. 1989: Incidence and prevalence of child sexual abuse. In Ouston, J. (ed.), *The Consequences of Child Sexual Abuse.* London: Association for Child Psychology and Psychiatry.

Vizard, E. 1998: Operational criteria for sexual arousal disorder of childhood. Paper given in the forensic session of the Residential Conference of the Child and Adolescent Psychiatry Faculty of the Royal College of Psychiatrists, Bristol, 24–26 September.

Vizard, E. and Usiskin, J. 1999: Providing individual psychotherapy for young sexual abusers of other children. In Erooga, M. and Masson, H. (eds), *Children and Young People Who Sexually Abuse Others: Challenges and Responses.* London: Routledge, 179–210.

Vizard, E., Monck, E. and Misch, P. 1995: Child and adolescent sex abuse perpetrators: a review of the research literature. *Journal of Child Psychology and Psychiatry* **36**: 731–56.

Vizard, E., Wynick, S., Hawkes, C., Woods, J. and Jenkins, J. 1996: Juvenile sexual offenders. *British Journal of Psychiatry* **168**: 259–62.

Watkins, B. and Bentovim, A. 1992: The sexual abuse of male children and adolescents: a review of current research. *Journal of Child Psychology and Psychiatry* **33**: 197–248.

Woods, J. 1997: Breaking the cycle of abuse and abusing: individual psychotherapy for juvenile sex offenders. *Clinical Child Psychology and Psychiatry* **2**: 379–92.

18

Arson and property offending

CARLY SMITH, DEANNE BENNETT AND NATHAN WHITTLE

INTRODUCTION AND DEFINITIONS

Property offences are deemed in law as notifiable offences and, if crime statistics are to be considered reliable, such offences account for the bulk of recorded crime figures. The definition of what constitutes a property offence is not homogeneous when we consider that theft, for example, may incorporate a host of offences ranging from theft of a motor vehicle to theft from a home/shop/business. Some offences may incorporate violence against the person as well as a property offence – for example aggravated burglary or robbery. Property offences may be expressive – for example criminal damage and arson.

Many children and young people will, at some time, engage in a form of property offending, such as attempting to acquire a favourite item from a shop or destroying their sibling/friend's belongings. There is a need for all individuals who are in contact with the child or young person to differentiate between the child who has not yet learnt the social or moral code in relation to such behaviour, and the young person who engages in 'youthful crimes'.

There have been numerous studies examining the biological, sociological, cultural, socio-economic and psychosocial factors that increase an individual's propensity to engage in criminal behaviour and the factors involved in both development or remission of a 'criminal career'. This chapter examines a range of literature regarding the nature, occurrence and intervention strategies used with adolescents who engage in property offending.

Definitions

Arson
Prior to the Criminal Damage Act of 1971, arson was cited as a common law offence. Under the Act it is now classed as follows:

Section 1(1):
'[A] person who without lawful excuse destroys or damages any property belonging to another, intending to destroy or damage any such property or being reckless as to whether such property is destroyed or damaged shall be guilty of an offence ... punishable with imprisonment of 10 years.'

Section 1(2):
'[An] offence committed under this section by destroying or damaging property by fire shall be charged as arson; the offence is punishable by life imprisonment.'

Section 1(3):
'[If] a person endangers the life of another through such activity, this shall be punishable with a maximum of life imprisonment.'

Theft
The 1968 Theft Act states:

'A person is guilty of theft if he dishonestly appropriates property belonging to another with the intention of permanently depriving the other of it.'

Robbery
'A person is guilty of robbery if he steals ... , and immediately before or at the time of doing so ..., and in order to do so, he uses force ... on any person or puts or seeks to

put any person ... in fear of being then and there ... subjected to force...'.

Burglary

'A person is guilty if (A) he enters ... any building ... or part of a building ... as a trespasser ... and with intent ... to commit any such offence [and] (B) having entered ... any building ... or part of a building ... as a trespasser ... he steals or attempts to steal anything in the building or that part of it or inflicts or attempts to inflict on any person therein grievous bodily harm'.

Aggravated burglary

'A person is guilty of aggravated burglary if he commits any burglary and at the time has with him any firearm or imitation firearm, any weapon of offence or any explosive'.

Deception

'A person who by any deception dishonestly obtains property belonging to another with the intention of permanently depriving the other of it [is guilty of deception]'.

Blackmail

'A person is guilty of blackmail if with a view to gain for himself or another, or intent to cause loss to another, he makes any unwarranted demand with menaces; and for this purpose a demand with menaces is unwarranted unless the person making it does so in the belief (a) that he has reasonable grounds for making the demand; and

(b) that the use of the menaces is a proper means of reinforcing the demand'.

Going equipped

'A person shall be guilty of an offence if, when not at his place of abode, he has with him any article for use in the course of or in connection with any burglary, theft or cheat'.

The literature

Tables 18.1 and 18.2 describe the features and some conclusions of various studies of firesetters and property (acquisitive) offenders.

However, there is a dearth of literature examining *why* young people engage in delinquent or antisocial behaviour, and there is a paucity of literature examining why young people *cease* engaging in delinquent or antisocial behaviour. Research needs to address whether young people desist from offending or move on to experiment with other types of criminal activity that have lower detection rates.

The age of onset of offending has to be examined in order to examine changes in offending and the juncture at which participation decreases. On a global level it has been well documented that the earlier a person engages in offending behaviour, the more likely it is that the behaviour will become entrenched (Tolan and Lorion

Table 18.1 *Classifications*

Author(s)	Classification
Fineman (1980)	Firesetting: interaction involving personal and familial factors predisposing the young person to the behaviour; e.g. positive/negative arousal, family problems, educational difficulties.
Vreeland and Levin (1980)	Firesetting is the culmination of difficulty/fear of direct expression of aggression.
Patterson (1982)	Firesetting occurs at the end of a continuum of antisocial behaviours.
Kolko and Kazdin (1992)	Attraction to fire, heightened arousal, impulsivity and limited social competence.
Muckley (1994)	*Curiosity* Fires accidental, young person lacks judgement of consequences, often admits behaviour and experiences guilt. *Problem* Fires often set alone, are in response to adverse family events and as a means of gaining attention or expressing anger. The young person often admits the behaviour and experiences guilt. For the older problem firesetter, peer pressure is often a factor. The behaviour promotes feelings of power, excitement and may be the result of anger or disturbed behaviours.
Fineman (1995)	*Curiosity* Young person does not understand the consequences, therefore no intent to harm. Such behaviour often the result of 'seeing' qualities of flame and how objects burn. *Accidental* Carelessness and experimentation usually involving children. *'Cry for help'* Conscious/subconscious desire for attention to an intrapersonal dysfunction without intent to harm. *Delinquent* The behaviour may be used for crime concealment or profit.
Williams (1996)	Serious fires are often the result of poor judgement. Fires are often set in delinquent groups/peer. Likely to mature out of this behaviour.

1988). Farrington (1994) observed that the peak age of offending (not conviction) for a first offence was between 13 and 15 years, and that such behaviour coincided with a peak of other delinquent behaviour(s).

A Home Office study (1995) related to young people and crime found that expressive offences such as vandalism and arson were prevalent between the ages of 14 and 17 in males and females. Property offences – particularly the visible forms such as shoplifting and theft – were prevalent between the ages of 18 and 21 in males and between 14 and 17 in females. The propensity to engage in more sophisticated forms of property offending such as fraud and theft from work increased during the early twenties for males. For all types of offending there was an observed decrease in offending levels following the mid teenage years.

The study also revealed that, when the frequency of offending *by gender* was examined, the ratio between males and females in relation to property offences *per se* was 7:3, but for expressive offences it was 1:1. When age

was included the ratio increased further still. Property offences amongst the 14- to 17-year-old age group were equal at 1:1 but rose to 3:1 in the 18- to 21-year-olds. For expressive offences the ratio for males and females was 1:0 in the 14- to 17-year-olds, rising to 3:7 in the 18- to 21-year-olds.

Graham and Bowling (1995) conducted a self-report study examining offending behaviour. In the 2500 young people surveyed, property offences were the most common form of offending (for young males) and, in contrast to other research results, the numbers of males involved escalated rather than declined. The number of females reporting involvement in property offending (in line with other research) declined with age. For expressive offences such as vandalism, graffiti or arson, both males and females reported decreased involvement in line with increased age.

Criminal Statistics for England and Wales (HMSO 1995) indicates that a high proportion of all offences committed by young people are offences of theft and burglary. Other

Table 18.2 *Clinical features (firesetters)*

Author(s)	Study	Conclusions
Tennent *et al.* (1971)		Criminal justice system reluctant to prosecute mentally ill firesetters. Such offenders often demonstrate high levels of psychopathology, suicide and self-mutilation. Psychotic episodes were apparent in 57.8% of cases examined.
Virkkunen (1974)	30 arsonists diagnosed with schizophrenia	Hallucinations/delusions were the principal motive in 30% cases. Fires were set in empty buildings rather than residential/occupied buildings.
Herjanic *et al.* (1977) Hill *et al.* (1982) Harmon *et al.* (1985) O' Sullivan and Kelleher (1987)		Firesetters and arsonists demonstrate a high degree of psychopathology.
Bradford (1982)		The label of psychopathy is more frequently attached to arsonists than controls. There may be a tendency to over-diagnose antisocial personality disorder when assessing firesetters.
Geller (1984)		Firesetting episodes often accounted for by reasons other than psychosis. Firesetting in response to hallucinatory experiences less common than those due to delusional ideation.
Jackson (1994)		Psychotic symptoms not necessarily playing a causal role in firesetting. Illness a setting condition rather than a direct precursor.
Leong (1992)		Firesetters and arsonists often demonstrate high degree of psychopathology and high rates of substance abuse.
Rice and Harris (1991)	243 arsonists admitted to maximum-security psychiatric institution	Firesetters less assertive. Mentally ill firesetters had greatest difficulty in expressing anger, disappointment and feelings of hurt.
Rix (1994)	153 adult arsonists referred for pre-trial psychiatric reports	13% no formal diagnosis; 8% diagnosed with schizophrenia. Psychosis/depressive disorders most common in women. Alcohol/substance abuse most common in men. 45% had diagnosis of personality disorder with a prominence of paranoid and passive–aggressive characteristics.
Puri *et al.* (1995)	36 firesetters referred to a forensic psychiatry service	56% men had psychiatric history. 70% women had psychiatric history. 66% of total had organic brain disorder.

property offences saw a decline in the number of young people found guilty or cautioned. Where the offence was identified as criminal damage the percentage of males found guilty or cautioned was 6% at 10–14 years, 4% at 14–18 years and 3% at 18–21 years. For females, data indicated a lower rate across all ages recorded – at 1%. As with all statistics of crime, the true extent of offending regardless of the type of offence cannot be measured 'exactly' owing to a number of factors – for example underreporting by the 'victim' or lack of detection.

Historical background

Firesetting and arson are devastating behaviours impacting both on a micro level (the victims) and a macro level (wider society). From a historical perspective firesetting is not a modern phenomenon. Fire has typically been seen as a powerful symbol evident in mythology. Bronowski (1976), in his scientific epic *The Ascent of Man*, underlined the fact that 'fire has been known to early man for about 400,000 years'.

The ancient Egyptians believed in an association between fire and eternal life – that the Phoenix was believed to live for hundreds of years, burn itself to death and then rise from the ashes of its funeral pyre. Within Greek mythology, Prometheus (having stolen fire from the gods) was condemned to the everlasting torment of having his liver torn out by vultures. Fire was also used to destroy the bodies of those who had committed suicide – burning the hand that committed the act separately from the rest of the body. The Roman culture believed in the goddess of the domestic hearth named Vesta, who was worshipped by virgin priestesses.

There are numerous references to the use and abuse of fire in the Bible; for example fire guided the Israelites through the Wilderness and served as making a sacrifice to the Lord. Fire has been associated with the notion of punishment. Its use in the Christian era was as a purifier of souls – in the burning of witches and heretics (Topp 1973).

Within the Hindu religion, use of fire can be seen in the practice of *Suttee* – the symbolic ritual of self-immolation, performed by widows on the funeral pyres of their husbands.

Throughout the Middle Ages fire was viewed as the means through which alchemist's gold could be obtained. From early times physicians sought the use of fire for healing, and true 'believers' were thought to be sanctified and protected by fire. Early rituals and beliefs may in part be responsible for the use of 'ordeal by fire', a means of establishing truth or falsehood in those accused of criminal acts.

By the middle of the nineteenth century, doctors became interested in what they termed 'pathological forms of firesetting'. Marc, a Frenchman, first described 'pyromania' in 1833 (Topp 1973). Later, the German school of thought suggested fireraising was seen in sexually frustrated males. Freud and Jung saw it as a symbolic and archetypal outlet for sexual impulses.

Today, there are less extreme sexual connotations to firesetting as research has been undertaken into the aetiology and treatment of the problem. The reasoning behind the choice to engage in property offences may appear clear – a personal need for money or food. For others the need may evolve from obtaining items for their monetary value or to attain status with peers. Further reasoning behind the choice to commit property offences may include threats, as a dare or as an act of rebellion.

The aetiology of offending

Why do young people engage in offending? The Cambridge Study of Delinquent Behaviour used self-report and official data to follow 411 Caucasian 'working-class' males born in 1953 (West and Farrington 1973, 1977). The results indicated that one in five of these adults had been convicted of offences prior to the age of 17. The authors suggested that a number of factors appeared to predispose the young people to offending behaviour patterns – not least their socio-economic status, the experience of dysfunctional parenting, a history of parental/sibling criminality, schooling difficulties and a history of antisocial behaviour. The authors argued that in relation to delinquency, the highest predisposing factor was dysfunctional behaviour exhibited at under 10 years of age. The research has since been criticized as it did not examine other social classes, female offending patterns, or offending patterns of members of ethnic minorities.

As stated previously, a number of theories have been proposed to explain the onset of offending behaviour and the engaging in of delinquent and antisocial behaviour.

Social learning theory examined the effect of the environment on the acquisition and maintenance of behaviour. In relation to conditioning, individuals were deemed to be motivated to achieve particular goals, such as status or the possession of objects of desire. Where the individual achieved his or her goal the behaviour was rewarded regardless of whether that behaviour was good or bad. The behaviour, now reinforced, could be reverted to when or if the need arose again. Bandura (1973) stated that the motivators of behaviours were attitudes and observed that not all behaviours were learned via direct experience; rather they were modelled on observed behaviour (real or fictitious) and consequences. The individual's interpretation of behaviour and consequences was ultimately responsible for eliciting/extinguishing the behaviour.

For an individual engaged in an expressive act such as criminal damage or arson, cognitive and normative factors may influence the individual's interpretation of the event and the person's subsequent reaction. There may be deficits in the individual's ability to process whether events (particularly aversive consequences) were malevolent, accidental, foreseeable or well-intentioned.

Functional analysis examined what function a particular behaviour had for the individual. This theory proposed that events do not occur in a vacuum; rather they are constructed from antecedents, behaviours and consequences. Any behaviour, therefore, became part of the learning theory and the antecedent to another set of behaviours.

ASSESSMENT OF OFFENDERS

Introduction

Mental health practitioners are ideally placed to examine psychosocial, psychological, psychiatric, physical, developmental and historical factors that aid identification of the emergence and maintenance of delinquent or antisocial behaviours. Practitioners acknowledge that the majority of individuals who engage in minor acts of property offending are rarely referred for psychiatric examination, so the incidence of morbidity in this population remains unknown. Other acts of property offending (e.g. arson) may not be perceived as providing the perpetrator with a direct source of gain. Such acts are typically covert and do not result in conviction or referral for psychiatric examination. For some individuals the offending and motive of gain may be subsidiary to deep-seated tensions that are beyond the control of the individual and pathological in origin.

From a mental health perspective, the assessment of individuals cautioned/charged or convicted of property offences is in essence the same as an assessment undertaken with any individual suspected of demonstrating a psychiatric illness. The heterogeneity of behaviours demonstrated alongside the idiosyncratic characteristics of individuals engaged in such behaviours often prevent a standardized assessment process revealing all the potential risk factors. Assessments must therefore encompass a broad-based conceptual framework acknowledging situational, contextual, social, personal, historical and functional variables.

As with any antisocial or offending behaviour, an accurate and thorough assessment is essential to establish domains that represent both the risk and protective factors. No one theory will encompass all possible tenets of behaviour, so a number of assessment theories may be utilized to suit the needs of the individual engaged in such behaviour, the environment where the assessment takes place, and the experience of staff undertaking the assessment. A number of factors have been identified to represent standards for assessment procedures.

Practitioners have highlighted the need for assessments that demonstrate how the offending behaviour relates to an individual's overall psychopathology. The psychopathology must be recorded in a format that is clear on both a multi-disciplinary and multi-agency level. The assessment must define the background, precursors, motives and processes of the behaviour(s) and provide risk indicators. The assessment must facilitate the individual's empowerment by defining the most appropriate treatment approach (medical/psychosocial) reflecting the needs and opinions of the individual whilst at the same time outlining the resources needed to undertake global assessment and treatment. Finally, any assessment procedure must advise the individual/practitioners and the purchaser as to the whole picture and be an appropriate audit tool for progress (evidence-based practice).

A global assessment must be undertaken that does not just consider the property-offending behaviour. The information gathered must be consistent, standardized and coded to facilitate data analyses.

PERSONAL DEVELOPMENT

Information is needed about the individual's progress through developmental stages, the possible impact of physical trauma (e.g. details about the birth – normal, delayed confinement, caesarean section, forceps delivery, handicap), and the birth order and number of siblings or step-siblings. Within this section of the assessment there should also be a detailed description of psychosocial adjustment – attachment style, coping with peers, moral development, and so on.

FAMILY PROBLEMS

This section of the assessment considers the possible impact of family and carers' behaviour on the individual, looking for any suspected or documented history of neglect, or witnessed or experienced abuse – physical, emotional or sexual. Where there has been separation from carers, it is appropriate to establish the point in time, the number of surrogate parents (relative and non-relative) and the number and type of placements (local authority, open/foster/secure/special school).

EDUCATIONAL HISTORY

This section of the assessment may be completed with the assistance of teachers and educational psychologists. It considers the number and type(s) of school attended – mainstream/special/residential/college. Where concerns have been raised, the academic record alongside the intelligence quotient (via standardized assessment such as the WISC) should be sought. A record of periods of truancy or exclusion (and in some cases details of behaviour during such periods, such as time spent alone, engaged in criminal activity) may be documented. Parents and carers may provide further insight into the young person's relationships with peers. Was the individual a bully or bullied, easily led or isolated? Were the relationships with individuals of a similar age? Were the relationships same-sex or mixed?

Table 18.3 *Clinical features (acquisitive offenders)*

Author(s)	Study	Conclusions
Gibbens *et al.* (1971)		10–15% of shoplifters presented with psychiatric disorder.
Gibbens (1981)		By 1981 he reduced this figure to 5%.
Depression		Examples include:- isolated individuals under stress, older adults, bipolar disorder and acute grief reaction states e.g. bereavement.
McDaniels-Wilson (1998)	436 incarcerated females	Females high incidence of mania (early onset of abusive experience), ↑ property offences.
Lamontagne *et al.* (2000)	106 adult first offenders	Depression most common disorder associated with shoplifting. Subjects with depression present greatest number of irrational beliefs related to shoplifting.
Anxiety		Examples include states where the individual is distracted via heightened anxiety.
Compulsive state Wiedman (1998)	12 subjects aged 21–58	This clinical state is referred to as 'kleptomania' and incorporates a host of states including heightened tension, compulsive urge followed by sense of relief once the act has been committed. This type of offending typically serves little purpose as the goods stolen are often worth little and the behaviour is not in response to anger. Weidman: some indications that kleptomania may be associated with affective spectrum disorder.
Psychosis Wessley (1997)	First episode cases extracted from Camberwell Case Register	The main criteria here is that an individual can be guided by delusions when choosing to engage in offending; e.g. following 'voices'. By contrast individuals may be in a state of mania (grandiose mood) and commit offences believing that everything is all right. Wessley observed no increased risk of criminality *per se* in males, but increased rates in females.
Brain damage		For some individuals a serious head trauma may result in noticeable changes in personality, including heightened anger/aggression, impulsivity, lack of awareness and risk taking. Where the damage impacts upon cognitive capacity the individual may lack the ability to plan, follow through actions, recognize danger; e.g. taking cars without consent.
Substance misuse		Increased offending behaviour may result from substance dependency or the need to maintain status. Offending may be committed in a 'state of disinhibition'.
McDaniels-Wilson (1998)	436 incarcerated females	↑ incidence of property offending.
Stewart *et al.* (2000)	1075 clients aged 16–58 years	Frequency of illicit substance misuse ↑ levels of criminal behaviour.
Other 'states'		There are a number of states that may be temporary or permanent; e.g. confusion arising from medication such as sedatives, antidepressants, antiepileptic medication and steroids. Physical states may induce confusion; e.g. hypoglycaemia.

Property offences

It is clear that property offending may be delineated into two distinct types:

- those that involve acquisitive offences, such as robbery or theft
- those that involve destruction of property.

From this viewpoint it is possible to examine the psychopathology of acquisitive versus destructive behaviour. From a 'motivation' perspective, acquisitive offences can be further defined to examine intent and psychiatric/psychological abnormality. As with firesetting, the bulk of recorded crime in relation to acquisitive offences demonstrates a population that would be considered as psychiatrically 'normal' individuals.

Within recognized diagnostic criteria, property offending by young people may be classified within the remit of 'conduct disorder'.

Conduct disorder and antisocial personality disorder

The features of conduct disorder are multifarious, but in relation to both firesetting and property offending they incorporate the individual's capacity to engage in acts that are deemed to violate social norms and the basic rights of others. Where the conduct is not aggressive the young person may be engaged in acts of destruction against property, deceitfulness and theft. Whilst the destruction of others' property include firesetting and vandalism, behaviours such as deceitfulness and/or theft includes breaking into property (residential, public, business or motor vehicles), stealing goods that are of little or no value and where there is no confrontation of the victim – shoplifting and obtaining goods by deception.

Where the onset of conduct disorder is in early childhood there must be at least one of the criteria present prior to the age of 10 years; when this criterion is fulfilled, the prognosis may be for an increased propensity to develop antisocial personality disorder. Where the onset is in adolescence and no criteria were present under the age of 10, the prognosis is better in that such individuals are less likely to experience persistence of the conduct disorder or develop antisocial personality disorder.

Conduct disorder may be further defined as mild, moderate or severe.

- Where it is mild, the problems/behaviours demonstrated are not in excess of those required to make a diagnosis and result in relatively minor behavioural problems.
- Where it is moderate, the problems are intermediate and may involve causing some harm to others, such as through shoplifting or acts of vandalism.
- Where it is severe, the problems are in excess of the criteria for diagnosis and may result in significant harm to others, such as confronting the victim to steal property or breaking and entering.

Fineman (1980) argued that firesetting is rarely a single problem. Kuhnley et al. (1982) suggested that firesetters were more frequently diagnosed as being conduct disordered or having attention deficit disorder than were non-firesetting children. Kolko et al. (1985) observed that children who set fires and who were diagnosed as having conduct disorder demonstrated more extreme behaviours than did children with the same diagnosis who did not set fires. Firesetters were also more likely to engage in property destruction, lying, stealing, vandalism and cruelty to animals. Walker (1983) stated that firesetters achieved higher scores in externalizing behaviours and lower scores in internalizing behaviours than did non-firesetters.

The incidence of diagnosed conduct disorder has increased. Current estimates suggest that for males under 18 years the rate is 6–16%, whilst for females it is 2–9%. It is therefore one of the most common diagnoses (DSM-IV).

Antisocial personality disorder encompasses a range of behaviours that violate social norms and demonstrate a disregard/violation of the rights of others. Whilst this diagnosis cannot be attached to individuals under 18 years of age (within the legal provisions of English law), a young person may demonstrate features of antisocial personality and a criteria for diagnosis in adulthood is the presence of conduct disorder under the age of 15. In relation to property offending, individuals engage in acts that may lead to arrest, such as destroying property or

stealing. They may be involved in deceitful or manipulative behaviour in order to obtain money and demonstrate little or no remorse and minimize the effect on their victims. The incidence of antisocial personality disorder ranges from 3% for males to 1% for females – a lower incidence than that recorded for conduct disorder.

The prognosis may be dependent upon maturational processes. It is not unknown for professionals to see a remission in the antisocial behaviour demonstrated by young adults; by the time a person matures into his or her forties, practitioners would expect to record a remission in all antisocial behaviours (DSM-IV).

TREATMENT INTERVENTIONS

Introduction

There is a distinct lack of comprehensive literature examining the efficacy of 'programmes' dealing with adolescent or mentally disordered adolescent offenders. In some cases offences such as arson and criminal damage are afforded a high media profile and appear to have 'victims', whilst other offences considered minor in terms of 'the victim' are submerged into society's economic statistics. Crimes that have severe impact on their 'victims' – such as theft of a motor vehicle and driving without due care or attention resulting in a pedestrian's death – merit the development of treatment programmes for the perpetrator at both community and institutional level; whereas those convicted of repeated acts of firesetting are not diverted to such intervention programmes – rather they are 'contained'.

Education for the child and the family can be an important preventative measure. Research has shown that children who are predisposed to be curiosity firesetters (or repeat stealers) often received less supervision and education about the consequences from the family network. Some fire services have developed short intervention programmes that incorporate education regarding the consequences of firesetting.

Stewart (1993) identified a number of factors in relation to firesetting (although it would be feasible to transfer the ideas for other offender populations) that could be identified and targeted for treatment, including psychological and behavioural antecedents to offending. She suggested that the 'relapse prevention model' could be useful in the management of recidivists. This model reviews details of the offence cycle in order to assist the offender to identify the emotional, cognitive and circumstantial antecedents to the firesetting behaviour. Practitioners, she suggested, could then target treatment to facilitate the development of coping behaviour(s) – for example, escape from or avoidance of high-risk situations, relaxation techniques, assertiveness training, and cognitive reconstructing.

Jackson (1994) argued that, for pathological arsonists, the 'only viable option theory' promoted treatment interventions that helped the individual to attain greater psychological insight into his or her motives for firesetting (again it would be feasible to transfer the ideas to other offender populations). This theory promotes the development of problem-solving strategies alongside helping the individual to overcome inhibitions that may previously have prohibited the use of alternative strategies. The theory thus redirects the individual's efforts towards attainable goals. Jackson commented that this approach highlighted that the prediction of future risk lay within the underlying psychological factors that led to distress, rather than in any specific psychiatric disorder. The 'only viable option' model was essentially the first stage in the development of more appropriate coping strategies that influenced the immediate environment and an individual's subsequent social integration.

Approaches to recidivism

For some young people their offending behaviour has become entrenched. Whilst practitioners would envisage that maturational and/or lifespan transitional processes would have some impact, for some young people the roots of the behaviour are far more psychological in nature. As with other behaviour(s) that may be deemed a 'risk to self or others', the factors that precipitate the onset of offending are not necessarily the obverse of factors that precipitate desistance. Adolescents engaged in offending, regardless of the nature of the offence, require a wide range of intervention options incorporating some or all of the initiatives outlined below.

Where it is possible, a multi-disciplinary and multi-agency approach will reduce the potential for the individual to relapse, but such an approach requires coordinated and consistent methods of operation alongside acknowledgment of each profession's own 'vocabulary' and 'agenda'.

Skills training
Skills training aims to develop a wide range of social skills, to build or enhance self-esteem and assertiveness. It also aims to promote the individual's ability to use adaptive coping mechanisms as an alternative to offending. Such training promotes self-awareness of potential abilities, thus serving to increase mental health and ultimately quality of life. For some individuals – especially those with early-onset psychiatric illness, or certain cognitive disabilities such as poor attention, impaired thought processes, problem-solving and conceptualisation – there may be limitations to the type of work that can be undertaken. In those cases, practitioners can seek positive outcomes in terms of awareness and the maintenance of current cognitive capacity, as opposed to alteration.

Understanding of environmental factors
Here the practitioner aims to facilitate the identification of triggers that promote the risk of firesetting. Examples are substance abuse, stressful social situations, peer pressure, academic failure or a dysfunctional home environment. Like skills training, the objective is to provide the individual with strategies to manage or avoid environmental trigger situations.

Regardless of the counselling approach adopted, the ultimate aim is to reduce psychological distress.

Behavioural therapy
Behavioural techniques involve the modification of behaviour without attempting to discuss any underlying illness. Such therapies have their roots in behaviourism and examine how behaviours are acquired, their nature, frequency, triggers and consequences. Then the assessment may indicate the stages of intervention to be used, such as desensitization to stressors, or 'flooding' to elicit desired behaviour and extinguish undesirable behaviour.

Such approaches may be used in the early stages of intervention whilst the individual becomes aware of his or her cognitive capacity. However, they are limited as they are typically viewed as a means to an end because of their focus on modification of behaviour without the cognitive changes that can be achieved by challenging attitudes, beliefs and thoughts.

Supervision and support
Within an institutional setting, support comes from the team responsible for 'care' – the core group that may be derived from health, social or penal services. There may be extended teams providing support – social services, educational, pastoral and community clinical teams. Finally there may be support available via family and other carers, voluntary organizations or support groups.

Within the remit of cooperation with intervention and a good prognosis, positive support and positive role models have been advocated to increase global life chances. By contrast, where negative behaviour is reinforced by carers or others, the prognosis is poor. Support, whether provided by professionals or other carers, requires supervision to promote coping strategies in an effort to avoid role conflicts, decreased motivation and personnel/carer 'burnout'.

Fire education
This intervention may be administered in a number of situations including school, care home or hospital environment. The ultimate aim is to promote an individual's understanding of the causes and effects of his or her behaviour and to accept responsibility for it. A number of courses designed by fire authorities have a structured approach to dealing with serious offenders. At a more conventional level, the fire service delivers education to primary school children in an effort to promote fire safety and awareness.

Education about the victims
Victim education aims to promote awareness on two levels: providing insight into why a particular victim was selected, and developing a sense of empathy through

moral development. The precursors to victim selection, planning, the level of offence (e.g. deceit, violence) and its impact are important factors that outline attributional styles and the level of 'criminal competence'. Alongside such an analysis there have been increased moves to promote 'mediation' or facing up to the personal consequences of the offence, by hearing the victim recount the experience and the person's subsequent need for an explanation of why he or she was selected.

Approaches to mentally ill offenders

Where mental illness has been formally diagnosed, an assessment of needs (educational, social, physical, psychiatric, developmental and emotional) alongside an assessment of risk to the self and others is essential to explore whether the offending behaviour is a consequence of the symptomatology of illness or correlational and derived from other aspects of the individual's psychopathology.

Firesetters and property offenders are heterogeneous groups presenting with a range of developmental, familial, interpersonal, behavioural, social, legal and clinical needs. Any intervention programme undertaken should to some extent be individualized but should always be based on an accurate and thorough clinical and risk assessment. Relevant treatment approaches and environmental controls/adaptation can then be used to promote functioning and reduce the individual's need to engage in offending. The need to consider the impact of the illness – the degree of insight, responsibility, empathy, remorse and willingness to cooperate with the programme – are confounding variables with any group of offenders but may be more pronounced in individuals demonstrating mental illness.

Practitioners may be faced with multifarious problems that have exacerbated either the illness or the offending behaviour, and so may need to have greater involvement with the family and carers. Treatment, whilst similar to programmes offered to other offenders, may also involve removal from carers and/or the family, or therapy within the terms of restrictions on the person's liberty. Treatment may, for individuals who present with early-onset mental illness, involve a period of hospitalization for assessment; for others it may involve the use of medication.

Consideration of which treatment approach to use will ultimately be based on the practitioner's assessment of the individual and the person's present situation. Selection of methods of treatment will incorporate a decision-making process.

- Will treatment intervention affect the individual's immediate level of risk?
- According to the degree of risk, will treatment be implemented in the community or within inpatient/secure settings?
- Will the individual's degree of risk at the time of assessment be immediately reduced?
- What are the intervention priorities?
- How will intervention be evaluated?

Treatment resistance

Treatment resistance is borne of a multiplicity of factors. Such factors may be static (e.g. related to historical factors in the young person's life), whereas others may be transient (e.g. related to an event perceived as hostile or adversive) occurring at a particular point in time. Such factors have to be considered in relation to the risk factors that precipitated the offending behaviour. Practitioners have acknowledged that tentative risk factors incorporate historical, developmental, situational, psychosocial and familial factors.

With early modelling (vicarious) experiences, the young person indirectly imagines the experiences of firesetting – the impact of the flames, the potential physical injuries. This may or may not be related to early exposure to related phenomena, such as witnessing fireplay/firesetting or visual media. The vicarious experiences may be heightened with certain familial occupations, such as when a family member deals with combustible products (e.g. drivers, construction workers) or where there is direct involvement (e.g. medical professionals with casualties and fire service personnel).

Engaging in antisocial behaviours and aggressive response patterns fulfils some of the criteria for conduct disorder and may also increase the propensity to participate in risk-taking activity or offending behaviour.

Limited judgement skills may be the result of delayed development, a low intelligence quotient, poor social skills (e.g. assertiveness), a lack of positive role models or limited opportunities. Low academic achievement may result in social isolation from peers, and it may lead to externalizing behaviours that result in suspension or exclusion, or to a sense of failure and the need to achieve some notoriety. Whilst young people are still developing their personality traits, some demonstrate traits of callousness, jealousy and revenge-seeking.

For some individuals the experience of limited parental/carer supervision provides opportunities to test the boundaries. For others, erratic punishment schedules present the young person with mixed messages about what is acceptable at any point in time. Where parents/carers are absent, neglecting or abusive or where there is evidence of parental/sibling psychopathology (a history of psychiatric illness, personality disorder, substance abuse, criminality), there may be an increased propensity for the young person to become involved with delinquent individuals, or to feel neglected or 'scapegoated', and to externalize feelings through challenging or offending behaviour.

Whilst the above list is not exhaustive, nor are the factors mutually exclusive, it helps to illustrate the diversity of factors that may impede successful intervention.

A number of studies with adult offenders have examined the frequency of previous acts of firesetting (Hurley and Monahan 1969; Hill *et al.* 1982; Harmon *et al.* 1985; Leong 1992; Stewart 1993; Rix 1994). Other studies have examined the rate of relapse in convicted arsonists at follow-up (Inciardi 1970; Soothill and Pope 1973; Sapsford *et al.* 1978; Repo and Virkkunen 1997). Reported relapse rates range between 4% (Soothill and Pope 1973) and 35% (O'Sullivan and Kelleher 1987). Sapsford *et al.* (1978) observed that harsher sentences resulted in higher reconviction rates. Few studies have indicated the relapse rates for specific psychiatric hospital inpatient populations, but estimates of 35% have been proposed (Tennent *et al.* 1971; Geller 1984; Rice and Harris 1991). In relation to children and adolescents, the relapse rates observed have ranged between 23% (Stewart and Culver 1982) and 33% (Repo and Virkkunen 1997).

One difficulty in predicting future dangerousness and arson recidivism lies in the nature of the offending behaviour, in that it is often a covert activity that is difficult to detect. A second difficulty lies in the fact that many individuals are diverted from prosecution.

Management of firesetting behaviour

When considering the question of future dangerousness, practitioners are considering the likelihood of an individual repeating an offending behaviour in a variety of situations. Faulk (1988) argued that the practitioner's judgement was influenced both by the dynamics of the individual case and by the potential effect(s) that therapeutic and other interventions were likely to achieve in both the short and long term.

Prins (1994) argued that throughout the process of the assessment of risk, behaviour needed to be examined holistically under a number of specific headings that included past behaviour, previous and index offence(s), trigger factors, mental disorder, vulnerability, self-percep-tions, anger management, acceptance or denial, and the ability of the individual to work with a practitioner to challenge antisocial or delinquent behaviour. Where such a methodology was imposed it would be feasible to codify and operationalize information and intervention strate-gies. This approach would provide a framework to estab-lish standardized collection of information and enrich both knowledge and the implementation of evidence-based practice.

Any assessment should examine the individual's psychopathology and how or whether it is related to the offending behaviour, in order that potential causal links can then be promoted as an indicator(s) of risk. Then there is the need for repetition of the assessment to evaluate the degree of change. Practitioners acknowledge the need to undertake wherever possible a needs-led assessment in an effort to increase the potential for successful intervention by appropriately matching resources required and reflect-ing the opinions of the individual. Again such an assess-ment cannot be viewed as static; rather it must be consistently and routinely administered to be effective.

Finally, there must be an acknowledgement that simply placing an individual within a restrictive environment without treatment intervention might in the short term reduce risk by removing opportunity or access, but this is a false reading. In a similar vein, in an effort to meet the 'needs' of young people, simply placing them in a caring environment will not fulfill all their needs at all points in time.

FUTURE DIRECTIONS

Whilst there is a paucity of longitudinal studies of ado-lescents engaged in property offending *per se*, practition-ers and policymakers have to exercise caution. They need to take into consideration the fact that such offending is notoriously difficult to detect and that even when detected some individuals are diverted from prosecution. Also, firesetters and property offenders do not present as homogeneous groups, so using one standard treatment approach is unlikely to be appropriate for all individuals in a particular offending group. Practitioners need to consider how a proposed treatment will affect the imme-diate level of risk an individual poses. The extent to which more recent therapeutic interventions will impact on recidivism rates has yet to be clarified.

Bailey *et al.* (2001) examined the case histories of 20 females referred to an adolescent forensic service, in Greater Manchester, England. The aim was to describe a cohort of offenders in an attempt to develop an empirically based assessment and intervention strategy. The authors concluded that certain characteristics - such as prevalence of conduct disorder, previous psychiatric contact, poor socialization, care pathways and experience of sexual abuse – were in line with previous studies. The investigation provided the focus for future research. In 1995 the research team developed a pre-coded proforma for the collection of data on 76 variables. The proforma was used to collect retrospective case-note data on 107 male and female adolescents referred to an adolescent forensic service. The initial results of this study confirmed the heterogeneity of adolescent firesetters, high conduct-disorder prevalence rates, poor peer relationships, high levels of previous offending (criminal versatility), poor home environment and educational attainment. The study highlighted the need for clearer analysis of sequence of thoughts and affect to establish possible responses to treatment. Alongside the study other members of the department were involved in the development of an empirically based assessment/treatment protocol. The protocol provided clinicians and non-clinical staff with a comprehensive picture of adolescent fireplay/firesetting across situational and contextual factors.

The implementation of assessment and intervention packages is limited by human and financial constraints. Such programmes are also limited where an individual has been placed within conditions of security, thus restricting their mobility and access to potential targets. In those circumstances a true measure of risk cannot be achieved. What can be developed is a 'picture' of all factors that contributed to or maintained the behaviour as well as potential routes for intervention.

Practitioners selecting the method of intervention therefore need to consider whether the intervention can take place within a community setting, a hospital or a secure environment. There are physical, psychological and emotional consequences for both the offender and the community of where the treatment takes place.

Finally, if we are to move forward in our understanding of the aetiology, assessment and management of all offending behaviour, we need to adopt a knowledge/evidence-based practice approach and remain focused on the fact that, as well as preventing an escalation in such behaviour, early intervention may reduce the risk of such behaviour emerging.

APPENDIX: CASE STUDIES

VIGNETTE 1

Notes: Female referred by social services. Normal developmental milestones. Early history indicated sexual abuse by father. Relationships with both parents poor. Attended mainstream school – no learning difficulties. Was bullied and truanted. Previous contact with psychiatry/psychology services. History of alcohol abuse. Criminal history included property, violence and criminal damage. Firesetting started at 9 years, lighting grass. At age 14, handcuffed self to car park and attempted to set fire to self; barricaded self in room and set fire to mattress. Frequent episodes of absconding. Final act: drank alcohol with friend; left home early in morning; walked to modern open barn; struck match, placed it in hay and ran away. Placed in secure accommodation.

Intervention: Following assessment it was noted that features of mixed disorder of conduct and emotion and concerns were raised in relation to borderline state personality. Difficulties in expressing emotions and in linking this to behavioural difficulties was the main emphasis of first intervention. It was established that the firesetting did not promote arousal or excitement, nor was it a pattern of displaced anger. The firesetting did appear to be linked to intentions of self-harm.

Recommendations were made detailing the need for commitment from agencies over a lengthy period to provide care and intervention packages. It was suggested that

movement to a therapeutic environment that offered cognitive therapy would be of benefit. Where such procedures were in place the young person would be able to gradually move forward and not become over-dependent upon one service.

VIGNETTE 2

Notes: Male referred by child and adolescent psychiatrist. Normal developmental milestones. Early history indicated sexual abuse by a male that was known. No history of substance abuse. Attended special school – no learning difficulties. Normal peer relationships and no truancy. Previous contact with psychology service. Previous criminal history included sexual offences (both contact and non-contact). Relationships with both parents good. Firesetting started at age 14, fire set in his own home. Aged 15, again set three fires in own home causing £14,000 worth of damage. Took batteries out of smoke alarms and threw them on the fire. Left pet in the house. Overwhelming urge to destroy. Summoned help. Placed in secure accommodation.

Intervention: During examination the youth denied feeling angry but could not explain the urge to destroy things. He has had intensive work both as inpatient and day patient regarding previous abusive experience and abusing behaviour alongside offending behaviour. He demonstrated little motivation to confront his problems which ultimately increased his potential for engaging in subsequent 'risky' behaviours. The recommendation was for continued support within a secure environment with urgent and intensive work being undertaken. A 12-month inpatient stay was undertaken followed by discharge to another secure environment.

VIGNETTE 3

Notes: Male referred by child and adolescent psychiatrist. Normal developmental milestones. Early history indicated physical abuse by father. History of polysubstance misuse. Attended mainstream school – no learning difficulties. Normal peer relationships and no truancy. Previous contact with psychology service. Previous criminal history included property and criminal damage. Relationships with mother good, with father neutral. Fireplay started aged 7, melting heads off toys, burning matches on carpet, grass fires. Following move to open local authority unit became discontent. Peers suggested set a fire then they could move. Pressurised to act, set fire to mattresses then waited in another room while fire alarms activated. Moved to secure accommodation.

Intervention: At examination this adolescent presented as angry and frustrated, rejected and a 'scapegoat' for family and peers. A diagnosis of socialized conduct disorder was made. When placed in an environment lacking structure he was unable to modify his behaviour and was open to suggestions from peers regarding destruction of property. The recommendations were a period of stay in an

PART 5

Treatment approaches

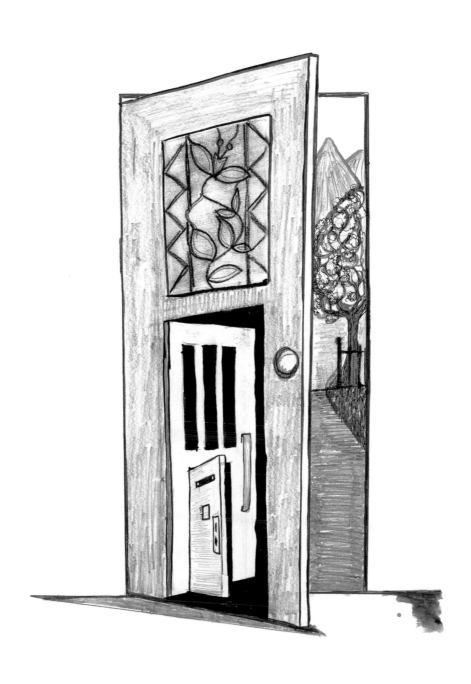

PART

19

Cognitive–behavioural therapies

KEVIN EPPS AND TRACEY SWAFFER

FROM THEORY TO THERAPY

'Cognitive–behavioural therapy' (CBT) is an umbrella term which refers to intervention techniques and strategies which have their roots in three psychological theories: behavioural theory, social learning theory, and cognitive theory. Kendall (1991) defines CBTs as those which 'use enactive performance-based procedures as well as cognitive interventions to produce changes in thinking, feeling and behaviour' (p. 5). One of the defining characteristics of CBT is the explicit emphasis placed on learning. Factors that influence learning can be located within the individual ('internal factors') and within the surrounding environment ('external factors'). Internal factors include perceptual, emotional and cognitive functioning which, in turn, are influenced by biological and developmental variables that are intrinsic to the individual. External factors include the type of stimuli to which the individual is exposed, in addition to the manner in which stimuli are presented. Learning is also influenced by the interaction of individual and environmental factors. Thus, two people exposed to an identical situation may retain different information, and subsequently react differently because of their different learning experiences.

Unfortunately, there is a growing tendency to divorce cognitive and behavioural theory from practice. A recent study found that whilst many probation officers had been trained in the use of particular CBT techniques and strategies, many were unclear about the theoretical underpinnings of the techniques (Home Office 1997). This places limitations on the ability to use theory to create solutions to novel problems, an important skill in clinical practice. There is also growing concern that the term 'CBT' is sometimes used over-inclusively. This is a worrying trend, and may undermine evaluations of treatment effectiveness and outcome. With this in mind it seems important to provide a brief overview of the three psychological theories that underpin CBT.

Behaviourism

Behaviourism has its roots in learning theory, driven by scientific enquiry into discovering the 'laws of learning' and their influence on behaviour (Catania 1992). There are various types of learning, making the term difficult to define. However, in clinical practice changes in patterns of behaviour and thinking are accepted as evidence that learning has occurred. Modern behavioural theory recognizes that learning plays an important role in helping to shape human behaviour; that it involves an interaction between the individual and the environment; and is mediated by the sensory, perceptual and cognitive characteristics of the individual (Blackman 1981; Catania 1992). Behavioural interventions, however, emphasize the influence of the external environment on behaviour, especially features of the immediate situation (environmental cues) that trigger problem behaviour.

Research into learning has established that some events are more likely to enhance or strengthen learning, whilst others inhibit or reduce the likelihood of learning. The principles of *reinforcement* and *punishment*, and the term '*three-term contingency*' are fundamental to developing an understanding of behavioural theory and its applications in therapeutic settings.

REINFORCEMENT

A behaviour that is followed by an event which *increases* the probability of that behaviour occurring again is considered to have been reinforced. Behaviours that are reinforced during the course of childhood development have a greater chance of surviving and of becoming a feature of the individual's habitual way of responding to particular events in the environment. It is important to point out that reinforcing events often escape conscious attention: people are not always aware of the positive events which influence their behaviour. Further, not all reinforcers appear to be rewarding from the viewpoint of an observer. It is well known, for example, that pain may serve as a reinforcer (Miller 1960), and that the experience of pain can be a reinforcer in some incidents of deliberate self-injury (Epps 1997a).

There are two types of reinforcement: *positive reinforcement* and *negative reinforcement.* The former refers to events in which something is applied or given to an individual; for example, giving praise or material goods as a consequence for desirable behaviour. In contrast, negative reinforcement requires something to be removed from the individual, usually something undesirable that the person would rather avoid or escape ('escape learning'). For example, a child who is excused from doing much-hated homework after complaining of feeling unwell has been negatively reinforced and is more likely to use this complaint again.

Positive and negative reinforcement often work in tandem. Consider, for example, a parent who gives a child sweets to put an end to a noisy temper tantrum. If this tactic is successful, the child has been positively reinforced and is more likely to use a temper tantrum as a way of obtaining sweets. The parent, on the other hand, has been negatively reinforced and is more likely to use the same tactic again to avoid the noise and inconvenience of a temper tantrum. Through this mechanism it is sometimes possible to explain how negative patterns of social interaction are established. In looking at the parent–child behaviour of conduct-disordered children, Patterson and his colleagues (Patterson 1986; Patterson and Stouthamer-Loeber 1984) found that many were locked into 'coercive patterns' of behaviour. Negative, antisocial behaviour had attracted parental attention, such as scolding and shouting, at the expense of positive, prosocial behaviour. Over a period of time this resulted in an increase in antisocial behaviour, an escalation in ineffective parental attempts to discipline the child, and a feeling of hostile antagonism between parent and child.

PUNISHMENT

In behavioural theory, the term 'punishment' has a very specific meaning. A behaviour which is followed by an event which *decreases* the probability of that behaviour occurring again has been punished. In common with the concept of reinforcement, there are positive and negative forms of punishment.

Positive punishment refers to events which are applied or given to an individual. The use of interventions which produce physical pain, such as smacking or slapping, frequently spring to mind. However, these types of behaviours are associated with a variety of legal and ethical problems. Further, there is little research supporting their effectiveness in producing behaviour change (Walters and Grusec 1977). More acceptable forms of positive punishment include verbal reprimands and extra chores or work.

Negative punishment, in contrast, involves removing reinforcers from the individual, something desirable that the person would rather keep. Thus, a child may be prevented from playing with a favourite toy, or an adolescent may be denied access to some or all of his or her pocket money.

Discontinuing reinforcement for a particular behaviour results in the process known as *extinction*. Although there is usually some degree of resistance to extinction (e.g. the child more frequently complains of feeling unwell to avoid homework), extinction ultimately results in a decrease in the target behaviour. An extinction procedure commonly used with children is 'time-out' from positive reinforcement. This usually involves removing the child from sources of social reinforcement, such as attention from peers. Used correctly, in conjunction with reinforcement, punishment can help to reduce undesirable behaviour (Marshall 1965). However, punishment is likely to be less effective with children with very low self-esteem, especially those that have been subject to abuse and harsh treatment.

THREE-TERM CONTINGENCY

Any behaviour that produces consequences in the physical or social environment (operant behaviour) can be subject to analysis. It has already been noted that the extent to which a behaviour produces reinforcing or punishing *consequences* will have some bearing on the likelihood of the behaviour occurring again. However, analysing consequences is only part of the equation. It is also important to examine events which precede behaviour, known as *antecedents*. Some antecedents serve as triggers for particular kinds of behaviour. For example, a teacher leaving a classroom for a few minutes may serve as a trigger for the class bully to intimidate a vulnerable pupil.

The notion of *three-term contingency* involves placing a behaviour (B) in the context of its antecedents (A) and its consequences (C). The three-term contingency is central to *applied behavioural analysis* and to the school of behavioural treatment known as 'behaviour modification'. Manipulation of the environmental antecedents and consequences surrounding a particular target behaviour is central to most behavioural interventions that seek to modify and shape behaviour. For example, behavioural approaches to depression help the individual to structure a daily routine in an effort to trigger behaviours that will be positively reinforced (Fennell 1989). Rewards for achieving specific behavioural targets may take the form of approval, access to desired activities, or points or tokens which can be used to gain access to such activities or purchase material goods. Behavioural contracts may also be used, whereby the individual agrees to behave in certain ways and receives rewards for doing so (DeRisi and Butz 1975).

Behavioural modification approaches have been used in the treatment of aggressive adolescents (Varley 1984), and in residential settings, where there is greater control over the environment (Cullen and Seddon 1981; Milan 1987). The term 'behaviour therapy' is also used, although use of this term tends to be restricted to individualized behavioural interventions focused on improving behavioural competence and performance – for example, helping someone to become less anxious by teaching them how to relax, or how to be more assertive by teaching assertiveness skills.

Cognitive theory

Although behavioural practitioners do not deny the existence of an inner psychological world of thought and feeling, there has been considerable debate about the influence of these factors in determining behaviour (Blackman 1981). This debate has been central to the development of CBTs. Traditionally, many behavioural practitioners considered the inner psychological world to be less important than external events in determining behaviour, and therefore focused their interventions on external factors (Jones et al. 1977). Thus, whilst counselling a young male offender to help him to develop a positive self-image may be useful and desirable, it could be argued that a more powerful intervention would be to teach him social and personal skills that evoke positive responses from other people. This positive feedback would, in turn, reinforce and encourage further episodes of effective social behaviour and help the offender to develop a positive self-image.

However, the role of cognition was subject to considerable attention during the 1970s and 1980s as part of the information-processing paradigm (Bower 1975; Klahr and Wallace 1976). Cognitive psychology soon established itself as a respected discipline and clinical practitioners began to incorporate ideas and techniques into their own brands of therapy, sometimes independently of mainstream cognitive psychology (Brewin 1988). The work of Ellis (1962), who developed rational–emotive therapy (RET), and Beck's (1976) cognitive therapy, have had a major impact on clinical practice.

The term 'cognition' refers to various processes that enable us to gain information about, and an understanding

of, our environments (Goswami 1998). It is not a unitary concept, but refers to a wide range of mental structures, processes and products, including attention, perceptions, appraisals, beliefs, attitudes, memories, goals, standards and values, expectations, and attributions, in addition to current thoughts and self-statements (Kendall 1991; Reinecke et al. 1996). Thus, it is not only the cognitive contents that are of interest to the clinician, but the ways in which information is represented in memory and the mediational processes by which information is processed and used.

A fundamental assumption of cognitive therapy is that cognitions influence emotions and behaviour. Thus cognitions, not overt behaviour, are the primary target of therapy, although behavioural change is obviously a desired outcome. The role of faulty, dysfunctional, unhelpful styles of thinking in criminal behaviour has a long tradition (Yochelson and Samenow 1976). Thus, offenders are frequently reported as having 'concrete' or 'impulsive' styles of thinking (Hollin 1990a). It is not surprising, therefore, that cognitive techniques were incorporated into treatment programmes for offenders. Recent years have seen the development of specific types of cognitive therapy, such as the thinking-skills programmes, geared specifically to offender populations (Ross et al. 1989).

Social learning theory

Social learning theory is associated with the work of Rotter (1954) and Bandura (1977, 1986). It has its roots in behaviourism, recognizing that much of human behaviour is learned and is influenced by the behaviour of others. However, while the environment remains a key factor in learning, the impact of the environment on behaviour is mediated by cognition. Bandura drew particular attention to the role of observational learning. Individuals do not learn everything from direct physical experience; rather they learn through observing others. He described various stages in the process of observational learning: attention, retention, and motor reproduction.

Bandura found that the strength of observational learning, in terms of whether the observer retains information and is likely to copy the behaviour, is dependent upon motivational variables. He identified three main influences on motivation:

- *external reinforcement*, which refers to the extent to which behaviour is reinforced or punished (as in operant theory)
- *self-reinforcement*, which is the sense of pride and achievement experienced when an individual satisfies a particular goal
- *vicarious reinforcement*, which is the observation of other people's behaviour (the model) being reinforced or punished.

Thus, one child is more likely to imitate another child if the child model has been observed to be rewarded for a behaviour.

Self-regulatory processes have a central role in social learning theory, recognizing that individuals are selective about the aspects of the environment to which they attend. Bandura's concept of *self-efficacy* is particularly important to the issue of self-regulation and has an important influence on clinical practice. Self-efficacy refers to a belief that one can perform the behaviours necessary for a given outcome in a specific situation. This competency belief is distinct from knowledge about what behaviour is needed to produce the outcome.

Although at first sight social learning theory seems to be an integration of cognitive and behavioural theory, it was developed independently of modern cognitive theory. In terms of its application in therapeutic settings, it places emphasis on the manipulation of environmental factors rather than cognitive factors.

THERAPEUTIC APPLICATIONS

The application of interventions derived from the three theoretical models described above to the management and treatment of young offenders has been practitioner-led, using case-study research (Edwards 1996) and the scientist–practitioner model of practice (Long and Hollin 1997). This model was developed to bridge the gap between psychological research and clinical practice, with the goal of ensuring that the profession of clinical psychology was strongly rooted in empirical research. Although not without its problems and critics (Peterson 1985; Shakow 1978), the model encouraged clinicians to undertake and publish research. Research into the use of CBT in clinical settings was also facilitated by the extensive behavioural and cognitive experimental research literature. There is now a substantial literature on the use of CBT in applied settings, including those for antisocial, delinquent adolescents (see Hollin 1990a, 1993). Unfortunately, there has been a recent decline in empirical research into the use of CBT with juvenile offenders (Milan 1996), despite their usefulness in reducing recidivism (Lipsey 1992).

Prevention approaches (Kirschenbaum and Ordman 1984) and school-based interventions (Burchard and Lane 1982) are not covered in the present chapter, and only passing reference is made to family approaches (Alexander and Parsons 1973; Bank *et al.* 1987; Welch 1985) and multi-systemic therapy (Henggeler 1999). The main focus is on the use of CBT with adolescents who have already offended, especially the significant minority who place most demand on services owing to the persistent and serious nature of their criminal behaviour. Many of these adolescents present with a complex variety of social, psychological and behavioural problems in addition to their offending, including substance abuse, self-injury, learning difficulties, and psychiatric illness (Bailey *et al.* 1994).

The relevant literature can be categorized in several different ways, according to location (community, institutional or residential), focus of the intervention (for example, sexual deviancy, anger, problem-solving, assertiveness), target population included in the programme (at-risk children, low-tariff delinquent adolescents, adolescents convicted of serious or persistent offending), type of offence (violent, sexual, property, mixed-offender groups), and the way in which the intervention is delivered (individual, group, family). Intervention programmes can generally be described according to these various categories.

GROUP PROGRAMMES

Although all CBT interventions seek to change the behaviour of the individual, some programmes are delivered to groups of offenders. The use of small groups as a form of therapy has a long history within adolescent psychiatry (Brown 1992). Group work is cost-effective, and is a natural extension of the school classroom environment. It can be used to facilitate learning through peer pressure, group discussion, modelling, and skill-building exercises, such as role-play, in a way that is difficult in individual therapy. The social context and use of group activities also reduces boredom and opting-out. Consequently, group work has become the preferred medium for delivering some CBT interventions to young offenders.

Traditionally, most offender programmes were targeted at mixed groups of young offenders, using either exploratory, psychodynamic group techniques, or the structured, skill-training CBT techniques described later in the chapter. However, interest in the treatment of adolescent sex offenders during the 1980s, initially in the USA (Becker *et al.* 1993), led to the development of offence-focused small-group work (Margolin 1984). This type of work, which is addressed by Eileen Vizard in Chapter 17 on juvenile sex offenders, was deemed necessary because many sex offenders have problems and needs that cannot easily be addressed through traditional generic group work.

However, although offence-specific group work is particularly associated with the treatment of sexual offenders, other types of offences and problems have been singled out for special attention, usually on the basis that the type of offence has powerful compulsive or 'addictive' elements which require focused, in-depth attention. Offence-focused group programmes have been described for adolescents with an extensive history of car crime (Chapman 1995; Kilpatrick 1997; McMurran and Whitman 1997), shoplifting (MacDevitt and Kedzierzawski 1990), firesetting (Barnett and Spitzer 1994; Hollin and Epps 1996;

Kolko 1988), and crime related to substance abuse (McMurran 1991, 1996; McMurran and Hollin 1993). Whilst the content and nature of the work varies according to the focus of the group, drawing from the various CBT methods outlined in the present chapter, the group generally functions in a similar way to those for sex offenders, with an emphasis on active participation, skill-building, and relapse prevention.

INDIVIDUAL INTERVENTIONS

For a variety of reasons, group work is sometimes not feasible. There may be insufficient numbers, or organizational or logistical problems preventing group work. Alternatively, the young person in question may be too disruptive or violent to make effective use of group work; have problems that are too personal or sensitive to discuss in a group setting; or may simply refuse to participate. It has also been suggested that group work is not suitable for some types of offender on the grounds that it may actually encourage criminal behaviour (Andrews *et al.* 1990). Consequently, individual work may therefore be the only available option. It is probably the case that some of the most difficult, violent and dangerous young offenders, such as those seen in residential secure units, are not suited to offence-focused group work, at least not until a considerable amount of individual work has been carried out (Epps 1997b).

Individual assessment

One of the hallmarks of cognitive–behavioural interventions is the use of structured, objective methods of assessment. Individualized assessment is especially important when planning individual interventions. It seems sensible to invest more time and resources into those adolescent offenders who have committed the most serious offences and who may be at risk of re-offending in similar, or more serious, ways. In addition, the problems presented by many high-risk offenders are long-standing and particularly complex.

Individual clinical assessment has three main objectives:

1 to collect relevant information about the individual and the problems of interest
2 to make sense of the information in an effort to understand the factors which contribute to the problem behaviour
3 to decide how best to intervene.

CBT assessment proceeds on the assumption that the individual lacks appropriate behavioural skills, or has beliefs (cognitive contents) or problem-solving capacities (cognitive processes) that are in some way deficient or distorted.

To overcome the limitations of any one method of assessment, *multi-modal assessment* is encouraged. Information is drawn from a variety of sources (self-report, direct behavioural observation, indirect or third-party behavioural observation, psychometric assessment, and archival background documentation) using a variety of techniques (interviewing, diary-keeping, self-monitoring, paper-and-pencil questionnaires and rating scales, structured behavioural observation schedules, informal observation reports, approved psychometric tests).

Specific problematic behaviours and cognitions are targeted for particular attention within a CBT approach. Several psychometric measures have been developed to facilitate the cognitive assessment of some problem areas. For example, the Adolescent Cognition Scale (Hunter *et al.* 1991) and the Multi-Phasic Sex Inventory (Nichols and Molinder 1984) are sometimes used to assess the beliefs, attitudes and cognitions in adolescent sex offenders. Where behavioural data are collected, good clinical practice dictates that a *baseline* should be established before intervention begins, in which data about the problem are plotted graphically for either visual or statistical inspection. A stable baseline is one in which the identified problem (in terms of frequency or intensity, for example) remains constant over the assessment period. The establishment of a baseline enables the effects of intervention to be more easily determined.

Making sense of the information gathered during an assessment is perhaps the most complex task. An underlying assumption of behavioural assessment is that behaviour, both adaptive and maladaptive, serves some kind of function for the individual, and that behaviours which survive over the course of time are those with the greatest functional utility. Individuals are not necessarily aware of the functional significance of particular behaviours. The use of cognitive assessment is especially useful in this respect, helping to provide information about the thoughts (including fantasies) and feelings which are associated with the problem behaviour and which may in themselves serve as powerful sources of reinforcement. Assessment of offence-related fantasies is particularly important in young people who commit sadistic, bizarre and inexplicable acts of sexual or physical violence (Bailey 1996, 1997; Duncan and Duncan 1971; Hardwick and Rowton-Lee 1996).

The technique of *functional analysis* provides a useful framework for analysing and understanding problem behaviour (Sturmey 1996) and has increasingly been applied to individuals who offend (Gresswell and Hollin 1992; Hollin 1990a, 1992). This technique uses Skinner's (1938, 1953) three-term contingency, in which behaviours (B) are placed in the context of their antecedents (A) and consequences (C). Functional analysis seeks to use the available information to form a hypothesis about the factors serving to maintain the behaviour. Using this model, it is equally possible to subject cognitions to the same analysis, construing them as 'private behaviours'. Thus, it becomes possible to explore the reciprocal relationship that exists between thoughts, emotion and behaviour, such as that developed by Novaco (1978) in his model of anger.

According to the functional analytic model, interventions designed to change problem behaviour constitute a form of hypothesis testing. This framework sits easily within the scientist–practitioner model referred to earlier and helps to explain why functional analysis has been applied across a diversity of clinical settings. The technique is especially useful with adolescents who present with extremely challenging behaviours of an antisocial or self-destructive nature (Epps 1997a; Hollin *et al.* 1995). Functional analysis, combined with regular reviews of programme effectiveness, can help to provide a clear rationale for clinical decision-making and problem-solving (Nezu and Nezu 1989).

Cognitive–behavioural interventions

CBT practitioners working with individual young offenders have at their disposal a range of intervention techniques and strategies (Camp and Ray 1984; Hollin 1990a,b; Kendall 1991; Kennedy 1984; Reinecke *et al.* 1996; Wilde 1996). As an approach to working with offenders, CBT assumes that offending behaviour has been shaped by the social environment (family, peers, neighbourhood, subculture, culture); that the offender has failed to acquire, or fails to use, certain cognitive skills; or has learnt inappropriate ways of behaving. One of the strengths of CBT is its ability to bridge the gap between behaviour modification and traditional insight-oriented therapies. The use of cognitive techniques in addition to behavioural approaches provides the means to engage the young person in meaningful dialogue about the problem, to explore possible explanations for its origin, and to develop effective cognitive coping strategies. Cognitive techniques may prove to be particularly useful in treating the symptoms of post-traumatic stress disorder (PTSD) (Pynoos and Nader 1993) which may contribute to the development of some types of violent behaviour (Dodge *et al.* 1990a; Perry 1994), particularly in children who have been subject to traumatic experiences, such as sexual or physical abuse (Falshaw *et al.* 1996).

Recent years have seen a marked increase in the use of CBT with offenders, both juvenile and adult. Although CBT has been used with offenders for many years, their use was often confined to clinical psychologists working in psychiatric settings with mentally disordered offenders (Howells 1982; Perkins 1986). Expansion in the use of CBT from hospital to community settings owes much to reviews of the treatment literature which provided evidence for the effectiveness of CBT interventions for reducing criminal recidivism among delinquents (Andrews *et al.* 1990; Garrett 1985; Gendreau and Ross

1979; Hollin 1993; Lipsey 1992, 1995; Losel 1995; Palmer 1975; Whitehead and Lab 1989). Interventions employing behavioural, cognitive and multi-modal CBT methods, focused on criminogenic factors, showed the largest and most consistent effects. Further, programmes that addressed cognitive problems had significantly better outcomes than the ones which did not (Gendreau and Andrews 1990; Izzo and Ross 1990). Lipsey (1992) estimated that CBT treatment programmes can produce reductions in recidivism of 20% or more in juvenile offenders. A recent study by the Offenders and Corrections Unit of the Home Office (1997) provided data on the use of cognitive skills programmes in 39 probation areas in England and Wales. A total of 191 programmes were on offer.

Most of the interventions described in the remainder of this chapter have two goals:

- to increase and strengthen self-control
- to enhance the capacity of the offender to understand the perspective of others.

ANGER MANAGEMENT TRAINING

A variety of CBT interventions have been used to deal with the problems of anger and aggression in children and adolescents (Lochman *et al.* 1991), including cognitive modelling (Goodwin and Mahoney 1975), social problem-solving training (Chittenden 1942; Robin *et al.* 1976; Spivak and Shure 1974; Zahavi and Asher 1978), social perspective-taking training (Chandler 1973), self-instructional techniques (Meichenbaum 1977; Meichenbaum and Goodman 1971), rational–emotive behaviour therapy (REBT) (Wilde 1996), and anger management (or control) training (Dangel *et al.* 1989; Deffenbacher 1988; Feindler and Ecton 1986; Kaufman and Wagner 1972; Schlichter and Horan 1981). Of these, anger management training is probably the best known and frequently used technique. This technique owes much to the work of Novaco (1975, 1985, 1994), whose cognitive–behavioural model of anger led to the development of anger management programmes designed to reduce angry arousal and improve coping strategies.

Based on Meichenbaum's (1975) stress-inoculation model, Novaco (1985) construes anger as a stress reaction with three response components: cognitive, physiological and behavioural. CBT interventions assume that an angry, aggressive state is mediated through a person's perceptions, expectations and appraisals and that the likelihood of violence is increased or decreased as a result of this process. Studies have identified the presence of social–cognitive difficulties among violent adolescents (Davis and Boster 1992; Dodge 1980; Dodge *et al.* 1990b; Feindler 1991; Kendall *et al.* 1991; Lochman and Dodge 1994; Munro 1995; Slaby and Guerra 1988; Swaffer and Hollin 1997). These include deficiencies in abstract reasoning and problem-solving, and the presence of cognitive distortions (dysfunctional thinking processes) leading to hostile appraisal of neutral situations.

Use of anger management training with offender populations has been driven by the desire to reduce angry aggression. A typical programme consists of several modules devoted to helping the offender to recognize the emotion of anger and its associated physiological and cognitive sequelae; explore and challenge beliefs supporting aggression; identify triggers that lead to the experience of anger; develop techniques to enhance self-control, such as relaxation and breathing exercises, and cognitive strategies, such as counting from one to ten; and strengthen motivation to avoid angry aggression by exploring the negative consequences of angry aggression to self and others (Feindler and Ecton 1986).

Unfortunately, the terms 'violence' and 'aggression' are often used interchangeably in the literature, making it difficult to interpret research findings. An intervention that is successful in modifying the aggressive behaviour of school children, for example, may not have the same effect when used with recidivistic delinquents with a history of serious violent assaults. Furthermore, some studies do not distinguish physical violence from sexual violence, whilst others draw distinctions between serious, chronic and antisocial violent offenders (Tate *et al.* 1995).

Most studies have used anger management training with mixed groups of aggressive and violent adolescents in community, institutional and psychiatric settings (Dangel *et al.* 1989; Feindler and Ecton 1986; Feindler and Fremouw 1983; Feindler *et al.* 1984; Tate *et al.* 1995). In one of the few books devoted to this area, Feindler and Ecton (1986) provide the most convincing account of its effectiveness, sometimes with extremely violent, explosive adolescents displaying severe behaviour disorders.

Anger management programmes are now widely used with young offenders in a variety of contexts, including those detained in custodial settings (McDougall *et al.* 1987). McDougall and associates found that their anger management programme was associated with a reduction in institutional offending in the 18 young offenders in their study.

INTERPERSONAL TRAINING IN PROBLEM-SOLVING SKILLS

For some time it has been recognized that many persistent offenders are poor at solving interpersonal problems (Bandura 1973; Sarason 1978). Frequently they are inflexible in their approach to problem-solving, and do not have access to the various cognitive and behavioural skills and strategies that most people take for granted. In essence, they are poor at thinking on their feet, the result of a variety of cognitive problems reported in the research literature on delinquency, including deficits in means-to-an-end thinking, alternative thinking, and perspective-taking (Platt *et al.* 1973, 1974; Spivack and Levine 1963).

In extreme instances, there may be poverty of thought and impaired verbal reasoning skills. Poor verbal intelligence, often in the context of an average IQ, is consistently reported in the research literature on juvenile delinquency (Camp 1966; Prentice and Kelly 1963; Quay 1987a).

Problem-solving training was first introduced into the behavioural literature by D'Zurilla and Goldfried (1971), who suggested five steps for its use in clinical practice:

1 Develop a general orientation or set to recognize the problem.
2 Define the specifics of the problem and determine what needs to be accomplished.
3 Generate alternative courses of action that might be used to resolve the problem and achieve the desired goals.
4 Decide among the alternatives by evaluating their consequences and relative gains and losses.
5 Verify the results of the decision process and determine whether the alternative selected is achieving the desired outcome.

The first, and most extensive, clinical application of problem-solving training to children was undertaken by Spivack and Shure (1974). Among other findings, they found that it was successful in facilitating adjustment in kindergarten children and in preventing maladaptive behaviour when these children entered first grade. Problem-solving training has since been used in a variety of applied settings, including those treating antisocial adolescents (Guerra and Slaby 1990; Hains 1984), where the aim has been to enhance the development of cognitive strategies to increase the adolescent's self-control and social responsivity.

The Viewpoints Training Programme (Guerra and Panizzon 1986), which focused mainly on violent adolescents, made extensive use of problem-solving training. The programme was designed to effect changes in beliefs and attitudes about the legitimacy of violence in response to conflict and emphasize specific social problem-solving skills. In a controlled evaluation of this project, Guerra and Slaby (1990) looked at a sample of 120 adolescents incarcerated for violent crimes. Those who attended a 12-session workshop on social problem-solving showed increased skills in solving problems and decreased endorsement of beliefs supporting aggression. Further, they were rated by staff as less aggressive and impulsive than an attention-only control group and a no-treatment group. Unfortunately, there were no group differences in the number of parole violators 24 months after release.

SELF-INSTRUCTION TRAINING

Self-instruction training (SIT) was introduced in the early 1970s by Meichenbaum (1974, 1975, 1977) and developed by Goldstein and Keller (1987), drawing on the language-developmental branch of cognitive-developmental psychology, especially the ideas of Luria (1961) and Vygotsky (1962). Based on the notion that children gradually move away from a social world regulated by adults, to one in which they regulate their own behaviour through overt and then covert speech (what they say to themselves), Meichenbaum and Goodman (1971) developed a self-instruction programme to teach impulsive children how to control their own behaviour. This programme required the instructor to model the overt behaviour and the appropriate self-statements. The child then imitated the target behaviour while first self-instructing aloud, then whispering, and finally covertly rehearsing the self-statements. Since this initial application, SIT has been successfully applied to a variety of clinical problems, including problems commonly found in antisocial adolescents, such as impulsivity, aggression, hyperactivity, academic under-achievement, and poor social competence (Craighead *et al.* 1978; Kendall and Williams 1981; Snyder and White 1979; Williams and Akamatsu 1978).

Another type of SIT, termed 'thought-stopping' (Wolpe 1969), has also been used successfully to reduce the frequency and intensity of aggression in a 16-year-old boy with a long history of aggressive outbursts (McCullough *et al.* 1977). Unfortunately, this technique was less useful when applied to delinquent boys incarcerated in a state training school (Huntsinger 1976). Kendall and Braswell (1985), reviewing the literature in this field, concluded that there was significant evidence of treatment effectiveness. However, they recommended that more attention should be given to adapting self-instructional procedures to suit the age and verbal ability level of individual children.

SELF-MANAGEMENT TRAINING

Self-management training, also known as 'behavioural self-control training' (BSCT) (Mahoney and Thoresen 1974) or 'self-regulation training' (Bandura 1978; Mahoney and Arnkoff 1978), has been used extensively in clinical practice. It has its origins in Skinner's (1953) suggestion that individuals control their own behaviour in the same fashion that they control others' behaviour; that is, through operant procedures. However, more recently the role of internal, cognitive factors in self-control has been emphasized (Goldfried and Merbaum 1973; Kanfer 1970, 1971; Kanfer and Karoly 1972; Mahoney and Arnkoff 1978; Mahoney and Thoreson 1974; Reinecke *et al.* 1996; Ronen 1997).

Deficits in self-control, especially in the ability to delay gratification, have been reported in delinquents (Unikel and Blanchard 1973). It is generally accepted that there are four important components to self-control: goal-setting, self-monitoring, self-evaluation, and self-reinforcement or, alternatively, self-punishment. Failures in one or more of these factors may help to undermine self-control. For example, it seems that delinquents

often fail to set goals or lack confidence in their ability to achieve conventional goals, choosing alternative antisocial goals (Sarason 1978). They are also more likely to have an external locus of control, believing that they have little influence over events (Beck and Ollendick 1976).

Numerous studies have shown that children and adolescents (O'Leary and Dubey 1979) and delinquents (Ayllon and Milan 1979; Gagne 1975; Seymour and Stokes 1976; Snyder and White 1979; Stumphauzer 1976; Wood and Flynn 1978) can be helped to improve their self-regulatory skills. The emphasis in treatment programmes for delinquents is on training in educational, vocational and interpersonal skills in the hope that this will increase their expectations that they can achieve conventional goals through socially acceptable behaviour and therefore begin to regulate their own behaviour more effectively (Fixsen *et al.* 1976).

TRAINING IN PERSPECTIVE-TAKING

The idea that some individuals are able to violate the rights of other people with little compunction or guilt because of an inability or failure to assume the perspective or point of view of the victim has a long history in psychology (Gough 1948; Hogan 1973; Sarbin 1954). Numerous studies have since found that delinquents and adult prisoners score lower on various perspective-taking tasks than do non-criminal comparison groups (Chandler 1973; Kennedy *et al.* 1980; Little and Kendall 1979; Rotenberg 1974; Widom 1976). Deficits in perspective-taking appear to be especially severe among delinquents and adult criminals labelled as 'psychopathic' (Jurkovic and Prentice 1977; Kennedy *et al.* 1979).

Although various perspective-taking tasks, such as role-play, are included in treatment programmes for delinquents, Chandler's (1973) study is usually cited in support of the usefulness of perspective-taking as an intervention for delinquents. In this study, 15 delinquent boys were required to work in small groups to develop short scenarios about real-life situations, which they then had to role-play and videotape, with each boy taking turns to play each role. All the videotapes were then viewed by the group, ostensibly in an effort to improve the scenarios. The boys who took part in this perspective-taking exercise showed greater improvement in perspective-taking than either an attention control group or a no-treatment group. Compared to the control groups, the treatment group also had almost 50% fewer incidents of delinquency during an 18-month follow-up.

A related technique developed by Feshbach (1984) is known as 'empathy skills training'. This intervention involves teaching offenders to identify another person's emotional state (affect identification), understand the situation from the other person's point of view (perspective-taking), and experience in themselves the emotions and distress felt by the victim (emotional responsiveness).

SOCIO-MORAL REASONING TRAINING

A number of studies indicate that delinquents are characterized by delayed or impaired moral reasoning, resulting in lack of concern for others and a preoccupation with satisfying their own needs (Blasi 1980; Jurkovic 1980; Lee and Prentice 1988). Gibbs (1991) suggests that antisocial juveniles are particularly prone to self-centred cognitive distortions, associated with a tendency to blame others for their own transgressions. Several attempts have been made to enhance socio-moral reasoning in delinquents in the belief that facilitation of the development of the cognitive processes involved in the evaluation and resolution of moral issues would lead to less antisocial behaviour (Arbuthnot 1992; Gibbs et al. 1984).

The intervention programme by Gibbs and associates involved small-group discussions on a variety of socio-moral issues, in which participants were required to justify their thoughts and engage in the process of reaching a group consensus on the best solution. Compared to a no-treatment control group, the intervention produced a significant improvement in moral reasoning. Using a similar procedure with male and female 'behaviour disordered' adolescents who were at risk for delinquency, Arbuthnot (1992) reported a similar finding. However, he also found that enhancement in moral reasoning resulted in a reduction in antisocial behaviour. He notes, however, that to be maximally effective socio-moral reasoning training needs to be combined with training in social and interpersonal skills to improve empathy, and communication and listening skills. Unfortunately, as yet there has been no systematic evaluation of socio-moral reasoning training with serious and persistent young offenders.

MULTI-MODAL INTERVENTIONS

Although all of the above interventions have at some time been delivered using individual or group-work techniques, several CBT intervention programmes have been developed specifically for groups which incorporate a range of behavioural and cognitive components, termed 'multi-modal programmes'. Some of these programmes have been subject to considerable development and evaluation and are delivered only by trained practitioners according to programme guidelines. Three programmes that warrant particular attention are the Think Aloud programme (Camp et al. 1977a; Camp 1980; Camp and Bash 1980), Aggression Replacement Training (ART) (Goldstein and Glick 1987), and Reasoning and Rehabilitation (Ross and Fabiano 1985; Ross et al. 1988).

THE THINK ALOUD PROGRAMME

This multi-component training package, based on an assessment of the mediational skills of aggressive boys, utilizes self-instructional training and interpersonal problem-solving techniques. Although it has mainly been used for the treatment of young aggressive boys, rather than adolescent offenders with a history of serious violence, many of the ideas and techniques paved the way for later programmes. The programme was targeted at two problems frequently found in aggressive boys (Camp 1977; Camp et al. 1977b): impulsive, excessive task-irrelevant speech during problem-solving; and a deficit in appropriate self-guiding speech when confronted with both cognitive and social problems.

Think Aloud was designed as a structured psychoeducational training programme that could be carried out by teachers. A training manual was prepared, with lesson plans, covering approximately 40 sessions. The programme employed a variety of techniques, helping the child to pass through several phases of skill development. Initially teachers modelled cognitive responses to specific problems, which children were encouraged to copy. Children were then prompted to generate their own cognitions, and taught and encouraged to develop independent verbalizations of plans, self-monitoring and evaluation. The type of problems addressed progressed from concrete tasks such as puzzles and mazes, to abstract interpersonal and social problems encountered in real life. Emphasis was particularly placed on understanding the notion of cause and effect, and on generating alternative courses of thought and action. For example, one lesson examined the kinds of criteria that can be used to evaluate whether an action was a good idea or not a good idea.

AGGRESSION REPLACEMENT TRAINING (ART)

ART is a multi-modal, psychoeducational intervention designed to alter the behaviour of chronically aggressive young people. It incorporates skill-streaming (designed to teach a broad range of social behaviours), anger management training (a curriculum for modifying anger responses), and moral reasoning training (designed to enhance awareness of the damaging consequences of violence) (Goldstein and Glick 1987). The use of a multi-modal approach enables ART to tackle the wide range of problems that are commonly found in persistently aggressive young people (McGuire 1997). Adolescents whose aggression has persisted throughout childhood have often failed to develop the perspective and role-taking skills and empathy associated with a reduction in aggressive behaviour from the age of about 4 or 5 years, when childhood aggression is usually at its peak (Matthews and Brooks-Gunn 1984). Chandler (1973), for example, found marked deficits in the ability of delinquents to differentiate their own and others' point of view. A common mistake was for them to assume that others possessed information that was available only to themselves. Anger management training alone is not sufficient to overcome these serious deficits in cognitive and emotional functioning.

ART has been used widely with aggressive and violent juveniles in correctional institutions in the USA (Goldstein and Glick 1987) and in the community, with juvenile gangs (Goldstein and Soriano 1994). Goldstein and Glick found that violent youths who received ART, compared with those who did not, showed significant increases in constructive, prosocial behaviours, more advanced moral reasoning, and decreases in rated levels of impulsivity, within the institutional setting. However, ART youths did not differ from controls in either the number or intensity of acting-out behaviours. In a review of treatment effectiveness of violent juvenile delinquents, Tate *et al.* (1995) conclude:

> 'ART shows promise because of its multi-modal approach, its ability to be delivered within secure juvenile correctional facilities, and its production of some cognitive–behavioural changes in violent adolescents. However, its effectiveness for reducing violent behaviour both before and after release of the youth from a correctional facility has yet to be demonstrated' (p. 779).

THE REASONING AND REHABILITATION PROGRAMME

In addition to the multi-modal programmes developed specifically to deal with anger and aggression, a variety of combined CBT interventions have been used to tackle the various social–psychological problems frequently found in persistent and serious juvenile offenders, especially those that are considered to be criminogenic.

One of the most thoroughly developed is the Reasoning and Rehabilitation (R&R) programme developed in Ontario by Ross and his colleagues (Ross and Fabiano 1985; Ross *et al.* 1988). This is a cognitive-skills training package, which has since been used by the Correctional Services of Canada in a number of prisons (Fabiano and Porporino 1992; Robinson *et al.* 1991), and is now being piloted by a number of probation areas and prison establishments within the UK (McGuire 1995; Raynor and Vanstone 1994). R&R has also given rise to several similar programmes, including the Thinking Skills programme operated in some British Young Offender Institutions (YOIs) (Blud and Whitehead 1995), the Straight Thinking on Probation (STOP) programme established by the Mid-Glamorgan Probation Service (Knott 1995), the Cognitive Self-Change programme (Bush 1995), and the EQUIP programme (Gibbs 1996; Gibbs *et al.* 1995).

The R&R programme consists of 35 two-hour group sessions, which are designed to teach not only various cognitive skills, such as problem-solving techniques, but also a range of social and self-control skills, negotiation skills, creative or lateral thinking skills, and critical reasoning. Initial evaluation was extremely promising. Ross *et al.* (1988), for example, found that 30% of the standard probation group were reincarcerated, compared to 0% for the R&R group. The STOP programme described by Knott (1995) also significantly reduced rates of re-offending. The R&R programme has subsequently been modified

and extended to various settings (Fogg 1992; Garrido and Redondo 1993; Robinson *et al.* 1991; Ross and Ross 1995). As yet, however, there are no reports of its effectiveness specifically on young offender populations.

INSTITUTIONAL AND RESIDENTIAL PROGRAMMES

Introduction

Residential care, including secure accommodation, is still the only option for the most difficult, disruptive and dangerous adolescents (Bullock *et al.* 1990; Epps 1997b; Harris and Timms 1993). During the year ending 31 March 1996, 829 young people were detained in Local Authority Secure Accommodation Units in England and Wales (Department of Health 1996). At any one time a significant number of young offenders are detained in YOIs, run by the prison service, and the Secure Training Centres. In addition, a small number of difficult and dangerous young people are looked after in adolescent mental health facilities, usually under the 1983 Mental Health Act (Bailey *et al.* 1994). The role and function of these different types of facility varies, especially in the extent to which they are able to provide an environment that facilitates desirable behavioural and cognitive change. Moos (1974) noted that the psychological climate within correctional institutions can either help or hinder the development of prosocial behaviour. Young Offender Institutions, for example, are primarily custodial establishments, and are not designed to promote personal change.

For a variety of reasons there are now very few residential facilities for difficult and dangerous adolescents that offer a structured CBT approach to treatment. In Britain residential practice is now largely determined by legislation and guidance under the 1989 Children Act (DoH 1991) and suffers from a lack of trained and experienced staff (Utting 1991, 1997). Nevertheless, there are reports in the literature of several successful residential programmes for difficult and delinquent adolescents informed by social learning theory, operated in both community and secure settings.

Of the community residential programmes, the most well-known and influential is the Achievement Place programme, which began in Kansas but was replicated across the USA (Braukmann and Wolf 1987; Phillips *et al.* 1971). Each Achievement Place project typically consists of a family-style home managed by a specially trained couple ('teaching-parents'), for about six offenders per home. Each group home uses a variety of intervention approaches based on social learning theory, and seeks to modify existing behaviour using a variety of techniques, including use of a token-economy programme (TEP), a merit system, skills-training and a self-government system (Burchard and Lane 1982). New teaching-parents spend a year training in the use of CBT, using a comprehensive training manual (Phillips *et al.* 1974).

Although there have been attempts to replicate elements of the Achievement Place programme in Britain (Brown 1975, 1977; Hoghughi 1979; Reid 1982; Reid *et al.* 1980; Yule and Brown 1987), these were sometimes confined to secure residential units, where the restrictions imposed by security limited programme delivery. For more than twenty years social learning theory also informed practice at the Department of Health's Glenthorne Youth Treatment Centre (Barlow 1979; Hollin *et al.* 1995), which offered care, education and psychosocial treatment in secure conditions to some of the most difficult and challenging adolescents in Britain (Browne *et al.* 1995). The social learning framework seems to have survived because of its breadth and its compatibility with a range of other conceptual and therapeutic models, such as CBT and humanistic counselling. More importantly, it has a clear focus on behaviour and provides techniques and strategies which are successful in fulfilling core residential tasks: care, safety, behavioural management, and behavioural and attitudinal change.

Two areas worthy of further discussion are the use of behavioural treatment regimes to maintain a stable living environment, and the provision of a conceptual framework for making sense of challenging behaviour.

Behavioural treatment regimes

In residential childcare settings, especially in secure units, staff and young people are in close proximity for much of the time, with high levels of social contact. Central to the social learning model is the notion that individuals are influenced by, and influence, their social environment, through the process of reciprocal determinism (Bandura 1986). The model provides a framework for analysing interactions between staff and residents, with a view to using contingency management techniques to engineer a social environment that is more likely to promote desirable behavioural and cognitive change.

The development of the Level System at Glenthorne YTC was one product of the social learning model (Ostapiuk and Westwood 1986). This system replaced the token-economy programme (TEP) originally used, and is now used in several other secure units. It operates by allowing the young person a structured, graded access to increasingly higher levels of privileges contingent upon meeting appropriate behaviours – for example, access to electrical items, computer games, and late-night television. This contingency management system helps to create a stable, predictable, daily living environment, with clear behavioural expectations and consequences. In turn, new admissions to the unit are more likely to model the positive behaviour of established residents and less likely to display the types of disordered, disruptive

behaviour often seen in other settings. Indeed, peer pressure may be applied to discourage disruptive behaviour. The influence of peers in effecting behavioural change has been well documented in the research literature (Cohen and Przybycien 1974; Hartup 1970; Kendall 1977; McGee *et al.* 1977).

The creation of a stable living regime also promotes opportunities for positive interactions between staff and young people, and allows more time for other activities such as education and vocational training. Young people, including the most difficult and challenging, benefit from recognition and praise from adults. Exposure to a wide range of activities provides young people with opportunities for achievement, and opportunities for staff to deliver praise, which together help to build self-esteem and a sense of self-efficacy. Young people who achieve at a consistently high level on the Level System can be taken off it and placed on a behavioural contract. Similarly, those who perform at an unacceptably low level, who lack the ability or motivation to improve their performance, can also be taken out of the system and placed on an individualized behavioural reinforcement programme targeted at specific problem behaviours. Young people particularly deficient in self-control, such as those with learning and attention difficulties, and high levels of anxious arousal, who are often overactive and distractible, sometimes benefit from a higher rate of feedback and reinforcement, perhaps on an hourly basis.

It is inadvisable to manage or treat mentally ill adolescents as part of their peer group within a behaviourally oriented treatment regime. An underlying assumption of this type of regime is that young people can be held responsible for their behaviour and subject to rewarding or punishing consequences in an attempt to modify their behaviour. Young people experiencing an acute mental illness cannot always be held responsible for their behaviour. Furthermore, they may be oblivious to the consequences of their behaviour and therefore fail to learn from their experiences. Nevertheless, CBT has increasingly been used with individual adult psychiatric patients displaying acute symptoms of mental illness (Chadwick and Lowe 1990; Fowler and Morley 1989) and those detained under the Mental Health Act 1983 due to personality disorder, including those with a history of offending (Hughes *et al.* 1997). There are few reports describing use of CBT with mentally ill juvenile offenders, although problem-solving and self-management techniques have been used successfully with children and young people suffering from pervasive developmental disorder (autism) (Hare and Paine 1997; Litrownik 1982, 1984; Visconti *et al.* 1996).

Understanding challenging behaviour

Staff working in residential settings for adolescents sometimes feel perplexed and anxious when confronted with extreme types of disturbed and difficult behaviour. Self-destructive behaviours, rather than violence toward others, are particularly likely to result in a psychiatric referral (Hatfield *et al.* 1996). Social learning theory can provide a useful explanatory framework for understanding challenging behaviour, and promotes an optimistic problem-solving approach to treatment. Staff behaviour can also be incorporated into the functional analysis of the young person's problem behaviour. This can help staff to recognize that their own behaviour (what they say and what they do) exerts an important influence over the behaviour of the young people in their care. As a consequence they are more likely to consider themselves as agents of change, rather than attributing responsibility for change solely to the young person. Staff who feel in control are also less likely to experience a sense of hopelessness and helplessness when confronted with challenging behaviour. Further, staff who share a common understanding of problem behaviour will be more supportive of the treatment programme and less likely to undermine or sabotage it.

STRATEGIES FOR TACKLING TREATMENT OBSTACLES

Not all young offenders are suitable for CBT. Furthermore, although cognitive–behavioural analysis is often useful as an explanatory framework, and can be used to prescribe interventions that theoretically should reduce the risk of re-offending, it is not always possible to put theory into practice. Failure to consider the limitations of CBT approaches will result in treatment failure, which may undermine confidence in this type of approach. If this is to be avoided it is important that techniques be used appropriately and that programmes be properly evaluated. Unfortunately, insufficient attention has been given to factors which limit usefulness, or the extent to which it is possible to overcome obstacles to change. Consideration especially needs to be given to two sets of factors: motivation to change, and programme management.

Motivation to change

All psychological therapies, including CBT, require active participation. Individuals in treatment are expected to use their time and energy completing tasks and exercises in an effort to produce personal change, addressing problems they would often rather avoid. Most people find personal change difficult, especially when trying to change habitual behaviours. It takes a lot of practice to learn to handle situations differently, and requires compliance and cooperation with the treatment programme. Unfortunately, many offenders, especially those with a chronic history of offending associated with serious social and psychological problems, are particularly deficient in these areas (Gudjonsson 1990). Adolescents are especially noted for their ambivalence. It is not altogether surprising, therefore, that young people with a history of personal failure, low self-esteem and low self-efficacy – characteristics frequently found in serious and persistent juvenile offenders – are often resistant to treatment. This poses a significant dilemma for practitioners: should young offenders who show no interest in addressing their problem behaviour be excluded from treatment? Unfortunately there is no simple solution to this dilemma. Willingness to comply with treatment is difficult to assess and is open to change. Some young offenders who are excluded from treatment may be denied the opportunity to change, resulting in further offending and victimization. On the other hand, attempting to treat young offenders who are unlikely to benefit is a waste of resources and may prevent treatment being offered to individuals who have more to gain.

The 'stages of change' model developed by Prochaska and colleagues can be useful when assessing motivation to change (Prochaska and DiClemente 1982; McConnaughy *et al.* 1983). The model describes the stages and processes that individuals pass through when changing their behaviour, beginning with 'precontemplation', and progressing through 'contemplation', 'preparation', 'action', and 'maintenance' stages. However, there is no research into the use of this model with young offenders.

Some young offenders referred for CBT are not consulted, on the assumption that they can somehow be persuaded to participate in treatment. The referral may reflect only the wishes of the referring agent: they want the young person to change and they want the therapist to do it. Accepting this type of referral can place the therapist under considerable pressure, especially where there is a risk of serious offending. Ultimately, the referring agency may hold the therapist, and CBT, accountable for failure. This issue can cause problems in residential contexts, where psychological treatment using CBT is often confused with residential behavioural treatment using contingency management. Wherever possible, therapists should proceed with caution when accepting a referral, and at the outset should make some estimation of likely treatment outcome. It may be desirable to offer the young person a fixed number of sessions to assess motivation to change.

The technique of *motivational interviewing* (Miller 1983, 1985; Miller and Rollnick 1991) has also provided a useful framework for analysing and enhancing motivation to change. Miller's insight was to identify poor motivation as a problem in and of itself, which can sometimes be analysed and treated like any other problem. Motivational interviewing particularly appealed to practitioners working with sex offenders (Laws 1989), where failure to comply with treatment may increase the risk of further victimization. Keeping the offender in treatment, and developing and maintaining motivation to change, are fundamental to this type of work. An engaging, flexible therapeutic style, and the use of praise and reinforcement, is preferable to an overbearing, judgemental, confrontational style which is aversive and threatening.

Historically, CBT has sometimes been reduced to a set of techniques and procedures, with little consideration of the interpersonal aspects of this type of work. Delinquent adolescents are especially sensitive to therapist characteristics (Edelman and Goldstein 1984; Holmes 1993). Although use of motivational techniques can never guarantee compliance and cooperation with treatment, they can help to foster a positive approach to working with individuals resistant to the idea of personal change.

Programme management

A variety of features associated with the delivery and management of CBT interventions have a bearing on effectiveness. Consideration should be given to identifying suitable treatment targets and desirable outcomes; client characteristics (age, gender, type of problems, treatability, motivation to change); programme content; programme delivery; organizational problems; and the generalization of behavioural and cognitive change. CBT programmes, especially multi-modal programmes delivered over many months to large numbers of offenders, and complex residential behavioural treatment programmes, require careful planning, hard work and commitment. It is especially important to avoid 'programme drift', in which programmes are not delivered as planned and are therefore less effective. The problem of programme drift has often not been considered in much of the outcome research. Discovering that an intervention does not produce the desired change tells us little if the intervention was used inappropriately or carried out incorrectly.

Hollin (1993) describes a variety of strategies that can be used to avoid programme drift. Central to this task is the use of methods to monitor and measure integrity, and a system for managing this task. If treatment integrity is to be maintained programmes should be delivered by trained staff, with adequate time and resources.

A consistent research finding in studies looking at the effectiveness of CBT is the failure of interventions to *generalize* (Abikoff 1979; Braukmann and Wolf 1987; Feindler 1991; Meichenbaum and Asarnow 1979; Stokes and Baer 1977). Not only do gains typically fail to transfer to other areas of cognitive functioning and to other settings, they also tend to dissipate over time. It is generally accepted, however, that such failures of maintenance and transfer result not from any inherent deficiency in CBT, but from the manner in which interventions are generally conducted (Glenwick and Jason 1984). Specifically, interventions are often delivered in an artificial environment

detached from the real world (e.g. in a clinic, inpatient or residential setting), often by individual practitioners using non-real-world tasks, such as role-play.

It has been suggested that more attention should be given to providing continuity in care and treatment, with aftercare and follow-up, to prevent relapse (Mulvey *et al.* 1993). The use of support networks and paraprofessionals should also be explored (Hartman 1979). Moore and Cole (1978), for example, used modelling, role-play and close supervision to train undergraduate volunteers to work successfully with hyperactive children aged 8–12 years. Behavioural parent-training has also been used with some success (Thoresen *et al.* 1979). However, these components are often lacking in many CBT programmes, especially in residential and institutional settings. Treatment is often carried out in isolation from external resources, and there may be no provision for aftercare and support owing to lack of funding, despite the fact that they deal with some of the most difficult and dangerous adolescents who present with chronic, long-term difficulties requiring long-term interventions.

Multi-systemic therapy

Multi-systemic therapy (MST), developed in the USA by Henggeler and colleagues (Henggeler and Borduin 1990; Henggeler *et al.* 1998; Henggeler 1999), is the name given to an intensive and comprehensive strategy designed to overcome many of the limitations of traditional interventions for young people with behavioural and mental health problems. Essentially, MST recognizes that to successfully intervene in the lives of young people it is necessary to direct interventions not only at the young people themselves, but also at the social contexts in which they live. The aim is to create a cohesive and integrated network of interventions around young people in their natural community habitat. Thus, interventions, including traditional forms of CBT, behavioural parent training, and other empirically based treatment approaches, are directed at the young person, the family, the school, the peer group and the neighbourhood. Problem behaviour is considered to be a function of difficulty within any of these systems and/or difficulties that characterize the interfaces between these systems (e.g. school–home and family–neighbourhood relations).

Henggeler has outlined nine MST treatment principles, shown in Table 19.1, whilst Henggeler *et al.* (1998) have recently published specific guidelines for implementing MST. Key service-delivery characteristics include low caseloads (five families per clinician); delivery of services in community settings (e.g. home, school); time-limited duration of treatment (4–6 months); constant access to therapists to provide crisis intervention (24 hours/day, 7 days/week); and the provision of comprehensive services. Adherence to the MST principles and guidelines has been

Table 19.1 *MST treatment principles*

1 The primary purpose of assessment is to understand the fit between the identified problems and their broader systemic context.

2 Therapeutic contacts should emphasize the positive and should use systemic strengths as levers for change.

3 Interventions should be designed to promote responsible behaviour and decrease irresponsible behaviour among family members.

4 Interventions should be present-focused and action-oriented, targeting specific and well-defined problems.

5 Interventions should target sequences of behaviour within or between multiple systems that maintain identified problems.

6 Interventions should be developmentally appropriate and fit the developmental needs of the youths.

7 Interventions should be designed to require daily or weekly effort by family members.

8 Intervention effectiveness is evaluated continuously from multiple perspectives, with providers assuming accountability for overcoming barriers to successful outcomes.

9 Interventions should be designed to promote treatment generalization and long-term maintenance of therapeutic change by empowering caregivers to address family members' needs across multiple systemic contexts.

Reproduced from Henggeler (1999) with permission.

shown to predict favourable long-term outcomes for violent and chronic juvenile offenders, whereas poor adherence predicts high rates of re-arrest and incarceration (Henggeler *et al.* 1997).

CONCLUSIONS AND FUTURE DIRECTIONS

Over the past decade there has been a radical rethink about 'what works' with offenders (McGuire 1995), associated with the development of psychological frameworks for understanding offending behaviour (Blackburn 1993; Hollin 1989). There are strong financial and ethical arguments supporting the use of techniques that have some proven efficacy in reducing the risk of re-offending. Although CBT interventions are only part of the solution to reducing crime among young people, they have a very important role to play. Unfortunately, there has been insufficient financial investment in the development and evaluation of community CBT programmes. The MST programme developed by Henggeler and colleagues looks particularly promising, and serves to illustrate the kind of intensive, comprehensive service delivery required to reduce recidivism in persistent young offenders.

It seems somewhat paradoxical that, at a time when tremendous inroads are being made into understanding the origins of psychosocial problems and antisocial behaviour in children and young people (Rutter and

Smith 1995; Rutter *et al.* 1998), there is minimal investment in the UK into the development and evaluation of community CBT interventions. Instead, there has been heavy investment into the building of secure accommodation, which will only ever serve the needs of the minority of extremely difficult and problematic young people.

In terms of research, investigation is needed into the relationship between patterns of cognitive and behavioural problems, response to treatment, and recidivism. Some time ago Kennedy (1984) noted that many treatment programmes use various CBT interventions with undifferentiated groups of offenders. These groups probably include individuals with only mild deficits, or no deficits at all, in all or some of the various skills being taught. Kennedy suggested that interventions should instead be targeted at those in greatest need. In a similar vein, Hersen (1981) and Lazarus (1976) advised that interventions should be tailored to the pattern of behavioural and cognitive strengths and deficits of the target group. For example, the various patterns of cognitive deficits often found in aggressive adolescents (Akhtar and Bradley 1991; Kendall 1993) are likely to require different types of intervention.

Traditional classification systems, such as those based on personality or psychiatric assessment, are not suited to the delivery of CBT programmes (Beker and Heyman 1972; Cavior and Schmidt 1978). The classification system developed by Quay (1987b) seems to have some utility. Quay suggested, for example, that 'immature-attention deficit' offenders might benefit from CBT more than 'socialized-aggressive' offenders. As yet, however, there have been no controlled studies looking at factors affecting treatment suitability.

Unfortunately, programme integrity often seems to be compromised by economic and political motives. It is easier to justify public expenditure if large numbers of offenders are put through CBT treatment programmes at low cost, regardless of whether the treatment is maximally effective. Burnett (1996) found that the probation system for assessing and matching offenders to programmes is far from satisfactory. The criminal justice system is not organized or designed to take into account the treatment needs of individual high-risk offenders. However, the Psychological Inventory of Criminal Thinking Styles (PICTS), an 80-item questionnaire developed by Walters (1995), shows some promise as a measure for assessing cognitive styles and deficits in offenders.

The role of CBT in mainstream education, as a way of preventing antisocial behaviour, also needs to be explored. Commenting on their work with young aggressive boys, Camp and Ray (1984) suggested that if long-lasting clinical effects are to be expected it may be equally, or more, important to improve cognitive functioning than it is to decrease aggressive behaviour. One of the strengths of CBT is that it equips young people with thinking and behavioural skills that may be utilized at a later point in life. Children and adolescents who lack interest and motivation when the CBT programme is delivered may nevertheless retain information and skills that are useful later in life.

REFERENCES

Abikoff, H. 1979: Cognitive training interventions in children: review of a new approach. *Journal of Learning Disabilities* **12**: 123–35.

Akhtar, N. and Bradley, E.J. 1991: Social information processing deficits of aggressive children: present findings and implications for social skills training. *Clinical Psychology Review* **11**: 621–44.

Alexander, J.F. and Parsons, B. 1973: Short-term behavioural intervention with delinquent families: impact on family process and recidivism. *Journal of Abnormal Psychology* **81**: 219–25.

Andrews, D.A., Zinger, I., Hoge, R.D. *et al.* 1990: Does correctional treatment work? A clinically relevant and psychologically informed meta-analysis. *Criminology* **8**: 369–404.

Arbuthnot, J. 1992: Sociomoral reasoning in behaviour-disordered adolescents: cognitive and behavioral change. In McCord, J. and Tremblay, R.E. (eds), *Preventing Antisocial Behaviour: Interventions from Birth through Adolescence*. New York: Guilford.

Ayllon, T. and Milan, M. 1979: Correctional Rehabilitation and Management: a Psychological Approach. New York: John Wiley.

Bailey, S. 1996: Adolescents who murder. *Journal of Adolescence* **19**: 19–39.

Bailey, S. 1997: Sadistic and violent acts in the young. *Child Psychology and Psychiatry Review* **2**: 92–103.

Bailey, S.M., Thornton, L. and Weaver, A.B. 1994: The first 100 admissions to an Adolescent Secure Unit. *Journal of Adolescence* **17**: 1–13.

Bandura, A. 1973: *Aggression: a Social Learning Analysis*. Englewood Cliffs, NJ: Prentice-Hall.

Bandura, A. 1977: *Social Learning Theory*. Englewood Cliffs, NJ: Prentice-Hall.

Bandura, A. 1978: The self system in reciprocal determinism. *American Psychologist* **33**: 344–58.

Bandura, A. 1986: *Social Foundations of Thought and Action: a Social Cognitive Theory*. Englewood Cliffs, NJ: Prentice-Hall.

Bank, L., Patterson, G.R. and Reid, J.B. 1987: Delinquency prevention through training parents in family management. *Behaviour Analyst* **10**: 75–82.

Barlow, G. 1979: United Kingdom: the Youth Treatment Centre. In Payne, C.J. and White, K.J. (eds), *Caring for Deprived Children: International Case Studies of Residential Settings*. London: Croom Helm.

Barnett, W. and Spitzer, M. 1994: Pathological fire-setting 1951–1991: a review. *Medicine, Science and the Law* **34**: 4–20.

Beck, A.T. 1976: *Cognitive Therapy and the Emotional Disorders*. New York: International Universities Press.

Beck, S.J. and Ollendick, T.H. 1976: Personal space, sex of experimenter, and locus of control in normal and delinquent adolescents. *Psychological Reports* **38**: 383–7.

Becker, J.V., Harris, C.D. and Sales, B.D. 1993: Juveniles who commit sex offenses: a critical review of research. In Hall, G.C.N., Hirschman, R., Graham, J. and Zaragoza, M. (eds), *Sexual Aggression: Issues in Etiology, Assessment, Treatment, and Policy*. Washington, DC: Taylor & Francis.

Beker, J. and Heyman, D.D. 1972: A critical appraisal of the California differential treatment program. *Criminology* **10**: 3–59.

Blackburn, R. 1993: *The Psychology of Criminal Conduct: Theory, Research and Practice*. Chichester: John Wiley.

Blackman, D.E. 1981: The experimental analysis of behaviour and its relevance to applied psychology. In Davey, G. (ed.), *Applications of Conditioning Theory*. London: Methuen.

Blasi, A. 1980: Bridging moral cognition and moral action: a critical review of the literature. *Psychological Bulletin* **88**: 1–45.

Blud, L., and Whitehead, B. 1995: Cognitive skills programmes. Paper presented at the What Works with Young Prisoners? Conference, HMYOI and RC Glen Parva, Leicester.

Bower, G.H. 1975: Cognitive psychology: an introduction. In Estes, W.H. (ed.), *Handbook of Learning and Cognitive Processes*, Vol. 1. Hillsdale, NJ: Lawrence Erlbaum.

Braukmann, C.J. and Wolf, M.M. 1987: Behaviourally based group homes for juvenile offenders. In Morris, E.K. and Braukmann, C.J. (eds), *Behavioural Approaches to Crime and Delinquency: a Handbook of Application, Research and Concepts*. New York: Plenum Press.

Brewin, C.R. 1988: *Cognitive Foundations of Clinical Psychology*. London: Lawrence Erlbaum.

Brown, A. 1992: *Groupwork*, 3rd edn. Aldershot: Ashgate.

Brown, B.J. 1975: An application of social learning methods in a residential programme for young offenders. *Journal of Adolescence* **8**: 321–31.

Brown, B.J. 1977: Gilbey House: a token-economy management scheme in a residential school for boys in trouble. *British Association for Behavioural Psychotherapy Bulletin* **5**: 79–89.

Browne, K., Falshaw, L. and Hamilton, C. 1995: Characteristics of young people involved with the Glenthorne Youth Treatment Centre during the first six months of 1995. *Youth Treatment Service Journal* **1**: 52–71.

Bullock, R., Hosie, K., Little, M. and Millham, S. 1990: Secure accommodation for very difficult adolescents: some recent research findings. *Journal of Adolescence* **13**: 205–16.

Burchard, J.D. and Lane, T.W. 1982: Crime and delinquency. In Bellack, A.S., Hersen, M. and Kazdin, A.E. (eds), *International Handbook of Behaviour Modification and Therapy*. New York: Plenum Press.

Burnett, R. 1996: *Fitting Supervision to Offenders: Assessment and Allocation Decisions in the Probation Service*. Home Office Research Study 153. London: Home Office.

Bush, J. 1995: Teaching self-risk management to violent offenders. In McGuire, J. (ed.), *What Works: Reducing Offending*. Chichester: John Wiley.

Camp, B.W. 1966: WISC performance in acting-out and delinquent children with and without EEG abnormality. *Journal of Consulting Psychology* **30**: 350–3.

Camp, B.W. 1977: Verbal mediation in young aggressive boys. *Journal of Abnormal Psychology* **86**: 145–53.

Camp, B.W. 1980: Two psychoeducational treatment programs for young aggressive boys. In Whalen, C.K. and Henker, B. (eds), *Hyperactive Children: the Social Psychology of Identification and Treatment*. New York: Academic Press.

Camp, B.W. and Bash, M.A. 1980: Think Aloud: improving self-control through training in problem solving. In Rathjen, D.P. and Foreyt, J.P. (eds), *Social Competence: Intervention for Children and Adults*. New York: Pergamon Press.

Camp, B.W. and Ray, R.S. 1984: Aggression. In Meyers, A.W. and Craighead, W.E. (eds), *Cognitive Behaviour Therapy with Children*. London: Plenum Press.

Camp, B.W., Blom, G.E. Hebert, F. and van Doorninck, W.J. 1977a: 'Think Aloud': a program for developing self-control in young aggressive boys. *Journal of Abnormal Child Psychology* **5**: 157–69.

Camp, B.W., Zimet, S.G., van Doorninck, W.J. and Dahlem, N.W. 1977b: Verbal abilities in young aggressive boys. *Journal of Educational Psychology* **69**: 129–35.

Catania, A.C. 1992: *Learning*, 3rd edn. Englewood Cliffs, NJ: Prentice-Hall.

Cavior, H.E. and Schmidt, A.A. 1978: A test of the effectiveness of a differential strategy at the Robert F. Kennedy Center. *Criminal Justice and Behaviour* **5**: 131–9.

Chadwick, P.D.J. and Lowe, C.F. 1990: The measurement and modification of delusional beliefs. *Journal of Consulting and Clinical Psychology* **58**: 225–32.

Chandler, M.J. 1973: Egocentrism and antisocial behaviour: the assessment and training of social perspective-taking skills. *Developmental Psychology* **9**: 326–32.

Chapman, T. 1995: Creating a culture of change: a case study of a car crime project in Belfast. In McGuire, J. (ed.), *What Works: Reducing Reoffending*. Chichester: John Wiley.

Chittenden, G.E. 1942: *An Experimental Study in Measuring and Modifying Assertive Behaviour in Young Children*. Monographs of the Society for Research in Child Development, VII (1, serial no. 31).

Cohen, S. and Przybycien, C.A. 1974: Some effects of sociometrically selected peer models on the cognitive style of impulsive children. *Journal of Genetic Psychology* **124**: 213–20.

Craighead, W.E., Wilcoxon-Craighead, L.W. and Meyers, A.W. 1978: New directions in behaviour modification with children. In Hersen, M., Eisler, R.M. and Miller, P.M. (eds), *Progress in Behaviour Modification*, Vol. 6. New York: Academic Press.

Cullen, J.E. and Seddon, J.W. 1981: The application of a behavioural regime to disturbed young offenders. *Personality and Individual Differences* **2**: 285–92.

Dangel, R.F., Deschner, J.P. and Rasp, R.R. 1989: Anger control training for adolescents in residential treatment. *Behaviour Modification* **13**: 447–58.

Davis, D.L. and Boster, L.H. 1992: Cognitive–behavioural expressiveness interventions with aggressive and resistant youths. *Child Welfare* **71**: 557–73.

Deffenbacher, J.L. 1988: Cognitive-relaxation and social skills treatments of anger: a year later. *Journal of Counselling Psychology* **35**: 234–6.

DeRisi, W.J., and Butz, G. 1975: *Writing Behavioural Contracts*. Champaigne, IL: Research Press.

Dodge, K.A. 1980: Social cognition and children's aggressive behaviour. *Child Development* **51**: 162–70.

Dodge, K.A., Bates, J.E. and Petit, G.S. 1990a: Mechanisms in the cycle of violence. *Science* **250**: 1678–83.

Dodge, K.A., Price, J.M., Bachorowski, J. and Newman, J.P. 1990b: Hostile attributional biases in severely aggressive adolescents. *Journal of Abnormal Psychology* **99**: 385–92.

DoH (Department of Health) 1991: *The Children Act 1989: Guidance and Regulations: 4. Residential Care*. London: HMSO.

DoH (Department of Health) 1996: *Children Accommodated in Secure Units: Year-ending 31 March 1996, England*. London: Government Statistical Service.

Duncan, J.W. and Duncan, G.M. 1971: Murder in the family: a study of some homicidal adolescents. *American Journal of Psychiatry* **127**: 74–8.

D'Zurilla, T.J. and Goldfried, M.R. 1971: Problem solving and behaviour modification. *Journal of Abnormal Psychology* **78**: 107–26.

Edelman, E. and Goldstein, A.P. 1984: Prescriptive relationship levels for juvenile delinquents in a psychotherapy analogue. *Aggressive Behaviour* **10**: 269–78.

Edwards, D.J.A. 1996: Case study research: the cornerstone of theory and practice. In Reinecke, M.A., Dattilio, F.M. and Freeman, A. (eds), *Cognitive Therapy with Children and Adolescents*. London: Guilford Press.

Ellis, A. 1962: *Reason and Emotion in Psychotherapy*. New York: Lyle Stuart.

Epps, K.J. 1997a: The use of secure accommodation for adolescent girls who engage in severe and repetitive self-injurious behaviour. *Clinical Child Psychology and Psychiatry* **2**: 539–52.

Epps, K.J. 1997b: Looking after children in secure settings: recent themes. *Educational and Child Psychology* **14**: 42–52.

Fabiano, E.A. and Porporino, F. 1992: Rational rehabilitation. Paper presented at the What Works? conference, Salford University, Manchester, UK.

Falshaw, L., Browne, K. and Hollin, C.R. 1996: Victim to offender: a review. *Aggressive and Violent Behaviour* **1**: 389–404.

Feindler, E.L. 1991: Cognitive control strategies in anger control interventions for children and adolescents. In Kendall, P.C. (ed.), *Child and Adolescent Therapy: Cognitive–Behavioural Procedures*. London: Guilford Press.

Feindler, E.L. and Ecton, R.B. 1986: *Adolescent Anger Control: Cognitive–Behavioural Techniques*. Elmsford, NY: Pergamon Press.

Feindler, E.L. and Fremouw, W.J. 1983: Stress inoculation training for adolescent anger problems. In Meichenbaum, D. and Jaremko, M.E. (eds), *Stress Reduction and Prevention*. New York: Plenum Press.

Feindler, E.L., Marriott, S.A. and Iwata, M. 1984: Group anger control training for junior high school delinquents. *Cognitive Therapy and Research* **8**: 299–311.

Fennell, M. 1989: Depression. In Hawton, K., Salkovskis, P.M., Kirk, J. and Clark, D.M. (eds), *Cognitive Behaviour Therapy for Psychiatric Problems: a Practical Guide*. Oxford: Oxford University Press.

Feshbach, N.D. 1984: Empathy, empathy training and the regulation of aggression in elementary school children. In Kaplan, R.M., Konecni, V.J. and Novaco, R.W. (eds), *Aggression in Children and Youth*. Lancaster: Martinus Nijhoff.

Fixsen, D.L., Phillips, E.L., Phillips, E.A. and Wolf, M.M. 1976: The teaching family model of group home treatment. In Craighead, W.E., Kazdin, E.A. and Mahoney, M.J. (eds), *Behaviour Modification: Principles, Issues and Applications*. Boston: Houghton-Mifflin.

Fogg, V. 1992: *Perspectives: Implementation of a Cognitive Skills Developmental Program*. American Probation and Parole Association, Winter, 24–26.

Fowler, D. and Morley, S. 1989: The cognitive-behavioural treatment of hallucinations and delusions: a preliminary study. *Behavioural Psychotherapy* **17**: 267–82.

Gagne, E.E. 1975: Effects of immediacy of feedback and level of aspiration statements on learning tasks for delinquent youngsters. *Journal of Abnormal Child Psychology* **3**: 53–60.

Garrido, V. and Redondo, S. 1993: The institutionalisation of young offenders. *Criminal Behaviour and Mental Health* **3**: 336–48.

Garrett, C.J. 1985: Effects of residential treatment on adjudicated adolescents: a meta-analysis. *Journal of Research in Crime and Delinquency* **22**: 287–308.

Gendreau, P. and Andrews, D.A. 1990: Tertiary prevention: what the meta-analyses of the offender treatment literature tells us about 'what works'. *Canadian Journal of Criminology* **32**: 173–84.

Gendreau, P. and Ross, B. 1979: Effective correctional treatment: bibliotherapy for cynics. *Crime and Delinquency* **25**: 463–89.

Gibbs, J.C. 1991: Sociomoral developmental delay and cognitive distortion: implications for the treatment of antisocial youth. In Kurtines, W.M. and Gerwirtz, J.L. (eds), *Handbook of Moral Behaviour and Development: 3. Application.* Los Angeles: Lawrence Erlbaum.

Gibbs, J.C. 1996: Sociomoral group treatment for young offenders. In Hollin, C.R. and Howells, K. (eds), *Clinical Approaches to Working with Young Offenders.* Chichester: John Wiley.

Gibbs, J.C., Arnold, K.D., Ahlborn, H.H. and Cheesman, F.L. 1984: Facilitation of sociomoral reasoning in delinquents. *Journal of Consulting and Clinical Psychology* **52**: 37–45.

Gibbs, J.C., Potter, G.B. and Goldstein, A.P. 1995: *The EQUIP Program: Teaching Youth to Think and Act Responsibly through a Peer-helping Approach.* Champaign, IL: Research Press.

Glenwick, D.S. and Jason, L.A. 1984: Locus of intervention in child cognitive behaviour therapy: implications of a behavioural community psychology perspective. In Meyers, A.W. and Craighead, W.E. (eds), *Cognitive Behaviour Therapy with Children.* London: Plenum Press.

Goldfried, M.R. and Merbaum, M. (eds) 1973: *Behaviour Change through Self-control.* New York. Hold, Reinhart & Winston.

Goldstein, A.P. and Glick, B. 1987: *Aggression Replacement Training: a Comprehensive Intervention for Aggressive Youth.* Champaign, IL: Research Press.

Goldstein, A.P. and Keller, H. 1987: *Aggressive Behaviour: Assessment and Intervention.* Elmsford, NY: Pergamon Press.

Goldstein, A.P. and Soriano, F.F. 1994: Juvenile gangs. In Eron, L.D., Gentry J.H. and Schlegel, P. (eds), *Reason to Hope: a Psychological Perspective on Violence and Youth.* Washington: American Psychological Association.

Goodwin, S.E. and Mahoney, M.J. 1975: Modification of aggression through modelling: an experimental probe. *Journal of Behaviour Therapy and Experimental Psychiatry* **6**: 200–2.

Goswami, N. 1998: *Cognition in Children.* Hove: Psychology Press.

Gough, H.G. 1948: A sociological theory of psychopathy. *American Journal of Sociology* **56**: 359–66.

Gresswell, D.M. and Hollin, C.R. 1992: Towards a new methodology for making sense of case material: an illustrative case involving attempted multiple murder. *Criminal Behaviour and Mental Health* **2**: 329–41.

Gudjonsson, G.H. 1990: Psychological treatment for the mentally ill offender. In Howells, K. and Hollin, C.R. (eds), Clinical approaches to working with mentally disordered and sexual offenders. *Issues in Criminological and Legal Psychology* **16**: 15–21 (Leicester: British Psychological Society).

Guerra, N.G. and Panizzon, A. 1986: *Viewpoints Training Program.* Unpublished training manual. Santa Barbara: Center for Law-Related Education.

Guerra, N.G. and Slaby, R.G. 1990: Cognitive mediators of aggression in adolescent offenders: 2. Intervention. *Developmental Psychology* **26**: 269–77.

Hains, A.A. 1984: A preliminary attempt to teach the use of social problem-solving skills to delinquents. *Child Study Journal* **14**: 271–85.

Hardwick, P.J. and Rowton-Lee, M.A. 1996: Adolescent homicide: towards an assessment of risk. *Journal of Adolescence* **19**: 263–76.

Hare, D.J. and Paine, C. 1997: Developing cognitive behavioural treatments for people with Asperger's syndrome. *Clinical Psychology Forum* **110**: 5–8.

Harris, R. and Timms, N. 1993: *Secure Accommodation in Child Care: Between Hospital and Prison or Thereabouts?* London: Routledge.

Hartman, L. 1979: The preventive reduction of psychological risk in asymptomatic adolescents. *American Journal of Orthopsychiatry* **49**: 121–35.

Hartup, W. 1970: Peer interaction and social organization. In Mussen, P.H. (ed.), *Carmichael's Manual of Child Psychology,* Vol. 2. New York: John Wiley.

Hatfield, B., Harrington, R. and Mohamad, H. 1996: Staff looking after children in local authority residential units: the interface with child mental health professionals. *Journal of Adolescence* **19**: 127–39.

Henggeler, S.W. 1999: Multisystemic therapy: an overview of clinical procedures, outcomes, and policy implications. *Child Psychology and Psychiatry Review* **4**: 2–10.

Henggeler, S.W. and Borduin, C.M. 1990: *Family Therapy and Beyond: a Multisystemic Approach to Treating the Behaviour Problems of Children and Adolescents.* Pacific Grove, CA: Brooks/Cole.

Henggeler, S.W., Melton, G.B., Brondino, M.J., Scherer, D.G. and Hanley, J.H. 1997: Multisystemic therapy with violent and chronic juvenile offenders and their families: the role of treatment fidelity in successful dissemination. *Journal of Consulting and Clinical Psychology* **65**: 821–33.

Henggeler, S.W., Schoenwald, S.K., Borduin, C.M., Rowland, M.D. and Cunningham, P.B. 1998: *Multisystemic Treatment of Antisocial Behaviour in Children and Adolescents.* New York: Guilford Press.

Hersen, M. 1981: Complex problems require complex solutions. *Behaviour Therapy* **12**: 15–29.

Hogan, R. 1973: Moral conduct and moral character. *Psychological Bulletin* **79**: 217–32.

Hoghughi, M.S. 1979: The Aycliffe token economy. *British Journal of Criminology* **19**: 384–99.

Hollin, C.R. 1989: *Psychology and Crime: an Introduction to Criminological Psychology.* London: Routledge.

Hollin, C.R. 1990a: *Cognitive–Behavioural Interventions with Young Offenders.* Oxford: Pergamon Press.

Hollin, C.R. 1990b: Social skills training with delinquents: a look at the evidence and some recommendations for practice. *British Journal of Social Work* **20**: 483–93.

Hollin, C.R. 1992: *Criminal Behaviour: a Psychological Approach to Explanation and Prevention.* London: Falmer Press.

Hollin, C.R. 1993: Advances in the psychological treatment of delinquent behaviour. *Criminal Behaviour and Mental Health* **3**: 142–57.

Hollin, C.R. and Epps, K.J. 1996: Adolescent firesetters. In Hollin, C.R. and Howells, K. (eds), *Clinical Approaches to Working with Young Offenders.* Chichester: John Wiley.

Hollin, C.R., Epps, K.J. and Kendrick, D.J. 1995: *Managing Behavioural Treatment: Policy and Practice with Delinquent Adolescents.* London: Routledge.

Holmes, J. 1993: Attachment theory: a biological basis for psychotherapy? *British Journal of Psychiatry* **163**: 430–8.

Home Office 1997: *Changing Offenders' Attitudes and Behaviour: What Works?* Research Study 171. London: Home Office.

Howells, K. 1982: Mental disorder and violent behaviour. In Feldman, P. (ed.), *Developments in the Study of Criminal Behaviour: Vol. 2. Violence.* Chichester: John Wiley.

Hughes, G., Hogue, T., Hollin, C.R. and Champion, H. 1997: First-stage evaluation of a treatment programme for personality disordered offenders. *Journal of Forensic Psychiatry* **8**: 515–27.

Hunter, J.A., Becker, J.V. and Goodwin, D.W. 1991: The reliability and discriminative utility of the Adolescent Cognition Scale for juvenile sexual offenses. *Annals of Sex Research* **4**: 281–6.

Huntsinger, G.M. 1976: Teaching of self-control of verbal and physical aggression to juvenile delinquents. Unpublished manuscript, Virginia Commonwealth University.

Izzo, R.L. and Ross, R.R. 1990: Meta-analysis of rehabilitation programs for juvenile delinquents: a brief report. *Criminal Justice and Behaviour* **17**: 134–42.

Jones, R.T., Nelson, R.E. and Kazdin, A.E. 1977: The role of external variables in self-reinforcement. *Behaviour Modification* **1**: 147–78.

Jurkovic, G.J. 1980: The juvenile delinquent as moral philosopher: a structural – developmental approach. *Psychological Bulletin* **88**: 709–27.

Jurkovic, G.J. and Prentice, N.M. 1977: Relation of moral and cognitive development to dimensions of juvenile delinquency. *Journal of Abnormal Psychology* **86**: 414–20.

Kanfer, F.H. 1970: Self-regulation: research, issues, and speculations. In Neuringer, C. and Michael, J.L. (eds), *Behaviour Modification in Clinical Psychology*. New York: Appleton Century Crofts.

Kanfer, F.H. 1971: The maintenance of behaviour by self-generated stimuli and reinforcement. In Jacobs, A. and Sachs, L.B. (eds), *The Psychology of Private Events*. New York: Academic Press.

Kanfer, F.H. and Karoly, P. 1972: Self-control: a behaviouristic excursion into the lion's den. *Behaviour Therapy* **3**: 398–416.

Kaufman, L.M. and Wagner, B.R. 1972: Barb: a systematic treatment technology for temper control disorders. *Behaviour Therapy* **3**: 84–90.

Kendall, P.C. 1977: On the efficacious use of verbal self-instructional procedures with children. *Cognitive Therapy and Research* **1**: 331–41.

Kendall, P.C. 1991: Guiding theory for therapy with children and adolescents. In Kendall, P.C. (ed.), *Child and Adolescent Therapy: Cognitive–Behavioural Procedures*. London: Guilford Press.

Kendall, P.C. 1993: Cognitive–behavioural therapies with youth: guiding theory, current status, and emerging developments. *Journal of Consulting and Clinical Psychology* **61**: 235–47.

Kendall, P.C. and Braswell, L. 1985: *Cognitive–Behavioural Therapy for Impulsive Children*. New York: Guilford Press.

Kendall, P.C., Ronan, K.R. and Epps, J. 1991: Aggression in children/adolescents: cognitive–behavioural treatment perspectives. In Pepler, D.J. and Rubin, K.H. (eds), *The Development and Treatment of Childhood Aggression*. Hillsdale, NJ: Lawrence Erlbaum.

Kendall, P.C. and Williams, C.L. 1981: Behavioural and cognitive approaches to outpatient treatment with children. In Craighead, W.E., Kazdin, A.E. and Mahoney, M.J. (eds), *Behaviour Modification: Principles, Issues and Applications*, 2nd edn. Boston: Houghton Mifflin.

Kennedy, R.E. 1984: Cognitive–behavioural interventions with delinquents. In Meyers, A.W. and Craighead, W.E. (eds), *Cognitive Behaviour Therapy with Children*. London: Plenum Press.

Kennedy, R.E., Kirchner, E.P. and Draguns, J.G. 1979: Perspective-taking in adult criminal psychopaths. Unpublished manuscript, Pennsylvania State University.

Kennedy, R.E., Kirchner, E.P. and Draguns, J.G. 1980: Perspective-taking, socialization, and moral judgement in adult criminals and noncriminal controls. Unpublished manuscript, Pennsylvania State University.

Kilpatrick, R. 1997: Joy-riding: an addictive behaviour? In Hodge, J.E., McMurran, M. and Hollin, C.R. (eds), *Addicted to Crime?* Chichester: John Wiley.

Kirschenbaum, D.S. and Ordman, A.M. 1984: Preventative interventions for children: cognitive–behavioural perspectives. In Meyers, A.W. and Craighead, W.E. (eds), *Cognitive Behaviour Therapy with Children*. London: Plenum Press.

Klahr, D. and Wallace, J.G. 1976: *Cognitive Development: an Information Processing Approach*. Hillsdale, NJ: Lawrence Erlbaum.

Knott, C. 1995: The STOP programme: reasoning and rehabilitation in a British setting. In McGuire, J. (ed.), *What Works: Reducing Reoffending*. Chichester: John Wiley.

Kolko, D.J. 1988: Community interventions for juvenile firesetters: a survey of two national programs. *Hospital and Community Psychiatry* **39**: 973–9.

Laws, D.R. (ed.) 1989: *Relapse Prevention with Sex Offenders*. New York: Guilford Press.

Lazarus, A.A. 1976: *Multi-modal Behaviour Therapy*. New York: Springer.

Lee, M. and Prentice, N.M. 1988: Interrelations of empathy, cognition, and moral reasoning with dimensions of juvenile delinquency. *Journal of Abnormal Child Psychology* **16**: 127–39.

Lipsey, M.W. 1992: The effects of treatment on juvenile delinquents: results from meta-analysis. Paper presented at the NIMH Meeting for Research to Prevent Youth Violence, Bethesda, MD.

Lipsey, M.W. 1995: What do we learn from 400 research studies on the effectiveness of treatment with juvenile delinquents? In McGuire, J. (ed.), *What Works: Reducing Offending*. Chichester: John Wiley.

Litrownik, A.J. 1982: Special considerations in the self-management training of the developmentally disabled. In Karoly, P. and Kanfer, F.H. (eds), *Self-management and Behaviour Change: From Theory to Practice*. New York: Pergamon Press.

Litrownik, A.J. 1984: Cognitive behaviour modification with psychotic children: a beginning. In Meyers, A.W. and Craighead, W.E. (eds), *Cognitive Behaviour Therapy with Children*. London: Plenum Press.

Little, V.L. and Kendall, P.C. 1979: Cognitive–behavioural interventions with delinquents: problem-solving, role-taking, and self-control. In Kendall, P.C. and Hollon, S.D. (eds), *Cognitive Behavioural Interventions: Theory, Research and Procedures*. New York: Academic Press.

Lochman, J.E. and Dodge, K.A. 1994: Social–cognitive processes of severely violent, moderately aggressive, and non aggressive boys. *Journal of Consulting and Clinical Psychology* **62**: 366–74.

Lochman, J.E., White, K.J. and Wayland, K.K. 1991: Cognitive-behavioural assessment and treatment with aggressive children. In Kendall, P.C. (ed.), *Child and Adolescent Therapy: Cognitive–Behavioural Procedures*. London: Guilford Press.

Long, C.G. and Hollin, C.R. 1997: The scientist–practitioner model in clinical psychology: a critique. *Clinical Psychology and Psychotherapy* **4**: 75–83.

Losel, F. 1995: Increasing consensus in the evaluation of offender rehabilitation? Lessons from recent research syntheses. *Psychology, Crime and Law* **2**: 19–39.

Luria, A.R. 1961: *The Role of Speech in the Regulation of Normal and Abnormal Behaviors*. New York: Liverwright.

MacDevitt, J.W. and Kedzierzawski, G.D. 1990: A structured group format for first offense shoplifters. *International Journal of Offender Therapy and Comparative Criminology* **34**: 155–64.

Mahoney, M.J. and Arnkoff, D.B. 1978: Cognitive and self-control therapies. In Garfield, S.L. and Bergin, A.E. (eds), *Handbook of Psychotherapy and Behaviour Change: an Empirical Analysis*, 2nd edn. New York: John Wiley.

Mahoney, M. and Thoresen, C. 1974: *Self-control: Power to the Person*. Monterey, CA: Brooks.

Margolin, L. 1984: Group therapy as a means of learning about the sexual assaultive adolescent. *International Journal of Offender Therapy and Comparative Criminology* **28**: 65–72.

Marshall, M.H. 1965: The effects of punishment on children: a review of the literature and suggested hypothesis. *Journal of Genetic Psychology* **106**: 23–33.

Matthews, W.S. and Brooks-Gunn, J. 1984: Social development in childhood. In Meyers, A.W. and Craighead, W.E. (eds), *Cognitive Behaviour Therapy with Children*. London: Plenum Press.

McConnaughy, E.A., DiClemente, C.C., Prochaska, J.O. and Velicar, W.F. 1983: Stages of change in psychotherapy: measurement and sample profiles. *Psychotherapy: Theory, Research and Practice* **20**: 368.

McCullough, J.P., Huntsinger, G.M. and Nay, W.R. 1977: Case study: self-control treatment of aggression in a 16-year old male. *Journal of Consulting and Clinical Psychology* **45**: 322–31.

McDougall, C., Barnett, R.M., Ashurst, B. and Willis, B. 1987: Cognitive control of anger. In McGurk, B.J., Thornton, D.M. and Williams, M. (eds), *Applying Psychology to Imprisonment: Theory and Practice*. London: HMSO.

McGee, C., Kauffman, J. and Nussen, J. 1977: Children as therapeutic change agents: reinforcement intervention paradigms. *Review of Educational Research* **47**: 451–77.

McGuire, J. (ed.) 1995: *What Works: Reducing Reoffending*. Chichester: John Wiley.

McGuire, J. 1997: Psycho-social approaches to the understanding and reduction of violence in young people. In Varma, V. (ed.), *Violence in Children and Adolescents*. London: Jessica Kingsley.

McMurran, M. 1991: Young offenders and alcohol-related crime: what interventions will address the issues? *Journal of Adolescence* **14**: 245–53.

McMurran, M. 1996: Substance use and delinquency. In Hollin, C.R. and Howells, K. (eds), *Clinical Approaches to Working with Young Offenders*. Chichester: John Wiley.

McMurran, M. and Hollin, C.R. 1993: *Young Offenders and Alcohol: a Practitioner's Guidebook*. Chichester: John Wiley.

McMurran, M. and Whitman, J. 1997: The development of a brief intervention for car theft. In Hodge, J.E., McMurran, M. and Hollin, C.R. (eds), *Addicted to Crime?* Chichester: John Wiley.

Meichenbaum, D. 1974: *Cognitive Behaviour Modification*. Morristown, NJ: General Learning Press.

Meichenbaum, D. 1975: Self-instructional methods. In Kanfer, F.H. and Goldstein, A.P. (eds), *Helping People Change*. New York: Pergamon Press.

Meichenbaum, D. 1977: *Cognitive–behaviour modification: an integrative approach*. New York: Plenum Press.

Meichenbaum, D. and Asarnow, J. 1979: Cognitive–behaviour modification and metacognitive development: implications for the classroom. In Kendall, P.C. and Hollon, S. (eds), *Cognitive–Behavioural Interventions: Theory, Research and Procedures*. New York: Academic Press.

Meichenbaum, D. and Goodman, J. 1971: Training impulsive children to talk to themselves: a means of developing self-control. *Journal of Abnormal Psychology* **77**: 115–26.

Milan, M.A. 1987: Basic behavioural procedures in closed institutions. In Morris, E.K. and Braukmann, C.J. (eds), *Behavioural Approaches to Crime and Delinquency: a Handbook of Application, Research and Concepts*. New York: Plenum Press.

Milan, M.A. 1996: Working in institutions. In Hollin, C.R. and Howells, K. (eds), *Clinical Approaches to Working with Young Offenders*. Chichester: John Wiley.

Miller, N.E. 1960: Learning resistance to pain and fear: effects of overlearning, exposure, and rewarded exposure in context. *Journal of Experimental Psychology* **60**: 137–45.

Miller, W.R. 1983: Motivational interviewing with problem drinkers. *Behavioural Psychotherapy* **11**: 147–72.

Miller, W.R. 1985: Motivational interviewing: a review with special emphasis on alcoholism. *Psychological Bulletin* **98**: 84–107.

Miller, W.R. and Rollnick, S. 1991: *Motivational Interviewing: Preparing People to Change*. New York: Guilford Press.

Moore, S.F. and Cole, S.O. 1978: Cognitive self-mediation training with hyperkinetic children. *Bulletin of the Psychonomic Society* **12**: 18–20.

Moos, R.H. 1974: *The Social Climate Scales: an Overview*. Palo Alto, CA: Consulting Psychologists Press.

Mulvey, E.P., Arthur, M.W. and Reppucci, N.D. 1993: The prevention and treatment of juvenile delinquency: a review of the research. *Clinical Psychology Review* **13**: 133–57.

Munro, F.M. 1995: Social skills differences in aggressive and non-aggressive male young offenders within an unfamiliar social situation. *Medicine, Science and the Law* **35**: 245–8.

Nezu, A.M. and Nezu, C.M. (eds) 1989: *Clinical Decision Making in Behaviour Therapy: a Problem-Solving Perspective*. Champaign, IL: Research Press.

Nichols, H.R. and Molinder, I. 1984: *Multiphasic Sex Inventory*. Tacoma, WA: authors.

Novaco, R.W. 1975: *Anger Control: the Development and Evaluation of an Experimental Treatment*. Lexington, MA: D.C. Heath.

Novaco, R.W. 1978: Anger and coping with stress. In Foreyt, J.P. and Rathjen, D.P. (eds), *Cognitive Behavior Therapy*. Lexington, MA: D.C. Heath.

Novaco, R.W. 1985: Anger and its therapeutic regulation. In Chesney, M.A. and Rosenman, R.H. (eds), *Anger and Hostility in Cardiovascular and Behavioral Disorders*. New York: Hemisphere.

Novaco, R.W. 1994: Anger as a risk factor for violence among the mentally disordered. In Monahan, J. and Steadman, H. (eds), *Violence and Mental Disorder*. Chicago: University of Chicago Press, 21–59.

O'Leary, S.G. and Dubey, D.R. 1979: Applications of self-control procedures by children: a review. *Journal of Applied Behaviour Analysis* **12**: 449–65.

Ostapiuk, E.B. and Westwood, S. 1986: Glenthorne Youth Treatment Centre: working with adolescents in gradations of security. In Hollin, C.R. and Howells, K. (eds), *Clinical Approaches to Criminal Behaviour*. Leicester: British Psychological Society.

Palmer, T. 1975: Martinson revisited. *Journal of Research in Crime and Delinquency* **12**: 133–52.

Patterson, G.R. 1986: Performance models for antisocial boys. *American Psychologist* **41**: 432–44.

Patterson, G.R. and Stouthamer-Loeber, M. 1984: The correlation of family management practices and delinquency. *Child Development* **55**: 1299–307.

Perkins, D.E. 1986: Sex offending: a psychological approach. In Hollin, C.R. and Howells, K. (eds), *Clinical Approaches to Criminal Behaviour*. Leicester: British Psychological Society.

Perry, B.D. 1994: Neurobiological sequelae of childhood trauma: PTSD in children. In Murray, M. (ed.), *Catecholamines in Post-traumatic Stress Disorder: Emerging Concepts*. Washington, DC: American Psychiatric Press.

Peterson, D.R. 1985: Twenty years of practitioner training in psychology. *American Psychologist* **40**: 441–51.

Phillips, E.L., Phillips, E.A., Fixsen, D.L. and Wolf, M.M. 1971: Achievement Place: the modification of the behaviours of pre-delinquent boys with a token economy. *Journal of Applied Behaviour Analysis* **4**: 45–59.

Phillips, E.L., Phillips, E.A., Fixsen, D.L. and Wolf, M.M. 1974: *The Teaching Family Handbook*, revised edn: Lawrence, KS: University of Kansas.

Platt, J.J., Scura, W. and Hannon, J.R. 1973: Problem-solving thinking of youthful incarcerated heroin addicts. *Journal of Community Psychology* **1**: 278–81.

Platt, J.J., Spivack, G., Altman, N., Altman, D. and Peizer, S.B. 1974: Adolescent problem-solving thinking. *Journal of Consulting and Clinical Psychology* **42**: 787–93.

Prentice, N. and Kelly, F.J. 1963: Intelligence and delinquency: a reconsideration. *Journal of Social Psychology* **60**: 327–37.

Prochaska, J.O. and DiClemente, C.C. 1982: Transtheoretical therapy: towards a more integrative model of change. *Psychotherapy: Theory, Research and Practice* **9**: 276–88.

Pynoos, R.S. and Nader, K. 1993: Issues in the treatment of post-traumatic stress in children and adolescents. In Wilson, J.P. and Raphael, B. (eds), *International Handbook of Traumatic Stress Syndromes*. New York: Plenum Press.

Quay, H.C. 1987a: Intelligence. In Quay, H.C. (ed.), *Handbook of Juvenile Delinquency*. New York: John Wiley.

Quay, H.C. 1987b: Patterns of delinquent behaviour. In Quay, H.C. (ed.), *Handbook of Juvenile Delinquency*. New York: John Wiley.

Raynor, P. and Vanstone, M. 1994: *Straight Thinking on Probation: Third Interim Report*. Bridgend: Mid Glamorgan Probation Service.

Reid, I. 1982: The development and maintenance of a behavioural regime in a Youth Treatment Centre. In Feldman, M.P. (ed.), *Developments in the Study of Criminal Behaviour: Vol 1. Prevention and Control of Offending*. Chichester: John Wiley.

Reid, I.D., Feldman, M.P. and Ostapiuk, E.B. 1980: The Shape Project for young offenders: introduction and overview. *Journal of Offender Counselling Services and Rehabilitation* **4**: 233–46.

Reinecke, M.A., Dattilio, F.M. and Freeman, A. 1996: General issues. In Reineck, M.A., Dattilio, F.M. and Freeman, A. (eds), *Cognitive Therapy with Children and Adolescents: a Casebook for Clinical Practice*. London: Guilford Press.

Robin, A., Schneider, M. and Dolnick, M. 1976: The turtle technique: an extended case study of self-control in the class room. *Psychology in the Schools* **13**: 449–53.

Robinson, D., Grossman, M. and Porporino, F. 1991: *Effectiveness of the Cognitive Skills Training Program: From Pilot Project to National Implementation*. Ottawa: Correctional Services of Canada.

Ronen, T. 1997: *Cognitive Developmental Therapy with Children*. Chichester: John Wiley.

Ross, R.R. and Fabiano, E.A. 1985: *Time to Think: a Cognitive Model of Delinquency Prevention and Offender Rehabilitation*. Ottawa: Institute of Social Services and Arts.

Ross, R.R. and Ross, B. (eds) 1995: *Thinking Straight*. Ottawa: Cognitive Centre.

Ross, R.R., Fabiano, E.A. and Ewles, C.D. 1988: Reasoning and rehabilitation. *International Journal of Offender Therapy and Comparative Criminology* **32**: 29–35.

Ross, R.R., Fabiano, E.A. and Ross, B. 1989: *Reasoning and Rehabilitation: a Handbook for Teaching Cognitive Skills*. Ottawa: Cognitive Centre.

Rotenberg, M. 1974: Conceptual and methodological notes on affective and cognitive role taking (sympathy and empathy): an illustrative experiment with delinquent and nondelinquent boys. *Journal of Genetic Psychology* **125**: 177–85.

Rotter, J.B. 1954: *Social Learning and Clinical Psychology*. Englewood Cliffs, NJ: Prentice-Hall.

Rutter, M. and Smith, D. (eds) 1995: *Psychosocial Disorders in Young People: Time Trends and their Causes*. Chichester: John Wiley.

Rutter, M., Giller, H. and Hagell, A. (eds), 1998: *Antisocial Behaviour by Young People*. Cambridge: Cambridge University Press.

Sarason, I.G. 1978: A cognitive social learning approach to juvenile delinquency. In Hare, R.D. and Schalling, D. (eds), *Psychopathic Behaviour: Approaches to Research*. New York: John Wiley.

Sarbin, T.R. 1954: Role theory. In Lindzey, G. (ed.), *Handbook of Social Psychology*. Cambridge, MA: Addison-Wesley.

Schlichter, K.J. and Horan, J.J. 1981: Effects of stress inoculation on the anger and aggression management skills of institutionalized juvenile delinquents. *Cognitive Therapy and Research* **5**: 359–65.

Seymour, F.W. and Stokes, T.F. 1976: Self-recording in training girls to increase work and evoke staff praise in an institution for offenders. *Journal of Applied Behaviour Analysis* **9**: 41–54.

Shakow, D. 1978: Clinical psychology seen some 50 years later. *American Psychologist* **33**: 148–58.

Skinner, B.F. 1938: *The Behaviour of Organisms*. New York: Appleton Century Crofts.

Skinner, B.F. 1953: *Science and Human Behaviour*. New York: Free Press.

Slaby, R.G. and Guerra, N.G. 1988: Cognitive mediators of aggression in adolescent offenders: 1. Assessment. *Developmental Psychology* **24**: 580–8.

Snyder, J.J. and White, M.H. 1979: The use of cognitive self-instruction in the treatment of behaviourally disturbed adolescents. *Behaviour Therapy* **10**: 227–35.

Spivack, G. and Levine, M. 1963: *Self-regulation in Acting-out and Normal Adolescents*. Washington, DC: National Institutes of Health.

Spivack, G. and Shure, M.B. 1974: *Social Adjustment of Young Children: a Cognitive Approach to Solving Real-Life Problems*. San Francisco: Jossey-Bass.

Stokes, T.F. and Baer, D.M. 1977: An implicit technology of generalization. *Journal of Applied Behaviour Analysis* **10**: 349–67.

Stumphauzer, J.S. 1976: Elimination of stealing by self-reinforcement of alternative behaviour and family contracting. *Journal of Behaviour Therapy and Experimental Psychiatry* **7**: 265–8.

Sturmey P. 1996: *Functional Analysis in Clinical Psychology*. Chichester: John Wiley.

Swaffer, T. and Hollin, C.R. 1997: Adolescents' experiences of anger in a residential setting. *Journal of Adolescence* **20**: 567–75.

Tate, D.C., Reppucci, N.D. and Mulvey, E.P. 1995: Violent juvenile delinquents: treatment effectiveness and implications for future action. *American Psychologist* **50**: 777–81.

Thoresen, K.E., Thoresen, C.E., Klein, S.B. *et al.* 1979: Learning House: helping troubled children and their parents change themselves. In Stumphauzer, J.S. (ed.), *Progress in Behaviour Therapy with Delinquents.* Springfield, IL: Charles C. Thomas.

Unikel, I.P. and Blanchard, E.B. 1973: Psychopathy, race, and delay of gratification by adolescent delinquents. *Journal of Nervous and Mental Disease* **156**: 57–60.

Utting, W. 1991: *Children in Public Care: a Review of Residential Child Care.* London: HMSO.

Utting, W. 1997: *People Like Us: Report of the Review of the Safeguards for Children Living away from Home.* Norwich: The Stationery Office.

Varley, W.H. 1984: Behaviour modification approaches to the aggressive adolescent. In Keith, C.R. (ed.), *The Aggressive Adolescent: Clinical Perspectives.* New York: Free Press.

Visconti, P., Caretto, F., DeAngelis, D., Piptone, E.E. and Sepe, D. 1996: Cognitive–behavioural treatment in autism. *Developmental Brain Dysfunction* **9**: 39.

Vygotsky, L. 1962: *Thought and Language.* New York: John Wiley.

Walters, G.C. and Grusec, J.E. 1977: *Punishment.* San Francisco: Freeman Press.

Walters, G.D. 1995: The Psychological Inventory of Criminal Thinking Styles: 1. Reliability and preliminary data. *Criminal Justice and Behaviour* **22**: 307–25.

Welch, G.L. 1985: Contingency contracting with a delinquent and his family. *Journal of Behaviour Therapy and Experimental Psychiatry* **16**: 253–9.

Whitehead, J.T. and Lab, S.P. 1989: A meta-analysis of juvenile correctional treatment. *Journal of Research in Crime and Delinquency* **26**: 276–95.

Widom, C.S. 1976: Interpersonal and personal construct system in psychopaths. *Journal of Consulting and Clinical Psychology* **85**: 330–4.

Wilde, J. 1996: *Treating Anger, Anxiety, and Depression in Children and Adolescents: a Cognitive–Behavioural Perspective.* Washington, DC: Accelerated Development.

Williams, D.Y. and Akamatsu, T.J. 1978: Cognitive self-guidance training with juvenile delinquents: applicability and generalization. *Cognitive Therapy and Research* **2**: 285–8.

Wolpe, J. 1969: *The Practice of Behaviour Therapy.* New York: Pergamon Press.

Wood, R. and Flynn, J.M. 1978: A self-evaluation token system versus an external evaluation token system alone in a residential setting with predelinquent youths. *Journal of Applied Behaviour Analysis* **11**: 503–12.

Yochelson, S. and Samenow, S.E. 1976: *The Criminal Personality: 1. A Profile for Change.* London: Jason Aronson Inc.

Yule, W. and Brown, B.J. 1987: Some behavioural applications with juvenile offenders outside North America. In Morris, E.K. and Braukmann, C.J. (eds), *Behavioural Approaches to Crime and Delinquency: a Handbook of Application, Research, and Concepts.* New York: Plenum Press.

Zahavi, S. and Asher, S.R. 1978: The effect of verbal instructions on preschool children's aggressive behaviour. *Journal of Social Psychology* **16**: 146–53.

Psychodynamic therapies

CHRISTOPHER CORDESS

INTRODUCTION

In 1916, Freud published *Some Character Types Met With in Psycho-Analytic Work*. Within a brief discussion of what he calls 'The Exceptions', he quotes the tragedy of Shakespeare's King Richard III. Richard feels himself to have been cheated by nature, by being born deformed, and feels that this permits him to behave as if exempt from the moral laws by which others must abide, in particular those of incest and parricide. He thinks of himself as an exception and resolves to become murderous, rapacious and a confirmed villain:

'But I, that am not shaped for sportive tricks,
Nor made to court an amorous looking-glass;
I that am rudely stamp'd, and want love's majesty
To strut before a wanton ambling nymph;
I, that am curtail'd of this fair proportion,
Cheated of feature by dissembling Nature,
Deform'd, unfinish'd, sent before my time
Into this breathing world, scarce half made-up,
And that so lamely and unfashionable,
That dogs bark at me as I halt by them;
...
And, therefore, since I cannot prove a lover,
To entertain these fair well-spoken days,
I am determined to prove a villain,
And hate the idle pleasures of these days.'

If we accept that Richard speaks consciously, by a dramatic device, what for others is less conscious or unconscious, the speech is packed with some of the psychological ingredients of the juvenile offender's mind and behaviour which this chapter addresses. We need not assume that Richard refers only to physical, rather than psychological, deformity.

At the risk of being reductive, we can identify Richard's knowledge of himself and his internal world in analytic terms. The sense of trauma and deprivation, which gives him – so he believes – the moral right to take what does not belong to him, whether by killing, rape or theft, is familiar to those working with offenders and is described in much of the psychodynamic literature: It is behaviourally evident, for example, in those cases of the abused becoming the abuser. The law of *talion* of the Old Testament – 'an eye for an eye' – and the same of the unconscious, applies. Winnicott (1982[1956]) has written of the formation of the 'antisocial tendency' as a consequence of deprivation – that is, of a privation of something which has been experienced and lost, but has not been able to be mourned. In this view, if the loss could be taken in to the psyche and 'worked through' – or psychologically metabolized – then, after a period, there can be a development of emotional acceptance with the generation of new attachments. The antisocial posture will be obviated.

There is in Richard's speech the description of having been 'cheated by dissembling nature' – and, therefore, apparently, of being given permission to cheat back. Also, envy of those who can 'entertain these fair, well-spoken days', and the determination, since that cannot be, 'to prove a villain' and ('wanting love's majesty') instead to hate, take revenge and prove, literally, to be 'offensive'.

But Richard does not escape from either the external, but more significantly for us, from his internal world of guilt and persecution. In the monologue of the play's last Act there are descriptions of his relentless suffering at the hands of his 'conscience' which we can equate with '*super-ego*':

'O coward conscience, how doest thou afflict me!

...

What! do I fear myself? There's none else by:
Richard loves Richard; that is, I am I.
Is there a murderer here? No, Yes, I am:
Then fly: what! from myself? Great reason why:
Lest I revenge. What! myself upon myself?
Alack! I love myself. Wherefore? for any good
That I myself have done unto myself?
O! No: alas! I rather hate myself.
I am a villain, Yet I lie; I am not.
My conscience hath a thousand several tongues,
And every tongue brings in a several tale,
And every tale condemns me for a villain.
All several sins, all us'd in each degree,
Throng to the bar, crying all, 'Guilty! guilty!'
I shall despair. There is no creature loves me;
And if a die, no soul will pity me:
Nay, wherefore should they, since that I myself
Find in myself no pity to myself?'

Richard provides a precise description of his realization of his preoccupation with self – his 'narcissism' – and of the inwardly turned murderousness which threatens to revenge 'myself upon myself', that is, by suicide. He elaborates the fragmented voices of persecution – of 'a thousand several tongues' – of his super-ego and ends with a final realization that his narcissism is in fact a 'destructive narcissism' – to use Herbert Rosenfeld's term (Rosenfeld 1987) – or 'malignant narcissism' (Kernberg 1992). Richard continues, pitilessly dissecting the inexorable bleakness and emptiness that is his fate – we could say, by now, that in psychoanalytic terms he realizes the absence of any good 'internal' objects. By 'objects' here we mean *functioning* mental representations of interacting, significant past figures, primarily parents, or those *in loco parentis*, which allow good feeling and capacity to think. 'I shall despair. There is no creature loves me' and 'I myself find in myself no pity to myself'.

GENERAL BACKGROUND

Young offenders have been particularly in the news in recent years. They stir strong emotions within society, with polarizations of views from extreme demands for more and more punishment to the frankly sentimental. To quote Winnicott (1984), 'what is needed is something that is neither sentimental nor revengeful'. It is no surprise that this polarization – the 'splitting' – of different views and responses to the young offender mirrors the feelings and responses of the institutions, carers and therapists who deal with these young people, which in turn can be seen to reflect the disparate and frequently confused and split internal mental worlds of the young offenders themselves.

However, we should be on our guard against furthering a 'them and us' view of this subject. One of the major strengths of the psychodynamic view is that it offers an alternative to some theories which attempt to ascribe criminal behaviour to a linear and simple causation, and to a categorical rather than a dimensional difference between delinquents and non-delinquents. Minor acts of delinquency are part of normal adolescence (and for that matter adulthood), and 'the delinquent' or juvenile offender needs to be seen in this context. Social and political policy tends towards defining core high-risk groups. Thus the danger, for example, of the new 'Antisocial Behaviour Order' (Crime and Disorder Act 1998) is that it confirms an identity especially of young people who may have been going through a developmental 'phase'.

As Winnicott (1984) said, the criminal act 'compels the environment to be important'. We, as representatives of society, and policymakers on our behalf, are compelled to respond.

To work with juvenile offenders is necessarily to become involved in the politics of our response – politics with a small 'p', but also, particularly at the present time, Politics with a large 'P'. In 1993, a series of newspaper articles claimed that the state is not to blame for the problems of the children it takes care of as they have often already been affected by adverse experiences of their family life. The individuals working with these children achieve great success through their devotion, however, they often work in poor conditions with low pay and with little recognition from the public, and the children suffer as a consequence. The editorial posits that the Government needs to reform the state care system as it has come to be associated with neglect, abuse and irresponsibility.

The situation has not changed since that was written. Although the editorial does not refer specifically to the juvenile offender, these comments are even more true for this group. There is frequently a progression from failed early attachments, via disrupted family life and then – especially for boys – the adoption of a delinquent pattern of offending behaviour leading in some cases to detention in secure facilities. The populations of young offender institutions, as well as adult prisons, have a high incidence of having been in 'care'. It is an interesting question why we tend to be punitive to this already disposed group rather than rehabilitative, habilitative or therapeutic. Possibly, they are further 'hated' because of their very 'failure' and vulnerability which confronts society with the unbearable. This has been described as the failure of society to meet the delinquent with an appropriate 'depressive position' (Copley 1994).

The case of the murder of 2-year-old James Bulger by two young boys in 1993 provides an example of a challenge to our understanding which may provoke a response such as that of former Prime Minister John Major, 'that we need to condemn a little more and understand a little less'. There is a danger that a false polarity is thereby set up – not unlike the false oppositional categories of the 'mad or bad?' debate – in which 'understanding' carries a pejorative weight. Because understanding and condemnation in this view are placed in opposition, there is the assumption that the more we understand, then the more we necessarily exonerate or condone – the 'soft option', so feared especially at the present time, but also at other times in contemporary history. There is not much new in our societal responses: There is a cyclical motion in the relative emphases placed upon punishment, deterrence, retribution, and rehabilitation and treatment, from one historical period to the next. Insofar as this seems to be especially true for society's response to the young delinquent, it may be seen to reflect the vulnerability of this age group, both to themselves but also to the changing perceptions and policymaking of adults. The internal dynamics of the particular interplay of forces of progression and regression which is characteristic of the adolescent period – and is reflected in our response to adolescents – is described by many authors, but particularly well by Deutsch (1968).

Developmental theories, and psychoanalytic theory in particular, have emphasized that the adolescent period demands an integration of fundamental biological and psychological changes, as a crucial stage in the organization of libidinal and aggressive forces into the individual's later psychical life. Disruptions in this development may lead to breakdown; for example, the adolescent may attack his or her own body – as described by Laufer and Laufer (1989); or it may lead to acts of delinquency, including acts of violence and sexual violence. From Klein's (1927) point of view, the internal world of the infant and child is indeed one (partly) inhabited with much hate and violent phantasy. The phantasy may be enacted in play or in the external, real world. It is, however, in fact (fortunately) far less commonly enacted as actual murder.

In recent years, young males between the ages of 10 and 20 years have accounted for approximately half of all recorded crime; per capita of population, the peak age of offending is in 14- to 17-year-olds. The trend is for more minor offences in the younger age groups, with violence and sexual offences in the middle and later teenage years. Although few juvenile offenders have yet attracted a clear *psychiatric* diagnosis, many of them have been emotionally neglected and damaged, if not frankly physically and sexually traumatized with the consequent likelihood of the failure of personality development. There is evidence of frequently gross failure of attachment to parental or other significant figures, as discussed by de Zulueta (1993). Many will be found to be depressed or to be using their offensive

actions to defend against depression, as described by Williams (1978). Some will have major difficulties and confusions of identify and of gender identity. They have the features of a dispossessed group not only in emotional, but also in familial, social, economic and educational terms. A sizeable minority will go on to careers in recidivism; many will develop disorders of character and personality and will develop psychiatric disorders of various types. From a psychodynamic point of view their juvenile offending may be seen as a symptom or warning of later more obvious personality difficulties, or at least as a marker of something having gone wrong in the developmental process.

A number of authors (e.g. Robins 1966, 1979) have shown how adult behaviour disorders, and specifically criminality, can be predicted from child conduct disorder. Rubenstein *et al.* (1993) have shown how the long-term criminal outcome of specifically adolescent sex offenders is extremely poor in terms of future adult sexual offending, but also for future adult non-sexual violent offending (for example, murder, kidnapping, robbery and assault) compared with adolescent non-sexual offenders. These authors confirm also the association between sexual abuse in childhood and repetitive adult sexual offending, and recommend – since sexually assaultative delinquents are at particularly high risk of subsequent sexual and non-sexual violence and serious offending – that special efforts should be made to treat them in adolescence.

These studies and findings make an overwhelming case for the provision of better services for adolescents, and specifically adolescent offenders. Within our current system, however, denial operates at all levels and all adolescent groups remain largely relatively neglected. Hope – an essential prerequisite in helping the troubled young – can easily be abandoned by the adolescent and by professionals too. By contrast, as Winnicott (1982 [1956]) makes clear, delinquency also carries with it a sense of potential 'hope', since it represents an attempt at action on the objective world, in contrast to giving up and of demoralisation in the face of the adolescent task. Our way of understanding the communication and our response to the early delinquent act is therefore crucial.

There was an approximate halving of the number of young persons and young offenders sentenced to immediate custody in the years 1985 to 1990, largely as a result of sentencing policy, and there was hope that the Children Act 1989 and the Criminal Justice Act 1991 would further this move away from locking up children in 'youth custody'. Cautioning, both recorded and unrecorded, was seen to be a good thing. Although these policies did not signify any positive therapeutic position, they did represent an acknowledgement of the frequently negative effects upon young people of punitive institutional detention. But the present political instinct appears to be one of greater locking up, largely to allay anxiety and to appease the demands of voters as a short-term response to a perceived (but not substantiated) rise in youth crime. Proposals in Britain for new 'secure training units' for delinquent 12- to 15-year-olds, at massive economic expense and undoubted emotional cost, without predictable benefit, are an alarming prospect. A change of government in 1997 has not brought with it any discernible sense of enlightenment or change of policy. All knowledgeable professionals advise against locking up more juveniles – except where serious danger to self or others dictates – on the basis of both effectiveness and cost, not to speak of humanity. At best it provides protection for society, but only for the duration of custody.

THEORETICAL BACKGROUND

Some of the pioneering work and publications in the understanding and management of the juvenile offender began impressively early. An example is Stanley Hall (1916[1905]) – although not from a psychodynamic perspective – in his classic text with the splendidly baroque Edwardian title (which says it all) *Adolescence: Its Psychology and its Relations to Physiology, Anthropology, Sociology, Sex, Crime, Religion and Education*. Aichorn (1925) applied psychoanalytic understanding to the education of delinquents which he described in his classic text *Wayward Youth*. Cyril Burt (1925) provided fundamental data of much psychodynamic interest. Kate Friedlander (1947) wrote of 'the scientific knowledge which has brought about the change from retribution and deterrent punishment to the idea that the individual offender needs to be re-educated'.

Within psychoanalysis the various theoretical emphases *broadly* agree upon the developmental importance of early infantile experience, of attachment, and of the experience of emotional containment as a crucial grounding for later maturation.

Overview of a psychodynamic schema of development

Following Freud, we can view *adolescence* as the fourth and predominantly *genital* stage of psychosexual development after the so called 'oral', 'anal' and 'phallic' stages. This provides a helpful basis, although the terminology can be off-putting at first, and so long as it is realized that psychodynamic ideas have developed and elaborated – variously – round this 'bare-bones' model. For schematic purposes (after Blos 1966), we may in turn divide adolescence itself into four substages.

PRE-ADOLESCENCE

Pre-adolescence, at the onset of puberty, is characterized by increased instinctual pressure which tends to the indiscriminate investment of the libidinal and aggressive modes of early and infantile life. (The fact that 'aggression' can no longer be thought of simply as instinctual, and unitary, does not need to detain us at this point of the overview.) Erotic life is undeveloped, but physical manifestations such as erections and nocturnal emissions occur as the consequence of non-specific experiences of arousal, for example of anger, fear or shock.

This stage follows on from a period, classically called 'latency', in which, amongst other tasks, intellectual linguistic and conceptual developments have occurred, and the '*ego*' – or (broadly) the sense of self – has become more established and strengthened. Precocious sexualization by adults (i.e. sexual abuse) during this phase, as indeed in later phases of adolescent development, can have disastrous consequences for the very active psychological changes – progressions, digressions and regressions – which are part of this, hopefully, flexible and pliable organic series of stages of development.

During the pre-adolescent phase, groups and 'gangs' are especially popular. Blos (1966) speaks of such groups as functioning for the 'socialization of guilt'. In this way the *super-ego* (or conscience) conflict with regard to instinctual gratification, and the consequent guilt, can be unburdened on to the group in general or on to a leader (who is frequently older) as the instigator of the consequent acts of transgression.

EARLY ADOLESCENCE

If all went well in pre-adolescence, the emotional life then becomes wider and richer. Friendships are formed which at first tend to be idealized and narcissistic. It is not uncommon that, as the adolescent is turning away from primary (parental) objects, he or she experiences 'lows' of mood: 'I'm bored' will frequently be heard, as the young person seeks, but has not yet found, new 'objects' (persons or activities) for emotional investment. The child knows fairly clearly what he does *not* want, but has not yet found what he *does* want. Indeed, this can be a life-long predicament. It is well described by Phillip Larkin (1988).

ADOLESCENCE PROPER

In adolescence proper a turn occurs toward heterosexual object choice with renunciation of the incestuous, parental, 'Oedipal object'. It may also be a phase of increased intellectualization, asceticism and religiousness with concern for philosophical and social issues. This period frequently covers an age range for boys between 14 and 16 years, and for girls somewhat younger, although no hard-and-fast rule applies and 'normal' development allows for great variation.

LATE ADOLESCENCE AND AFTER

In late and post-adolescence, momentous new departures are put through 'trials' and experimentations towards the eventual establishment of a fairly coherent structure of character by the end of adolescence – at around age 21 years: not a finished product but a formed one.

Deviations within the idealized schema

The foregoing brief, and simplistic, summary of 'normal' adolescent development and the adolescent task may be contrasted with the major difficulties which many juvenile offenders suffer and which they eventually present to professionals. It offers a model which we can use in order to try to understand, and to respond to, their predicament in a helpful way. The delinquent act – across a range from the not so serious to the major violent or sexual act – commonly represents a deviation, a blockage, a failure in this idealized version of development.

Increasingly, psychodynamic thinking in Britain focuses upon 'object relations'. This refers to infantile and later interpersonal relations, and to relationships within the mind of the individual between innumerable internalized 'objects' (persons). This includes the 'internalization' of capacities of relating, of thinking and of reflection; see, for example, Fonagy (1991). The adequacy of the initial infant–caregiver relationship is seen as crucial, and is summarized in Winnicott's phrase of 'good-enough mothering'. Psychodynamic thinking has returned to an emphasis upon the various possible disruptions in early relationships and to the centrality of trauma in the genesis of abnormal development. Delinquency and violence are seen as the consequences of traumatic infantile, child, adolescent or, indeed, adult psychological experience. The increasing recognition of post-traumatic stress disorder and its consequences in children and in adults reflects a similar trend. Trauma for these purposes is defined as a particular experience of emotional loss or rejection, which may take the forms of (a) an absence or withdrawal of emotional warmth and affection by parents (indifference), or (b) overt hostility, aggression, physical neglect or violence. Attachment between 'carer and cared for' (Bowlby 1984) is thereby prevented, aborted or distorted.

There has been much recent empirical validation of these theories. For example, Stern (1985) has demonstrated the consequences of the failure of attachment, or normal 'attachment' and 'reciprocity', between infant and caregiver, and of the later building up of 'affiliative bonds' of affection. These failures lead to deficient development of self-esteem and a failure of the development of a capacity for empathy for others, and generally to failed socialization.

One consequence – 'violence as attachment goes wrong' – has been described by de Zulueta (1993). Failure of attachment is a common denominator of many young and adult offenders. Frequently these young people have spent most of their lives 'in care', with serial placements and numerous substitute parents. It can be said that they have suffered from a surfeit of different types of parents – foster parents, house parents, various surrogate

parents – but rarely one with whom attachment and the growth of attachment could reasonably proceed.

Williams (1978) distinguished between two types of adolescent 'acting out' – for which we may substitute the word 'offending' – according to the degree of working through which has occurred of 'the depressive position', following the formulation of Melanie Klein. Both, however, can become overladen with secondary gain, whereby the initial 'cause' (the primary 'gain') becomes established, and lends certain additional (secondary) psychological advantages. Put in other words, the 'acting out' may become part of an individual's identity, and 'ego sytonic' rather than causing distress ('ego dystonic').

In Williams' first type of 'acting out'/offending, the negotiation of the depressive position is central. According to Kleinian theory, this development normally begins in the first year of life, but needs reworking, particularly at the stage of adolescence and other times of change and potential crisis. If this stage – which effectively turns on the relationship of the infant to the 'primal' object, usually the mother, and of the adolescent to the parental figures – has been relatively successful, and a good relationship has been maintained, 'acting out' may then – when it occurs – take a relatively benign form. A child may, for example, steal money from his mother's handbag. Winnicott gives examples of being able to help such children, and thereby their mothers, with relatively short or even single consultations. Winnicott suggests that the child steals in symbolic form only what once belonged to him by right. The child is unwittingly trying to make up for a deprivation experienced in the original commonwealth of his or her relationship with the mother, and is alerting the environment to this fact. For Winnicott, this minor antisocial act, like a regression in psychoanalysis, is a return to the point at which the environment was felt to fail the child.

The second type of 'acting out'/offending is far more serious in what it represents and possibly in its consequences. If there has been a bitter, hateful renunciation of the 'primal' object – the mother – then there will be a paranoid mode of relating to the world. There will have been little working through of the 'depressive position' or, to use Winnicott's term, the 'stage of concern'. This form of 'acting out' is primarily destructive, and may escalate to actual violence if it cannot be contained in phantasy and in thinking.

Sometimes with adolescent offenders, libidinal and so-called 'aggressive' (destructive) drives (as described by Freud) come together in a most dramatic and catastrophic way. We do not need to enter the debate of whether the aggressive drive is 'primary' (innate), or 'secondary' (consequent upon the internalization of trauma), or a mixture of both. We may be shocked and horrified, but *consciously* not half so much as the offending adolescent: *post hoc*, it is frequently not difficult to understand the mental state behind the escalation – from apparently minor acts or destruction to the possibly cataclysmic. In the present author's experience, young offenders can commonly be helped to acknowledge the peculiar and intensely painful mental states which accompanied their offences; but, being emotionally painful, it is also common that this acknowledgement is only temporary. 'Healing' (the longer-term recognition of the unhappy well-springs of their behaviour) – and therefore the prevention of recidivism – is a more difficult matter.

Most delinquents or juvenile offenders are troubled children, but mostly they do not know it consciously and deny the fact. The psychoanalytic or psychodynamic approach allows us to know it by a particular form of listening – with a 'third ear' – to the communication behind the act. If the communication can be received and understood, that is a beginning towards the delinquent act no longer being necessary.

However, the response of our penal system for juveniles is generally to ignore such a mode of understanding. Not only does it not address and attempt to repair the developmental failures, but it also effectively prevents the completion of the developmental tasks of adolescence. The age of locking up young offenders in our system, from 12 years to 21 years, corresponds quite precisely with the stages of development in adolescence which have been described above. Young people are locked up, frequently for 23 hours a day in the worse scenarios, and have little hope of 'practising' the tasks of relatively successful separation from parental figures – both real (objective, parents) and the internal images of them. Nor do they have opportunity for developing attachments to new 'heterosexual' objects, and of negotiating adolescent homosexual anxieties and experiences – without, for example, the primitive defensive recourse to the 'macho', 'queer bashing' culture of the prison. Intellectual and social concerns are even more restricted than frequently they already have been. The oppressive regimes induce only compliance or, marginally more hopefully – for future development – defiance.

In brief, premature foreclosure of the adolescent task is very likely to be exaggerated, and emotional growth stunted by the response of parts of our system. It is a system which demands compliance by authoritarian force. To quote Winnicott (1984) again: 'I like to think that there is a way of life that starts from the assumption that morality that is linked with compliance has little ultimate value.'

LIMITATIONS OF PSYCHODYNAMIC UNDERSTANDING IN CLINICAL MANAGEMENT

All the foregoing is easily said, but what is to be done? In looking to psychodynamic knowledge for help we should be clear that – as Freud wrote in 1925 in his introduction to Aichorn's *Wayward Youth*:

'... delinquent children demand (literally) much more than the analytic method alone can provide, but psychoanalytic understanding is necessary for house parents, therapists, social workers, teachers and all those professionals who are bold enough to take on this difficult work. In the case of children, young delinquents and, as a rule, criminals dominated by their instincts, the psychoanalytic method must be adapted to meet the need.'

This view is reiterated by Kate Friedlander (1947). She writes:

'I do not wish to convey the impression that psychoanalysis can do more than explain certain manifestations of delinquency. This field is one which by its very nature needs the co-operation of sociology, criminology, penology and psychology (including psychiatry) if it is to achieve valuable results.'

The psychodynamic viewpoint can help the individual, but perhaps more importantly other staff, to understand some of the dynamic reasons behind the frequently puzzling – but also communicative – behaviour of offending adolescents. The work involves many of the insights and skills of the psychoanalyst: it is demanding in its currency of raw and (so-called) 'primitive' emotions and in the countertransference experience. It taxes one's sensitivity of when just to listen, when to aim only to support psychologically, and when to make a verbal statement (an 'interpretation'). It is never comfortable but it can be immensely rewarding, although frequently chastening. Hope and trust need to be fostered, where they are commonly nearly absent. Therapeutic zeal needs to be tempered with a realistic appreciation of the frequently dire emotional and psychological predicament of the young person.

Only in favourable, and less malignant cases, can the 'acting out' be kept within an individual therapeutic relationship. At the beginning there will be some hopelessness that the internal traumatized state can be repaired, and the young person's demeanour and behaviour may be relatively compliant. As a therapeutic relationship grows – as an 'object relationship' is made – then the delinquency, benign or malignant, will come into the transference and tend to be acted out within it. Mostly in this situation several workers with different roles – as adjuncts to family or school – are necessary. Glover (1960) wrote of 'the distributive transference', where several professionals take the brunt of the transferential pressure – and the tendency for 'cutting off' emotionally by staff is therefore less necessary or likely. For the individual therapist cannot be expected to struggle alone with the emotional demands of some of these young people. To attempt to do so, and to 'close down' emotionally out of self-protection, is likely to add to the emotional traumatization which in their earlier lives they have come to expect, and, indeed, which they are trying to break through by escalation of their 'acting out'.

It is unavoidable, indeed it is necessary, that the seriously out-of-control cases require and receive residential and secure management; however, the danger, and the present likelihood, is of loss of individuality and of coercion into compliant uniformity. It is easy to deprecate but sometimes difficult in practice to avoid.

THE INSTITUTIONAL SETTING

When we consider the juvenile offender, his or her behaviour, and our response, making use of aspects of psychoanalytic understanding, we are then necessarily in the realm of applied psychoanalysis, and of a major adaptation to the classical two-person analytic setting.

Developmentally, after the first experience of the dyadic infant–mother relationship, the next experience of 'social' life occurs inside the group which constitutes the family. Where this process has gone awry it may be that another 'family' (e.g. a foster or adoptive family) or another group (a children's home, a community home, a therapeutic community, or secure institution) has the formidable task of trying, for shorter or longer duration, to undo and provide repair for these initial failures.

This section gives a brief account of the present author's experience of consulting to a young offenders' institution, which is a prison for young people – previously called youth custody and before that Borstal. The chapter appendix offers some vignettes of individual young offenders.

As in all therapeutic interventions with offenders, there is always a 'third party' present – the criminal justice system – represented by prison, by prison officers or by ourselves: one cannot exclude oneself from a part in this triangle.

Although at different times I have felt it was not worthwhile – indeed, at times hopeless – I have tried, using a psychodynamic understanding, to hang on to the belief that the 700–800 young people (aged between 14 and 21 years) detained there so very much need to be listened to receptively. The Dr Barnardo's poster slogan 'What this boy needs is a good listening to' (rather than 'talking to') comes to mind – and listened to with a receptive psychodynamic ear, and to be understood. I have attributed my feelings of sometimes near total exasperation to the profound defensiveness and psychological impenetrability of the organization. But it is all too easy to blame 'the institution'. Although antisocial behaviour may not in some of these cases have become firmly established as a repetitive habit, change as we all know is a difficult and slow process. Individual staff members – including several enthusiastic prison governors who have come and gone – have been most welcoming. A number of staff have shown themselves hungry for the sort

of understanding that psychodynamic insights give: unsurprisingly, too, many feel greatly threatened.

The predominant culture is now custodial. There is psychiatric input from prison medical officers and visiting psychiatrists only for those young people who are either obviously psychiatrically very disturbed, or whose offences are serious enough for the criminal justice system to have to take notice and to request a psychiatric evaluation and psychological explanation of their particular offences. From a life of relative disinterest from others, the young serious offender may become the centre of much inter-disciplinary professional attention. As Winnicott remarks, the easiest way to get help is provocatively and through violence.

Prison officers particularly, but also other staff, frequently choose to work with adolescents, and it is good that some do. Frequently they have strong personal views about young people and identify strongly with deprived and severely damaged individuals. Obviously, this can lead to what a psychoanalyst regards as 'acting out' in the countertransference, either from an excessively sympathetic and colluding stance, or from an excessively punitive or correctional approach. This is likely to be largely unconscious and the staff member remains unaware. Staff need help and support in order to use their feelings about these young people creatively.

Nevertheless, I have learned how much individual offenders, when given the opportunity, want to be listened to and to have their point of view – as well as their offence behaviour – understood, if that is possible. Often contact is intense and immediate, and very brittle: defences are primitive and fragile. For example, a common initial account is of a 'wonderful', 'magic' mother and a related version of father, either equally idealized or of a profoundly bad version. Very soon this idealization falls away. Probably the boy relates that he last saw his mother when he was 3 years old when she placed him in care. He frequently has no memories of her, only 'images': to use a photographic metaphor used by one boy, he had 'stills' of a chaotic, abusing mother, of a traumatizing childhood; he lives in an essentially persecutory and terrifying world. Was it possible, this lad wanted to know in our second session – expressing a capacity which gave hope – that these 'stills' could ever become a movie?

The concept of the 'moral defence' (Fairbairn 1952[1946]) – in essence – is poignantly exemplified by the attempt at psychological protection of the (actually) 'bad' parents by this brittle idealization. There is a defensive denial of an acknowledgement that their parents were, in reality, seriously deficient: The idealization is a crude, but emotionally impoverishing, denial.

It is as if these children and adolescents have never been listened to before and had (almost) given up hope that talking could be of any consequence: They rush at the opportunity, often to find themselves confronting, with me, their 'internal' worlds which they had come – with more or less success – hitherto to keep locked out of mental experience. Awful histories of abuse are not uncommon, often divulged for the first time. It is still an awful shock to me to see a big 'macho' (possibly tattooed) young man collapse into the terribly distressed 'infant' within. This frequently brings great initial relief but is provocative because necessarily short term. Frequently, as a I drive away from the institution, I feel very sad, but smugly, wonderfully unburdened – like some cowboy (so the pejorative image has struck me) riding out of town – having had close, genuine and very moving contact with a disturbed and very troubled adolescent, and knowing that at the very least he must wait one week before I see him again. Worse, it is quite likely that our contact may have been a 'one off'; since he may next week have been sent to a prison cell, another young offenders' institution or some other place.

One tries to be prepared for such emotional exposure – the individual adolescent's and one's own – in the face of the degree and intensity of suffering and pathology, and the inadequacy of what one offers. I try to prime staff about particularly vulnerable youngsters so that they can be with them when I am gone. The question persists; is it better to offer something, however inadequate, than nothing at all? I have a working viewpoint that it is, and that making oneself available and leaving the possibility of contact largely open-ended, is worthwhile for at least some of these young men. In many cases I offer to see them after their release and a few do make contact at this later stage. For others, no doubt, one becomes a bad, neglecting figure or, alternatively, an idealized helper whom they will never see again.

Clearly the omission here is of any concept of a 'therapeutic community', where a socio- and psycho-therapeutic culture provides the underlying ethos of the institution. However, therapeutic communities appear to be undergoing a resurgence, as seen in the planned growth in new 'Henderson Hospital' and HMP 'Grendon Underwood' units. In the present author's view they offer the single best environment for the sufficiently motivated patient/client.

CONCLUSION AND FUTURE DIRECTIONS

What sort of setting is most suitable for a helpful and therapeutic engagement with the young delinquent? Clearly the least restrictive environment which allows for the maximum of personal and varied human engagement is preferable. The therapeutic community must be the model to be aimed at, whereby sociotherapy and psychotherapy go hand in hand with education, and responsibility and forms of self-government are encouraged. Some examples are sketched briefly in this conclusion.

Past models of therapeutic communities for adolescents included Peper Harow in Godalming and Dartmouth House in Greenwich, both now closed. It is not the 'fashion' of the times to work so thoroughly with traumatized and traumatizing young people; rather to go for more 'quick fix' and coercive methods. But human nature is not so easily changed, and short-term economies are likely to be long-term expenses – certainly in human, but also in economic, terms. Earlier community 'experiments' included the Ford Republic in America and the Little Commonwealth in Britain set up by Homer Lane; and those of the psychoanalytically informed 'Hawkspur Experiment' or 'Q Camps' set up by Marjorie Franklin, and the 'Barns Experiment' of W. D. Wills. An LCC school (Bredinghurst) was described by Robert Shields (1971), a psychoanalyst, in *A Cure for Delinquents*' (1971) – a challenging if possibly over-optimistic title for us to consider and to conjure with.

One current working model in Britain is the Henderson Hospital for young adults suffering from personality disorder. However, patients contract voluntarily to be admitted and to participate in the community. For a forensic population of serious offenders, forms of compulsory detention are unavoidable. But there are major difficulties in establishing a therapeutic community ('TC') where young people are compulsorily detained, and the whole idea of the 'TC' may thereby be seriously diluted. The alternatives to such attempts at therapeutic facilities have grown largely 'piecemeal'.

Secure facilities for juvenile delinquents sit mainly within justice and social care with varying but usually inadequate levels of input from psychotherapists in the critical roles of consultation, liaison and staff support in addition to individual or group work with young people.

National commissioning of medium secure adolescent psychiatric in-patient services was introduced in April 2002. Although a welcome development, its primary emphasis is on those adolescents with serious mental illness. Many young offenders have other significant and multiple unmet needs (Bailey and Thornton 1994) meriting a structure and ethos as exemplified in the therapeutic community model. Overall there is a particular lack of therapeutic facilities for 17- to 20-year-old offenders who have not yet developed a major psychiatric illness but where intervention in late adolescence could prevent a trajectory into antisocial, borderline and/or psychopathic personality disorder in adulthood. This group includes adolescents displaying violent and sexualised behaviours, many of whom have themselves experienced earlier trauma, violence, abuse and loss.

Whatever the setting, there is a case for the application of psychodynamic ideas in the understanding of the young offender, and in helping those across many disciplines – from teaching, social work, and child and adolescent psychiatry amongst them – who are working hard to provide for these very demanding young people. Psychiatrists have a role to play also in the politics of child provision – and the promotion of child health as a preventative measure – as well in the provision and planning of services for the mentally unwell and the delinquent young person. Young offenders have frequently had traumatized lives, but the anxieties that they provoke often lead policymakers to precipitate decisions which are in the best interest of neither society nor the young offender.

APPENDIX: CASE STUDIES

A criminal action may be regarded as a rich source of information about the 'inner state of affairs' of the offender's mind, like a dream sequence, revealing much that remains consciously unknown. Just as Freud considered the manifest dream to be a compromise – like a symptom – so, too, can we regard the criminal act. Another analogy is that of 'play' in the analysis and therapy of children. Reference has been made already to Klein's (1927) paper in which she describes the violent, destructive and murderous phantasy life of the infant and child, which, however, remains only partially enacted in the child's play. Later she emphasized also the loving and reparative aspects of the child's inner world. Murderousness is not in the usual way enacted in fact. Given an adequate or 'good enough' relationship with parents or their substitutes, such phantasies and impulses are contained (Bion 1962, 1965) and mitigated by parental care and love. However, where such containment has failed these phantasies (unconscious) or fantasies (conscious) may be acted out in the criminal act.

VIGNETTE 1

Michael was first seen by me the day after he had been charged with attempted murder: he was a white, British, 16-year-old secondary school pupil and had no previous record of offending behaviour, although later he was able to tell me – shame-faced – of perverse, quasi-psychotic sexual experimentation in his early teens with a male infant cousin.

For three months preceding this offence he had felt mentally tortured by homosexual desire and anxiety. This took the form of a very concrete split in his mind between 'homosexual = bad' and 'heterosexual = good'. His sleep was disturbed, as were his waking hours, by his intrusive sexual fantasies of homosexual acts; he felt tormented. He resolved to injure or kill a homosexual man by way of achieving 'cure' for his awful dilemma. He visited a men's lavatory on three occasions in the week preceding his offence: On the latter visits some form of masturbatory sexual contact took place, but his partners did not know of his largely murderous intent. In a sense these were felt like 'rehearsals', and had some similarity to 'grooming' for the major criminal and psychological act.

On the day of the offence he picked up a man from the same public lavatory and took him home. During sexual 'play' he attacked the man viciously. Only the proximity of a casualty department prevented the man's death. My patient/client felt horrified by what he had done, but he was no longer tormented by his sexual conflict: he felt relieved and remained so for a longer time than I predicted. He was desperate to talk to me to try to understand how he could have done such a thing. However, after some six weeks, the same persecuting dilemma returned and with it a rage at me which was hardly bearable and which continued – *mutas mutandi* – some years on.

He is contemptuous, witheringly dismissive and arrogant, and I experience most clinical sessions with him as emotional and intellectual 'killings'. I have been, I think, largely unable so far to help him but he is required (by law) to come to see me. He has found a religious solution for the time being, but feels that no-one, other than God, has ever helped him. He does not feel himself to have suffered a seriously traumatized life, although there were early and apparently 'managed' separations from parents in his early life as a result of family illness. I see him in the hope that some part of his violent mind is mitigated by his contact with me. This young man illustrates – in the most crude and concrete way – the fantasy of 'cure' by the psychodynamically described mechanism of 'projection identification', and then its enactment. That is to say that he had – and acted upon – a phantasy that he could rid his mind of unbearable contents by mentally pushing (and punching) them into his victim, and then by killing them off within his victim. Now – without (fortunately) the actual physical enactment – he does the same to me.

VIGNETTE 2

Robert has nightmares. He has a long history of violent assaults, first on teachers, then on staff in a residential home. He has not assaulted staff in the penal institution – he has not been allowed the opportunity. Instead he breaks up his cell from time to time and sometimes cuts his own arms or thighs with any sharp instrument that comes to hand. This is not uncommon behaviour in violent young men who lose the psychologically stabilizing opportunities of 'acting out' in the community, and frequently of violence towards others.

I wish to focus only on Robert's dreams. They are, without exception, violent, bleak, brutal and lacking a narrative sequence whatsoever. They are not untypical of this group of young men and share some of the qualities of those who suffer the nightmares of post-traumatic stress disorder (PTSD); they are repetitive and unchanging. Predominantly there is a recurrent dream/nightmare of being mown down by a gang in advancing gunfire and of the death throes he suffers, which, however, never end in death. It is as if he is the victim of continual nocturnal torture, whilst, during his waking hours, he would pretend that he can be only the perpetrator. A particular, and to him very troubling daytime fantasy, however, is one of leaving the institution, only to be shot by marksmen as soon as he leaves the gates.

Robert's is an extreme – and clear – version of what is common in my experience to many of these boys. They are very much victims as well as perpetrators. The description by Herbert Rosenfeld of the 'internal mafia gang' in the persecuted, paranoid mind is an accurate description of the internal world of these superficially 'normal', anti-social adolescents. Rosenfeld (1987) describes the internal worlds of his patients in analysis, but this can be applied, too, to the *actual* formation of gangs by many young people. They may be relatively benign or, as in these cases, malignant. 'The destructive narcissism of these patients,' writes Rosenfeld, 'appears often highly organised, as if one were dealing with a powerful gang dominated by a leader who controls all the members of the gang to see that they support one another in making the criminal, destructive, work more effective and powerful … [they] dream of being attacked by members of the Mafia or other adolescent delinquents.' He continues: '… to change, to receive help, implies weakness and is experienced as wrong or as failure by the destructive narcissistic organisation which provides the patient with his sense of superiority.'

VIGNETTE 3

A quite different expression of 'the dream' – more a day-dream serving a partially defensive purpose – was that of a boy who had killed but denied that it had happened: 'It was a dream'. 'Tell me the dream,' I suggested. He responded with a long and accurate narrative of the sequence of events preceding, during and after the homicide. Only later was he able to accept – albeit partially, and with editing of the most horrific detail – the reality of his mostly accurately registered and remembered 'dream'. Those who live in such awful, persecuted internal worlds – and who sometimes act it out in fact – potentially know far more than they can fully bear to acknowledge. We, too, as therapists need to struggle to bear to think the 'unthinkable' in order to help these patients to do so, too.

REFERENCES

Aichorn, A. 1925: *Wayward Youth*. New York: Viking Press.
Bailey, S. and Thornton, L. 1994: The first 100 admissions to an adolescent secure unit. *Journal of Adolescence* 17: 207 20.
Bion, W.R. 1962: *Learning from Experience*. London: William Heinemann.
Bion, W.R. 1965: *Transformations*. London: William Heinemann.
Blos, P. 1966: *On Adolescence: A Psychoanalysis Interpretation*. London: Free Press/Collier Macmillan.
Bowlby, J. 1984: Violence in the family as a disorder of the attachment and caregiving systems. *American Journal of Psychoanalysis* **44**: 9–27.
Burt, C. 1925: *The Young Delinquent*. London: University of London Press.
Copley, B. 1993: *The World of Adolescence: Literature, Society and Psychyoanalytic Psychotherapy*. London: Free Associations.
Deutsch, H. 1968: *Selected Problems of Adolescence: Psychoanalytic Study of the Child*. London: Hogarth Press/Institute of Psychoanalysis.
Fairbairn, R. 1952[1943]: The repression and the return of bad objects (with special reference to the 'war neuroses'). In *Psychoanalytic Studies of the Personality*. London: Tavistock/Routledge.
Fonagy, P. 1991: Thinking about thinking: some clinical and theoretical considerations in the treatment of the borderline patient. *International Journal of Psychoanalysis* **72**: 639–56.
Freud, S. 1916: *Some Character Types Met With in Psycho-Analytic Work*, standard edn, 14. London: Hogarth Press/Institute of Psychoanalysis, 309.
Friedlander, K. 1947: *The Psycho-Analytical Approach to Juvenile Delinquency*. New York: International Universities Press.
Glover, E. 1960: *The Roots of Crime: Selected Papers on Psychoanalysis*, Vol. II. New York: International Universities Press.
Hall, S.G. 1916[1905]: *Adolescence: Its Psychology and its Relations to Physiology, Anthropology, Sociology, Sex, Crime, Religion and Education*, 2 Vols. New York: Appleton.
Kernberg, O. 1992: *Aggression in Personality Disorders and Perversions*. New Haven, CT: Yale University Press.
Klein, M. 1927: Criminal tendencies in normal children. In *Love, Guilt and Reparation*. London: Hogarth Press.
Larkin, P. 1988: The life with a hole in it. In *Collected Poems*. London: Faber & Faber, 202.
Laufer, M. and Laufer, E. 1989: *Developmental Breakdown and Psycho-Analytic Treatment in Adolescence: Clinical Studies*. New Haven, CT: Yale University Press.
Robins, L.N. 1966: *Deviant Children Grown Up*. Baltimore: Williams & Wilkins.
Robins, L.A. 1979: Sturdy childhood predictors of adult outcomes: replications from longitudinal studies. In Barrett, J.E., Rose, R.M. and Klerman, G.L. (eds), *Stress and Mental Disorders*. New York: Raven.
Rosenfeld, H. 1987: Destructive narcissism and the death instinct. In *Impasse and Interpretation*. London: Routledge.
Rubenstein, M., Yeager, M., Goodstein, B. and Lewis, D. 1993: Sexually assaultative male juveniles: a follow-up. *American Journal of Psychiatry* **150**: 262–5.
Shields, R. 1971: A cure for delinquents. In *The Treatment of Maladjustment*. London: William Heinemann.
Stern, D. 1985: *The Interpersonal World of the Infant: A View from Psychoanalysis and Developmental Psychology*. New York: Basic Books.
Williams, A. H. 1978: Depression, deviation and acting out in adolescence. *Journal of Adolescence* **1**: 309–17.
Winnicott, D. 1982[1956]: The antisocial tendency. In *Through Paediatrics to Psycho-Analysis*. London: Hogarth Press.
Winnicott, D.W. 1984: *Deprivation and Delinquency*. London: Tavistock.
de Zulueta, F. 1993: *From Pain to Violence: the Traumatic Roots of Destructiveness*. London: Whurr.

21

Arts therapies

LYNN P. AULICH

INTRODUCTION

'Arts therapies' is a term which for the purposes of this chapter encompasses:

- art therapy
- dance movement therapy
- dramatherapy
- music therapy.

The arts therapies have evolved gradually since the early twentieth century, with postgraduate training courses, professional associations; and state registration with the Council for Professions Supplementary to Medicine, for qualified practitioners.

Art, drama, dance movement and music therapies have developed their own bodies of theory, as separate disciplines, based on practice. The developmental history of each discipline is documented and disseminated in specialist journals devoted to theory and practice and in a growing number of theoretical and practical books.

Arts therapists are psychotherapists whose art form is the primary means of expression, while verbal expression frequently arises as a precursor or a consequence of the art, action, music or dance and is an important part of the therapeutic work.

THE ARTS IN HEALTH

General issues

The arts in the broadest sense have an intrinsic therapeutic value for individuals and society as a whole. The importance of the arts to the evolution of human life is undisputed; it is through archaeological evidence of ritual, pictures and artefacts that we come to know anything of the lives of our ancient ancestors. It could be said that the arts are evidence of the connections between individuals, with their own personal experiences and interpretations, and the societies in which they live. Individual personal experience is unique, but resonates with many other people. The need for people to be creative individually and to generate culture collectively in the service of mental and physical well-being is recognized in the fields of anthropology, philosophy, history of art, and psychology and medicine.

Arts activities – drama productions, music, writing, drawing and painting – which take place in hospitals, prisons, schools and institutions for the care of young people have an important therapeutic role in providing a means of self-expression and community cohesion. Professional dancers, actors, writers, artists and musicians 'in residence' or employed by education departments in services for young people have designed programmes to address specific problems such as offending behaviour. An example is structured workshops in collaboration with probation services and youth justice to work with young people who set fires (Fine and Macbeth 1996). The actors, artists, dancers, musicians and writers employed for this purpose are not offering therapy. Rather, arts therapists are trained to undertake the development and understanding of a specifically therapeutic relationship between the patient, the therapist and their creative work as a vehicle for psychological change.

Training in the art therapies

The majority of arts therapists are trained to degree level in visual art, drama and literature, music or dance prior to undertaking a postgraduate training specific to the therapeutic use of each art form. A thorough experiential training, theoretical and practical training in the application of psychodynamic principles provides arts therapists with common ground. These therapists are also required to undergo personal psychotherapy twice a week for two years during training. The overall purpose of training is to enable practitioners to harness the inherent therapeutic qualities of creative expression into the service of effecting permanent positive change in individuals who engage in therapy.

Arts therapists are employed as clinicians in a wide variety of institutions and organizations providing health and social services. As institutions become increasingly specialized, arts therapists are beginning to identify and develop specific approaches in response to the difficulties of their patients (Wood 1999). One of the areas of specialization that has evolved in the arts therapies since the 1980s is in forensic psychiatry.

There are an increasing number of established posts in adult and adolescent forensic services. Arts therapists are often employed part-time or for a few sessions a week. In practice this means they have a heavy caseload of young people with complex difficulties. Shortage of time and lack of status within the institution does not afford the opportunity to build research into the timetable. This partly accounts for the paucity of published research by arts therapists in forensic psychiatry.

In adolescent forensic psychiatry the arts therapist's task is to contribute to multi disciplinary assessment and to provide treatment of young people in secure facilities and in the community. The arts therapy assessment offers a young person the opportunity to inform the assessment team about current thoughts, feelings and experiences. It can also provide information about the young person's needs in terms of psychological intervention and appropriate placement, the risk a young person presents to himself or herself and others, the management of those risks, and the suitability of the particular form of art therapy as a treatment.

The facilitating environment

Arts therapists working with individuals or groups of people with identified mental health problems provide a facilitating environment whereby the young person feels comfortable and safe enough to begin therapeutic work. An uninterrupted, regular time, in a calm, properly equipped room with a therapist whose whole attention is focused on them alone, enables young people to rediscover, or sometimes to discover for the first time, the capacity to play and communicate through play. The physical aspects of the facilitating environment allow therapists to concentrate on providing mental containment. The young person is held in the mind of the therapist through her (or his) attention, her capacity for thought, and her ability to feel empathy.

The facilitating environment is necessary for the development of a relationship between patient and therapist based on trust that is essential to therapeutic work. An important aspect of the facilitating environment in forensic psychiatry is the personal physical safety of therapists and patients, which requires an extra level of containment in the form of co-therapists and staff with a supporting role.

The physical environment is very important to arts therapists. For optimum effectiveness, drama, dance, music and art therapy sessions need generously sized, private, uncluttered space with secure storage.

Creativity

The creative process is shared by all the arts therapies, as an underlay to whatever theoretical approach is employed as a framework to understand the therapeutic relationship (see later). Definition of this process proves elusive, but a breakdown of the different stages involved may be useful here.

The beginning of a creative cycle is the recognition of a problem to be solved or an idea to be explored. A period of intellectual and emotional immersion in the subject follows, requiring a search through a combination of internal resources such as memory and imagination and external sources such as observation, pictures, books, music, plays, papers and discussion and conversation. A period of incubation experimentation or processing follows where ideas are tried out and played with to explore the possibilities. Illumination and inspiration arise from this form of play, leading to insight, and making new unforeseen connections between thoughts, feelings and ideas and actions. A period of evaluation tests out new insights to find out whether they make sense, communicate and fit the situation (Meekums 1993).

Young people who are mentally disordered, distressed and traumatized frequently experience difficulties in using their capacity for communicating thoughts and feelings in a creative and constructive manner. Arts therapists work to engage their patients in a discovery or a rediscovery of the creative process.

Collaborative work

Art, music dance movement and drama therapists working in forensic psychiatry frequently collaborate with other professionals – psychiatric nurses, occupational therapists, speech and language therapists, teachers, clinical psychologists and psychiatrists in a team approach to assessment and treatment. It is important not to work in isolation with this group of young people. Institutional dynamics mirroring the difficulties of the patient group mitigate against good communications between staff from different disciplines. The isolation of one therapist, or all the therapists from each other, through failures in communication is a dynamic that arts therapists continually strive against.

The arts therapists on the team are often able to offer their fellow professionals valuable information about patients' perceptions of their predicament, otherwise unavailable. For arts therapists, it is vital that they be able to translate their medium of exchange between themselves and patients into language other professionals will understand. Failure to communicate what happens in art, drama, music or dance to other members of the staff team results in an arts therapist becoming isolated or marginalized.

In adolescent forensic psychiatry, practice demonstrates the effectiveness of therapeutic work undertaken by a therapist using a verbal, cognitive approach and an art therapist or music therapist working in collaboration (Bailey and Aulich 1996). The psychodynamics underlying an intervention structured in two or more parts can be problematic and need frequent discussion in the treatment team. In some cases the benefits of offering two different forms of therapy outweigh the problems caused by defence mechanisms such as 'splitting'. The therapists and the young person aim to understand how and why they came to be in their current predicament and have a means to prevent a recurrence. However, case-study evidence suggests that music therapy and art therapy with young people in forensic psychiatry are effective as the sole form of individual psychotherapy within a structured programme of education, occupational therapy and directed, offence-related work (Flower 1993; Aulich 1994).

THE THEORETICAL BASIS OF ARTS THERAPIES

Arts therapists working with young people are familiar with the works of Freud, Jung, Melanie Klein, Anna Freud and Donald Winnicott whose theories of early infant experience, object relations, symbol formation and the concept of transitional space are especially relevant. Art, drama, dance, music and literature take place in and embody the space between the real and the imaginary described by the notion of the transitional object and transitional space (Winnicott 1971). The production or art object can be understood as a transitional object, the product of phantasy and imagination.

Many arts therapists are aware of and use John Bowlby's attachment theory as a framework for understanding the nature of the therapeutic relationship, especially in their work with forensic patients. The influence of failed or problematic attachments in early life on the young person's capacity to reflect on his or her own or other people's states of mind – which in turn influences aggressive, violent and self-harming behaviour – has been extensively researched and documented (Zulueta 1996; Fonagy and Target 1996; Fonagy 2001). The dynamics of attachment are manifest in a tangible, visual, physical form in the arts therapies in addition to being present in the struggle to reach and maintain a therapeutic relationship.

The arts therapies are highly successful in engaging young people and adults to make connections between thoughts, emotions, the physical body and actions. Through experience of therapeutic relationships it is possible to form new healthy attachments, giving young people another chance. The role of arts therapies in assisting healthy brain development in children whose brain development is physically damaged by continual exposure to trauma is intuitively important and needs to be researched.

Many young people who are referred to forensic services have suffered deprivation, neglect and a combination of physical, sexual and emotional abuse. They have frequently experienced a lack of emotional stability, insecurity and inadequate parenting.

The novelty, sensuality and richness of arts therapists' tools, the art materials, instruments, props and costumes can be overwhelming to deprived young people. Lethargy, boredom and oppositional, hostile and destructive behaviour are common responses to the prospect of creative activity. Young people who have experienced privation need time to adjust to working therapeutically; art materials and instruments or unaccustomed physical movement can be over-stimulating, resulting in an inability to concentrate, or inhibiting, making it very difficult to know how to begin work. In the arts therapies, privation and deprivation can be seen in limited imagination – emptiness, impoverished, sparse and stereotypical imagery in young people's products. In these situations therapists offer various ways to warm up and relax, or to settle and focus. Young people with little access to cultural knowledge or experience often need to be given stimuli and encouragement to develop the capacity to have ideas and be inspired.

Arts therapists are frequently active participants in the therapeutic process, playing in an interactive, responsive way, as a parent would with a child. For the art therapist this means painting and drawing with, or experimenting with, the materials in order to engage a young person in handling them and making images. For a music therapist it means providing a carefully attuned accompaniment to engage and encourage the young person to use the instruments in making sound reciprocally. In drama, the therapist becomes an interactive participant, supporting and playing roles with and for the young person. The dance movement therapist moves in response to the patient's improvised dance.

Many of the young people in forensic services have learning disabilities, developmental delay and emotional and behavioural disorders and mental illness, making conversational approaches to therapy impossible. Problems in communicating feelings in a comprehensible form frequently leads to frustration and 'acting out'. Young people in this predicament frequently experience difficulty in articulating thoughts and feelings as a consequence of a limited vocabulary for describing emotions or an inability to distinguish between different emotions. Some young people are too anxious and agitated to speak coherently or become easily distracted, overactive or destructive. Feelings of shame and guilt and embarrassment can seriously inhibit young people's capacity to talk about themselves and their actions. In these situations a primarily non-verbal therapy provides a means of communication.

At the other end of the spectrum, arts therapies can assist highly articulate young people from obscuring their feelings, especially painful shameful and guilty feelings rationalized and intellectualized through words. Young people in forensic mental health service frequently have a history of therapeutic intervention, have learned the art of pleasing therapists with familiar jargon phrases while continuing to avoid expression of their feelings.

Arts therapies are active, action-oriented ways of thinking, feeling and communicating with others where therapists and patients are not necessarily face to face with each other. The therapist's attention is on the state of the therapeutic relationship with the patient and on the process and production of the work. Qualities of the therapeutic relationship or aspects of it can be embodied within the art form; the music, dance, play or painting. The art form acts as a third party: attention is focused on the mask or the song in addition to the patient's words and body language. Art forms contain projected, externalized feelings, often unmanageable, shameful, murderous feelings which might otherwise be overwhelming. Projection into an art form creates a distance between the art object, piece of music or dramatic sequence, as a container of projected feelings and the artist who cannot acknowledge those feelings. This distance affords the therapist and the patient time to reflect and consider the possible meanings of the work. This aspect of arts therapies makes them accessible to people finding face-to-face work in verbal psychotherapy too threatening and confrontational. Young people who have rejected verbal psychotherapy are often willing to work in music, art, drama or dance movement therapy.

A major task for young people is developing the ability and the courage to take responsibility for their actions and the consequences. Participation in drama, art, music and dance assists them in understanding the links between feelings, intention, action and consequences. For a young person who is so distanced from personal feelings and actions that he or she is dissociated, cut off from the emotions or in denial, the art object or sound sequence can help the individual to move gradually towards understanding and acceptance of traumatic events.

Arts therapists understand that issues arising from interpersonal interactions between the therapist and the patient in the present resonate and provide insight into past relationships and past trauma. Relationships formed in the present can lead back to those in the past and return to influence the present where difficulties can be addressed. The dynamics of past trauma re-enact or play themselves out in offensive behaviour, a repeat trauma which re-traumatizes the perpetrator and spreads the trauma to new victims – and, if we fail to look after ourselves through supervision, to the therapists.

Each art form has the capacity to encapsulate the particularity of a person's predicament. If the mind is a terrain then all forms of communication are means of describing and documenting the view. Words provide one viewpoint, a drawing, a piece of music, a series of movements describe the same place from entirely different perspectives. Each of the arts therapies has the capacity to help individuals find new means of self-expression. This leads on to the development of self-esteem, confidence and more satisfactory ways of interacting with other people. The therapeutic alliance provides a model of a non-exploitative, reliable relationship opening up the possibility of being able to form good relationships in the future.

Therapy is not a way to take pain, sadness and anger away; it cannot cure or mend the past. The focus in treatment is on nurturing a young person's strengths and capabilities, not to expunge the past but to reduce and neutralize its capacity to distort the present. Resilience is important if a young person is to be able to manage feelings in adverse circumstances without harming the self or others in the future.

Young people who have suffered chronic trauma often defend themselves by becoming cold – emotionless and dissociated from their emotions. When a young person does not feel, he or she cannot recognize feelings in others. Some young people in this position go on to commit acts of extreme violence and sadism. Therapy offers the means to begin to acknowledge emotions, accept them as part of the self, then to learn how to use those feelings to recognize distress in others, transforming painful experiences into the capacity to reflect and empathize. This is a slow, labour-intensive process. The damage caused by chronic trauma, abuse and neglect can be ameliorated only in long-term therapy (Bailey and Aulich 1996).

ARTS THERAPIES IN FORENSIC SETTINGS

The provision of arts therapies in forensic settings is steadily developing as their value to people in this situation is increasingly recognized (Teasdale 1997a). Joyce Laing's pioneering work in art therapy began in 1973 with an invitation to establish an art therapy programme in the special unit for extremely violent and disturbed men in Barlinne prison (Carrel and Laing 1982). Many adolescents who attended her art therapy sessions were able to address the emotional and behavioural difficulties leading them into antisocial criminal behaviour. Laing (1984) says:

'While labelled as deviants many offenders are inventive, ingenious, quick-witted, and have great vitality. It may be that the creative aspects of the criminal have, for reasons of background experience or psychological make-up, been misdirected towards destructive ends. If the art therapist can channel these talents in a positive creative direction, the offender will experience a new perception of the self and where he belongs in society.'

Art therapy

Art therapy has been used in the probation service with young people (Liebmann 1990). The work is initially focused on the offence by encouraging the young people to use the 'comic strip' format, a series of sequential drawings to describe what happened, before, during and after an offence. Through the process of expansion and exploration of the comic strip it is possible to work therapeutically with the emotional issues arising.

In the USA, links between delinquency, serious criminal offences, murder and childhood trauma have been researched using a young person's drawings of the crime scene (e.g. Burgess *et al.* 1990). The drawings were used to access the young person's memory of what occurred and his or her perceptions about the offence; that is, what the individual thought was happening at the time. The study recognized the value of the drawings in identifying attachment difficulties, and sexual/physical abuse, with the attendant distortion of dynamics relating to the need to have power and be in control. The insights gained from the crime-scene drawings provided a guide to the most appropriate form and direction of treatment.

The introduction of therapy into a traditional prison environment is fraught with difficult paradoxical situations constantly challenging therapists, inmates and the philosophy of the institution (e.g. Cronin 1994; Edwards 1994; McCourt 1994). The provision of art therapy in young offender institutions gives inmates the opportunity to address some of the emotional issues that led them into offending, this being an important aspect of preventing recidivism (e.g. Baillie 1994). In regional secure units, the relationship between mental disorder and offending behaviour are recognized and are the focus of assessment and treatment. Art therapy makes a significant contribution to the therapeutic regime in adult secure facilities (Karban and West 1994; Innes 1996, 1997) and in the adolescent forensic mental health service (Aulich 1994).

Art therapy as an analytical investigative process is part of the assessment and treatment programme in the therapeutic community model used in Grendon Underwood. Art therapy is an effective component of the group therapy programme for personality disordered offenders (Teasdale 1995) in which participants are gradually able to understand the antecedents of their violent acts and the consequences to themselves and others. Case studies demonstrate how the art therapy group provides the opportunity to assimilate and incorporate new insights and ways of thinking and feeling into daily interactions with others:

'What the art therapist can offer is a focus for mutually reflective review which aims to aid the offender-client in bringing issues together through visualization. My argument is that this process of bringing points together provides a challenging contrast to the criminal actions which have left the offender's own and others lives in pieces.' (Teasdale 1997b)

Art therapists working within a cognitive–behavioural framework contribute to group treatment programmes for adolescent sexual abusers developed by voluntary agencies, probation services and social services (Gerber 1994; Hargood 1994). Art therapy has an effective role in group work, using directed art-based exercises to identify cycles of abuse and other factors contributing to sex offending. Art therapy is also used to alert group workers to mental health issues, such as suicidal feelings arising in the course of group work (Gerber 1994).

Dance therapy

Dance movement therapists use movement to encourage self-expression and to stimulate communication between patient and therapist. This work is founded on the recognition that the body is used constantly in the process of non-verbal communication from the time the fetus begins to move in the womb. Physical movement continues to be our primary means of developing a sense of self, of being a separate body and experiencing secure intimate relationships with others. Although western culture emphasizes verbal and written language to communicate, people respond continually and subconsciously to non-verbal information about personality, life experience and emotional states through gesture, posture and movement (Blatt 1996).

Dance movement therapy has been used in the US penal system with sex offenders (Blatt 1996) and is beginning to be developed in forensic mental health services in the UK.

Dramatherapy

Dramatherapy has gained a high profile in the treatment of patients in special hospitals and regional secure units. Jennings and Minde (1993) delineated dramatherapy practice into three main areas with relevance to people in forensic services: as development, as ritual, and as theatre art.

Dramatherapy as development
Dramatherapy as development is based on the premise that people are able to engage in dramatic activity in its simplest form from birth. The earliest communications between babies and adults occur through an exchange of

sounds, actions and movements. Dramatherapy also looks at the use of the voice and physical coordination from a developmental perspective. In common with dance movement therapy, drama therapy provides a means of helping people gain control over, and feel at ease with, their bodies both physically and psychologically. In a forensic setting, a developmental approach would encourage people to experience imaginative play and take part in drama games within a group.

Dramatherapy as ritual

Dramatherapy as ritual explores humans' need to symbolize and structure their experiences through forming rituals to mark important events. Ritual ceremonies and festivals are shared community events allowing the expression of common human needs in symbolic form. At the same time, rituals provide participants with dramatic distance from their own personal experience. The formation of rituals can be creative and helpful, or they can be destructive, as in humiliating, dangerous initiation rites in street gangs and racist groups. Drama therapy approaches that explore ritual formation are useful with mentally disordered offenders, to contain and distance destructive feelings to prevent impulsive 'acting out'.

Dramatherapy as art

Dramatherapy as theatre art centres on the dramatic performance, either improvised or with a text, rehearsed and performed to an audience. It is possible for the actor to recognize aspects of his or her own personality and behaviours in a character and give expression to feelings through choosing a character with a particular role. The expression of grief, for example, through a character can lead to the actor recognizing and expressing personal grief in a way that may have been impossible otherwise.

Drama uses symbols and metaphors to arouse powerful emotional states resonating between the actors and the audience. Important human life events – birth, death, transitions, journeys, love affairs – are explored and contained in art forms people can identify with, such as plays, stories, myths and legends. The structure of these art forms often provides a framework of 'introduction, exploration and resolution', making it possible to address very powerful emotions and remain safe and contained.

Works by Shakespeare, Homer, Virgil, Ibsen and the Greek tragedians explore taboos: difficult subjects such as incest, rape, the murder of close relatives, rivals, friends, enemies and strangers, suicide, transvestism, racism, violence, jealousy, megalomania, and madness. Drama therapy offers a vehicle for the expression of these feelings while remaining supported, and in control.

Music therapy

In music therapy, a range of musical instruments is made available which are not dependent on skill or musical experience to produce sound. The instruments are selected for accessibility and suitability for free improvization and spontaneous expression. Music therapy is highly interactive as the therapist accompanies and responds to the patient directly through sound. Melodies, harmony, rhythm, pace and their opposites can produce or reflect affective states, so these aspects of music making are the primary means of expressing emotional experience.

THE ISSUE OF CONTROL

The need to exert control and power over other people as a defence against being and feeling helpless and powerless is a dynamic underlying many violent and sexual offences. The need to deny vulnerability and control others through abusive behaviour is a dynamic frequently leading the patient to persecute the therapist. The power relationship between patient and therapist is thus a fundamental concern. It is important to find a balance between the amount of control retained by the therapist and the degree of freedom allowed by the patient in the session (Flower 1993). Music therapy affords the opportunity to make small but genuine choices, such as whether or not to play, which instruments to use, and whether or not to record the session. The consequences of choices made in the safe and contained environment of the music therapy session are observable and can be explored through music, telling the story of the music and through discussion.

Young people have very different reasons for wanting to participate in the emotionally demanding process of therapy. Clinical experience in therapy demonstrates how particular and individual the experience of therapy is for each young person. The need for the therapist to be clear in explanations, and sensitive and highly observant towards the patient during non-verbal and verbal interactions, is vital to effective and safe work with this group of young people.

OUTCOMES

Research undertaken at Broadmoor into the benefits of dramatherapy with adults reports a significant measure of change for the better. Drama and dramatherapy in custodial settings has been shown to be exciting, moving, motivating and effective in creating permanent change in the treatment of people in forensic services (Cox et al. 1992). A group of patients in a secure psychotherapeutic environment have been found to have reduced levels of anger and an increase in attempts to control their expression of anger following a short period of group dramatherapy (Reiss et al. 1998).

Dramatherapy and its close relative psychodrama are also used in a non-clinical context where therapists and professional actors work together; an example is the Geese

Theatre Company who work with adults and young people in custodial settings on specific issues such as violence, aggression and sexual offending. Drama workers are trained to offer drama workshops in prisons and young offender institutions (Thompson 1996). This work can be beneficial and has therapeutic effects – but it is not arts therapy.

Music therapy in adult forensic mental health services and prisons is well documented and researched (e.g. Hoskins 1995; Loth 1996; Slobada 1997). In contrast, music therapy with adolescents in forensic mental health services has suffered from lack of resources for research, although it is long established in particular services. Research in music therapy with emotional learning and behavioural disorders (Montello and Coons 1998) and with destructive adolescents (Lehtonen and Shaunessy 1997) demonstrated significant positive changes on the ratings scales for hostility and aggression following a period of group music therapy.

CONCLUSIONS

Possibly the most important aspect of the arts therapies is the opportunity for transformation. Powerful, uncomfortable feelings such as anger, frustration, aggression, destructiveness, hostility, jealousy and envy can be harnessed in creating something which did not exist before, which informs and communicates thoughts and feelings to others and opens up a space for reflection. Using the body in dance and drama, making a sculpture or a passage of sound is about using the emotions, about recognition, mastery, self-control and a constructive form of agency.

Interest in the value of arts therapies' contributions to adult forensic mental health services is growing, but few services for adolescents make full use of the unique therapeutic skills of arts therapists with young people. Given the interest young people frequently have in the arts, in culture and in creative self-expression, and their reluctance to participate in verbal therapy, the scarcity of arts therapists in these services reveals a fundamental distrust of the value and validity of the modality. This obstacle can be overcome through arts therapists' continued engagement in research, in participating in the debate about what constitutes valid research, and through involvement in the education of arts therapy trainees and fellow professionals.

Arts therapists are rarely employed full time. The consequence of this is a full caseload of young people with complex difficulties, leaving little time to offer arts therapy trainees a properly supervised placement, and scarce time to undertake essential research projects necessary to contribute to the evidence base for practice and to develop and refine theory. Many forensic services for young people employ only one or two of the arts therapy disciplines, if any. The consequence is that they lag behind many more progressive mental health and community services in providing therapies accessible and acceptable to young people in distress.

As a small group of professionals working in forensic psychiatry, and especially few working with adolescents, arts therapists struggle to establish and maintain their practice. As with most groups of people who work on the periphery of services, we can be susceptible to feelings of grandiosity to compensate: 'Arts therapies can do all things for all people, and arts therapies can reach lost people when all else has failed.' The desperation and impotence felt by many clinicians in this field when they encounter young people who are challenging to treat can lead to premature exhaustion and feelings of failure. There is a need for all forms of therapy to recognize the limits as well as the possibilities provided by their methods.

Arts therapies are an important part of assessment and treatment services for mentally disordered young people in forensic mental health, not as the 'icing on the cake' but as the 'bread and butter' of the service.

REFERENCES

Aulich, L. 1994: Fear and loathing: art therapy, sex offenders and gender. In Liebmann, M. (ed.), *Art Therapy with Offenders*. London: Jessica Kingsley.

Bailey, S. and Aulich, L. 1996: Adolescents who murder. In Welldon, E. and Van Velsen, C. (eds), *A Practical Guide to Forensic Psychotherapy*. London: Jessica Kingsley.

Baillie, C. 1994: Art as therapy in a young offenders institution. In Liebmann, M. (ed.), *Art Therapy with Offenders*. London: Jessica Kingsley.

Blatt, J. 1996: Dance movement therapy. In Cordess, C. and Cox, M. (eds), *Forensic Psychotherapy: Crime Psychodynamics and the Offender Patient: 2. Mainly Practice*. London: Jessica Kingsley.

Burgess, A.W. *et al.* 1990: Juvenile murderers: assessing memory through crime scene drawings. *Journal of Psychosocial Nursing and Mental Health Services* 28(1): 26–34

Carrell, C. and Laing, J. 1982: The Special Unit at Barlinnie Prison – Evolution Through its Art. Glasgow: Third Eye Centre.

Cox, M.C., Berry, S., Hewish, M. *et al.* 1992: Drama in custodial settings. In Cox, M. (ed.), *Shakespeare Comes to Broadmoor: the Actors are Come Hither*. London: Jessica Kingsley.

Cronin, P. 1994: Ways of working. In Liebmann, M. (ed.), *Art Therapy with Offenders*. London: Jessica Kingsley.

Edwards, S. 1994: Out of line. In Liebmann, M. (ed.), *Art Therapy with Offenders*. London: Jessica Kingsley.

Fine, N. and Macbeth, F. 1996: Playing with fire. In Liebmann, M. (ed.), *Arts Approaches to Conflict*. London: Jessica Kingsley.

Flower, C. 1993: Control and creativity: music therapy with adolescents in secure care. In Heal, M. and Wigram, T. (eds), *Music Therapy in Health and Education*. London: Jessica Kingsley.

Fonagy, P. 2001: Attachment and personality disorder. *Journal of the American Psychoanalytic Association* 48: 1129–46.

Fonagy, P. and Target, M. 1996: Personality and sexual development, psychopathology and offending. In Cordess, C.

and Cox, M. (eds), *Forensic Psychotherapy: Crime, Psychodynamics and the Offender Patient: 1. Mainly Theory.* London: Jessica Kingsley.

Gerber, J. 1994: The use of art therapy in juvenile sex offender specific treatment. *The Arts in Psychotherapy* **21**(5): 367–74.

Hargood, M. 1994: Group art therapy with adolescent sex offenders: an American experience. In Liebmann, M. (ed.), *Art Therapy with Offenders.* London: Jessica Kingsley.

Hoskyns, S. 1995: Observing offenders: the use of simple ratings scales to assess changes in activity during group music therapy. In Gilroy, A. and Lee, C. (eds), *Art and Music Therapy and Research.* London: Routledge.

Innes, R. 1996: An art therapist's inside view. In Cordess, C. and Cox, M. (eds), *Forensic Psychotherapy: Crime Psychodynamics and the Offender Patient: 2. Mainly Practice.* London: Jessica Kingsley.

Innes, R. 1997: Auto-erotic asphyxia and art psychotherapy. In Welldon, E. and Van Velsen, C. (eds), *A Practical Guide to Forensic Psychotherapy.* London: Jessica Kingsley.

Jennings, S. and Minde, A. 1993: *Art Therapy and Dramatherapy: Masks of the Soul.* London: Routledge.

Jennings, S. and Minde, A. 1996: Dramatherapy. In Cordess, C. and Cox, M. (eds), *Forensic Psychotherapy: Crime, Psychodynamics and the Offender Patient: 2. Mainly Practice.* London: Jessica Kingsley.

Laing, J. 1984: Art therapy in prisons. In Dally, T. (ed.), *Art as Therapy: An Introduction to the Use of Art as a Therapeutic Technique.* London: Tavistock.

Lehtonen, K. and Shaunessy M. 1997: Music as a treatment channel of adolescent destructivity. *International Journal of Adolescence and Youth* **7**(1): 55–65.

Leibmann, M. 1990: It just happened: looking at crime events. In Liebmann, M. (ed.), *Art Therapy in Practice.* London: Jessica Kingsley.

Loth, H. 1996: Music therapy. In Cordess, C. and Cox, M. (eds), *Forensic Psychotherapy: Crime Psychodynamics and the Offender Patient: 2. Mainly Practice.* London: Jessica Kingsley.

McCourt, E. 1994: Building up to a sunset. In Liebmann, M. (ed.), *Art Therapy with Offenders.* London: Jessica Kingsley.

Meekums, B. 1993: Research as an act of creation. In Lee, C. and Payne, H. (eds), *Handbook of Inquiry in the Arts Therapies: One River, Many Currents.* London: Jessica Kingsley.

Montello, L. and Coons, E. 1998: Effects of active versus passive group music therapy on pre-adolescents with emotional, learning and behavioural disorders. *Journal of Music Therapy* **35**(1): 49–67.

Reiss, D., Quayle, M., Brett, T. and Meux, C. 1998: Dramatherapy for mentally disordered offenders: changes in levels of anger. *Criminal Behaviour and Mental Health* **8**: 139–53.

Slobada, A. 1997: Music therapy and psychotic violence. In Welldon, E. and Van Velsen, C. (eds), *A Practical Guide to Forensic Psychotherapy.* London: Jessica Kingsley.

Teasdale, C. 1995: Reforming zeal or fatal attraction: why should art therapists work with violent offenders? *Inscape* Winter Edition: 2–9.

Teasdale, C. 1997a: Art therapy as part of a group therapy programme for personality disordered offenders. *Therapeutic Communities Journal* **18**(3): 209–22.

Teasdale, C. (ed.) 1997b: *Guidelines for Arts Therapists Working in Prisons.* London: Home Office/HM Prison Service for England and Wales.

Thompson, J. 1996: Stage fights: violence, conflict and drama. In Liebmann, M. (ed), *Arts Approaches to Conflict.* London: Jessica Kingsley.

Winnicott, D.W. 1971: *Playing and Reality.* Harmondsworth: Penguin.

Wood, C. 1999: Gathering evidence: expansion of art therapy research strategy. *Inscape* **4**: No. 2.

de Zulueta, F. 1996: Theories of aggression and violence. In Cordess, C. and Cox, M. (eds), *Forensic Psychotherapy: Crime, Psychodynamics and the Offender Patient: 1. Mainly Theory.* London: Jessica Kingsley.

22

Physical treatments

ANDREW CLARK

INTRODUCTION

Physical treatments play a limited but important role in the management of some adolescent psychiatric disorders, so familiarity with their usage is an essential part of the clinical practice of the adolescent psychiatrist (Jaffa 1995). However, they should not be viewed in isolation but rather as one component of a treatment programme which encompasses physical, psychological and social measures. They can be divided into three broad groups:

- non-biological
- biological but non-pharmacological
- pharmacological.

Holding, restraint, seclusion and physical punishment are non-biological physical treatments sometimes applied to young people. Electroconvulsive therapy (ECT) is a non-pharmacological biological treatment which may be considered on occasion in specific cases. Re-feeding is a biological intervention which in some circumstances can also be regarded as an integral part of the medical treatment for a mental disorder, particularly anorexia nervosa. Powerful pharmacological agents can be instrumental in major improvements in a young person's behaviours, emotions, cognitions and overall level of functioning when used appropriately to treat particular disorders.

Each of these interventions carry significant risks and adverse side effects which are capable of misuse and inappropriate prescription where there may be no benefit to the young person but actual harm may result. Each of them is considered in this chapter. For greater detail, particularly about practical prescription of psychopharmacological agents specifically to children and adolescents,

readers may wish to consult the textbooks by either Green (1995) or Kutcher (1997) – although do bear in mind that they are both written from a North American rather than a European perspective.

Examination of prescribing practices or attitudes both in the UK and in the USA shows that the extent to which adolescent mental health professionals use biological treatments varies considerably and that this seems unlikely to be solely related to variations in the populations or disorders treated (Adams 1991; Bramble and Dunkley 1992; Parmar 1993; Kaplan *et al.* 1994; James 1996; Bramble 1997; Walter and Rey 1997). Physical treatments have been regarded as controversial not merely by the lay community but also by child mental health professionals, and concerns about the over use of medication as a form of social control and the use of ECT as punishment continue to be expressed (Kaplan and Hussain 1995; Oxlad and Baldwin 1995). Empirical research on which to base adequate conclusions about appropriate evidence-based practice is still lacking for many treatments, due in part to the complexity of the issues involved (Fava 1996).

GENERAL PRINCIPLES

There are a number of general principles which should underlie prescription of any treatment intervention.

1 It should follow and be based upon an appropriate assessment and formulation.
2 It should be targeted to diagnosis and/or symptoms and it should be based upon evidence for its efficacy in so doing.

3 It should be at the least interventionist level necessary for efficacy and it should attempt to minimize the risks of adverse effects where possible.

4 It should be based upon appropriate informed consent from the young person and his or her family.

5 Any prescription should be accompanied by arrangements for monitoring and review both of treatment efficacy and of side effects, possibly including the use of appropriate rating scales.

Full achievement of these aims is not always possible. At times urgency may necessitate treatment before full assessment and formulation – such as in the case of an acutely psychotic young person in need of rapid tranquillization to ensure the safety of the person or others. Evidence of efficacy may be limited to extrapolation from adult practice and to uncontrolled reports of child and adolescent usage. The practitioner may even be using a drug beyond its product licence. (So long as it is based upon a body of accepted professional opinion and practice, and the awareness of this fact and the particular reasons for it are documented, this is not of itself grounds for concern.) Minimal dosages and prescription of only one psychotropic agent may not be possible in more complex or resistant cases. Full consents may not be readily obtainable; a duty of care is still owed to the young person presenting in an acute disturbed state with no-one holding parental responsibility immediately available. Notwithstanding practical difficulties such as these, the broad principles remain desirable goals.

CONSENTS

The prescription of any form of intervention should require either appropriate informed consent or a legal mandate making that unnecessary. Precise legal definitions and practices vary within different jurisdictions, although the broad considerations remain similar. This chapter considers the current position within England and Wales; readers in other countries will need to refer elsewhere for particular advice. In adulthood, only the individual concerned can legally give consent to treatment, whilst in childhood it is those holding parental responsibility for the child. In adolescence, the position of the young person in giving consent *vis-à-vis* the parents is more complex and requires assessment of the individual's particular capacity, maturity and understanding. Ideally consents need to be sought both from parents and from young people, and practitioners should be wary in proceeding with treatments based solely upon consent from either parents alone or young people alone (Pearce 1994).

For consent to be valid it is necessary that the individual giving that consent is able to understand the nature, purpose and likely effects of the proposed treatment.

They must be provided with adequate information, must be free from duress, must be capable of understanding the information given, and must be capable of making or exercising choice. Each of these considerations applies to children and young people, though with certain important riders (McClellan and Werry 1994; Pearce 1994). It is important that the language and terminology used be tailored to the developmental stage and intellectual ability of the young person. Information must include not merely the benefits but also the potential side effects of treatment, particularly those of a more serious or enduring nature (Brabbins *et al.* 1996).

The differential and position of influence of the adult doctor *vis-à-vis* the child patient means that care should be taken not to exert undue persuasion or coercion. This may be especially so in forensic mental health practice when the young person concerned may already be subject to some degree of restriction of liberty or practice and there is the consequent danger of *implicit* duress. Where it is not possible to obtain valid consent from parent or young person it may be necessary to consider compulsory treatment through the appropriate legislation – within England and Wales, the Mental Health Act 1983 (Nicholls *et al.* 1996).

HOLDING, RESTRAINT AND SECLUSION

Physical punishment has no place in the management of psychiatric disturbance at any age. However, physical containment and ensuring of safety may play an important part in the overall management of a disturbed adolescent. The nature of the physical environment and the ratio of staffing to young people are integral to this.

Building design should include consideration of needs for privacy, space, light and access to the outside. Staffing ratios should be concerned not merely with absolute numbers but also with experience, expertise and maturity. The separation of the young person from others, and from any instrument with which the individual might self-harm or injure others, may on occasion be necessary – even, on rare and extreme occasions, to the point of formal seclusion (Angold and Pickles 1993).

It is important that units have clear stated policies on the use of restraint, holding techniques and seclusion and that these do not become used as a form of physical punishment. It is further important to consider carefully the legal status of any individual whose liberty is to be restricted. Different countries have their own legal frameworks, but within England and Wales use of the Mental Health Act 1983 or of the secure accommodation provisions in s25 of the Children Act 1989 is likely to be necessary beyond the immediate need to ensure safety (which would probably be covered under common law).

PHARMACOLOGICAL AGENTS

Antipsychotic medications

Antipsychotic medications are specifically indicated in the treatment of schizophrenia and manic disorders, and in the symptomatic management of acute organic brain syndromes (including drug-induced psychotic states). There is at times pressure for their symptomatic prescription as a means of managing serious aggressive behaviours occurring in the absence of psychiatric illness but this should be resisted as a solution.

Until recently the only drugs available were the traditional neuroleptic agents (butyrophenones, phenothiazines, etc.), examples of which in common usage include haloperidol, thioridazine and chlorpromazine. These predominantly act upon dopaminergic transmission pathways but do also affect cholinergic, alpha-adrenergic, histaminergic and serotoninergic receptors.

In recent years there has been significant change in options and practice with the development of a new group of agents, based upon the older agent clozapine (see below), and called 'atypical antipsychotics'. This group of newly developed drugs do not possess the typical D_2 receptor selectivity which characterized the older neuroleptic agents. Examples currently include risperidone, quetiapine, olanzepine and sertindole, with others due to be released or in development. These appear to be relatively devoid of both immediate and longer-term side effects and yet have at least equal antipyschotic efficacy and may be becoming the first-line treatment of choice, particularly in younger patients (Thomas and Lewis 1998; Clark and Lewis 1998). Those side effects which have been reported do include sedation, weight gain, headache and some extrapyramidal effects, but all at lower levels than the older conventional agents. This reduction in side effects is likely to be translated both into better compliance and into consequent longer-term greater cost-effectiveness, despite the initial extra costs of the medication itself (Knapp 1997).

Whilst there are a large number of case reports and open studies of the use of antipsychotics in the treatment of psychotic disorder in adolescents, there are only four controlled trials of their usage. A double-blind controlled study of 75 adolescents with schizophrenia showed the conventional antipsychotic drugs haloperidol and loxapine to be superior to placebo (Pool *et al.* 1976). Lower-potency agents such as chlorpromazine or thioridazine have fewer extrapyramidal side effects but are more likely to produce anticholinergic effects and sedation (Realmuto *et al.* 1984). A controlled double-blind study in 16 children with schizophrenia also showed haloperidol to be superior to placebo (Spencer and Campbell 1994). The efficacy of clozapine over haloperidol in otherwise treatment-resistant cases has recently been demonstrated in a double-blind trial of 21 cases of childhood-onset schizophrenia (Kumra *et al.*

1996). There are as yet no controlled trials of the newer atypicals, although many of the case reports and open studies do relate to these.

Much of the systematic work concerning the side effects of antipsychotic medication in children and adolescents has been with older agents and in a wide variety of underlying conditions. Higher-potency dopaminergic blockers such as haloperidol or trifluoperazine tend to produce dose-related parkinsonian symptoms, and non-dose-related acute dystonias. There are reports of dyskinesias, akathisias and (rarely) neuroleptic malignant syndrome, all occurring amongst children and young people, although there may be some differences in dosage sensitivity from when similar events occur in adults (Richardson *et al.* 1991; Casey 1993). Many side effects, particularly those of drug-induced motor disorders and of behavioural toxicity, can easily be missed unless specifically sought; symptoms such as flattening of affect or response, amotivation and impaired cognitive functioning may even be attributed to manifestations of the underlying illness (Spencer and Campbell 1994; Dorevitch *et al.* 1995). Overall, children appear to be at increased risk of common and uncomfortable side effects from antipsychotic medication – especially dystonias – although further age-specific studies are needed (Sachdev 1995). In adult mental health practice these side effects are often treated symptomatically by concomitant prescription of an antimuscarinic agent (e.g. procyclidine or benzhexol); in younger patients the preferred initial strategy should be to switch to one of the atypical antipsychotics less likely to cause such effects (Clark and Lewis 1998).

As there is no evidence – with the exception of clozapine (see below) – to suggest that any individual antipsychotic is most effective in treating psychotic symptoms, the choice of agent is primarily based upon its side-effect profile (e.g. is sedation a desirable effect for this patient?). In recent years there has been considerable concern about the excessive dosages of antipsychotic medication being prescribed and the associated dangers (Kane 1994; Thompson 1994; Will *et al.* 1994; Lowe *et al.* 1996). Low-dosage regimens appear as effective as higher dosages and produce fewer adverse effects. Recommended dosages for children and adolescents are cited as 0.5–9.0 mg/kg daily of chlorpromazine equivalent (McClellan and Werry 1994), 0.02–0.12 mg/kg daily of haloperidol (Spencer and Campbell 1994), or up to 10 mg daily of haloperidol (Clark and Lewis 1998). Any individual agent should be continued for at least six weeks before concluding it to be ineffective.

Clozapine is the only antipsychotic drug with a demonstrated effectiveness in otherwise treatment-resistant cases of schizophrenia. This efficacy of clozapine over haloperidol in otherwise treatment-resistant cases has been clearly established in adults: about 40% of patients unresponsive to adequate treatment with conventional drugs have shown improvement on clozapine, albeit sometimes only after some months of treatment (APA 1997), and it has been demonstrated in a double-blind trial of 21 cases of childhood-onset schizophrenia (Kumra *et al.* 1996). However, clozapine is also known to cause agranulocytosis and is consequently only prescribable in treatment-resistant cases of schizophrenia (usually defined as inadequate response to two antipsychotic agents in adequate dosage for adequate time) and subject to close haematological monitoring. In the UK this monitoring is an integral part of its product licence and prescription is dispensed only upon evidence of a recent satisfactory blood test. Other, mainly dose-related, side effects known to occur include drowsiness, excessive salivation and epileptiform seizures (Remschmidt *et al.* 1994; Kumra *et al.* 1996).

A number of young people suffering from schizophrenic disorders will fail to take oral antipsychotic medication regularly, even despite close supervision and monitoring of their medication. In many instances this may be overcome by psychoeducational approaches towards them and their families as to the benefits of medication, and by ensuring that side effects are kept to a minimum. Ensuring once-daily dosages when possible, and consideration with carers of the timing of these to be most convenient, are often helpful practical strategies. Even so, in a few patients compliance with oral medication will remain erratic. It may then be necessary to consider prescription of a depot preparation – oily long-acting preparations given by intramuscular injection at intervals of between a week and a month. At present only the traditional neuroleptics are available in depot form, so their usage does need to be balanced against the increased risk of immediate and longer term side effects. In some individuals the benefits of control of their illness is, nonetheless, likely to outweigh these risks (McClellan and Werry 1994; Remschmidt 1993; Lowe *et al.* 1996; Clark and Lewis 1998).

Antidepressants

Prescription of antidepressant medication remains relatively widespread despite limited evidence of its efficacy in adolescents and the evidence for the efficacy of psychotherapeutic intervention in mild-to-moderate depressions (Harrington *et al.* 1998). In adults the efficacy of antidepressants in treating major depressive disorders is well established. However, randomized controlled trials of a variety of tricyclic antidepressants amongst children and adolescents have consistently failed to demonstrate any clinically significant benefit over placebo (Hazell *et al.* 1995; Fisher and Fisher 1996) – but this research finding has not been translated into clinical practice for a variety of reasons (Eisenberg 1996; Pellegrino 1996). Small sample size of trials, heterogeneity of cases, different pharmacodynamics and metabolism in young people have all been posited as explanations (Remschmidt and Schulz 1995). Emslie *et al.* (1997) have reported a randomized controlled

trial amongst adolescents to demonstrate a clear benefit from prescription of fluoxetine, a selective serotonin reuptake inhibitor (SSRI). Other potential antidepressants either are not formally or satisfactorily evaluated for use with adolescents (e.g. venlafaxine, nefazodone) or may have significant problems in tolerability and dietary compliance (the monoamine oxidase inhibitor group of agents). There is also evidence of the effectiveness of both the older tricyclic antidepressant agent clomipramine and of the newer selective serotonin reuptake inhibitor fluoxetine (Riddle *et al.* 1992) in the treatment of obsessive–compulsive disorders.

The majority of young people with depressive disorders should therefore be treated psychotherapeutically in the first instance. Medication should be reserved for those with severe disorders where symptoms do not respond to such measures and where there is a pervasiveness of mood disturbance and of social functioning. Discussion prior to prescription with both the young person and the carers or family is important both in ascertaining attitudes and resistances to the initial prescription and in ensuring that treatment is not stopped prematurely because the delayed action of the drugs has not been appreciated.

In view of the lack of evidence for their efficacy and their higher side-effect profile (particularly their cardiotoxicity), the traditional tricyclic antidepressant agents can no longer be regarded as drugs of first choice when medication is considered appropriate. A selective serotonin reuptake inhibitor should rather be chosen, although there appears to be no intrinsic advantage in antidepressant activity as to which particular agent is prescribed. The side-effect profiles do differ across the various drugs and different individuals will tolerate different agents variably. Most can be given as once-daily dosages, thereby improving likelihood of compliance. Once prescribed, they should be continued for an adequate length of time (6–9 months), rather than stopped prematurely because the immediate depressive symptoms have resolved. It may be possible to reduce the dosage in the latter stages; for longer-acting agents such as fluoxetine this may mean alternate days (Monday, Wednesday, Friday and once at the weekend). This may also reduce the likelihood of a withdrawal syndrome.

Mood stabilizers

Both lithium and carbamazepine are used extensively in adult practice in the treatment of bipolar affective disorder in both its acute phases and as prophylaxis, and sodium valproate is finding increased usage – despite continuing controversy about the effectiveness of all three drugs (Post *et al.* 1997; Moncrieff 1997; Cookson 1997). As with elsewhere in child and adolescent pharmacotherapy, methodologically robust age-specific evidence is lacking. Arguments for continuities of treatment responsiveness between adulthood and childhood and adolescence need to be treated cautiously, especially where affective disorders are concerned. As noted earlier, there is evidence that treatments shown to be effective in adult-onset schizophrenia are also effective in early-onset cases, but there is also evidence in depressive disorders of the reverse. Reports of age-specific studies underway are urgently awaited (Geller and Luby 1997).

Lithium therapy requires close therapeutic monitoring with regular assessment of serum levels (at least every two months) if toxic levels are to be avoided. Blood levels should be kept at 0.7–1.0 mmol/L. Additionally, urea and electrolytes should be regularly checked and thyroid function should be checked annually. This may mean that its prescription is inappropriate for some individuals where non-compliance can be anticipated, whether with the treatment itself or with the accompanying monitoring. In these cases prescription of carbamazepine or valproate may be safer and more appropriate. These have greater safety in overdosage, and whilst serum levels can be informative they are not essential to monitoring of treatment. Typical carbamazepine dosage is 100–200 mg three times daily.

In treatment-resistant bipolar disorders, polypharmacy is almost inevitable. The usual strategy is of joint prescription either of an antipsychotic and a mood stabilizer or of two mood stabilizers in conjunction. There are few controlled studies of such combination therapies and none in children or young people. It would appear that lithium plus valproate is probably the safest and most effective combination, although further research is needed (Freeman and Stoll 1998).

Hypnotics and anxiolytics

The literature regarding usage of hypnotics and anxiolytics in young people is sparse. The anxiolytics and hypnotics, also sometimes termed 'minor tranquillizers', have been used in the treatment of anxiety and panic, of sleep disturbance and of other disorders where a calming or sedative effect is required.

Sleep disturbance is common amongst teenagers and may be reflective of an underlying psychiatric disorder meriting treatment in its own right (Morrison *et al.* 1992). Use of 'sleep hygiene' measures (regular routines, avoidance of alcohol, nicotine and stimulants, appropriate conducive environment) should be encouraged as an alternative to use of medication (Stores 1996). Benzodiazepines have been used in the past despite all their associated drawbacks of potential for dependency, daytime hangover effects and a rebound phenomenon on cessation. They may have benefit in the treatment of parasomnias such as night terrors by their reduction of time spent in stage-four sleep (e.g. diazepam 2 mg at night), but reassurance is usually sufficient alone in their management. Newer non-benzodiazepine hypnotics (e.g. zopiclone)

have fewer disadvantages but still cannot be recommended for use with young people (BMA/RPS 1998).

There is also little satisfactory evidence for the effects of medication to reduce levels of anxiety in children and adolescents despite the range of agents sometimes used in adult practice (Gadow 1992; Campbell and Cueva 1995; Nutt and Bell 1997). Benzodiazepines, antidepressants and low-dose propranolol have all been used although without proven benefit. Psychological approaches should remain first choice, possibly with the adjunctive prescription of propranolol (e.g. 10–20 mg three times daily) where somatic symptoms predominate and do not initially respond to behavioural and psychoeducational interventions.

Benzodiazepines may occasionally be useful in providing a short-term interim additional sedative effect in the treatment of psychotic disorders when used adjunctively to antipsychotic medication. Low regular dosages of diazepam (up to 10 mg three times daily) or of lorazepam (up to 2 mg four-hourly) for the first week only are typical examples (Clark and Lewis 1998).

Stimulants

The role of stimulant medication in the treatment of attention-deficit hyperactivity disorder in younger children is now well established (Sandberg 1996). They have demonstrable efficacy in increasing attention and on-task behaviours, in improving academic performance, and in reducing classroom disturbance. Concomitant behavioural and cognitive strategies are also an essential component of its management. Methylphenidate is the drug most commonly used (dosage titrated against response up to a maximum of 60 mg daily) with dextroamphetamine a secondary alternative.

The role of stimulants within the adolescent population remains less clear. New diagnosis of attention-deficit disorders during teenage years is difficult as it relies on much retrospective information with all its attendant potential unreliabilities. In addition, the features of conduct disorder, of history of educational failure and of substance misuse may all play further confounding influences. The decision regarding if, when and how to withdraw or stop the medication which has been prescribed for a younger child is also contentious, with some advocating that the disorder is life-long and therefore that medication should be continued through to adult life (Noone and van der Linden 1997). There are a number of references in the literature to the use of the drug pemoline being particularly useful with adolescents and young adults; However, the drug was withdrawn by the Committee on Safety of Medicines from use within the UK, other than on a named-patient-only basis, owing to concerns regarding its hepatotoxicity. Nevertheless, at the time of writing it remains available within the USA.

ELECTROCONVULSIVE THERAPY

Despite recurrent controversy, electroconvulsive therapy (ECT) is generally accepted as an effective treatment of severe depressive disorders in adults. It is also used on occasion in certain types of schizophrenia and in resistant manic disorder. Its effects and side effects have been extensively studied in a range of populations and disorders. In childhood and adolescence, however, its usage remains extremely infrequent, even in disorders which might be so treated in adult practice, and there are few studies of its effects. Expressed views as to its appropriateness may owe as much to polemic and prejudice as to any scientific rationale; for an example of this, see Baker (1994) and responses from Kellett (1994), Chattergee (1995) and Fink (1995).

The majority of the literature relates to single or multiple case reports of young people treated with ECT. Diagnoses have been surprisingly heterogeneous and included depressive disorders, schizophrenia, manic disorders, developmental disorders and catatonia. Attempts at systematic review and meta-analysis have produced conflicting findings, probably relating both to the nature of the questions asked and to the interpretations of the papers selected (e.g. Rey and Walter 1997; Baldwin and Oxlad 1996). Similarly it is difficult to be dogmatic about adverse effects of treatment.

This means that the practitioner should be cautious in its prescription but should not overlook it as a possibly effective treatment intervention in those severe cases of life-threatening major depressive disorders resistant to other interventions, or where the urgency of the situation necessitates a rapid response to treatment (e.g. stupor, determined suicidality, refusal to eat or drink). Severe and resistant manic disorders, catatonic states and treatment-resistant schizophrenias with high levels of affective symptoms may lead to similar consideration. A full reassessment of the young person, the disorder and all previous treatment interventions is mandatory. A second opinion from a colleague experienced in its use is usually advisable, although because of its rarity this will almost inevitably be a practitioner in adult mental health rather than one with particular expertise in child and adolescent psychiatry. Freeman (1995) goes so far as to suggest obtaining opinions from both a child/adolescent psychiatrist and an adult psychiatrist when considering treatment of a young person aged under 16 years.

Obtaining full consent or legal dispensation is mandatory; in England and Wales administration of ECT under the Mental Act 1983 without adequate consent requires a specific independent second opinion from a doctor appointed by the Mental Health Act Commission. Involvement of child and adolescent mental health professionals in the administration of the ECT is desirable, as is a physical separation from adults also receiving treatments. Regular review of the mental state of the young person should take place between treatments, and applications should not be prescribed as a set course or number of treatments to be completed.

RE-FEEDING

Food is not usually regarded as a medicine and the giving of food is not usually regarded as physical treatment. In certain circumstances, however, the giving of food by artificial means has been defined as medical treatment. This has primarily been in respect of anorexia nervosa, although it has also applied in cases of persistent vegetative state and in one instance psychopathic disorder with total food refusal (Mental Health Act Commission 1997). Decisions regarding nasogastric feeding, even in severe and life-threatening situations and particularly those without the individual's consent, should be carefully considered and regularly reviewed. The applicability of this guidance to those on 'hunger strike', as distinct from food refusal secondary to anorexia nervosa or severe depressive or psychotic conditions, seems particularly potentially contentious.

REFERENCES

Adams, S. 1991: Prescribing of psychotropic drugs to children and adolescents. *British Medical Journal* **302**: 217.

Angold, A. and Pickles, A. 1993: Seclusion on an adolescent unit. *Journal of Child Psychology and Psychiatry* **34**: 975–89.

APA (American Psychiatric Association) 1997: Practice guidelines for the treatment of patients with schizophrenia. *American Journal of Psychiatry* **154**(suppl.): April.

Baker, T. 1995: ECT and young minds (letter). *Lancet* **345**(8941): 65.

Baldwin, S. and Oxlad, M. 1996: Multiple case sampling of ECT to 217 minors: review and meta-analysis. *Journal of Mental Health* **5**: 451–63.

Brabbins, C., Butler, J. and Bentall, R. 1996: Consent to neuroleptic medication for schizophrenia: clinical, ethical and legal issues. *British Journal of Psychiatry* **168**: 540–4

Bramble, D. 1997: Psychostimulants and British child psychiatrists. *Child Psychology and Psychiatry Review* **2**: 159–62.

Bramble, D.J. and Dunkley, S.D. 1992: The use of antidepressants by British child psychiatrists. *Psychiatric Bulletin* **16**: 396–8.

BMA/RPS (British Medical Association and Royal Pharmaceutical Society of Great Britain) 1998: *British National Formulary*, no. 35. London: BMA/RPS.

Campbell, M. and Cueva, J.E. 1995: Psychopharmacology in child and adolescent psychiatry: a review of the past seven years: II. *Journal of the American Academy of Child and Adolescent Psychiatry* **34**: 1262–72.

Casey, D.E. 1993: Neuroleptic induced acute extrapyramidal syndromes and tardive dyskinesia. *Psychiatric Clinics of North America* **16**: 589–610.

Chattergee, A 1995: Electroconvulsive therapy (letter). *Lancet* **345**: 518–19.

Clark, A.F. and Lewis, S.W. 1998: Practitioner review: the treatment of schizophrenia in childhood and adolescence. *Journal of Child Psychology and Psychiatry* **39**: 1071–81.

Cookson, J. 1997: Lithium: balancing risks and benefits. *British Journal of Psychiatry* **171**: 120–5.

Dorevitch, A., Meretyk, I., Umansky, Y. and Galili-Weisstub, E. 1995: Antipsychotic drugs and tardive dyskinesia: preliminary results in an adolescent psychiatric ward. *Journal of Clinical Pharmacy and Therapeutics* **20**: 63–5.

Eisenberg, L. 1996: Commentary: what should doctors do in the face of negative evidence? *Journal of Nervous and Mental Disease* **184**: 103–5.

Emslie, G.J., Rush, J., Weinberg, W.A. *et al.* 1997: A double-blind, randomized, placebo-controlled trial of fluoxetine in children and adolescents with depression. *Archives of General Psychiatry* **54**: 1031–7.

Fava, M. 1996: Traditional and alternative research designs and methods in clinical pediatric psychopharmacology. *Journal of the American Academy of Child and Adolescent Psychiatry* **34**: 1292–303.

Fink, M. 1995: Electroconvulsive therapy (letter). *Lancet* **345**: 519.

Fisher, R.L. and Fisher, S. 1996: Antidepressants for children: is scientific support necessary? *Journal of Nervous and Mental Disease* **184**: 99–102.

Freeman, C.P. 1995: ECT in those under 18 years old. In Freeman, C.P. (ed.), *The ECT Handbook*. London: Royal College of Psychiatrists, 18–21.

Freeman, M.P. and Stoll, A.L. 1998: Mood stabilizer combinations: a review of safety and efficacy. *American Journal of Psychiatry* **155**: 12–21.

Gadow, K.D. 1992: Pediatric psychopharmacology; a review of recent research. *Journal of Child Psychology and Psychiatry* **33**: 153–95.

Geller, B. and Luby, J. 1997: Child and adolescent bipolar disorder: a review of the past 10 years. *Journal of the American Academy of Child and Adolescent Psychiatry* **36**: 1168–76.

Green, W.H. 1995: *Child and Adolescent Clinical Psychopharmacology*. Baltimore: Williams & Wilkins.

Harrington, R., Whittaker, J., Shoebridge P. and Campbell, F. 1998: Systematic review of efficacy of cognitive behaviour therapies in childhood and adolescent depressive disorder. *British Medical Journal* **316**: 1559–63.

Hazell, P., O'Connell, D., Heathcote, D., Robertson, J. and Henry D. 1995: Efficacy of tricyclic antidepressants in treating child and adolescent depression: a meta-analysis. *British Medical Journal* **310**: 897–901.

Jaffa, T. 1995: Adolescent psychiatry services. *British Journal of Psychiatry* **166**: 306–10.

James, A.C. 1996: A survey of the prescribing practices of child and adolescent psychiatrists. *Child Psychology and Psychiatry Review* **1**: 94–7.

Kane, J.M. 1994: The use of higher-dose antipsychotic medication. *British Journal of Psychiatry* **164**: 431–2.

Kaplan, C.A. and Hussain, S. 1995: Use of drugs in child and adolescent psychiatry. *British Journal of Psychiatry* **166**: 291–8.

Kellett, J. M. 1995: Electroconvulsive therapy (letter). *Lancet* **345**: 518.

Knapp, M. 1997: Costs of schizophrenia. *British Journal of Psychiatry* **171**: 509–18.

Kumra, S., Frazier, J.A., Jacobsen, L.K. *et al.* 1996: Childhood-onset schizophrenia: a double-blind clozapine–haloperidol comparison. *Archives of General Psychiatry* **53**: 1090–7.

Kutcher, S. 1997: *Child and Adolescent Psychopharmacology*. Philadelphia: W.B. Saunders.

Lowe, K., Smith, H. and Clark, A. 1996: Neuroleptic prescribing in an adolescent psychiatric inpatient unit. *Psychiatric Bulletin* **20**: 538–40.

McClellan, J. and Werry, J. 1994: Practice parameters for the assessment and treatment of children and adolescents with schizophrenia. *Journal of the American Academy of Child and Adolescent Psychiatry* **33**: 616–35.

Mental Health Act Commission 1997: *Guidance on the Treatment of Anorexia Nervosa under the Mental Health Act 1983*. Guidance note 3. Nottingham: MHAC.

Moncrieff, J. 1997: Lithium: evidence reconsidered. *British Journal of Psychiatry* **171**: 113–19.

Morrison, D.N., McGee, R. and Stanton, W.R. 1992: Sleep problems in adolescence. *Journal of the American Academy of Child and Adolescent Psychiatry* **31**: 94–9.

Nicholls, J.E., Fernandez, C.A. and Clark, A.F. 1996: Use of mental health legislation in a regional adolescent unit. *Psychiatric Bulletin* **20**: 711–13.

Noone, B.K. and Van der Linden, G.J.H. 1997: Attention deficit hyperactivity disorder or hyperkinetic syndrome in adults. *British Journal of Psychiatry* **170**: 489–91.

Nutt, D. and Bell, C. 1997: Practical pharmacotherapy for anxiety. *Advances in Psychiatric Treatment* 79–85.

Oxlad, M. and Baldwin, S. 1995: Electroconvulsive therapy, children and adolescents: the power to stop. *Nursing Ethics* **2**: 333–46.

Parmar, R. 1993: Attitudes of child psychiatrists to electroconvulsive therapy. *Psychiatric Bulletin* **17**: 12–13.

Pearce, J. 1994: Consent to treatment during childhood. *British Journal of Psychiatry* **165**: 713–16.

Pellegrino, E.D. 1996: Commentary: clinical judgement, scientific data and ethics: antidepressant therapy in adolescents and children. *Journal of Nervous and Mental Disease* **184**: 106–8.

Pool, D., Bloom, W., Miekle, D.H., Roniger, J.J. and Gallant, D.M. 1976: A controlled evaluation of loxitane in seventy five adolescent schizophrenic patients. *Current Therapeutic Research* **19**: 99–104.

Post, R.M., Denicoff, K.D., Frye M.A. and Leverich G.S. 1997: Re-evaluating carbamazepine prophylaxis in bipolar disorder. *British Journal of Psychiatry* **170**: 202–4.

Realmuto, G.M., Erickson, W.D., Yellin, A.M., Hopwood, J.H. and Greenberg , L.M. 1984: Clinical comparison of thiothixene and thioridazine in schizophrenic adolescents. *American Journal of Psychiatry* **141**: 440–2.

Remschmidt, H. 1993: Schizophrenic psychoses in children and adolescents. *Triangle* **32**: 15–24.

Remschmidt, H. and Schulz, E. 1995: Psychopharmacology of depressive states in childhood and adolescence. In Goodyer, I.M. (ed.), *The Depressed Child and Adolescent: Developmental and Clinical Perspectives*. Cambridge: Cambridge University Press, 253–79.

Remschmidt, H., Schulz, E. and Martin, P. 1994: An open trial of clozapine in thirty six adolescents with schizophrenia. *Journal of Child and Adolescent Psychopharmacology* **4**: 31–41.

Rey, J.M. and Walter, G. 1997: Half a century of ECT use in young people. *American Journal of Psychiatry* **154**: 595–602.

Richardson, M.A., Haughland, G. and Craig, T.J. 1991: Neuroleptic use, parkinsonian symptoms, tardive dyskinesia and associated factors in child and adolescent psychiatric patients. *American Journal of Psychiatry* **148**: 1322–8.

Riddle, M.A., Scahil, L., King, R.A. *et al.* 1992: Double-blind, crossover trial of fluoxetine and placebo in children and adolescents with obsessive–compulsive disorder. *Journal of the Amcrican Academy of Child and Adolescent Psychiatry* **31**: 1062–9.

Sachdev, P. 1995: The epidemiology of drug-induced akathisia: II. Chronic tardive and withdrawal akathisias. *Schizophrenia Bulletin* **21**: 451–61.

Sandberg, S. 1996: Hyperkinetic or attention deficit disorder. *British Journal of Psychiatry* **169**: 10–17.

Spencer, E.K. and Campbell, M. 1994: Children with schizophrenia: diagnosis, phenomenology, and pharmacotherapy. *Schizophrenia Bulletin* **20**: 713–25.

Stores, G. 1996: Practitioner review: assessment and treatment of sleep disorders in children. *Journal of Child Psychology and Psychiatry* **37**: 907–25.

Thomas, C.S. and Lewis, S. 1998: Which atypical antipsychotic? *British Journal of Psychiatry* **172**: 106–9.

Thompson, C. 1994: The use of high-dose antipsychotic medication. *British Journal of Psychiatry* **164**: 448–58.

Walter, G. and Rey, J.M. 1997: An epidemiological study of the use of ECT in adolescents. *Journal of the American Academy of Child and Adolescent Psychiatry* **36**: 809–15.

Will, D., Wrate, R.M., Bhate, S. *et al.* 1994: High-dose antipsychotic medication. *British Journal of Psychiatry* **165**: 269–70.

PART 6

Delivery of services

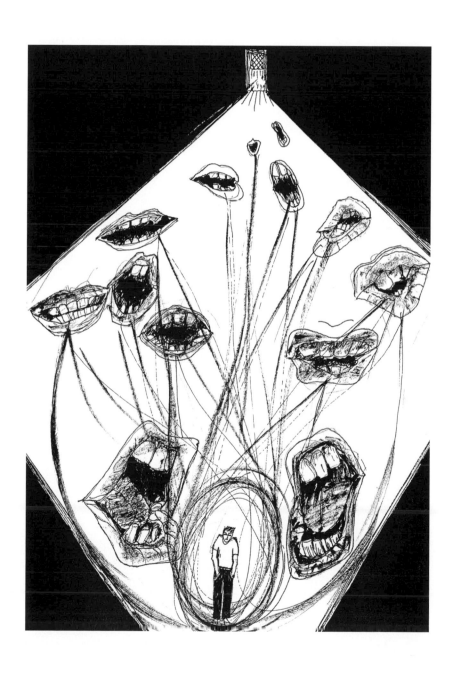

23

A strategic approach to commissioning and delivering forensic child and adolescent mental health services

RICHARD WILLIAMS

THE PLACE OF CHILDREN IN UK SOCIETY

Arguably, one of the most important features of the last century of the second millennium was the increasing importance of the welfare of children and adolescents in society. Now, in the twenty-first century, education, social care and healthcare for young people remain central political and societal issues in the UK about which most of us have opinions. Yet, this is an arena of paradox.

Definite improvements in the standing of minors, reflected in their improved survival, quality of life and opportunities, have been accompanied by increasing awareness of the continuing presence of powerful hazards to their development faced by young people, including those arising from family breakdown, their involvement in criminal and other antisocial activity, and the impact on them of a variety of forms of social deprivation, poverty, abuse and misuse. Exponential developments in our understanding of genetic influences on our development are paralleled by society's rising awareness of the importance of getting right the context in which children are brought up, educated and supported if they are to become effective and fulfilled adults (Longley *et al.* 2001).

But, all the while, progress brings in its wake new hazards to which we expose our children. For example, we are very concerned about the impact of the communications revolution on young people's development through radiation from mobile phones and other constructed risks. Also, many young people fail to benefit from recent advances. In some families, they look to becoming a third generation without work, and too many young people experience alienation or exclusion from the positive and creative aspects of society.

THE REQUIREMENT FOR FORENSIC MENTAL HEALTH SERVICES FOR YOUNG PEOPLE

This chapter covers three main themes that influence why forensic mental health services for young people should be developed in the UK. They are:

- the relationship between the law and children's mental health
- professional development and the growing potential capabilities of child and adolescent mental health services (CAMHS)
- developments in thinking about strategy for CAMHS.

The relationship between the law and children's mental health

The involvement of parliament in the affairs of young people, through legislation and the output of the select committees, and an increasing flow of government inspired or owned regulatory, guiding and advisory documents, supports a conclusion that there was increasing concern with the experiences, care and management of young people in the late twentieth century. The Children Act 1989 was revolutionary in reforming public and private law by bringing into a single statute much of the law relating to children and young people. More recently, there has been a review of the legislative framework relating to the involvement of young people in criminal and other antisocial activities, resulting in the Crime and Disorder Act 1998, reform of the adoption laws leading to the Adoption and Children Act 2002, and a review of mental health law. Thus, the last 20 years of the twentieth century and the beginning of the present century saw, in the UK at least, reviews of just about all aspects of the law relating to children and young people.

Alongside this, there has been a rising tide of public concern about misuse of children as well as growing concerns about risk and danger to young people within society and the crescendo of their involvement in criminal and antisocial behaviour in much the same time period (Audit Commission 1996). This raises many questions as to whether we are looking at both true increases in antisocial and criminal activity, misuse of, and disorder in young people as well as a greatly enhanced recognition of their problems. It also begs further questions, also addressed here, as to the complex interrelationships between the factors that lie behind these phenomena. Whatever the conclusions, there cannot be any doubt as to the continuing but rising importance and, in the opinions of some (e.g. Butler-Sloss 1998), of the increasingly crucial role that mental health professionals have to play in the welfare of children.

Looking back, there has also been increased involvement of mental health professionals employed by the statutory services at their interfaces with the law and about the welfare of children. In many cases, the history of CAMHS shows that the some services were developed at least partially at the instigation of the Courts which recognized their own needs for professional opinion in coming to effective judgements and the proper application of the law in respect of children and young people. Thus, forensic practice has been and remains a core element of all child and adolescent mental healthcare and it forms a recognized part of psychiatrists' training. Similarly, the role of child psychologists in this work is increasing. This is also recognized by the increasing number of texts for professionals in this field that offer guidance and expositions of the law as it relates to professional practice (e.g. Black *et al.* 1998; Williams *et al.* 2004).

Black *et al.* (1998) ascribe the substantial rise in medico-legal work in the last 30 years to two key factors. The first is the strong research tradition that has grown up in child and adolescent mental healthcare. The consequent and growing evidence-base enables child and adolescent mental health specialists to offer expert evidence as to the probabilities of outcome for many circumstances affecting children and adolescents. Their second major factor is society's evolving views of the rights of children that are now better protected by the Children Act 1989 and the Human Rights Act 1998.

Professional development and the growing potential capabilities of CAMHS

DEVELOPMENTAL CONCEPTS

But, another factor is also important in the growth of importance of forensic practice. This is the increasing recognition not only by children's professionals but also by professionals outside frequent practice with young people and in wider society of the importance of developmental concepts. There is increasing recognition of just how influential childhood experiences are on the lives of people not only as they grow up but also when they have grown up, increasing recognition of the linkages between childhood mental disorder and that in adulthood, and increasing recognition of the negative impacts on children's emotional lives and their development of living with a parent who has a sustained mental disorder. Examples of relevant recent literature include Council Reports from the Royal College of Psychiatrists (CR104, 2002 and CR105, 2002) Recent health economic evidence brings home these points (Knapp and Henderson 1999; Knapp *et al.* 1999; M.K. Knapp, personal communication 2000).

RISK FACTORS

Considerable knowledge has been gained of the range of risk factors and of how they operate during childhood on the present and future mental health of individuals affected (Rutter and Smith 1995; Wallace *et al.* 1997; Kurtz 1996; MHF 1999; ONS 1999). An area of recent and rapidly growing interest in this field is the study of resilience; that is, study of the factors that appear to protect individuals from developing disorder, and how to improve resilience rather than reducing risk factors (Rolf *et al.* 1990).

It is evident that the field described by interfaces between the law, legal practice, the rights and needs of young people and the work of mental health professionals relating to children and adolescents developed particularly rapidly in the second half of the twentieth century. But it is also clear that much more remains to be learned. As in many fields of health and social care practice, expanding knowledge and potential professional capability for intervention in children's mental ill-health have been accompanied by a lesser increase in resources and targeting of that resource within services. Generally, there is now an evident gap between potential expertise and the potential ability to deploy services offering that expertise in diagnosis, wider assessment and intervention with children and young people who have mental health problems and disorders. Consequently, many healthcare practitioners in the field now feel overwhelmed by the challenges.

Strategy

STRATEGY FOR DEVELOPING CAMHS

In 1995, the NHS Health Advisory Service (HAS) recognized this situation and made groundbreaking recommendations about how CAMHS in the UK should be developed (Williams and Richardson 1995). In 1999, the Audit Commission published its findings and recommendations as a follow-up to the HAS review. In 2001, the governments in England and Wales announced separately, at least in part in response to the Bristol Inquiry, that each will develop a National Service Framework (NSF) for childrens' healthcare that will include mental health and psychological wellbeing. As this book goes to press, both countries are making rapid progress with their children's NSFs.

More specifically, demands continue to rise rapidly for CAMHS to play a much greater role in advising the courts and in supporting the work of the Youth Justice Board. Thus, there is a particular rising demand for special expertise in the area of forensic mental health practice with certain children and young people who have more severe problems. But, increasingly, it is becoming difficult for all practitioners to have the necessary knowledge-base at their fingertips, and, so, it is likely that the tests set for the appointment of experts by the Courts and legal advisers will become more demanding.

So far, most child and adolescent mental health practitioners have sought to continue to be generalists within their specialism, combining elements of forensic practice alongside their work in the many other arenas. Some have been keener than others to take on forensic work. But demands are also rising significantly for a focus of special expertise in the arenas of forensic practice and research. This appears to be particularly so for expertise in interventions with very troubled young people and for the application of assessment and therapeutic techniques to the most difficult and disruptive of young people in circumstances of increased security. This raises key questions for policy-makers, service designers, commissioners, provider managers and practitioners. Should the professions enable and empower some of their members to develop special expertise in forensic mental health practice for children and young people, as has occurred in adult psychiatric practice? If so, what will be the future roles of the general child and adolescent mental health professionals in this regard and how will the interface between generalists and forensic specialists operate and be managed?

STRATEGY FOR FORENSIC CAMHS

This chapter explores these questions and some of the implications of the developments in potential professional capability on the design, delivery and management of mental health services for children and young people. It recommends that, rather than leaving the development of services to *ad hoc* processes, it would be better to develop coherent, deliberate and acknowledged strategic frameworks that will enable the development of services and new resources to be applied in rational, managed and verifiable ways in which the interrelationships between key service components can be progressed to avoid perverse incentives and to deliver better managed, cross-agency care.

The time is ripe for ideas on how this could be achieved. For example, in 2001, the National Assembly for Wales published its strategy for CAMHS, *Everybody's Business* (NAW 2001). That document includes a proposal to develop a network of forensic CAMHS and better services for children whose behaviour poses substantial challenges, as a part of a comprehensive, cross-sector approach to children's mental health.

The urgency for clarity of thinking in this field is exemplified not only by the rise of demand but also by recent legislation. In the UK, the implications at local and national levels of the Crime and Disorder Act 1998 and the subsequent policies of the Youth Justice Board created by that Act are that Youth Offending Teams (YOTs) should have improved access to health, education and social care resources for their clientele. Inevitably, these include specialist services for young people who use and misuse substances, and forensic mental health services as well as more generic CAMHS. But it is also evident that the concept of good access to mental health services for the relatively recently created YOTs is aspirational. This must be the case as, currently throughout much of the UK, access to Specialist CAMHS as a whole is limited and is offered on an *ad hoc* basis arising from service development around interested and charismatic figures, as the Audit Commission (1999) report appears to confirm.

Reality suggests that, currently, much of what is now demanded consequent on the Crime and Disorder Act 1998 cannot yet be delivered despite the earnest endeavours of local and health authorities to inject some new resources and of the providers to contribute. Indeed, experience in Wales from 1999 suggests that, while the health authorities made additional investments in the health services' contributions to the YOTs, this is not necessarily guided by clarity about the needs of the potential client group or the skills, training requirements and availability of the proposed new employees. Anecdotal information received by the author suggests that, in several areas at least, the baseline information on the health problems of young people who became clients of the YOTs early after their creation was poor and that initial estimates of need based on previous information did not fit with the demands that were actually being made on the YOTs' staff in respect of mental ill-health and substance misuse. Furthermore, different responses by different authorities in different areas appear to suggest a disparity of response to the new requirements and the possibility of increasing rather than reducing inequity. Therefore, the challenges for the future are:

- to develop effective services in predictable ways that meet actual need and which are informed by the views and preferences of young people and their families
- for forensic mental health services to be built upon established concepts of service design according to a strategic framework
- for the workforce requirements to be actively apprehended and met by longer-term planning and training.

RESTRUCTURING OR REDESIGN: DYNAMICS IN SERVICE COMMISSIONING AND DELIVERY

So far, this analysis leads to the conclusion that, presently, forensic CAMHS in the UK are in an embryonic state. More is delivered than is recognized by the Courts, by the responsible authorities and, indeed, by the practitioners themselves. But, this does not amount to provision of rational or comprehensive services. Nonetheless, professional interest and growing capability are such that rapid developments could be possible. This book brings together current knowledge and provides a solid platform. But, before setting out to develop services, it is important to take stock, recognize certain dynamics in service delivery and consider the direction in which we would like services to go. Already, this chapter has identified the availability of suitably trained and experienced staff supported by appropriate resources as the rate-limiting condition. The other dynamics selected for examination here are:

- need, supply and demand
- inter-agency boundaries
- the powers provided by legislation
- evidence-based practice
- the career routes of young people with problems.

Need, supply and demand

Currently, specialist CAMHS are often reported as overloaded by demand and this is not an uncomplicated situation. There is an untapped well of need for many health, special education and social welfare services. In general terms, experience suggests that when practitioners recognize the value, whether expressed anecdotally or in the form of harder evidence, of the provision of an aspect or element of service and begin to respond, demand rises leading once again to overload, experience of poor accessibility and recognition of the scarcity of the provision.

Not surprisingly, a first response to this situation is to demand greater service capacity; in effect, to seek more of the same. In other words, beginnings of new service provision, often made by enthusiastic people with a particular interest, provoke wider recognition of the value of the identified service element. This provokes increasing interest, greater demand, and recognition of scarcity and calls for increased investment. Arguably, much of the National Health Service has developed in this way around the emerging capability and expertise of enthusiastic and dedicated individuals, and forensic CAMHS provide a particular example of this dynamic. In forensic mental health, as in all healthcare fields, need, supply, demand and developing professional capability link inextricably.

Inter-agency boundaries

In similar terms, anecdotal experience of services leads to recognition of another source of pressure on service development in which professionals engaged in delivering services come to the opinion that there is deficiency of provision for patients or clients with particular problems and for which no agency has a solution.

Sometimes, limitations of current services lead their staff, reasonably, to define their legitimate core client groups, capabilities and capacities. Depending on the positions adopted by adjoining services or specialisms, gaps and overlaps may arise. As hypothetical examples, people with possible attention-deficit hyperactivity disorder (ADHD) may be considered legitimate parts of the client group by many paediatric and all specialist CAMHS in the same area, while neither might consider enuresis or behaviour problems as core. The former situation leads to challenges in ensuring complementary service quality while the second might lead to a gap in provision.

Put another way, the dynamic described here is that of gaps in service provision arising from all current services in an area coming to the view that they are unable to respond to the needs of a portion of the client group. At much the same time, there are temptations for these agencies to define, unilaterally, certain of these client problems into the zone of responsibility of the other services and not their own. Frequently, such scenarios are advanced by problems in inter-agency communication and planning. They become particularly contentious when one agency wishes to define the role of a partner in ways that do not fit the partner's internal determinations.

The demand for forensic mental health services for young people is a very good example of this situation. There is a common experience of the absence of specialized services in most parts of the country with a particular emphasis on the absence of services that are able to contain and then offer specific interventions to the most provocative and/or worrying of young people who are particularly difficult to engage. Often, in these circumstances, there may be a perception of a requirement for services that can offer a greater degree of security or a broader range of skills than those that are currently available in a particular area. In colloquial terms, this has led to the common conception of extremely difficult, disruptive and hard-to-place young people and searches for illusory out-of area and/or emergency placements. Locally, failure of fit between the external expectations of services and their internal opinions as to their zone of responsibility and abilities leads to case- and cost-shifting and inter-agency tension.

Rising above this to provide truly integrated child-centred services requires much cross-agency and personal maturity, sound communications and strong will. In recent years, the Dartington Social Research Unit has researched the barriers to effective inter-agency collaboration. Two recent papers (Salmon and Williams 2001; Williams and Salmon 2002) provide a contemporary summary that takes into account cooperation theory and examples of effective practice to produce a three-dimensional model for improving collaboration.

The powers provided by legislation

Within the field of forensic mental health services for young people, pressure on practitioners arises from application of the available legislation. Often, professionals talk of the gaps in the current legislation between the powers offered by the Children Act 1989 and those offered by the Mental Health Act 1983. There is a common conception in many parts of England and Wales and across a number of professions that the limitations of the Children Act 1989 and the particular strictures offered to securing young people are such that, when set beside the common (but arguably erroneous) conception that the Mental Health Act 1983 can be applied only in the circumstances of the most serious mental illness, there are gaps in the legislative framework. Whether or not there are gaps that really are insurmountable in present legislation, the perception is sufficiently powerful and widespread as to leave a number of particularly demanding young people, and the professions who care for them, in a state of uncertainty that gives rise to or results from attempts at case-shifting.

Evidence-based practice

A further contemporary dynamic concerns the application of evidence-based practice. While the phrase is new, the application of evidence to practice is not. Nonetheless, clinical governance is driving hard better use of evidence in clinical situations. Few practitioners now question the importance of applying the health economic concepts of effectiveness, cost-effectiveness, efficiency and cost–benefit analysis, among others, to mental health services, but there is a risk arising from basing both commissioning and service delivery on an over-rigorous or ill-informed application of the current evidence-base.

The essence of evidence-based practice is that of supporting investment in services that have neutral or better impact at the expense of services where the impact is at best doubtful or perhaps, even, negative. Taken to an extreme, there is a risk of this approach being applied to supporting interventions by services of known positive effectiveness over investments in services for which there is insufficient evidence. One result of too rigorous an application of this style of understanding of evidence-based practice could be that new or unproven treatments do not receive opportunities to be studied in depth, or they fail to attract support solely through lack of an evidence base. There is also a contemporary question as to what kinds of evidence will be admitted – should it be limited to that derived from carefully controlled quantitative research, or should opinion derived from qualitative research and from ethics and the humanities be admitted together (Graham 1999, 2000; Williams 2000)?

On this basis some very prevalent conditions, such as conduct disorder, about which the evidence base for the effectiveness of health service-based interventions has not been good, may also be regarded by some as not being at the core of NHS commitment. The risk of an appreciation of this kind would be to reduce over-greatly the priority attached to a group of disorders that are of high prevalence and where more research is required into developing effective management techniques and interventions. Thus, forensic mental health services have much to gain from evidence-based practice, though there are dangers in it for this emerging specialism from dismissing positive risks (Williams 1999). Similarly, awareness of the issues raised by evidence-based practice (EBP) (Graham 1999, 2000; Fish and Coles 1997) has led to development of the concept of values-based practice (VBP) to be applied alongside and in conjunction with EBP and reflective practice (Fulford and Williams 2003).

Career routes

In Chapter 24, Little and Bullock identify another challenging issue, that of accurately gathering information about the potential client group and, therefore, planning services which relate to the 'myriad of services' that has evolved 'to meet the needs of troubled adolescents' resulting in 'young people's problems being dealt with in any one or a combination of welfare and control systems'.

Little and Bullock point to five prominent 'career routes' taken by children in trouble that depend on 'life-route' decisions made by their families and 'process' decisions made by the agencies with which they come into contact. These process decisions may be affected by each of the dynamics identified in this section, but, significantly, their work reminds us all that commissioners and providers alike must also recognize the life-route decisions made by young people and their families.

Restructuring or redesign?

In summary, all of the dynamics identified here could have positive, but also restricting influences on the pace and direction of service development in forensic mental healthcare for children and adolescents through pressures to:

- solely provide more of the same
- fill the perceived gaps in the current pattern of services by simple uplift in volume
- respond uncritically to perceptions of gaps in the legislative framework
- apply rigorously a narrow view of the evidence base.

Approaches to planning services for the future on the basis of analysis of current service delivery problems may be styled 'restructuring', in which the new pattern of any new or developed services is built on adaptations to the present pattern. While each of the pressures identified here is legitimate and real, and we must recognise that responding to them could have service-enhancing impacts on the care offered to young people, there are also risks that they could be used as arguments for repackaging current services, applying any new resource in reactive ways or inadvertently perpetuating problems through failure to tackle deeper problems.

Alternatively, it is possible to take a rather more radical approach, here styled 'redesign', in which identification of the realistic functions required of particular services becomes the basis of investment for the future. Plainly, determining the functions required must take into account the processes and pressures identified here. It also requires analysis of the identified needs and views of an identified client group, and of the clinical realities. These matters should be considered with regard to:

- the scope of existing services
- the nature of current demands
- analysis of the gaps in the capacity of the existing services considered against the potential capability of the professionals engaged in those services and application of the evidence base
- awareness of the current growth points in professional practice, service development and research.

Some of the tensions, pressures and influences that should be taken into account in planning services are indicated by the two diagrams in Figure 23.1.

Bringing together these various contributions and sources of evidence about, what we call, 'equity gaps' is a demanding task. It requires input from a variety of different professional arenas and the coordinated activities of policymakers, service commissioners, practitioners, researchers and the managers of service delivery. Ideally, and particularly so in the case of forensic mental health services, this process requires active engagement of all the partner agencies (or stakeholders) that have an interest in the services that emerge.

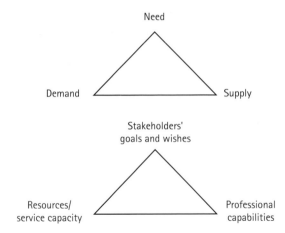

Figure 23.1 *Triangles of tension. (a) Tension between need, supply and demand. (b) Tension between the potential capability, the actual capacity of, and the aspirations of stakeholders for services.*

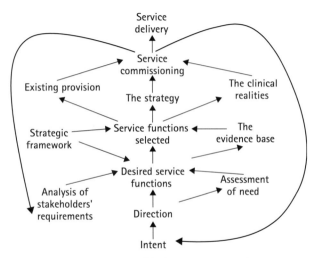

Figure 23.2 *The process of design as an approach to commissioning public sector services.*

Viewed in this way, the process of redesign underpins high-quality commissioning that is led by policy, driven through strategy, supported by applied research and informed by the stakeholders. The whole is likely to be more effective if the various contributions are brought and held together by application of a strategic framework for the disposition of services. This approach to strategy development and commissioning is illustrated by Figure 23.2, and the strategic framework recommended by the author is described later in this chapter.

This approach fits with the analysis presented by Little and Bullock, who call for:

- more research into young people and current impacts, risk factors, and effectiveness of interventions (individual needs assessment)
- greater thinking about and cross-boundary sharing of the concepts of need, understanding of mechanisms

and meanings of disorder, thresholds in decision-making, service patterns, outcome, perverse incentives, etc.

- corporate needs assessments based on these shared understandings
- a more rational cross-sectoral basis for decision-making
- provision according to predictions of need.

The concept of redesign also fits with recent re-examinations of the contribution of values to healthcare policymaking, strategy and delivery through their impact on priority setting and clinical decision-making. Thus, as we have noted, we now have values-based practice sitting alongside evidence-based practice and reflective practice as supports for improved decision-making (Fulford and Williams 2003).

Having established the case for design, this chapter examines next a number of inputs to the process of (re)designing forensic CAMHS.

THE NATURE OF CURRENT FORENSIC MENTAL HEALTH PRACTICE WITH YOUNG PEOPLE

The functions

One way of identifying the potential roles of forensic CAMHS is to start by considering the tasks that those relatively few experts in this field are being asked to take on now. While much of the evidence here is anecdotal, a qualitative survey conducted by the author suggests a list of tasks requested of professionals with a particular interest in forensic mental issues relating to young people. It is wide and includes:

- Providing assessments, diagnosis, advice on the management of and, in some cases, direct involvement in the care and treatment of young people who are:
  - involved in private law actions (as in the divorce of their parents, for example)
  - the subjects of public law applications
  - looked after by a local authority
  - patients of other healthcare specialists, particularly those patients who cause disruption to delivery of their own healthcare or that of other patients in paediatric and psychiatric settings
  - the subject of proceedings in the youth justice courts
  - the subject of criminal law proceedings relating to the most serious of disorders (including murder, manslaughter and arson)
  - offenders and/or those who are sentenced to reside in penal institutions.
- Providing assessments, diagnosis and treatment and other interventions for young people who are difficult to engage by virtue of the disruption they cause or the conditions they appear to require in order to contain

them or to make a care/intervention plan effective. This group of young people includes:
- certain young people with severe psychiatric disorders
- some young people who are mentally disordered offenders
- some severely suicidal and self-harming young people
- some young people, particularly adolescents, who exhaust staff, treatment regimens and the caring facilities provided by a range of other statutory and non-statutory agencies
- young people with mental disorders who are at substantial risk of absconding unless they are managed in a particular setting.
- Providing assessment, diagnosis and treatment, and other interventions, for young people who are the victims or perpetrators of certain particular forms of misuse and abuse.
- Providing certain services for some brain-injured adolescents.
- Providing diagnostic and therapeutic services for young people with severe organic psychiatric disorders.

Delivering forensic mental health services

Wide diversity is one of the striking features of the work requested of practitioners with a particular interest in forensic mental health issues in childhood and adolescence. Whether all of these tasks are legitimately those of the forensic mental health services is a matter for national, regional and local decision-making. Whatever the position taken, the breadth of current demand should be fully realized when designing forensic CAMHS.

It is tempting to extrapolate from the work undertaken by the forensic mental health services for adults to define the working responsibilities of forensic CAMHS. Doing so would certainly define a portion of the work required and a segment of the client group appropriate to these services. However, such an approach might also risk defining the tasks facing these specialist services too narrowly. Exploration of this issue points to one of the most important questions in planning the way forward which is that, so far, adequate definitions of the scope of responsibilities of these services (or their functions) have yet to be agreed across all agencies. This is at once both a challenge and an opportunity.

Part of the reason for the rather broad focus and long lists of tasks facing forensic mental health services for young people lies in the dependency of young people, the responsibilities of adults for their welfare and the theme of development that underpins the whole area.

The field does involve working with young offenders who may or may not be mentally disordered, and commissioners should be aware that the peak rates of offending occur in young people.

Much more frequently, the Courts and other legal services require psychiatric assistance with understanding children and their needs, mental states and behaviour. These understandings are required by the Welfare Checklists in civil circumstances covered by the public and private law in the Children Act 1989 and the Adoption and Children Act 2002 with a view to planning the most appropriate ways in which adults should discharge their responsibilities for them. These requests add substantial and important dimensions to the work of specialist practitioners and to the scope required of forensic CAMHS.

Additionally, some young people with particular problems that have defied intervention in more ordinary settings are referred to specialist forensic mental health services because of the expertise that referrers wish to enlist and because of the extent of the defiant and disruptive behaviours manifest by the young people. These referrals reflect behaviours that have rendered young people unmanageable in less specialized and/or secure settings, but also the dearth of services elsewhere in our health, social welfare, education, youth justice and penal services.

By their very nature, children and young people who manifest this range of problems are the source of concern to a wide variety of agencies in the UK. Troublesome behaviour can be the final common pathway of many differing processes and not all of these are related to disorders of health. The sectors of care into which young people with difficult, demanding and deviant behaviours, whether or not the result or cause of mental disorder, may find their way include:

- the local authorities through their:
  - social services departments
  - education departments
  - housing departments
- Youth Offending Teams
- the NHS
- the voluntary/non-statutory sector
- the police
- probation services
- youth and adult criminal justice services
- youth and adult penal services.

In reality, each of theses sectors of care has a contribution to make, of varying proportions, to the care and management of young people who present with particularly demanding problems, including persistent disruptions in their behaviour. On this basis alone, there should be excellent collaboration, good exchange of information and skills as well as well-organized coordination of responsibilities between all these agencies and sectors for the young people concerned.

A number of surveys have shown the high rates of referral between the agencies listed here, but have also demonstrated the very considerable problems that arise in collaboration between them. It is evident that, while the incidence and prevalence of symptoms of mental disorders may be particularly high in young people who: are persistent offenders; those who have been convicted of crime; those who are at risk of delinquency; and those who are looked after by local authorities; these are also the cases in which the sectors of care appear to experience particular difficulties in collaboration. Surveys in the UK have shown endeavours at collaboration across agency and sector boundaries but also how resources are lost in case-shifting between the agencies and, therefore, attempts to shift both responsibilities and costs between them.

In Chapter 24, Little and Bullock point out that offenders are marginal in most services but, when they are accompanied by notoriety or high perceived risk, their cases may lead to political and public sensitivity and to the responsible authorities being prepared to spend large sums on, often *ad hoc*, arrangements based on, sometimes, contradictory influences on decision-making. In these circumstances, there is an acquired risk that the solutions may also contribute to creating further problems.

The circumstances are particularly diverse, as reference to other chapters in this text shows, for young people within the community. Similarly, there are substantial challenges to the agencies with regard to providing services for young people who are considered to require care in greater security. Here, the major providers of the largest volume of secure residential services are:

- the secure units (previously the responsibility of the local authorities, many are now in the secure estate purchased by or the direct responsibility of the Youth Justice Board)
- the penal service through its young-offender institutions.

By comparison, the NHS funds and/or provides a relatively small volume of medium-secure inpatient beds.

Summary

The spread of the forensic mental health-related tasks listed in this section indicates that the following broad modalities of service are required:

- diagnostic and advisory services:
  - ambulatory, community and outpatient assessments
  - consultation within and between agencies in care planning
  - preparation and presentation of opinions, including report preparation
  - attendance at Courts to give professional evidence or expert opinion
  - advising other professionals in the course of their work
- therapeutic services:
  - ambulatory, community and outpatient therapeutic interventions

– residential and/or inpatient assessments, care, treatment and other interventions
• teaching, training, advising, supervising, consulting with and supporting other professionals
• research.

MOVING ON: COLLABORATIVE COMMISSIONING

The proposition of this chapter is that the way forward should be through developing comprehensive forensic CAMHS based on the processes of collaborative strategic planning and leadership and commissioning conducted by the statutory agencies acting together on the basis of an agreed strategic framework. The factors that appear to substantiate this proposition include:

• the considerable diversity of the potential client group (a matter to which this chapter will return)
• the impossibility, on present evidence, and, arguably, the inappropriateness of cleanly and appropriately separating a client group for each of the agencies alone, including the NHS.

The latter is based on:

• the broad spectrum of problems faced and presented by the most troubled and troublesome young people
• the most troubled young people having problems that fall into the arena of concern of more than one agency or sector of provision
• experience of the young people involved having problems that require the expertise of a range of agencies
• the high frequency of psychiatric symptoms in young people whose primary reason for residing in certain forms of statutorily provided provision, including secure facilities, may not necessarily lie in their having a primary diagnosable disorder for which treatment is the overriding priority
• the consequent need to offer services at a variety of levels of specialism and complexity
• the low volume of resources presently directed towards NHS-funded forensic mental health services at all levels of specialism.

In summary, it is evident that one of the key factors in developing forensic CAMHS is for all the relevant local agencies to agree between them their joint intent for the service and the contribution each will make to the provision of a comprehensive range of services sufficient to meet the wide range of needs of young people, their families, the agencies, and the youth justice, legal and court services.

Within that broad approach, inter-agency agreement is required to define the range of tasks to be laid before the local Specialist CAMHS and which should be taken on by

new Specialist Forensic CAMHS. This provokes an important question: What should be the proper role or intent for the more specialized forensic CAMHS within the wider spectrum of forensic services provided by the relevant agencies? Inevitably, this will be different in different geographical areas as it is influenced by the strategic and financial positions of the major sectors of care and their existing investments in elements of the wide spectrum of resources that might be summarized as impacting on child and adolescent mental health. This should also lead to deciding what specialist forensic mental health services may need to be procured from particular centres of expertise, very possibly at a distance.

Defining the client group

Already, reference has been made to the diversity of the potential client group for existing very specialized forensic CAMHS. Despite the evidence presented elsewhere in this book, it is difficult to speak with authority about the client group for forensic CAMHS because of:

• the limited research undertaken to date
• lack of a language to describe the young people's problems that adequately crosses the sectors of care and intervention
• lack of consistent agreement about the definition of the roles and functions of Specialist Forensic CAMHS and the other contributing agencies
• the restricted volume of Specialist Forensic CAMHS available at present.

In Chapter 2, Kroll has distinguishes between population and individual needs assessments. He describes epidemiological, comparative and corporate approaches to the former. In recent years, there have been a number of surveys in England and Scotland, mainly of the comparative type, that have contributed to population needs assessments. They were conducted by gaining reports from practitioners and by undertaking studies of groups of difficult, disruptive and hard-to-place adolescents or those who are already the subject of referral to the Specialist Forensic CAMHS that do exist. Additionally, there is a limited number of studies by questionnaire assessment of the mental health problems of samples of young offenders. Nicol et al. (2000) report an important comparative survey of this kind. It gets closer to identifying the individual needs of one component of the client group than most other previously published work. Nonetheless, various research projects conducted recently each give a different slant on the population of young people who meet certain core criteria (such as those of being considered to have mental health problems and acting in ways that are considered dangerous). Inevitably, different approaches to describing the client group confirm its broad diversity and illustrate a range of other features, including:

- the different methodologies of the research studies
- the very different opinions across the agencies as to what constitutes psychiatric disorder and mental health problems
- different opinions across the agencies as to the role of each of the other agencies
- the differing roles of the agencies as viewed by each from within
- research evidence of the high levels of psychiatric disorder even when consistent criteria are adopted across broad samples.

Nonetheless, it is clear that a rational approach to planning for the future of forensic CAMHS must recognize: the wide range of requirements and the broad spectrum of forensic inputs requested; the current lack of specialized expertise across the spectrum of need; the frailty of present services; and the current as well as the desired career routes of young people with problems.

Co-morbidity

Co-occurrence of developmental, health, education and social problems with other problems including, particularly, substance use is extremely common. Zeitlin argues that the 'co-morbid condition' is compounded by 'vulnerability, lack of family protection and exposure to a source of drugs' (Zeitlin 1999, 225). As we shall see, co-morbidity is an extremely important factor (Nicol et al. 2000; Williams et al., 2004) that must be recognised in planning realistic forensic CAMHS and this chapter summarises a survey that substantiates the significance of complexity of need in young people who use the current services.

Finding high levels of co-morbidity is not surprising as psychiatric disorders and many other health, education and social problems, including substance misuse and lower levels of access to and use of services, share overlapping risk and resilience factors. The triad of deprivation and poverty, psychiatric disorder and substance misuse stands together (Bushell et al. 2002). Recent studies investigating longitudinal predictors of drug use claim that the concurrent existence of social exclusion and psychiatric disorder provides a pathway to substance misuse (Kuperman et al. 2001; Pedersen et al. 2001; Mullen and Barry 2001). Ferdinand et al. (2001) claim that risk factors may form a chain or pathway that may first involve peer relationships, then delinquent behaviour, and finally drug use and/or psychiatric disorder. Social exclusion and psychiatric disorders can also be the cause of co-morbidity, non-attendance at services and non-recognition of substance misuse.

Co-morbidity is a professional concept that describes situations in which the single syndromes in present diagnostic classifications do not adequately describe the common experiences and needs of the population at risk. One response to this has been to provide more than one diagnosis (leading to the term 'dual diagnosis') and a second is offering a multi-axial formulation. However, patients/clients do not see or experience their problems as disjointed in any of these ways.

As Williams et al. (2004) have opined, the significance of co-morbidity to professional practice, service design and commissioning is that it emphasises the importance of: viewing people's needs from a broad perspective; directly involving young people and their carers; and providing articulated services that are able to respond to the real and inter-connected needs of the public. Furthermore, indicative findings from several recent studies in the substance misuse field show that where only substance misuse is treated, co-morbid behavioural conditions re-emerge in conjunction with higher levels of substance (Brown et al. 2001; Grella et al. 2001).

The wider client group

The evidence is thin on the definition and nature of *all* potential clients for forensic CAMHS. At one end of the spectrum described loosely by the list of functions summarized earlier is the increasing requirement of the Courts and other agencies for opinions relating to private, public and criminal law issues concerning children and adolescents. The author has found no estimate of the volume of this work that is required and no adequate survey of the needs of the young people involved. Yet, children's guardians and solicitors continue to plead for greater volumes and better availability of this kind of provision. In part, this reflects the sporadic availability of these services and, generally, non-existent planning for them. Perhaps we could base, albeit limited, estimates on statistics such as the numbers of young people looked after by local authorities, the number of divorce actions heard each year, and summary information provided by the YOTs?

At the other end of the spectrum of demand for forensic CAMHS lies the requirement for enhanced clinical services for the most troubled young people whose problems have already been described (Nicol et al. 2000). Many of them are to difficult to engage in ordinary CAMHS and they may, therefore, require not only special expertise but also a particular range of outpatient, day-patient and inpatient services, including some in medium-secure settings. Legitimately, a portion of these services should come from within the NHS or be funded by NHS monies.

Inevitably, much more has been reported about the most troublesome young people and it is to this extreme group that this chapter turns now.

CHILDREN AND ADOLESCENTS WHO ARE DIFFICULT, DISRUPTIVE AND HARD TO PLACE

In 1997, staff of the Health Services Management Centre (HSMC) in the University of Birmingham (Williams and

Barnes 1997) conducted an analysis of all the information that it could gain relating to groups of young people who had been referred to the existing healthcare services that offered very specialized forensic mental health services to young people. Most of the referred persons were adolescent boys. In addition, the HSMC staff visited many of the expert/highly specialized services and a variety of agencies to gain information, opinion and anecdotal experience. A description of this very troubled portion of the wider client group emerged.

Problems that influence referral

First, HSMC summarized the types of problem behaviours that seemed to influence referral patterns and, in particular, referrals to facilities that offer medium security. They included:

- self-harm – usually recurrent and conducted by physical methods
- serious antisocial behaviours
- bizarre and unpredictable behaviours
- behaviour that suggested substantial risk of serious aggression and violence to others
- failure to comply with or respond to treatment or management regimes in less intensive settings
- problem behaviours that challenge the capabilities, capacities, tolerance and/or staff morale of less-intensive and controlled local services
- substance use or misuse that is otherwise unmanageable.

Reasons for seeking a secure setting

In a second analysis, HSMC grouped the same adolescents according to broad sets of reasons for which more specialized opinion, care and treatment in secure settings had been sought. These included:

- discharging a sentence for offending – a secure setting had been directed as a punishment by the Courts but opinion was also presented to suggest that issues raised by mental disorder were also prominent features
- managing individuals who were considered dangerous to themselves or to others
- referring for assessment and treatment, individuals who had been unable to benefit from psychiatric assessment, care or treatment in less secure settings
- containing chaotic, unpredictable and uncontrollable behaviours that may or may not have reflected or stemmed from psychiatric illness
- responses to the anxieties of staff of the referring agencies.

Categories of problems

In its third analysis, HSMC endeavoured to group the young people by the nature of their most prominent

problems or major diagnoses. The broad categories that emerged from this analysis included:

- offenders – those young people who were required by the Courts to be cared for and/or treated in a setting of security as a part of their sentence or pending their trial in respect of alleged serious offences
- adolescents with severe mental illness – adolescents who had a serious and, possibly, an enduring mental illness and who required management in a secure setting in order to engage them in treatment and/or to protect them from harming themselves or others or from falling prey to serious exploitation
- mentally disordered offenders – adolescents who filled the criteria for both of the categories above (i.e. they had committed serious offences that required their care in a special, including secure, setting and they had a serious mental disorder that required them to be cared for and treated in a controlled setting). Individuals in this category may have:
  - committed an offence, including a serious offence, as a consequence of pre-existing mental disorder
  - developed a serious psychiatric disorder subsequent to committing an offence for which they had received a custodial sentence in a particular setting, including secure settings
- disordered and chaotic individuals – adolescents in this category were those whose behaviour presented containment, diagnostic and/or remedial challenges of such a marked degree that:
  - their needs and those of others around them had not been met by less secure settings or placements
  - the possible consequences of failing to restrict their behaviour were potentially very serious risks to the physical health of the individuals themselves or others (in some circumstances, this included risks arising from substance use or misuse of severe degree)
- adolescents who had serious learning disabilities coupled with problems in the other categories above but who were also considered to:
  - be at risk of serious exploitation; and/or
  - require specialized care and treatment that could not be provided in less-controlled settings.

HSMC drew attention to the greater frequency than often recognized of learning disabilities in the client group and also the very high levels of substance use (see also Nicol et al. 2000). The former could be conceived as unsatisfactory educational attainments that arose as a result of poor educational experience or poor learning potential, or both. There is insufficient evidence on this matter.

These analyses can be summarized graphically by way of Figure 23.3. This illustrates the common anecdotally reported finding of complex interactions between behaviours and disorder and the endemic use of substances by young people for whom secure settings are requested or directed.

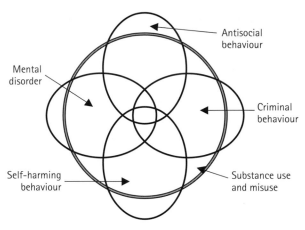

Figure 23.3 *The interacting problems of severely difficult and disruptive children and adolescents.*

Gender

HSMC found agreement that the populations described to it tended to have a considerable bias towards boys. This may reflect a variety of processes including:

- most surveys have considered the roles and activities of services as provided at the time rather than prospective samples taken from the community (thus, the HSMC survey reflected descriptions of the young people who occupied the places available in 1997)
- the performance of the criminal justice system in 1997 appeared to focus on offending in males
- youth offending institutions existed then for boys but not girls
- the apparently greater awareness and concern in society about violence in males
- the tendency for girls to be seen as in need of care and protection rather than punishment or psychiatric intervention.

There are other possible sources of evidence for believing that girls have, so far, been under-represented:

- There might have been a tendency to exclude females from consideration. Some may act dangerously towards themselves or others but, owing to their, generally, less overtly violent behaviour, they may not be included in returns in response to surveys.
- At the time of the HSMC's work in 1997, the staff of one hospital reported that most of its inpatients were girls who often presented a picture of chaotic and/or repetitive self-injurious behaviour together with poor socialization. The fact of that hospital being asked to provide services for females might well have reflected the lack of these services in other sectors of care.
- There was anecdotal information suggesting that a small but significant number of very difficult and dangerous female adolescents was receiving care in *ad hoc* and less-secure settings.

- HSMC staff were made aware of the high rates of eating disorders in adolescent females. Although young people with eating disorders are not traditionally considered as part of the client group and do not often require treatment in secure settings, they may present dangers to themselves and behaviours that are as difficult to manage as those that result in referrals to secure units.
- There have been tendencies in the past to underestimate the significance of sexual abuse in the aetiology of the problems experienced or produced by this client group and the nature of the needs that they present (see also Nicol *et al.* 2000).

Common features of young people in secure accommodation

Work conducted by a small number of groups, including that of Nicol *et al.* (2000), has drawn out features that many of the most troublesome adolescents have in common. Members of the client group at the most serious end of the spectrum appear to have certain features in common, including:

- high levels of expressed violence towards themselves or others
- dangerous behaviour that is provocative of recurrent concern in others about risk
- high levels of offending
- staff concern lest the individuals may have a psychiatric disorder.

Other features that emerge from recent research, including that of Nicol's group, on the most troubled and demanding adolescents, for whom specialized forensic mental health services appeared warranted, include their:

- very poor educational attainments and poor basic educational skills, including low levels of literacy
- chaotic relationships
- high levels of exclusion from school and from other services
- high levels of psychiatric symptoms and disorders – three quarters of the sample had a clinically significant psychiatric problem of some sort and young people who reached caseness showed the full range of diagnostic categories
- poor prospects of their needs for intervention having been met previously despite high levels of investment of professional time.

All too often, it appears that these young people come from backgrounds showing distorted and/or chaotic family relationships.

Necessarily, there must be circularity between the findings of recent surveys and the selection of the groups for study reflecting the career routes followed by the young people. Nonetheless, it is easy to see from the summarized picture presented here why it is that more-mainstream and less-specialized local agencies may find particular difficulty in coping with the problems presented by this group of young people. A feature that deserves reiteration is the very high levels of substance use and, in some cases, misuse in this very troubled group of young people. Given, the earlier section on co-morbidity, this finding is less surprising than the fact that very few surveys have demonstrated that issues relating to substance use and misuse are brought directly to the attention of services by the clients or their referrers. Also, problems arising from substance use appear to be much less frequently the core subject of concern than their pattern of use would suggest.

A STRATEGIC FRAMEWORK

The nature of strategy

This chapter has brought together analyses of what we know of the broad nature of demand for forensic CAMHS. They include views gained from staff who work in Specialist CAMHS and in the most specialized of forensic CAMHS and analyses of what is known of certain portions of the client group from their use of services. These substantiate the need for Specialist Forensic CAMHS. They also indicate the complexity of the domain and establish the need for a rational approach to delivering effective services that is led by policy, driven by strategy and actioned through effective collaborative commissioning.

This chapter has touched on many strategic issues. Strategy is a word that takes its origin from war fighting and acts of generalship and, in particular, the movement and management of large bodies of people prior to the fighting in order to gain advantage when it begins. So, at its root, strategy is about planning and positioning complex bodies of people engaged in more or less common tasks that have a longer-term agreed objective to achieve favourable positions. Strategy involves visioning the future but also brings with it a series of disciplines, patterns of thinking and behaviours that are intended to achieve identified future goals. In this respect, the assumption of this chapter is that the aim of the governments in the UK is to develop a pattern of forensic mental health services as a key part of the wider plan to deliver a better array of CAMHS (NAW 2001; DoH 2003).

The position taken in this chapter is that the best evidence must inform plans for forensic CAMHS. Also, generating greater trust between service agencies and sectors is one of the key tasks as the services must offer appropriate expertise for a very broad client group and the ability to discharge a range of identified functions through the combined efforts of a variety of agencies. In such a setting, a strategic framework can prove vital to achieving the understanding and integration of action required.

The current strategic framework for CAMHS

In 1995, the NHS Health Advisory Service published its report *Together We Stand* (Williams and Richardson 1995). That text offered a contemporary analysis of the state of CAMHS in England and Wales, took a multi-disciplinary, multi-agency and multi-sectoral approach to service development, and examined the knowledge-base and skills required by commissioners and staff who deliver child and adolescent mental healthcare. It has been received extremely positively by health and social care agencies and, within them, by managers and professionals alike. It is now widely accepted as the basis from which future developments in CAMHS are to be made and its recommendations on a four-tier strategic framework are now policy in England and Wales (DoH 1995; NAW 2001).

Since then, the Audit Commission's (1999) report has supported the findings of the HAS and added shape and depth to its recommendations. Central to the messages of both of these documents is the four-tier strategic framework for service design. Their detailed recommendations were pivoted around that framework.

It is pertinent to side-step for a moment to speculate about why it is that the strategic framework contained in *Together We Stand* has been so readily adopted. Doubtless, it had the enormous advantages of apparent simplicity and being launched into a strategic vacuum at a time when concern about the state of, and pressures on CAMHS in the UK was growing rapidly. It was developed by bringing together contributions from a number of academics and practitioners and from general managers in relevant sectors of care. As a result, it appears to have legitimized and resonated with political, professional and managerial determination to take action to develop CAMHS.

The four-tier strategic framework was intended to be applied to understanding the nature of services required to be deployed across agencies and within each of the sectors of care by them acting together. It created a 'language' to describe the field that is useable by professionals, general managers and policymakers, and it has broken free from the tensions that would have been inherent in adopting the existing terms and language of any one of the agencies or sectors of care. Previously, rising levels of concern about the nature, state and volume of CAMHS had failed to generate clarity in those responsible for the disposal of health, education and social care resources about how they might conceptualize the domain and tackle the evident problems. There is little doubt that the translatability of the language in the four tier strategic framework to the endeavours of a variety of different agencies, each of which had previously adhered to a different structure and language has been key to its impact. What the four-tier strategic framework has achieved so far is to bring together these streams of thought in such a

Nonetheless, elements of a more mature service do exist, mainly in England, but, as identified, they have no unifying or predictive framework. This leaves individual services and the care and case management of individuals to be guided by:

- local professional opinion and experience and the nature and quality of commissioner–provider relationships
- local inter-agency and intra-agency dynamics and pressures
- what is presently available.

It is also plain that this situation and the poverty of the present arrangements for commissioning and managing forensic mental health services for young people result in:

- poor planning and execution of care for individuals
- poor continuity of very specialized care for this client group
- many of the individuals who receive very specialized care doing so as a result of:
  - determined advocacy by particular members of service staff
  - the turbulence they create
  - the endurance of commissioners and/or service providers
- lack of proper external quality assurance and performance management of the kinds that might be required by an experienced commissioner for those services that do exist, due to:
  - commissioner inexperience
  - high rates of Out of Area Treatments (OATs) and out-of-county placements
  - long distances between the location of specialist services and many patients' homes
  - lack of performance management mechanisms for the existing services
  - inadequate mechanisms to enable local referrers to review their cases when admitted to more distant, very specialized services and, thereby, continue to contribute to high-quality care and case management.

The way ahead

Alternatively, the approach suggested here is one in which the agencies combine to collaboratively plan, fund, deliver and manage the performance of forensic CAMHS that are based on:

- multi-agency concepts
- cross-sector approaches and close working relationships between sectors and agencies
- expansion of NHS-funded local and outreach assessment and treatment capacity
- expansion of NHS-funded secure and other inpatient services.

One of the critical issues is that of how to determine or predict which of the young people exhibiting characteristics that bring them into the potential client group should follow each of the three avenues described by Little and Bullock in Chapter 24. This indicates the need to build up much better data in order to define more precisely which of the young people who are in the broad category of 'troublesome youth' will need input from forensic CAMHS.

While the number of young people requiring the most specialized services is relatively small, accurate prediction based on analysis of risk factors is difficult. Therefore, the primary purpose of comprehensive assessment should be to ensure appropriate early intervention. This might, in turn, prevent placement breakdowns which is one of the routes that can lead, inexorably, and over a long period in some cases, towards referral for secure psychiatric inpatient placement. Thus, comprehensive assessment is needed for young people who are considered to come within the broad categories defined by the characteristics that have been referred to earlier in this chapter. This includes some young people who are referred to CAMHS, a proportion of those who are clients of the social and/or education support services, and young people referred to the YOTs, and the other youth justice, probation and penal services.

The commissioning agenda

Moving forward is likely to be aided by an agenda for commissioning shared between individual healthcare agencies and local authorities exercising their responsibilities jointly together with more concentrated patterns of regional and national commissioning for some of the most expert services and especially those at Tier 4. Already, there are signs that in each of the National Health Services in the UK, there are moves towards identifying baselines for commissioning certain very specialized services on national and regional territories. Furthermore, there has been a shift of policy and commissioning practice to make individual regions in England and the separate countries of Scotland, Wales and Northern Ireland responsible for commissioning high- and medium-secure forensic mental health services for adults. The author of this chapter recommends that development of a similar template for children and adolescents and its coordination with the work of Strategic Health Authorities and Primary Care Trusts (in England) and Local Health Boards and Health Commission Wales (in Wales) could produce an appropriate commissioning mechanism. Within this vision, PCTs (England) and CAMHS Commissioning Networks (CCNs) in Wales would be responsible for commissioning Tier 3 services in a way that is harmonized with Tier 4 services that are commissioned nationally in Northern Ireland, Scotland and Wales and regionally in England.

In order to respond to this ambitious agenda, work is necessary at all tiers, supported by improved resources, staffing and staff training. In particular, a programme of commissioner training and development is vital. Achievement of such an ambitious agenda cannot be achieved unless particular commissioners are identified and given continuing and sustained responsibilities for forensic CAMHS. In addition, there is a need for a series of activities of a more general nature that will require collaboration and debate on a wide basis, including:

- work on defining the client group(s)
- more cross agency comprehensive needs assessments conducted against agreed common protocols
- mapping of the present array of services across all agencies
- agreement and implementation of a comprehensive plan for individual case assessment based on the best of present expertise
- a programme of targeted research and service evaluation
- collection of a more substantial database based on agreed cross-agency assessment criteria
- a programme of organizational development for service planners and providers.

TIER 3

At Tier 3, there is much to be done. Achieving an expanded capability in the forensic arena cannot be achieved easily or quickly, especially given the other demands on generic Specialist CAMHS and the existing staff and resource shortages. Nonetheless, the plan envisaged in this chapter is that of moving towards each local child and adolescent mental health service being the first port of call for requests for specialized forensic mental health service opinions delivered by teams of staff with identified responsibilities and training in this area. Each team should work in conjunction with the other local agencies to make recommendations as to the use of the other tiers of expertise guided through sustained relationships with the specialized centres of expertise. In this way, a local forensic mental health service could provide specialist back-up to the generic YOTs (at Tier 2) through outposted staff and by providing access to generic Tier 3 services and gateways to the more specialized tiers.

This requires:

- considerable multi-disciplinary expansion of the forensic capability of local CAMHS
- development of good local linkages between the peripatetic teams outreaching from the centres of special forensic expertise for young people with:
  - the Specialist CAMHS in identified local areas
  - services for young people who use and misuse substances
  - childcare agencies
  - Youth Offending Teams

  - local authority services of all types
  - secure units for children and adolescents in the area
  - medium-secure units for adults.

Children and adolescents who fall into the client group appropriate to a forensic CAMHS are often highly mobile and frequently known to more than one agency. Sometimes, their moves between agencies and sectors of care are planned, but, all too often, referrals are made by the processes of exclusion, result from exhaustion of the capabilities of particular services or, are made in desperation as a last ditch attempt to help (see Nicol *et al.* 2000 for a commentary on the burden experienced by carers and professionals). All too rarely does it seem that the care of individuals is subject to rigorously planned integrated care pathways. Therefore, a focus on analysing patient flows (the patients' journeys) and the design of appropriate care pathways is an important matter for appropriate R&D. The objective should be planned care, initiated at the local level, being the basis on which integrated services are delivered.

TIER 4

The outreach or peripatetic teams (working from centres of Special Forensic Expertise) should have the ability to cascade an increased volume of very specialized outpatient services and support to local services and, particularly, local Tier 3 forensic CAMHS teams in developing their knowledge and skill through teaching and consultation with local practitioners.

Application of developing information technology, including telemedicine, could bring the centres of special expertise into closer contact with the more distant local CAMHS. In this way, the present informal network of relationships between local services and a judiciously expanded number of specialist centres could be developed into an established and recognized pattern of planned care.

Currently, there is lack of mental health liaison services for consultation between the NHS and services provided by other sectors of care for children and adolescents who are very difficult to manage and hard to place. However, the accumulating evidence of the high level of psychiatric symptoms and/or disorders in these groups of young people makes the case for much improved liaison and consultative services provided not only to Tier 3 forensic CAMHS but also to probation services, YOTs, secure units and young-offender institutions. Also, there is a lack of targeted remedial, therapeutic and care programmes of tested efficacy for adolescent sexual offenders and for the victims of abuse. Thus, there is need for the peripatetic teams to develop effective programmes of care in conjunction with local services, and to teach and consult with practitioners in all sectors of care as well as the local specialist CAMHS.

It is inherent in this proposal that development of peripatetic outreach teams requires prior developments, locally, at Tier 3 and, nationally, at Tier 4. Each local service would need to be at an enhanced level of capability and each of the very specialized centres would need to have identified responsibilities for committing resources to the peripatetic teams. Each outreach team could then develop an awareness of services in all sectors of care so as to act as an information exchange.

Centres of special forensic expertise and the role of secure inpatient services

There is clear opinion held by many professionals and managers in the field that there is a need to expand in the number of centres of special expertise for adolescents who have severe mental illness and who require treatment in settings that offer security. The strategic framework presented here indicates that each should be capable of providing:

- very specialized inpatient care
- outreach clinical services
- teaching and research.

As identified earlier, the author believes that these centres of expertise should be developed into a complementary network. Thus, planning future services requires development of commissioning expertise.

The reviews summarized in this chapter indicate that there is a small yet definable group of young people within the overall client group of forensic CAMHS which might benefit from secure inpatient treatment in the healthcare system. Current evidence indicates that their problems cover the full range of psychiatric disorders.

A review of the Gardener Unit in Salford (NHS HAS 1994) produced an interim list of the kinds of young people for whom there may be a greater call for secure inpatient resources. This includes:

- mentally disordered offenders
- sex offenders and abusers
- severely suicidal and self-harming adolescents
- some severely mentally ill adolescents
- adolescents who need to begin psychiatric rehabilitation in secure circumstances
- brain-injured adolescents and those with severe organic disorders.

In addition, there are five other key matters. They are:

- the need to recognize the high levels of substance use and misuse in the client group
- the special needs of learning-disabled clients
- the challenges of differentiating those clients who require NHS-funded secure inpatient care within the overall client group, given the high prevalence of symptoms and disorders in the client group as a whole

- awareness that it is unlikely that each individual secure inpatient unit could deliver assessment, care and treatment effectively and appropriately to all of those who might benefit from such intervention and care (a matter of case-mix and specialization)
- the need to distinguish those young people who require secure inpatient care from those likely to benefit from lower levels of security.

While each of these matters needs further work, there appears to be a general consensus among those involved in this field that there is a need to increase the number of inpatient beds within very specialized forensic CAMHS, including those in secure settings, for a range of young people from the diverse potential client group.

The young people who appear to have the greatest immediate needs for an increase in secure NHS-funded provision include those with:

- very severe mental illnesses
- recurrent very severe self-harming behaviours
- serious brain-injury and some with other severe organic disorders.

Additionally, there is a need to develop and evaluate focused programmes of specialist intervention for adolescents who are:

- sex offenders and abusers
- mentally disordered offenders
- users, and particularly, misusers of substances
- in need of a secure setting in which to begin psychiatric rehabilitation
- learning-disabled as well as having other characteristics of the client group.

Given the profile of use of existing facilities, there is also a requirement for further research into the needs of both boys and girls and for young people from ethnic-minority origins for the most specialized resources in all sectors of care. Another important area for future development is the need to ensure liaison between secure inpatient facilities funded by the NHS and the secure residential facilities offered by other sectors.

Training professionals and managers for the future

One of the intentions of this chapter is to bring the contents of this highly specialized book together with the concepts of strategic leadership and management of public sector services to identify a way forward. The result generates a demanding agenda for action with considerable workforce and resource implications.

Such an ambitious programme cannot be delivered rapidly, but, unless deliberate planned action is taken, it is arguable that nothing coherent is likely to result and, despite their good intentions, local services will be left to react inadequately to crises. This chapter recognizes the contemporary pressures and contains a framework through which to plan developments rationally. A key feature that has emerged several times is the current lack of both the volume, and the levels of specialist expertise to deliver the kinds of services that could be supported by current capabilities or by those that are likely to emerge through continuing professional development and research.

Several themes have run close beneath the surface. Arguably, the most powerful of those relates to the agendas for recruitment and training that will be necessary to underpin any service advancements. The strategy proposed cannot be delivered without a longer-term workforce development plan.

The augmented four-tier strategic framework identified in this chapter indicates that different levels of specialist expertise are required. The author's opinion is that it is not feasible to base service planning around the provision of the full spectrum of forensic CAMHS by and from the most specialized centres. Nonetheless, they are critically important. We must build on the current circumstances in which it would appear that the most common and frequent demands for forensic mental health service expert capability are likely to require a defined level of expertise made available through local Specialist CAMHS. Equally, this chapter substantiates the notion that it is unlikely that this expertise can be developed or sustained without considerable training, additional recruitment and backing delivered by an expanded number of centres of special forensic expertise each with strong academic connections.

The framework proposed here envisages that patients could be moved through a more comprehensive and rational system according to need and negotiated, purposeful and evaluated care programmes. Knowledge, expertise and skill should also be key commodities that are moved purposely through the proposed network of forensic CAMHS. They are not simply a by-product of work with patients/clients. Thus, training and academic support, research and development should also be major matters for planning. They are required not only by professionals working within the various service tiers but also by those staff who manage service delivery and those who plan and commission services. Therefore, in parallel with the strategic framework offered here, this chapter also offers a four-level outline framework for training.

LEVEL 1: GENERAL SPECIALIST TRAINING

Basic knowledge about forensic mental health matters and the skills to assess and manage children and adolescents who might fall into the client group for forensic CAMHS should form part of the training for many professions. They include professionals who work within local generic Specialist CAMHS (including psychiatrists, nurses, social workers, psychologists, AHPs and teachers), the staff of YOTs, certain education service support staff, and children's teams in local authority social services departments.

In addition, workers in non-statutory sector projects which have a remit for work with young people, police officers and prison staff require familiarity at least with the concepts that are inherent in the work of forensic CAMHS.

LEVEL 2: ADVANCED TRAINING

Each local Specialist CAMHS should move in the direction of appointing a multi-disciplinary team of professionals who will lead on providing forensic CAMHS at Tier 3. They need to be more than averagely skilled in assessment techniques, report writing and in presenting themselves before Courts, as well as in the construction of programmes of care with a forensic focus. Additionally, many probation officers on the staff of YOTs will need advanced training that goes beyond that required on a day-by-day basis by the staff of the generic elements of Specialist CAMHS. These and other such staff require training at a level that is described as level 2 here.

LEVEL 3: VERY SPECIALIZED TRAINING FOR THE STAFF OF DAY-PATIENT AND INPATIENT SERVICES OFFERED BY THE CENTRES OF SPECIAL FORENSIC EXPERTISE

Staff who work at the centres of expertise, and particularly those who work with day-patients and inpatients, require a particularly high level of training in order to discharge their responsibilities. They should have thorough working knowledge of the law and be trained in techniques of control and restraint appropriate to young people as well as in more focused assessment and therapeutic techniques relevant to discharging particular programmes of care for, and intervention with some of the most troubled young people. Previous sections in this chapter have identified aspects of the client group and programmes that require staff to develop special expertise.

LEVEL 4: VERY SPECIALIZED TRAINING FOR THE PERIPATETIC STAFF OF THE CENTRES OF SPECIAL EXPERTISE

The model proposed in this chapter places particular responsibilities upon staff who offer outreach services. They require full training at all of the levels identified so far (1 to 3). Additionally, they should have advanced communication skills, the most effective of self-presentation skills, particular experience in mental health case consultation, and a high level of skill in teaching. Some of them should also be skilled in the techniques of service evaluation and in quantitative and qualitative research methodologies.

CONCLUSIONS

This chapter has moved from noting the historical context to identifying the challenges to be faced in effectively planning comprehensive forensic CAMHS for the UK. In so doing, the author has recommended moving from the present *ad hoc* system in which services have developed around the, often charismatic, advocacy of individuals, usually service providers, to a more rational commissioning and performance managed system that is led by policy, driven by strategy and based on need.

The challenge of more purposefully managing the professional process decisions and thereby influencing the career routes of the young people involved according to their needs lies at the heart of the strategic intent and direction proposed here. The advantages of a strategic framework in support of this task have been identified. The strategic framework presented here is capable of:

- containing an appropriately wide range of service activities
- enabling the healthcare contribution to forensic CAMHS to be developed in conjunction with the roles of other agencies
- identifying the roles of centres of special forensic expertise
- clarifying the functions of health-provided secure care.

Necessarily, the focus has been on improving the NHS-funded contribution to wider multi-sector services. Similar work is needed to identify the parallel service developments that are required within other sectors. The result that has emerged from these analyses and proposals sets an ambitious agenda for service development.

While services are currently thin and the volume of expertise required to move rapidly to delivering such a comprehensive array of services is missing now, this book ably demonstrates that the skills and knowledge do exist from which more effective services might be developed. Recruiting capable staff, training them and providing resources to support their work will be vital elements in moving forward. This calls for a coherent longer-term workforce development plan.

REFERENCES

Audit Commission 1996: *Misspent Youth: Young People and Crime.* London: Audit Commission.

Audit Commission 1999: *Children in Mind: Report on Child and Adolescent Mental Health Services.* London: Audit Commission.

Black, D., Harris Hendriks, J. and Wolkind, S. (eds) 1998: *Child Psychiatry and the Law.* London: Gaskell.

Brown, S.A., Amico, A.J.D., McCarthy, D.M. *et al.* 2001: Four-Year Outcomes from Adolescent Alcohol and Drug Treatment. *Journal of Studies on Alcohol* **62**: 381–88.

Bushell, H.D., Crome, I. and Williams, R.J.W. 2002: How can risk be related to interventions for young people who misuse substances? *Current Opinion in Psychiatry* **15**: 355-60.

Butler-Sloss, E. 1998: In Black, D., Harris Hendriks, J. and Wolkind, S. (eds) 1998: *Child Psychiatry and the Law.* 3rd edn. London: Gaskell, iii-ix.

DoH (Department of Health, Social Services Inspectorate of the Department of Health and the Department for Education) 1995: *A Handbook of Mental Health.* London: DoH.

DoH (Department of Health) 2003: *Getting the Right Start: National Service Framework for Children – Emerging Findings.* London: DoH.

Ferdinand, R.F., Blum, M. and Verhulst, F.C. 2001: Psychopathology in adolescence predicts substance use in young adulthood. *Addiction* **96**: 861–70.

Graham, P. 1999: Research and therapeutic interventions: bridging the chasm. The 1999 Rutter Lecture, given at the Faculty of Child and Adolescent Psychiatry of the Royal College of Psychiatrists Annual Residential Meeting, Manchester, UK, 22 April 1999.

Graham, P. 2000: Treatment interventions and findings from research: bridging the chasm in child psychiatry. *British Journal of Psychiatry* **176**: 414–19.

Grella, C.E., Hser, Y.-I., Joshi, V. *et al.* 2001: Drug treatment outcomes for adolescents with comorbid mental and substance use disorders. *The Journal of Nervous and Mental Disease* **189**: 384–92.

Knapp, M.K. and Henderson, J. 1999: Health economic perspectives and evaluation of child and adolescent mental health services. *Current Opinion in Psychiatry* **12**: 393–97.

Knapp, M.K., Scott, S. and Davies, J. 1999: The cost of antisocial behaviour in younger children: preliminary findings from a pilot sample of economic and family impact. *Clinical Child Psychology and Psychiatry* **4**: 457–73.

Kuperman, S., Schlosser, S.S., Kramer, J.R. *et al.* 2001: Risk domains associated with an adolescent alcohol dependence diagnosis. *Addiction* **96**: 629–36.

Kurtz, Z. 1996: *Treating Children Well: Guide to Using the Evidence Base in Commissioning and Managing Services for the Mental Health of Children and Young People.* London: Mental Health Foundation.

Longley, M., Williams, R., Furnish, S. and Warner, M. 2001. *Promoting Mental Health in a Civil Society: Towards a Strategic Approach.* London: The Nuffield Trust.

MHF (Mental Health Foundation) 1999: *Bright Futures.* London: MHF.

Mullen, L. and Barry, J. 2001: An analysis of 15–19 year-old first attenders at the Dublin Needle Exchange, 1990-97. *Addiction* **96**, 251–58.

NAW (National Assembly for Wales) 2000: *Everybody's Business: Consultation Document.* Cardiff: NAW.

NAW (National Assembly for Wales) 2001: *Everybody's Business: Strategy Document.* Cardiff: NAW.

NHS HAS (NHS Health Advisory Service, Mental Health Act Commission, Department of Health Social Services Inspectorate) 1994: *Review of the Adolescent Forensic Psychiatry Service based on the Gardener Unit, Prestwich Hospital, Salford, Manchester.* London: NHS Health Advisory Service.

Nicol, R., Stretch, D., Whitney, I., Jones, K., Garfield, P., Turner, K. and Stanion, B. 2000: Mental health needs and services for severely troubled and troubling young people, including young offenders in an NHS region. *Journal of Adolescence* **23**: 243–61.

ONS (Office for National Statistics) 1999: Mental health of children and adolescents. ONS (99) 409. London, Government Statistical Service.

Pedersen, W., Mastekaasa, A. and Wichtrom, L. 2001: Conduct problems and early cannabis initiation: a longitudinal study of gender differences. *Addiction* **96**: 415–31.

Rolf, J., Masten, A., Cicchetti, D., Nuechterlein, K. and Weintraub, S. (eds) 1990: *Risk and Protective Factors in the Development of Psychopathology.* Cambridge: Cambridge University Press.

Royal College of Psychiatrists 2002: *Council Report 104. Prevention in Psychiatry. Report of the Public Policy Committee Working Party.* London: Royal College of Psychiatrists.

Royal College of Psychiatrists 2002: *Council Report 105. Patients as Parents: Addressing the needs, including the safety, of children whose parents have mental illness.* London: Royal College of Psychiatrists.

Rutter, M. and Smith, D.J. 1995: *Psychosocial Disorders in Young People.* Chichester: John Wiley.

Salmon, G. and Williams, R. 2001: A strategic model for cooperation, partnership and teamwork. In *The Welsh Institute for Health and Social Care: the First Five Years.* Pontypridd: University of Glamorgan, 18–22.

Wallace, W.A., Crown, J.M., Berger, M. and Cox, A.D. 1997: Child and adolescent mental health. In Stevens, A. and Raftery, J. (eds), *Health Care Needs Assessment, The Epidemiologically*

Based Needs Assessment Reviews, 2nd series. Oxford: Radcliffe Medical Press.

Williams, R. 1999: Managing mental health care: risk and evidence-based practice. *Current Opinion in Psychiatry* **12**: 385–91.

Williams, R. 2000: A cunning plan: the role of research evidence in translating policy into effective child and adolescent mental health services. *Current Opinion in Psychiatry* **13**: 361–8.

Williams, R. and Barnes, M. 1997: Commissioning adolescent forensic mental health services. Health Services Management Centre of the University of Birmingham (unpublished).

Williams, R. and Richardson, G. 1995: *Together We Stand: the Commissioning, Role and Management of Child and Adolescent Mental Health Services.* London: HMSO.

Williams, R. and Salmon, G. 2002: Collaboration in commissioning and delivering child and adolescent mental health services. *Current Opinion in Psychiatry* **15**: 349–53.

Williams, R. (ed) 2004: *Safeguards for Young Minds.* Second edition London: Gaskell.

Williams, R., Gilvarry, E. and Christian, J. 2004: Developing an evidence-based model for services. In Crom, I., Ghodse, H., Gilvarry, E. and McArdle, P. (eds) *Young People and Substance Abuse.* London: Gaskell.

Zeitlin, H. 1999: Psychiatric comorbidity with substance misuse in children and teenagers. *Drug and Alcohol Dependence* **55**: 225–34.

24

Administrative frameworks and services for very difficult adolescents in England

MICHAEL LITTLE AND ROGER BULLOCK

INTRODUCTION

Some adolescents clearly have severe and sometimes chronic problems, usually manifested as some form of conduct or mixed emotional and conduct disorder. However, these conditions are only one part of the equation used to assess a young person's eligibility for a long-term placement in a secure unit. While the criteria for diagnoses are well established, quite as important are the professional, administrative and legal frameworks in which the young person's problems are addressed. For example, the young people may be too immature to be safely placed in prison, although his or her offending behaviour may make such a placement a legal possibility. Some display bizarre behaviour patterns, such as killing the family pets, but despite undergoing numerous assessments, are not found to be mentally ill – at least in the formal sense of displaying disorders of thought, speech or perception. Consequently they are not viewed as suitable for hospital treatment. A salient feature of young people who become candidates for long-term security is their tendency to present problems that cannot be effectively met by a single agency or intervention. Frequently, the result is an eclectic approach that attempts to incorporate the best features of several specialisms.

ADMINISTRATIVE STRUCTURES FOR PROVIDING SERVICES

In most western countries, a myriad of services has evolved designed to meet the needs of severely troubled adolescents. Consequently, young people's problems can be dealt with in any one of, or a combination of, welfare and control systems. For example, in England it is possible for a serious offender, such as a rapist, to be dealt with by social services within in the childcare system, but this is rare and most are sent by Courts to prison. In nearly all European Union states, the seriously violent adolescent can be sheltered either in prison custody, education, childcare or mental health provision; in England the latter has been viewed as a more benign and less stigmatizing option, often used by middle-class parents coping with their very difficult offspring.

In addition to a choice of services, there are several legal options available for very difficult young people. They may be looked after in residential or specialist foster care by the state, usually under a care order rather than under voluntary arrangements. In England this remains an option for young children convicted of serious crimes, such as arson, as well as for the small proportion of young people looked after away from home for welfare reasons who need to be placed in specialist secure accommodation because of the danger they present to themselves or others. However, such placements have to be ratified by a Court. Mental health orders offer another route to security but, although more common in the USA, they are rare in England. Serious offenders can be sentenced by a criminal court to custody, usually in a separate institution for young offenders, but those convicted of grave crimes can also be detained under mental health laws. In England, these offenders often elicit a s90 or s91 disposal. These refer to sections in the Powers of

Criminal (Sentencing) Act 2000 which replaced s53 of the Children and Young Persons Act 1933. Section 90 allows children convicted of murder to be detained indefinitely at 'Her Majesty's pleasure'. Section 91 allows children to be detained for a finite period when convicted of a crime which, were they adult, would merit a long sentence of 14 years or more.

The service and legal options for young people do not always coincide in a way that most observers would expect. For example, young people sentenced under ss90 and 91 can be placed wherever Her Majesty (or her representative) sees fit, such as a local-authority secure unit, a secure training centre or a young offenders' institution. In the past, some young people so sentenced went to open residential establishments, and some years ago it was rumoured that one offender was successfully rehabilitated in a private boarding school. Other grave offenders, particularly those long known to social services, may continue to be looked after by the state, while others in prison department custody clearly need and may benefit from the specialist help that education, mental health or social services can provide.

LIFE ROUTE, PROCESS, CAREER ROUTE AND PREDICTION OF OUTCOMES

Two dimensions of troubled children's lives have been used by the Dartington Social Research Unit in successive studies to understand what happens to young people passing through the administrative and legal systems just described (Bullock *et al.* 1998a). The first is *life route* – that is to say the decisions that a young person (and his or her family) makes that affect life chances. To make an accurate prognosis, it is necessary to build up a picture that begins at birth and covers all areas of a child's life. It is evident from previous research that choice in one area, such as living situations, can affect others, say family and social relations. The concept of life route also incorporates the individual's personality as this affects conduct. For very difficult young people, behaviour will reflect pathological conditions, such as conduct, emotional or mixed disorders. Thus, problems of running away, violence and offending which necessitate some form of intervention need to be taken into account in the assessment.

The second dimension is *process*, defined as the decisions made by professionals and/or Courts (in response to the young person's life route) that affect life chances. So, whether an adolescent is picked up by education, child guidance, social or health services will probably make a difference to long-term outcomes. Similarly, a Court's decision to make a s91 disposal is likely to influence the young person's psychological and social development and the way he or she is perceived by others.

Such an approach incorporates the background circumstances, needs and pathology of young people and their families as well as the interventions fashioned to ease difficulties. Thus it incorporates two streams of research that are rarely connected. These are clinical evidence on the effects of personality disorders, and studies of administrative processes. Getting into trouble with the law, which is one aspect of life route, clearly has an effect on long-term life chances, but so do the decisions of using the youth justice system – part of the process. Similarly, while key life events, such as the death of a parent or experience of sexual abuse, are likely to affect a child's functioning, so can the quality of the welfare agencies' responses to the problem: it is unlikely, for example, that several placement breakdowns while away in state care and loss of contact with relatives will do much to enhance a young person's life chances or behaviour in the long term.

With so many variables contributing to an outcome, it helps if the interaction between the decisions of child and family on the one hand and those of support agencies on the other is subsumed under the single term, *career route*. Decisions made at successive moments in a career will influence what happens subsequently. For example, an adolescent sentenced to youth custody is highly unlikely subsequently to gain a place in an elite public school, although one or two public school boys have secured a place in young-offender institutions. But there are more subtle connections; for instance, children in state care or accommodation suffering placement disruption also tend to experience disrupted schooling and so under-achieve academically. There is also a link between the unease generated in others by children who commit violent offences and the offenders' subsequent social isolation.

Career route, so defined, is a useful way of categorizing the situations of children and young people in need. The very difficult young people referred to welfare and control agencies for help will follow several different career routes. Five became evident in the research into young people requiring long stays in secure treatment settings described here. For example, those who interrupted apparently blameless lives with a one-off grave offence are clearly distinguishable from those long known to education and/or social services or those who are both seriously and persistently delinquent. The details of the each route will be given later.

But career route is more than just classification; its value is in *prediction*, encouraging us to say within a reasonable margin of error what a troubled adolescent's future life chances will be. Prediction is a notoriously complicated process and, when undertaken for a general population, very difficult (Rutter *et al.* 1998). The value of achieving correct predictions is somewhat reduced by the high number of 'false positives' that inevitably occur. These are individuals who display risk factors but do not succumb to the behaviour being predicted (Little and Mount 1999). They usually outnumber correct predictions on those who do. Unfortunately, this limits the value of results to practitioners seeking to identify who within the general population will need help in the future.

Predicting the future for young people known to be very difficult, however, is of a different order, since the starting point is the high-risk case already known to welfare or control agencies (Little 2002a). This makes it easier to make a prognosis of the future life chances. Moreover, while the starting point is the career route which the young person follows, the subsequent analysis can focus upon individual adaptations by predicting from research knowledge what can best be achieved from the point at which the label 'extremely difficult and disturbed' is applied, and, conversely, what is the worst scenario. This is likely to be helpful to those wishing to assess future needs and risks as for very difficult young people outcomes are generally predictable. Very few behave in unexpected ways, evidence that should hearten those undertaking therapeutic work with teenagers.

RELEVANCE OF RESEARCH INTO VERY DIFFICULT ADOLESCENTS

Research evidence about extremely difficult adolescents has not always played a part in the formulation of policy or the development of practice guidelines. As in so much that has been done on behalf of vulnerable children, provision tends to have developed piecemeal without much knowledge about the young people's needs: who they are, what they will respond to and what happens to them as they grow into adulthood. It is surprising that £150,000 per annum per young person can be spent on the most specialized interventions with so little known about outcomes.

Evaluating interventions for those in greatest need of help also has relevance for those working with more routine cases. Many developments in social work have been achieved because back-up facilities are available for those who strive to keep adolescents out of residential care, secure accommodation or youth custody. If community alternatives are to work, specialist facilities are necessary for the relatively small proportion who fail in such approaches. The messages learnt from these young people also help us understand the processes and factors associated with the need for expensive resources, such as long-term secure units. Despite some improvements in practice during the last 30 years, many of the young people in long-stay secure units are still casualties of the system and better care and control earlier on might have dispensed with much subsequent turmoil, upset, time and expense.

Such findings also have implications for wider child-care policy and practice. As the young people's situations partly reflect their responses to our interventions, a change in policy towards troublesome children will produce

fluctuations in the number of very difficult adolescents dealt with by means of specialized secure treatment units. If prison was felt to be unhelpful to those under the age of 21 years, the consequence for Youth Offending Teams and social services would be considerable, not least because they would find themselves responsible for caring for many more extremely difficult clients. On the other hand, if British psychiatrists were to follow their North American colleagues and admit more behaviourally disordered children to hospital, then the burden on other welfare services would ease.

PROCESSES FOR DEALING WITH DIFFICULT ADOLESCENTS IN ENGLAND

The young people in question are processed along a variety of avenues. Their problems may become manifest in school, requiring special education, child guidance or occasionally mental hospital. Difficulty associated with the family is more likely to result in the state looking after the young person, while juvenile offenders are processed through a separate juvenile justice system.

In addition to the legal and administrative categories, there are many informal decisions based on professional discretion that can influence the route taken by a difficult adolescent. A look at the routes taken by young people destined for long-stay secure units and the various by-ways along which some difficult children are diverted to other settings helps clarify the situation.

Although the heterogeneous nature of entrants to long-stay secure units is apparent from even the briefest scrutiny of the young people's background characteristics, arrivals will have followed one of three legal and administrative avenues already described. The high road is taken by children in state care or accommodation who display serious behaviour problems. Some of them, but not all, will also have committed offences. The second avenue involves serious offenders, a number of whom also display other behavioural difficulties. These are dealt with by Youth Offending Teams in each local authority and placements will follow either in local-authority secure units that sell places to the Youth Justice Board, secure training centres (mostly for younger lower-risk offenders), or young-offender institutions run by the prison department. A third route, frequently taken by children displaying disturbed behaviour from an early age, is special education and mental health. As young people get older, responses increasingly overlap. Children are transferred from special education to residential homes run by social services, children in care sentenced to prison custody and so on.

Looking at the three avenues in more detail, it can be seen that some very difficult young people may, if circumstances warrant and parents agree, be accommodated by local-authority social services under a voluntary agreement. Alternatively, they may be taken into care under a legal order if the Court is satisfied that the young person is suffering, or is likely to suffer, significant harm and that the harm is attributable to the care previously offered or to his or her being beyond parental control. Should the young person's behaviour continue to deteriorate to the point of needing secure accommodation, the Court must decide whether the criteria in s25 of the Children Act 1989 have been met (Ryan 1999). These state that '(i) he (or she) has a history of absconding and is likely to abscond from any other description of accommodation; and (ii) if he (or she) absconds suffering of significant harm is likely; or that if he (or she) is kept in any other description of accommodation he (or she) is likely to injure him or herself or other persons'.

For these young people, a number of options are available. Initially, placement in local-authority secure accommodation, usually for a short period, will be arranged. Should long-term treatment be entertained, a place might be sought in units that have traditionally provided for longer stays, although no official distinction is made with regard to their status. In 2001 in England, 432 places were available in these units but 75% of them were devoted to young offenders on remand or serving custodial sentences (Department of Health, annual). This is because many establishments 'sell' beds to the Youth Justice Board seeking places for young people under s90 and s91 sentences (currently 117) or detention and training orders (currently 126). So, the units will shelter a mixed population of serious offenders and disordered adolescents. Naturally, the greater the sophistication of the resource being sought, the greater will be the constraints on social workers' freedom of action; whether a place is available, whether the local authority will meet the cost and whether the secure setting considers they can help the child. All of this stands between the assessment of an adolescent's needs and the available placement.

Many very difficult adolescents are young offenders and enter the system via youth justice. Some, because of the persistence or the seriousness of their offending, will be sentenced to custody under a detention and training order for periods of between four months and two years. Others aged between 18 and 20 may be sentenced to youth custody for between three weeks and an unlimited period. For the minority of young people who commit grave offences, there will be an initial hearing in the magistrates' Court which, using another set of guidelines, will decide made whether or not to pass the case on to the Crown Court. If the child is found guilty in the Crown Court, the full range of custodial and community criminal disposals are available.

It is not only the disposal that determines the routes taken by serious offenders. A judge's decision to use the s90 or s91 option widens the range of placements in which the young person can be sheltered. Secure training centres and other childcare treatment settings as well as prison custody become possible. The judge's written recommendation to the Secretary of State also influences decisions made about the young person in future years, not least the duration and place of detention. The court decision is complemented by a set of formal procedures at the Home Office to determine appropriate placement. A horrendous murder by a juvenile will merit his or her case receiving careful and constant scrutiny at the highest levels in a way that a less emotive crime might not. But, even in this process, informal mechanisms operate.

The final set of avenues comes under the heading of education and mental health services. Most young people in this sector are behaviourally disordered or have severe special educational needs, rather than being mentally ill, and nearly all who continue to need help are referred on to the social services avenues. A tiny minority – no national figures are compiled – are diagnosed as mentally ill or have a borderline personality disorder. If the conditions laid out in the mental health legislation are met, then a place in a psychiatric hospital will be found. Some of the marginal cases will, on a psychiatrist's recommendation, be transferred to social services avenues and some pass on to youth custody. The Gardener Unit at Prestwich Hospital, for example, which undertakes observation and assessment on older adolescents, sees 40% of its leavers return home and 60% move on to other secure settings (Bailey et al. 1994).

OBSERVATIONS ON THE PROCESS

As was explained earlier, the processes just described have evolved in response to particular conditions existing at different moments in the history of services for children and young people in need. The separation of young from adult prisoners led to many initiatives and eventually to the creation of institutions which we today call youth custody. The closure of the reform schools, later known as approved schools, in the 1970s increased pressure for local-authority secure beds. The absence of provision for a young girl convicted of murder influenced the creation of the now defunct Youth Treatment Service. Given a *tabula rasa* on which to design a new service to meet the needs of difficult and disturbed young people, it is likely that the myriad of laws, routes and procedures, to say nothing of the institutions they serve, would be swept away. The complexity of the process contrasts with other parts of child welfare and juvenile justice systems where there is more logic and flexibility.

The effects of process

The overriding feature of available services is its tendency to be provision-led rather than needs-led (Harris and Timms 1993). If new treatment centres open, their beds fill with the rejects of the three sectors just described. If an institution closes, its catchment population switches seemingly effortlessly into other settings that have entirely different standards. The finding by Stewart and Tutt (1987) that in 1984 the North of England had twice the rate of young people in custody or secure accommodation than the South – including London – confirmed the provision-led nature of the system in the past. Among the reasons why the North had twice the rate of young people locked up was because it has twice the rate of secure beds available.

But young people's marginality within existing services does not mean that the process fails to influence their lives. Quite the contrary. More than most troubled young people, the interventions of statutory agencies have had a discernible effect on their lives. Many have lived away from home or been subject to specialist interventions for as long as they can remember. Those seemingly unproblematic until late adolescence might be thought of as exceptions to this rule, but watching somebody arrested for murder languish in the cell of a young offenders' institution, trying to make sense of the extraordinary chain of events set in process by the crime of which he or she is accused, rapidly revises one's opinions.

Marginality is frequently accompanied by notoriety. The grave offenders stand out by virtue of their crime. Murder, arson and rape are comparatively rare crimes and it is rarer still for a young person to be convicted of such an offence. On the other hand, those failing to evoke public scrutiny by virtue of their crimes often manage it on the basis of the high cost of sheltering them. One local authority, anxious to avoid spending the £2000 a week needed for a specialized, secure treatment bed, purchased a house on behalf of an extremely damaged youngster in their care and allocated four full-time social workers to look after him. Even those in less expensive prison department settings draw heavily on the public purse by virtue of the length of time they have to be incarcerated.

The fact that the state is prepared to shoulder the burden of such high costs reflects the particularly sensitive nature of the problems being tackled. A single individual can encompass both welfare and justice concerns. There is usually a consensus that the young person should be locked up and, where a crime has been committed, that he or she is seen to be punished. But the offender might also be a victim of abuse, neglect or disadvantage. Moreover, if he or she is very young, immature or has learning difficulties, it can be inappropriate, if not dangerous, to lock him or her up in an institution designed for older young offenders, such as youth custody. The response of the state reflects the natural urge to punish and deter others and an equally natural drive to offer young people opportunities for atonement, reform and treatment.

These influences on decision-making, which are often contradictory, are manifest in the apparently haphazard amalgam of processes described earlier. For every legal statute, there are several administrative channels to navigate, through Home Office, Department of Health, social services departments and education and health authorities. For every formal procedure, there are several informal mechanisms bound up in the traditions and practices of prison officers, social workers and mental health professionals. There is even a role in this process for the executive, although the involvement of the Home Secretary in the setting of sentences for ss90 and 91 grave offenders has been reviewed by the European Court of Human Rights, whose judgement may require revision of the legislation (Little 2002b).

None of the observations made above applies exclusively to processes for difficult and disturbed adolescents. The same provision-led features are apparent in child protection services (DoH 1995). The mix between legal, formal and administrative procedures can also be seen in services for children looked after away from home (Bullock *et al.* 1998b). But, each of these features is more marked for very difficult young people. The difference is that many of the new ways of thinking about welfare services – for example, of finding mechanisms to prioritize risk, setting out eligibility for services, ensuring that provision matches the needs of the child and identifying a single process leading to a continuum of interventions – have not been adequately adopted by those working with the most difficult young people in society.

The response of welfare and control agencies to a young person's difficulty is clearly going to influence young people's long-term life chances. The task ahead is to distil findings in a way that improves understanding of young people's career routes and to fashion predictive models that can be used by policymakers and professionals to refine and improve what is on offer for them.

Does it matter what is done?

Several research studies have explored the questions, 'What are the outcomes from different interventions?' and 'Can the same be achieved with less resource?'

Given the few young people who qualify for admission to long-stay secure units, it is difficult to make meaningful comparisons between outcomes from different establishments. We cannot simply compare reconviction rates because some long-stay units contain a significant proportion of young people who are both persistent offenders and very disturbed, a combination extremely rare in other secure settings. But what is clear is that there is no simple alternative to treatment that is outstandingly more effective. Evaluations of specialist regimes show some small but significant benefits but nothing dramatic (Bullock *et al.* 1998a; Bailey 2002; Ditchfield and Catan 1992; Marshall 1997).

On whatever dimension considered, the outcomes for very difficult young people appear to reflect the time, sophistication and effort taken by the institution selected to intervene. So, on the simple measure of conviction within two years of departure, for example, outcomes are best from the specialist centres, next best from the medium-intensive local-authority settings and worst from prison custody. These findings hold true even when young people's background characteristics, career route and protective factors are taken into account.

How can things be simplified?

To fashion an effective secure treatment service, the first exploration has to be the young people themselves. The complexity of their needs is at first mind-boggling. To start with, we know so much more about these youngsters than any other children in need. Seemingly, every profession takes an interest in them and the files rapidly expand. Every page explores another risk factor that interacts with one appearing in the previous section only to be ameliorated by a potential protective mechanism highlighted by somebody else. Each case takes professionals to the limits of their understanding and is usually beyond the ken of the typical lay person. No wonder the media take shelter behind words like 'evil'.

But there is an underlying pattern to all this misery. That much is evident when the young people's careers are analysed. For example, in the Dartington Unit's study of long-stay secure treatment units in England, five groups of young people were identified:

- those long in local-authority care who exceed the capabilities of good open residential provision
- those long dealt with by education, school psychology services and mental health services
- those previously unknown to control and welfare agencies whose behaviour deteriorates in mid-adolescence
- those who commit a one-off grave crime
- persistent delinquents who also commit a serious offence.

This classification would be of limited interest if the five groups had no predictive power but, within a reasonable degree of confidence, it is possible to say what a long-term state care case or an adolescent 'erupter' in the third group will be doing two years after referral, five years, and so on. There is some indication of where they will be living; what kinds of family and social relationships they will enjoy; how much trouble they will get into; whether they will go to school, get a job, fall ill or move about – and the same would be true for other groups of difficult young people.

Pattern and order are less apparent, however, in the response of the state to these young people. To say that the process is messy would not be far from the truth. Mess may not be a bad thing when dealing with adolescents, especially where flexibility and adaptability follow, but successive additions to legislation, national policy, local services and provider organizations have made the system very difficult to understand and has meant that long-stay does not necessarily guarantee that effective treatment is forthcoming. The exclusion of young offenders from the reforms that led to the Children Act 1989 did not help very difficult adolescents since it directed them to a system where the child's needs are not paramount. Similarly, the introduction of the national curriculum has restricted the type of education that can be offered to the young people. At an administrative level, the powers of the local child-protection service for teenagers in secure settings remain ambiguous. While each agency is probably satisfied with its approach to the majority of its users, some consolidation is necessary for these very difficult adolescents if each player in the process is to comprehend fully its role in relation to others.

This is not to say that current arrangements are without strengths. For many of the young people, the process produces results. The pragmatic English make it work but the system does not have its own internal logic. If we were starting from scratch, could we say with any certainty that the process we would design would look much like anything currently in place?

WHAT WOULD WE SEEK TO CHANGE?

Since the implementation of the Children Act 1989, child welfare in England has become increasingly a needs-led service; it is moving away from being driven by available provision. In this, secure accommodation and services for the most difficult and disturbed young people have moved much more slowly than other parts of children's services. Too often, the number of beds has determined the threshold defining extremely difficult or disturbed when it is the threshold that should determine the number of beds.

Increasingly – again using England as a benchmark – services are designed to meet the identified wide-ranging needs of children and young people referred for help. Once known to health, education and social services, most cases behave predictably and this information can be used to design an effective response to young people's problems. Too often the young people have been marginal to available interventions and the 'specialism' of the specialist places is their ability to pick up the pieces.

All this adds up to a failure to apply concepts that characterize a modern child welfare service to the most difficult cases. Much has been written about linking the concepts of need, threshold, services and outcome, and some research teams have worked closely with local authorities to put these ideas into practice. The aim has been to encourage agencies to move on from offering isolated initiatives to ones which prioritise risk, introduce eligibility criteria, encourage practitioners to respond creatively to the needs of children and families and adopt a perspective that sees all services as integral to a continuum, each part of which is useful to different cases at different moments in their care careers. All of this has become commonplace in the child protection arena but it is hardly entertained when it comes to very problematic adolescents. The end result is a piecemeal design that is no longer sufficient for the complexities it is intended to address.

MESSAGES FOR RESEARCH

The need on managers and practitioners is ever more pressing to explain outcomes and, therefore, to bring some additional rigour to the debate about 'what works' with very difficult young people. In order to facilitate this, we have used the terms 'life route', 'process' and 'career' and attempted to show how they are linked. The hope is that this will contribute to the achievement of a common language in child welfare; so that wherever difficult young people are discussed, there can be a surer sense that professionals are comparing like with like and that their responses are more consistent across the country. Clearly defined and widely accepted concepts also move research a little further forward towards what might be envisaged as a 'unified theory of children in need'. This concept refers to two types of connection; first between the concepts, methods and approaches, such as career, process, life route, risk indicators and protective factors, and, second, between the ideas that underpin research, the organization of welfare services and professional practice.

All of this represents a tall order and the image may, in retrospect, turn out to be little more than a chimera. The most contentious aspect is prediction. But however much the reader may quarrel with the evidence, it would be hard to dispute that for most of the young people discussed there are clear links between experiences prior to, during and after their stay in treatment. Would it not be beneficial if there were some place for the methods used to identifying these predictabilities in the organization of services and the processes applied to the young people?

In saying this, however, we have to be mindful that there are inevitably limits to what can be achieved. It is virtually impossible to forecast which ten of the several hundred thousand children in need each year will be convicted of a homicide. But we ought to be better than we are at predicting which 5000 of the 30,000 children looked after each year will stay long away from home and be vulnerable to 'drift', and we can be reasonably certain about the prospects of the 150 or so among the 5000 long-known children whose situation requires specialist interventions in long-term secure conditions each year.

OUTCOMES

The most important part of any process is obviously the outcome. Inevitably with these young people, there are

some shock and horror stories. There are also picture-book successes worthy of the glossiest magazine. Perhaps the most disappointing results are to do with outputs; that is to say measures of professional activity. The contrast between what these young people receive in specialist treatment centres and what they get after leaving is frequently sharp. Local authorities are capable of investing several hundreds of thousands of pounds on a long-term state care case up to the age of 18 years but often do very little thereafter, even to the extent of failing to allocate a social worker, despite requirements in the Children (Leaving Care) Act 1999. Prediction ought to extend to a reasonable sense of how much expenditure will be required from point of referral to achieve a reasonable outcome at 21 or, better still, 25 years.

There is also a contrast to be drawn between the progress made by the young people and development within their families. On the whole, the young people move on but their families do not; nor are there many changes in the environment in which the young person lives. More could be done to draw relatives into the treatment process and to link institutional and community intervention while the young person is away. At the every least, this finding is a reminder that treatment should teach strategies to help the young person cope with what has contributed to his or her difficulty in the past.

These messages are particularly important since most young people return home at some point to live with relatives and most of those who fail to get back have some contact with the family. There may be a continuing reliance on birth family since, on the whole, difficult and disturbed adolescents are not good at making enduring relationships, although some quickly become parents themselves.

The finding that the environment to which young people return remains depressingly constant is a reminder of the importance of education and employment opportunities to those who are disadvantaged. Yet, on the whole, attention to social functioning has been allowed to detract from attention to education so that, despite extended stays, few graduates from specialized treatment emerge with useful qualifications; and the consequence is that many never find work and some of those who do get employment lose it quickly because they do not have the wherewithal to cope with the ordinary stresses of the work environment.

In situations where the young person's living situation is relatively stable, some recent developments are tackling these problems. For example, Youth Offending Teams are multi-professional, employ consistent methods of needs assessment, and combine work with young people and families. Similarly, the detention and training order links institutional and community support. But for very difficult adolescents, the situation is less auspicious. There is movement between and within institutions and the agencies responsible for supervision bicker and change.

Placements deemed suitable may also be full so limiting other aspirations, such as proximity to the young person's home. In addition, many young people present complex needs that remain unmet however ambitious the new services might be. Surveys of the mental health of young people in residential institutions, for instance, show very high levels of illness and disorder, some of which far exceed the treatment capabilities of the settings in which the young people reside. Nichol *et al.* (2000) found that three-quarters of the young people living in all residential settings in a geographical region of England had significant problems, which included hyperactivity, conduct disorders, substance abuse and depression. A few inmates had even more serious conditions such as psychosis or suicidal tendencies.

In other areas, where efforts have been more concentrated, outcomes are more encouraging. The physical and psychological health of graduates is reasonable, given the poor expectations on entry to treatment. Their pattern of living arrangements usually reflects the pattern established prior to the treatment sojourn, which is a problem for those long in state care but reasonably favourable for those who are not. Offending outcomes are also positive. Naturally, the goal has to be no repeat serious offending, an objective not yet met. But, generally, conviction rates were lower than had been expected and, unusually for work in this area, the prospect of a relationship between different treatment strategies and improved offending behaviour was apparent.

While stressing that outcomes are moderately good and predictable, follow-up studies of leavers from long-stay secure treatment settings show that a positive situation at 18 or 21 is no indication of a life happy thereafter. Many have stored up problems of health or of isolation from work that will haunt them later on. Many have settled in happy domestic relationships that are supportive now but will come under strain in subsequent years. Most of the grave offenders have been law abiding but must be considered a long-term risk. Further interventions will almost certainly be necessary. Thus, the process will continue to be an important determinant of what happens to young people.

The relative lack of scientific and practice knowledge about what happens to disordered young people between, say, the ages of 18 and 25 or 30 is striking. In the past, researchers and professionals have tended to approach young adults as being merely extensions of adolescents. So, we complain about a task remaining unfinished, such as the failure to offer a good education, but are less concerned with a new task, such as encouraging late entry to continuing education or teaching social skills to stay in work. Working with young adults is not about doing more of the same.

So, existing research spawns further explanation. More evidence is needed on how careers develop, whether or not protective factors continue to operate and how long the effects of treatment last. It is, after all, only by looking at what happens in the very long term that we can know whether the cautious optimism resulting from achievements to date is well founded.

REFERENCES

Bailey, S. 2002: Treatment of delinquents. In Rutter, M. and Taylor, E. (eds) *Child and Adolescent Psychiatry.* Oxford: Blackwell, 1019–37.

Bailey, S., Thornton, L. and Weaver, A. 1994: The first 100 admissions to an adolescent secure unit. *Journal of Adolescence* XVII: 1–13.

Bullock, R., Little, M. and Millham, S. 1998a: *Secure Treatment Outcomes: the Care Careers of Very Difficult Adolescents.* Aldershot: Ashgate.

Bullock, R., Gooch, D. and Little, M. 1998b: *Going Home: the Re-unification of Families.* Aldershot: Ashgate.

Ditchfield, J. and Catan, L. 1992: *Juveniles Sentenced for Serious Offences: a Comparison of Regimes in Young Offender Institutions and Local Authority Community Homes.* London: Home Office Research and Planning Unit.

DoH (Department of Health) (annual publication): *Children Accommodated in Secure Units.* London: Government Statistical Service, www.doh.gov.uk/public/stats3.htm.

Harris, R. and Timms, N. 1993: *Secure Accommodation in Child Care: Between Hospital and Prison or Thereabouts.* London: Routledge.

Little, M. 2002a: *Prediction: Perspectives on Diagnosis, Prognosis and Interventions for Children in Need.* Dartington: Warren House Press.

Little, M. 2002b: The law concerning services for children with social and psychological needs. In Rutter, M. and Taylor, E. (eds) *Child and Adolescent Psychiatry.* Oxford: Blackwell, 1175–87.

Marshall, P. 1997: *A Reconviction Study of HMP Grendon Therapeutic Community.* London: Home Office Research and Statistics Directorate.

Nicol, R., Stretch, D., Whitney, I. *et al.* 2000: Mental health needs and services for severely troubled and troubling young people, including young offenders in an NHS region. *Journal of Adolescence* **23**: 243–61.

Rutter, M., Giller, H. and Hagell, A. 1998: *Anti-Social Behavior.* Oxford: Blackwell.

Ryan, M. 1999: *The Children Act 1989: Putting it into Practice.* Aldershot: Ashgate.

Stewart, G. and Tutt, N. 1987: *Children in Custody.* Aldershot: Avebury.

BIBLIOGRAPHY

Bullock, R. 2001: Juvenile offending: treatment in residential settings. In Hollin, C. (ed.), *Offender Assessment and Treatment.* Chichester: John Wiley, 537–50.

Department of Health 1995: *Child Protection. Messages from Research.* London: HMSO.

Department of Health 1998: *Caring for Children Away from Home: Messages from Research.* Chichester: John Wiley.

Department of Health 2001: *The Children Act Now: Messages from Research*. London: HMSO.

Hagell, A. and Hazel, N. 2000: *An Evaluation of Medway Youth Training Centre*. London: Policy Research Bureau.

Haggerty, R., Sherrod, L., Garmezy, N. and Rutter, M. 1995: *Stress, Risk and Resilience in Children and Adolescents: Processes, Mechanisms and Interventions*. Cambridge: Cambridge University Press.

Hollin, C. and Howells, K. 1996: *Clinical Approaches to Working with Young Offenders*. Chichester: John Wiley.

Kelly, B. 1992: *Children Inside: Rhetoric and Practice in a Locked Institution for Children*. London: Routledge.

Little, M. 1990: *Young Men in Prison: the Criminal Identity Explored Through the Rules of Behaviour*. Aldershot: Dartmouth.

Little, M. and Kelly, S. 1996: *A Life without Problems: the Achievements of a Therapeutic Community*. Aldershot: Arena.

Little, M. and Mount, K. 1999: *Prevention and Early Intervention with Children in Need*. Aldershot: Ashgate.

Little, M., Kogan, J., Bullock, R. and van der Laan, P. (forthcoming): ISSP: an experiment in multi-systemic responses to persistent young offenders known to children's services. *British Journal of Criminology* (in press).

Millham, S., Bullock, R. and Cherrett, P. 1975: *After Grace-Teeth: a Comparative Study of the Residential Experiences of Boys in Approved Schools*. London: Human Context Books.

Millham, S., Bullock, R. and Hosie, K. 1978: *Locking Up Children: Secure Provision within the Child Care System*. Farnborough: Saxon House.

Rutter, M. and Smith, D. (eds) 1995: *Psychosocial Disorders in Young People: Time Trends and their Causes*. Chichester: John Wiley.

25

Child protection in context: a systemic approach

ARNON BENTOVIM

INTRODUCTION

The consideration of child protection in adolescent forensic psychiatric practice is complex. Young people referred for assessment and treatment are at the confluence of so many systems, not only their family and social context, but often police services who have investigated criminal actions. Youth Offending Teams (YOTs) may be involved as a result. Social services teams may also be involved as often these are young people who may have given rise to earlier concerns, and there has often been extensive contact with families. Other community agencies may be involved playing a role in the young person's life, or may represent those individuals, families and communities against whom a young person may have offended against.

Not only are there many agencies and professional systems concerned with the young person, but there may well be also an inherent contradiction in the beliefs and attitudes of these agencies when young people whose behaviour is dangerous are investigated. The Institute of Child Health's programme of research on the development of abusive behaviour in young people who have been sexually abused (Skuse *et al.* 1998; Bentovim and Williams 1998) demonstrates that those young people who are most dangerous to other children are often the young people whose history demonstrates the greatest need for protection. Such children who are themselves highly dangerous have often been subject to extensive abuse, as well as exposure to physical violence perpetrated against a parent, and have been subject to physical abuse, rejection, disruption of care. The parents themselves may have been extensively abused.

These young people require therapeutic work directed at the impact of such abusive action perpetrated against themselves, and they may well require child-protection action to ensure that they do not continue to live in an environment which reinforces and perpetuates abusive action against them. Other children in the community need to be protected from their abusive actions. Thus such young people require a specific focus from professionals concerned with their offending behaviour, and from professionals who need to consider the young person's need for protection. Mental health professionals need to understand the current functioning of the young person, and to appreciate experiences which may have played a salient role in shaping and determining his or her current dangerous behaviour. Family contexts need to be understood, past and present. Such work needs to be carried out collaboratively between professionals and agencies working to the benefit of the young person. The potential for conflict and failure of working together is only too easy given the multiplicity of professional systems, workers, individuals and family members potentially involved.

A SYSTEMIC APPROACH

General issues

One approach to assist professionals in collaboration rather than conflict is to employ a systemic approach to the task. Systemic thinking arose in the 1960s when Von Bertalanffy (1962) set out the principles of general systems theory in response to then current dissatisfactions with a reductionist cause-and-effect tradition. The reductionist tradition attempted to explain complex multi-dimensional events in terms of simple cause-and-effect chains. General systems theory focused attention on pattern and form of the organization of biological systems. This type of analysis was later extended to psychosocial systems, including the family. A system is defined as 'an organized arrangement of elements consisting of a network of interdependent coordinated parts that function as a unit'. From a systems perspective the family was therefore seen as developing characteristic patterns and core ways of being and relating. Such patterns were thought to be carried forward in life in subsequent social contexts by family members.

Thus systems thinking encompasses a number of different issues, which include:

- a philosophy of observation which includes the context as well as the object concerned
- an approach to treating problems in context, which includes the individual, the family, and those concerned with them
- a number of methods of treatment, the best known being family therapy – there are far broader implications for treatment using a systemic prospective.

Such a perspective enables one to think of the way in which particular systems of relationships give rise to problematic behaviour. In addition, the way such problematic behaviour is defined in turn comes to organize relationships. So, 'problem-determined systems' are as important to consider as 'system-determined problems'.

Thus an important aspect of such an approach requires us to understand the way in which professionals have come to define the nature of social problems. The way we conceptualize problems has often arisen through a process of social construction. The nature of problems has been recognized as a result of the bringing together of different viewpoints, which results in a specific way of seeing a problem rather than being recognized as a 'pathological entity'.

Child protection: a systemic view

The child-protection system is a socially constructed entity. The current view of child protection emerged out of the dramatic response to the key article written by Henry Kempe *et al.* in 1962, 'The battered child syndrome'. There is ample evidence from other papers published earlier that severe physical abuse against children was recognized, but there was little professional notice or understanding of the processes involved. The publication of Kempe and associates's paper, and the marked professional response which followed, led to the widespread recognition that children were being 'battered', but they had not been perceived as such. Professional concern led

to the beginnings of child-protection systems in the USA, the UK and many other countries.

Kempe (1978) subsequently wrote of the sequence of recognition of different forms of abuse: severe physical abuse, neglect, emotional abuse and finally sexual and institutional abuse. Systems have been constructed to recognize, to manage, and to intervene to prevent such processes occurring. An elaborate inter-professional system of area child-protection committees have been established in the UK which consider the need of each local area. Relevant disciplines are represented, agency practice is developed. Strategy meetings are convened bringing police, social work and health professionals together when concerns about a specific child are raised. Case conferences are arranged to determine whether the child needs to be registered as in need of child protection and a protection plan devised to involve relevant community agencies. A legal process has developed to ensure that protection can be delivered at all levels of seriousness of threat to a child's or young person's well-being. Professional guidelines are produced by government departments to lay down standards of practice (e.g. DoH 2000a). This process led to the rewriting and bringing together of all law relating to children in the Children Act 1989.

Thus child protection is an entity, which has become elaborated around the recognition of the fact that children can be harmed within a family context. Society needs to develop ways of protecting children in their families, and of recognizing their rights to 'good enough care' rather than seeing children as parents' property. Child protection is therefore an aspect of attitudes which are developing within the societal context, where the rights of children, the rights of women, and the rights of families are argued and debated. Viewpoints change and influence each other in a systemic manner.

The nature of offending behaviour can also be constructed in a social context through definition of what offending acts are, the way such acts are perceived within the family, and the wider social context. There is a need to consider the intimate relationships between the young person who has offended, other family members, the history of those involved in such relationships, and the wider social network and context of which the family and the adolescent are part. An abusive act is defined differently by the perpetrating individual, the victim, the members of the family within the household, extended family, and institutions with whom such household members have daily contacts, whether these be in the spheres of education, health, social services or criminal justice.

Abusive behaviour perpetrated by young people has itself been the subject of developing thinking. Earlier there was a widespread belief that sexual activities perpetrated by young people were harmless sexual explorations. Those abused by young people gave very different stories – abusive action could be harmful, and young people who perpetrated sexually abusive acts should be considered as potentially dangerous young people and that such actions could continue into adult life. The confluence between young people whose behaviour is dangerous, and the fact that they have been subjected to damaging behaviour themselves, brings together the consideration of child protection in adolescent forensic psychiatry.

The child-protection framework

The child-protection framework in its current form derives from the Children Act 1989 which attempted to articulate a new approach to meeting the needs of children. This followed condemnation of professional intervention in family life as described in the Cleveland enquiry, where it was felt that too many children were removed from their parents' care because of suspicion that abuse had occurred. The Act was intended to create a new balance: children needed to be protected, but their long-term welfare also had to be promoted. It was felt that the family should be the best place for children to be raised, and that parents rather than local authorities should exercise responsibility for their children and decide what was best for them. Local authorities were therefore given responsibility (Part 3 of the Act) to provide support through services for families where children were defined as being in need, and to provide protection for children suffering or likely to suffer significant harm under Parts 4 and 5 of the Act. This followed investigation, if necessary applying to a Court for an interim-care or supervision order to provide adequate protection.

The key difference between the sections of the act focused on whether provisions could be made through cooperation with the parents (s17), versus the necessity for compulsion, through the acquisition of parental responsibility by a local authority, and the possibility of removing the child against parents' wishes (s31). There was also the important introduction of the concept of local authorities providing services to promote healthy development of children, either within the family, or by looking after children away from the family on a planned basis. The basic principles underpinning the Act reflect these ideas:

- Local authorities must work in partnership with parents and assist them to meet their responsibilities.
- There must be a minimal level of intrusion into family life; grounds for intervention need to be specific.
- It must be recognized that some parents *do* harm children, and the duty to investigate is strengthened. At all stages in the course of child-protection work, even if significant harm has occurred, consideration should be given to the possibility of working voluntarily with the family.
- Courts should not make orders unless doing so would be better for the child.

- If care orders are made by a Court, local authorities have a duty to return children to their families wherever this is possible.
- Health, education and other agencies have a duty to assist social services in the development and provision of both family support services and child protection.

Significant harm

An important construction introduced to the Children Act 1989 was 'significant harm', a concept which applied to duties to investigate, or make enquiries to the emergency protection system, and to care proceedings when required.

Harm was defined as either ill-treatment, or the impairment of health or development as a result of parents' failure to provide adequate care.

- Ill-treatment included all forms of abuse: sexual, physical and emotional.
- Impairment of health was focused on physical or mental health.
- Impairment of development was focused on physical, intellectual, emotional, social or behavioural developments.

Thus children were included who have or are likely to have impaired health or development within the definition of being a 'child in need' – the latter being defined as those children with disability (broadly defined) in the community who are unlikely to achieve or maintain a reasonable standard of health or development without the services of the local authority.

Local authorities have a statutory duty under s47/1 of the Children Act to make enquiries to decide whether action should be taken to safeguard or promote a child's welfare when they are informed that a child living or found in their area is suffering, or may be likely to be suffering, significant harm. There is a duty on local, educational, housing and health authorities to work together in such enquires. There have been a number of editions of guidance from government departments, such as *Working Together to Safeguard Children* (DoH 2000a), to help different agencies to develop best practice in such situations. Thus a strategy-meeting structure has developed to ensure that observations made about any child in the area can be brought together immediately by police, social work and health professionals. Decisions can then be made as to the nature of the concerns, how they should be investigated, and who should carry out the investigation. Such enquiries are brought together in the context of a child-protection conference to which representatives of all relevant agencies are invited, which includes the parents or children themselves if they are old enough to participate.

The most recent *Working Together* document spells out the roles and responsibilities to report and to take action, including local authorities, social services, educational services, youth services, health services, the police, probation services, and the wider community. Emergency protection can be applied for under s44 of the Children Act 1989, provided the Court is satisfied that there is reasonable cause to believe that the child is likely to suffer significant harm if:

- he or she is not removed to accommodation provided by or on behalf of the applicant, or
- the individual does not remain in the place where he or she is then being accommodated.

This is an important provision for those young people who it is felt are currently living in a context of considerable danger, or for those young people who may have left home and have found a safe venue to ensure that they can remain in such a placement, if there is a threat to a young person being removed from a context where he or she is considered to be safe. There is the possibility of a child being accommodated with the collaboration of parents under s20 of the Act. It is important that such issues be considered and the mechanisms to achieve safety be known.

The emphasis of the Act implies that at all times even when children are felt to be at risk, or to have been significantly harmed, there should be a working partnership between the authority and the family to provide services.

The criteria to take care proceedings – that is, for a local authority to take parental responsibility and to curb the parents' use of their responsibility – depends on whether the case reaches the threshold which includes:

- that the child concerned is suffering significant harm, or is likely to suffer significant harm
- the harm or likely harm is attributable to:
  - the care given to the child, or likely to be given to him if the order were not made, not being what it would be reasonable to expect a parent to give to him, or
  - the child is beyond parental control, 'rejecting' care offered and putting himself or herself in danger.

The child-protection process which developed as a result of social construction both before and after introduction of the Children Act 1989 has been the subject of considerable research and scrutiny (e.g. DoH 1995). A number of concerns have been raised, including the fact that professionals sometimes used statutory enquiries as a means of trying to obtain services for children, the state of the children not necessarily being attributable to the sort of care being given. It was noted that too often there was a narrow focus on abuse and whether abuse or neglect had occurred without considering the wider needs and circumstances of the child and family. Such enquires themselves could have highly stressful effects on families, family anxieties were not dealt with adequately, and there was a need for developing work in partnership rather than using authority when it was not required. Professionals

were too concerned about registering the children as having suffered significant harm without safeguarding the children and supporting the families afterwards. Inter-agency work, although often effective in times of crisis, did not continue adequately afterwards.

It was therefore felt it was necessary to refocus the aims of child welfare services.

- The focus should be on the benefits of intervention for the child's long-term well-being.
- Time and resources should be invested across agencies to plan and implement such interventions. It was essential to aim for good long-term outcomes in terms of health, development and educational achievement.
- It was important to develop services for children in need without triggering child-protection processes unnecessarily.
- It was important to ensure that children's views were taken into account, that parents and family members be fully involved. There should be a constructive tone for future interventions, and a realistic image of services to encourage and enable people to gain access to help and advice, rather than to fear revealing their problems.
- There should be skilled assessments, with multi-disciplinary provisions.
- There should be a growing awareness of the multiplicity of factors which affect the parents' ability to care. Family strengths should be built on.
- It was essential to work across boundaries to give due consideration not only for the child's safety and welfare, but the needs of all family members.
- Complementary roles should be recognized for adults and children, health and social care, with the pooling of expertise to strengthen parents' capacities to respond to their children's needs.
- It was essential to ensure that parents' problems and their effects on children should be adequately recognized and appropriate intervention provided.

The following more comprehensive definition of significant harm was adopted (Bentovim 1998a). Significant harm is:

'a compilation of significant events, both acute and longstanding which interact with the child's ongoing development, and interrupt, alter or impair physical and psychological development. Being the victim of significant harm is likely to have a profound effect on the child's view of [himself or herself] as a person and on [his or her future life]. Significant harm represents a major symptom of failure of adaptation by parents to their role, and also involves both family and society.'

In coming to this definition it was asserted that acts of family violence did not uniquely belong to the individual who perpetrates the violent act, or to the family within whose boundaries such violence occurred, or society which defined what was and what was not appropriate violence, but belongs to all three. Society contains attitudes, norms, rights and values about what degree of violence is permitted and against whom within the family and in what circumstances. Society legitimizes some violence and sees the violence or 'discipline' of family members as being approved in its proper place. Violent interactions and roles are an integral aspect of this process: individuals create families and regulate meanings within them, individuals are nurtured within the family, and their beliefs are organized about appropriate levels of violence. There is conforming or reaction against societal and family attitudes concerning violence and violent behaviour. Thus a cycle of violent actions is maintained or terminated in what has been termed a 'trauma-organized system' (Bentovim 1995). Violent actions evoke traumatic stress effects in the victims, and the repeated nature of such actions comes to organize the reality and perceptions of those participating, including potential protectors and professionals who become involved in the family's situation.

Child protection in specific circumstances

The most recent consultation document on working together to safeguard children (DoH 2000) has described a number of special circumstances which have particular relevance to the adolescent forensic psychiatric field.

It is recognized that children and young people who abuse others, including those who sexually abuse/offend, are likely to be children who have considerable needs themselves, and who may pose a significant risk of harm to other children. Research evidence suggests that children who abuse others may have suffered considerable disruption in their lives, will have been exposed to violence, will have witnessed or been subjected to physical and sexual abuse, will have problems in educational development, are likely to be children in need, and some will in addition be suffering or be at risk of significant harm and may be in need of protection at the time of professional concern as well as in the past (Skuse et al. 1998).

It is felt that such children and young people who abuse others should be held responsible for their abusive behaviour, whilst being identified and responded to in a way in which their needs are met, as well as protecting the public, by preventing the continuation or escalation of abusive behaviours amongst those young people who are likely to continue such a pattern. To achieve these goals, the following are suggested:

- There should be a coordinated approach on the part of youth justice, child welfare agencies, and health agencies.
- The needs of children and young people who abuse others should be considered separately from the needs of their victims.

- An assessment should be carried out in each case, appreciating unmet developmental needs, as well as specific needs arising from the offending child's behaviour.
- It is recommended that area child-protection committees who plan and coordinate services in each district, and YOTs, should ensure that there is a clear operational framework in place within which assessment, decision-making and case management takes place. It is recommended that neither child welfare, nor criminal justice agencies should embark upon a course of action that has implications for the other without appropriate consultation.
- It is essential that the health component of these young people's needs is fully explored.

These are important guidelines, and there is a requirement for extensive assessment of such young people to advise on the appropriate course of action. Specific decisions need to be made so that agencies such as the Crown Prosecution Service, YOTs, social services and those providing adolescent forensic services can decide:

- the most appropriate course of action within the criminal justice system, if the child is above the age of criminal responsibility
- whether the young abuser should be the subject of the child-protection system
- the mental health needs of the young person, and use of mental health provisions
- what plan of action should be put in place to address the needs of the young person, and what should be the involvement of all relevant agencies.

The view has been put forward that the young person who is responsible for abusive behaviour should not be the subject of a child-protection conference unless he or she is considered personally to be at continuing risk of significant harm. Whilst there may be no reason to hold a specific child-protection conference, there may still be a need for a multi-agency approach if the young abuser's needs are complex. Issues regarding educational and accommodation arrangements often require skilled and careful consideration. Where the young person has a specific psychiatric state, then the interface between mental health actions and orders may need to be put in the context of child-protection needs, as well as criminal action. Operational policies in each district, and roles and responsibilities, and the requirement to look at the individual young person's needs, are an important aspect of this particular process.

Children and young people living away from home

A further consideration in the consultation document *Working Together* is the protection of children living away from home. Revelations of widespread sexual, physical and emotional abuse of children living away from home have raised awareness of a particular vulnerability of children in such residential settings – to sexual, physical and emotional abuse and neglect, including peer abuse and bullying. Settings in which children live away from home should provide the same basic safeguards against abuse, and the development of an approach which promotes general welfare, and protects from harm of all kinds, and treats young people with dignity and respect. The child-protection procedures which are developed in each area must apply to children living away from home. It is advocated that there are a number of basic safeguards for all settings which include local authority, health and education settings, young-offender institutions and secure units.

- Children should be valued and respected, with self-esteem promoted as a basic principle.
- There should be openness to the external world and external scrutiny, openness with families and in the wider community.
- Staff and carers should be trained in all aspects of safeguarding children, alert to children's vulnerabilities and risks of harm, and knowledgeable about how to implement child-protection procedures.
- There should be regular and programmed access to trusted adults outside the institution: family members, social workers, independent visitors, advocates. Children should always be made aware of help they could receive from independent advocacy services, external mentors, and ChildLine.
- Complaints procedures should be clear, effective, user-friendly, readily accessible. The procedures should address informal as well as formal complaints. There needs to be an open communication about minor complaints as well as major complaints, and a register in each context.
- Recruitment and selection procedures should be rigorous, creating a high threshold of entry to deter abusers.
- Clear procedures and support systems should be in place to deal with expressions of concern by staff and carers about other staff or carers. A code of conduct needs to be established which instructs staff of their professional obligation to raise concerns, and procedures that do not prejudice whistle-blowers' positions and prospects.
- There should be a respect of diversity and sensitivity to race, culture, religion, gender and disability at all times.
- There needs to be an awareness of institutionalized and personally directed racism, active policies to prevent and confront all forms of racial abuse and harassment.
- There needs to be an alertness to risks to children from people exploiting them.

- Peer abuse must be taken as seriously as abuse perpetrated by adults, and should be subject to the same child-protection procedures. The importance of understanding differences between consenting, abusive, exploitative or inappropriate peer relationships needs to be recognized. There should not be high thresholds before taking actions.
- Bullying – defined as deliberately hurtful behaviour, repeated over a period of time – can take many forms, physical, verbal, or indirect. All settings need to have rigorously enforced anti-bullying strategies. Appropriate mechanisms and structures need to be developed to ensure that allegations of abuse committed by any professional, carer or volunteer are appropriately investigated.

CHILD PROTECTION IN THE CONTEXT OF ASSESSMENT AND THERAPEUTIC WORK

Assessment

There needs to be detailed assessment of the family context in which the young person presenting to an adolescent forensic mental health practitioner has grown up. A core assessment will often have been constructed prior to specialist referral following guidelines introduced by the Department of Health in 2000 – *The Framework for the Assessment of Children in Need and their Families* (DoH 2000b). This eco-systemic approach considers the domains of the child's needs, the capacity of the parents to meet them, and the family and social environment. Information needs to be gathered about psychiatric issues in the family history, and in addition there should be a focus on the parents' own experiences in childhood, the nature of their relationships, and attachment patterns which have resulted. An assessment needs to be made of both current and past domestic violence and abusive behaviour perpetrated against young people, and for which they are responsible. How aware are the parents of their children's problems? How do they understand the nature of their difficulties, and their motivation to protect if there is current abuse within the family context? Is there an understanding of the impact of past abusive patterns, and an assessment of a capacity to provide appropriate care currently and in the future?

There needs to be a detailed assessment of the young person, both of past and present psychiatric diagnosis and mental state, and a particular examination of the way in which his or her own experiences of violence and disruptive care have had an impact. It is important to make an assessment of the traumatic developmental effects of such experiences, and the way in which these have been transformed into current abusive patterns and potential.

The potential for therapeutic work needs to be tested actively, both for the child and for family members, in terms of motivation and some basic understanding of what is going to be required in the particular situation. There needs to be an assessment of whether there is an awareness of the need for therapeutic work that is focused on reversing the traumatic impact of family life, as well as supporting the safe behaviour of the young person and promoting the development of safe patterns of behaviour.

The prognosis for therapeutic work

Calder (1997) developed a model, based on Bentovim *et al.* (1987), to bring together the distinctive characteristics of cases to decide on the prognosis for therapeutic work, and whether statutory childcare proceedings were necessary to provide a safe context for care of the young person, and to reverse abusive family contexts and ensure future safety. It was found helpful to use the following categories:

1   *Hopeful prognosis* – a potential for working in partnership with the family without statutory intervention.
2   *Doubtful prognosis* – there not being sufficient information to be certain that it is possible to work in partnership, or that alternatively statutory intervention was required to work with the family.
3   *Hopeless prognosis* – there being no hope for working in partnership, so statutory intervention is required.

Silvester *et al.* (1995) tested the usefulness of these distinctions, showing that an attributional analysis of the statements made by family members correlated well with assessments. There is a parallel process in terms of assessment of dangerousness depending on the state of the young person, and the way in which his or her previous actions, and present patterns of impulsiveness and abnormal mental states, lead to a requirement to ensure safety for the young person, or for the environment.

THE HOPEFUL PROGNOSIS

There is a hopeful prognosis from therapeutic work when the young person accepts responsibility for any offending behaviour or abusive actions, both against family members and those outside. The individual is able to admit such activities to the family.

Family members do not take on a blaming or scapegoating attitude; for instance they do not blame the victim if that individual is within or close to the family. They understand and accept that offending dangerous behaviour has occurred, and that there is a requirement for protection both of the young person who has offended, and those who have been offended against.

Parents or appropriate family members are willing to take an appropriate level of responsibility for having

failed to protect victims, or to have been unaware of the state of the young person. There is some appropriate taking of responsibility, or capacity to reflect on previous family contexts, abusive action, the presence of destructive levels of domestic violence or abusive experiences. There is a willingness to engage in activities to deal with such experiences in the past and present. The family context is not one where such patterns are going to continue to a destructive level.

For a hopeful prognosis, parents are able to manage the protection of victims if they are within the family context, and also provide support for the young person who has offended. They are able to supervise contact, support work through a cooperative collaborative partnership with professionals, and make commitment to ongoing professional involvement, to ensure attendance at appropriate therapeutic care contexts. In addition, other relevant family members and siblings are willing to engage in appropriate family work, to develop self-protective skills.

In these situations where a hopeful prognosis is envisaged, it may be possible to work collaboratively with parents, provided that ongoing highly destructive or rigid family relationships do not predominate. Working in partnership may thus be feasible. There may be no necessity for statutory child-protection action.

When a young person's psychiatric state, or level of dangerousness to self or others, is high, there may be a requirement for a Court care order so that there can be sharing care between social services and the family if the young person is deemed to be 'beyond parental control'. For instance, secure accommodation can be provided, or other accommodation if it is acknowledged that levels of dangerousness are too high for the young person to remain within the community. Such an assessment may have a significant impact if the young person is within the criminal system as a result of the seriousness of any offending activities. The capacity of parents working reliably with professionals has an important impact on the planning for the young person. Alternatively action may need to be taken under the Mental Health Act 1983 to provide appropriate care.

CASES OF DOUBTFUL PROGNOSIS

The concept of doubtfulness is based on the view taken in the initial phase of assessments when it remains unclear whether the family and young person are going to work together with the professional system. There may be an initial denial of seriousness, and opposition to attempts to confront the nature of problems and to engage all family members in work to contain any dangerous and abusive behaviour.

Particular difficulties are noted where there is a multigenerational family culture of abuse which is denied. Such situations are commonly very doubtful in terms of possible work and change. Denial of abusive action, secrecy

If there has been a Court proceeding and the local authority is sharing parenting, then review meetings in which mental health therapeutic agencies report progress to the care agency can be a helpful way of prioritizing goals both for the young person who is abused, as well as victims and parents.

New information may emerge that there has been extensive victimization, having an important bearing on the young person's current status. Issues such as contact with the young person, and protection from ongoing harassments, may have to be considered. The process then needs to be re-configured as a crisis context, and strategy meetings between relevant police and social work professionals may be required to assess the young person's needs.

Similarly, when a young person within a residential or other context is demonstrating highly dangerous behaviours, the whole child-protection context must be reviewed. Assessment of the young person's needs should be kept under review, perhaps for more secure accommodation, a different mental health approach, or the protection of other children within the family.

Work with the family or other children may reveal that there has been major stresses within the family, such as widespread abuse and domestic violence, which perhaps have been denied or minimized in earlier phases of assessment.

The involvement of a social worker may be essential to maintain a child-protection perspective in the face of the often highly complex structure required to cope with the management of young people showing challenging or dangerous behaviours to themselves or others. There is a necessary questioning of the safety of procedures, of therapeutic approaches, of looking at issues of restraint, medication use, family contact, and both medium and longer-term planning. Social workers may be perceived as both helpful and obstructive because they have to challenge processes that are seen as helpful by one professional but potentially damaging by another. It is easy for conflict by proxy to occur. In this regard, a systemic perspective attempts to link together the different aspects of the work to ensure that appropriate solutions to the often intractable problems around a young person's needs can be achieved.

STAGE 4: RECONSTRUCTION AND REUNIFICATION

The fourth stage starts when the focus is on family and community reunification. The question has to be asked: 'Will it be safe for the young person to live within his family context or live within the community?'

Reunification within a protective context often involves the restoration of family or community relationships through a variety of meetings with the victim and family, spending increasing time together in supervised and unsupervised contexts. Reconstruction plans are often

worked out between family members, members of the mental health teams, together with care professionals who are looking always at balancing care needs with therapeutic needs.

Thus many young people are extremely keen to have a reunification meeting with appropriate family members, when they have been responsible for abuse against them. It is essential to ensure that nobody will be re-traumatized by such contacts, and that appropriate apology sessions can be arranged, ensuring that the victim's questions are going to be answered, as well as reflecting work done with the young person who has offended. The offender needs to take responsibility and provide appropriate explanations for abusive behaviour. Therapeutic work may sometimes run ahead of the child-protective context, and the capacity of the victim to cope. It is often helpful to confront a young person with the fact that the safety of younger victims is essential, so the offender has to demonstrate a capacity to behave in an appropriate non-abusive manner for contact to be re-established, and the issue of future reunification considered.

Planning of work, review meetings, review of care plans and statutory processes may seem cumbersome when a young person appears to have made good progress so that reunification with the family can be considered. However, the potential for reunification needs to properly thought out.

CONSENT TO TREATMENT

This topic is currently developing with the refinement of practice. Given that young people presenting with dangerous behaviour and associated psychiatric states may be highly resistant to acknowledging their actions and/or their illnesses, treatment might have to be provided against the individual's consent.

THE LEGAL CONTEXT

Williams and White (1996), in their wide-ranging review of young people and protective legislation, have provided a useful guide to consent to medical treatment. The principle in law has been enunciated that parental rights exist as long as they are needed for the protection of the child. The child has a right to make decisions once he or she reaches a sufficient understanding and intelligence. Children aged 16 or 17 are regarded as having the capacity to consent, and younger children who are 'Gillick-competent' (Gillick case [1986] AC112) may give consent without parental interference.

However, it has been judged that the converse is not the case. Individuals aged under 18 cannot withhold consent to treatment, so application to the Court should not be necessary. Thus it is established that treatment can be provided (e.g. medication) even if a young person does not wish to receive it, provided parental consent is obtained. A Court can make the decision if parental consent is not forthcoming. Court decisions also provide that a psychiatric assessment can be ordered, when a child is being assessed under the Children's Act regulation, even if the young person does not consent to such an examination.

The Mental Health Act 1983 may also be invoked, and young people can be detained under its provisions. However, a code of practice stresses the need to take parents' and the child's views into account, and any intervention should be the least restrictive. The question should always be asked as to whether a social services setting, educational contexts or therapeutic communities are preferable options, and whether care at home can be provided.

CHOOSING BETWEEN THE CHILDREN ACT AND THE MENTAL HEALTH ACT

William and White (1996) give clear guidance about the circumstances which allow for use of these legislations for children who manifest dangerous behaviour, associated with major mental health problems. There is considerable anxiety about how to identify the most appropriate choice, and few guidelines exist to assist professionals (see Chapter 30).

Williams and White point out that the Children Act 1989 may appear less stigmatizing as it reflects social and family failure rather than mental disorder. But there are no specific provisions to enforce medical treatments or to safeguard the rights of young people who are detained.

The Mental Health Act 1983 is not specifically orientated towards young people, their needs and circumstances, and there are insufficient safeguards to protect the interests of this group in all circumstances. The issue of stigmatization also needs to be addressed, set against the needs for specific treatment of a mental health problem.

The exact purpose of the proposed intervention needs to be evaluated. Williams and White (1996) point out that:

> 'a very seriously ill adolescent may require treatment within the Mental Health Act 1983, whereas a serious, self-harming offender with a psychiatric component to his or her problem may require detention (in secure accommodation) under the Children Act 1989. The balance lies between the need for containment and the need for medical treatment for mental disorder.'

In summary, providers of treatment should:

- understand the relevant legal provisions
- have easy access to competent legal advice
- keep in mind the importance of ensuring that care and treatment is managed with clarity, consistency and within a recognizable framework
- select the least stigmatizing and restrictive option consistent with care and treatment objectives.

CONCLUSIONS

This chapter has attempted to demonstrate that the issue of child protection is one that needs to be looked at continuously during assessment and treatment. Their needs have to be considered at all phases of the psychiatric work: during the crises which often surround the recognition of such young people's potentially dangerous behaviour, in the assessment of their mental health and experiences within their families, both in the past and currently, and during the process of assessment and delivery of services. Care has to be taken at all stages that the child-protection perspective is kept in mind, represented by social work professionals, and given appropriate authority and role within the mental health organization.

The protection role is key in considering training, appointment of staff, development of procedures for restraint, and therapeutic planning. The roles of child-protection agencies and their powers under the Children Act 1989 are essential to separate children from highly abusive contexts. The aim is to stabilize a young person sufficiently to make proper psychiatric assessments of states and needs, and to engage family members in therapeutic work to ensure a good outcome, using a method which fits the needs of the young person in the context of their particular family.

Staff who are providing care must be aware of their roles and of their responsibilities, and of the child-protection issues. Training, supervision and selection need to consider the issue of safety as well as skills. Child protection is not an 'add on', but an essential component of a best-practice approach to assessment and treatment in the adolescent forensic field.

REFERENCES

Bentovim, A. 1995: *Trauma Organised Systems: Physical and Sexual Abuse in Families*, revised edn. London: Karnac Books.

Bentovim, A. 1998a: Significant harm in context. In Adcock, M. and White, R. (eds), *Significant Harm: Its Management and Outcome*. Croydon: Significant Publications.

Bentovim, A. 1998b: Family systemic approach to work with young sex offenders. *Irish Journal of Psychology* **19**: 119–35.

Bentovim, A. and Kinston, W. 1991: Focal family therapy: joining systems theory with psychodynamic understanding. In Gurman, A. and Kniskern, D. (eds), *Handbook for Family Therapy*, Vol. 2. New York: Brunner/Mazel.

Bentovim, A., Elton, A. and Tranter, M. 1987: Prognosis for rehabilitation after abuse. *Adoption and Fostering* **11**: 26–31.

Bentovim, A. and Williams, B. 1998: Children and adolescents: victims who become perpetrators. *Advances in Psychiatric Treatment* **4**: 101–7.

Calder, M.C. 1997: *Juveniles and Children who Sexually Abuse: a Guide to Risk Assessment*. Dorset: Russell House Publishing.

DoH (Department of Health) 1995: *Child Protection: Messages from Research*. London: HMSO.

DoH (Department of Health) 2000a: *Working Together to Safeguard Children: Guide to Inter-agency Working.* London: HMSO.

DoH (Department of Health) 2000b: *The Framework for the Assessment of Children in Need and their Families.* London: HMSO.

Henggeler, S.W. 1999: Multi-systemic therapy: an overview of clinical procedures, outcomes and policy indications. *Child Psychology and Psychiatry Review* 4: 2–10.

Kempe, C.H. 1978: Recent developments in the field of child abuse. *International Journal of Child Abuse and Neglect* 2(4): 261–7.

Kempe, C.H., Silverman, F.N., Steele, B.F., Droegemueller, W. and Silver, H.K. 1962: The battered child syndrome. *Journal of the American Medical Association* 181: 17–24.

Silvester, J., Bentovim, A., Stratton, P. and Hanks, H. 1995: Using spoken attributions to clarify abusive families. *Child Abuse and Neglect* 19: 1221–32.

Skuse, D., Bentovim, A., Hodges, J. *et al.* 1998: Risk factors for development of sexually abusive behaviour in sexually victimised adolescent boys: cross-sectional study. *British Medical Journal* 317: 175–9.

Von Bertalanffy, L. 1962: General systems theory: a critical review. *General Systems* 7: 1–20.

Williams, R. and White, R. (eds) 1996: *Safeguards for Young Minds: Young People and Protective Legislation.* London: Gaskell/Royal College of Psychiatrists.

26

Clinical governance in an adolescent forensic inpatient service

MARIE BOLES

INTRODUCTION

The Gardener Unit was the first national adolescent forensic service to be established in the UK. The unit was commissioned in 1984 following the recommendations of the Butler and Glancy Report. It is located at the Bolton, Salford and Trafford Mental Health Trust just outside the city of Manchester. Some ten years later the service was the subject of a review, which was undertaken by the Mental Health Act Commission, the Social Services Inspectorate and the Health Advisory Service (NHS 1994). The outcome of the review made far-reaching recommendations for the future strategic development of the service. It concluded that the service offered a combination of facilities which was unique in the UK, as it provided an inpatient assessment and treatment function for adolescents, within a medium-level of security, combined with a community team which was able to offer secondary level services and outreach from the inpatient unit.

In essence the review concluded that the service should:

- reduce its bed capacity to 10 in order to provide a specialist service for adolescents with severe mental illness, unlike its previous remit of providing a service for adolescents with a mixed range of psychiatric conditions
- develop a peripatetic community Forensic Adolescent Consultation Team (FACT), working in close association with the inpatient unit and with the secure facilities for adolescents provided by other agencies and sectors of care

- become the model for the advisory teams recommended by the Reed Report (DoH 1992), and contribute to producing a better coordinated and planned spectrum of resources across agencies
- undertake a review of the accommodation of the service
- undertake a review of the management arrangements within the service, which included a review of the staffing skill mix and a training needs analysis.

MISSION AND PURPOSE OF THE SERVICE

The recommendations of the 1994 review did much to reinforce and underpin the principal functions of the unit. It was recommended that there should be provision of a specialist expertise in adolescent forensic psychiatry at a national level, within and along the spectrum of care, the objective being to provide coordinated and seamless packages of care.

The review recommended the provision of an inpatient resource at the Gardener Unit, for adolescents between the ages of 11 and 18 years, within medium security. These adolescents would present with serious mental illness with significant levels of risk and require psychiatric assessment and/or treatment and/or rehabilitation and could not otherwise safely receive this provision in a non-secure hospital setting.

The review recommended the provision of a national Forensic Adolescent Forensic Consultation and Treatment

Service (FACTS) to young people between the ages of 9 to 18 years who have severe disorder of conduct and emotion with significant levels of risk – this being primarily an assessment and outreach service. However, a small community North West regional treatment service is offered, in collaboration with statutory and non-statutory agencies.

Another recommendation was to maintain a focused research and development agenda to assist in maintaining an accurate awareness of the most appropriate service models, inform strategic development, ensure high quality and a service which is sensitive to the needs of its users.

Within the inpatient resource, care is provided within a safe, secure therapeutic environment which is delivered through a comprehensive multi-disciplinary team. Treatment approaches are comprehensive, integrated, client-focused and holistic. These are cognitive behavioural in emphasis but are supported by a range of psychodynamic approaches. There is continuous risk assessment and management. Where appropriate the service provides outreach work and advice after discharge. Ongoing health and social needs assessment is facilitated through the Care Programme Approach framework. This integrated approach requires the engagement of users, carers and significant others. The service also provides the adolescent with the opportunity to achieve through the provision of a specialist dedicated educational facility.

CLINICAL GOVERNANCE

Clinical governance is one of the major themes in the government's proposals to modernize the National Health Service in the UK. Clinical governance is set as a statutory duty for NHS Trust Boards in the NHS White Paper *The New NHS: Modern and Dependable* (DoH 1997a) and in the consultative document *A First Class Service: Quality in the NHS* (DoH 1998) This new corporate responsibility builds on the requirement in the *Health Service Guidance 97/17* (DoH 1997b) for trusts and health authority boards to have comprehensive controls assurance in place.

Clinical governance can be defined as:

'a framework through which the NHS organizations are accountable for continuously improving the quality of their services and safeguarding high standards of care by creating an environment in which excellence in clinical care will flourish.' (DoH 1998)

Prior to clinical governance there were varying degrees of success with quality assurance, clinical audit/effectiveness and clinical/non-clinical risk management. Clinical governance has emerged to address inequalities in clinical practice and in clinical outcomes; in other words, variations in performance and practice. It is a new model which marries clinical judgement with clear national standards. Clinical governance demands excellent systems for monitoring and improving the quality

of clinical care which should be linked to create a whole-systems approach. It is a process which assures the quality of effective service delivery by providing a renewed focus on quality by all. Since April 1999, clinical probity and quality improvement have been monitored and reported in the same way as financial probity and value for money.

The main components of clinical governance include:

- clear lines of responsibility and accountability for the overall quality of clinical care
- a comprehensive programme of quality-improvement activities
- clear policies aimed at managing risk
- procedures for all professional groups to identify and remedy poor performance.

Essentially it is a synthesis of important components, some of which are based in law, all of which require continuous attention for the effective delivery of high-quality clinical care.

THE BUSINESS EXCELLENCE MODEL

The 'business excellence model' is a self-assessment model which can be used by organizations to review performance. The model comprises nine quality criteria against which organizations can be assessed (Figure 26.1):

1 *Leadership* – the activities and behaviours of managers in driving the organization towards excellence
2 *Policy and strategy* – how planning activities, aims and objectives reflect the drive for continuous improvement
3 *People* – how, and the extent to which, the full potential of employees is realized
4 *Partnership and resources* – how the organization plans and manages its external partnerships and its resources in order to support its policy and strategy and the effective operation of its processes (including financial, information technology, information and knowledge and equipment and premises)
5 *Processes* – how the value-added activities are managed and monitored for continuous improvement
6 *Customer results* (patient, referrers and the stakeholders) – what is being achieved here compared with other organizational targets and best in-class performance
7 *People results* (staff) – what the staff feel about the organization (hard and soft measures)
8 *Society results* – perceptions of the organization in the community
9 *Key performance results* – what the organization is achieving in relation to its planned performance.

The model enables whole organizations, component parts or individual services within an organization to self-assess. The process is systematic with each of the nine criteria scored against approximately six sub-elements to indicate levels of achievement on a continuum.

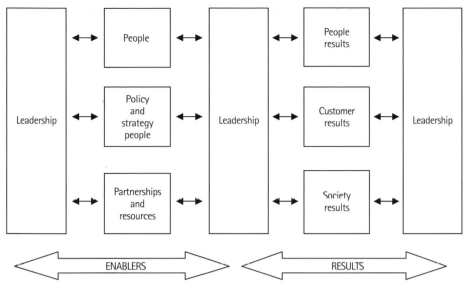

Figure 26.1 *Business excellence model.*

The assessment process is explicit in requiring trend data, evidence of quality issues, and organizations or services to encourage continuing improvement. The assessment process requires many forms of evidence including documentary evidence, interviewing key personnel and staff focus groups. The main benefit of self-assessment is that it facilitates systematic continuous quality improvement of the organization over the full range of activities and processes. The premise of the model is that *results* are achieved through the management of *processes* by *people*.

The business excellence model is potentially useful in supporting clinical governance in that it provides a means of integrating various quality initiatives, in a pragmatic whole-systems approach to improvement. It is a powerful diagnostic tool (helping to highlight blind spots), a means of measuring progress over time, a means of promoting and sharing best practice within an organization and externally, a basis of internal and external benchmarking, and a thorough and formalized approach to quality improvement based on objective data. Finally it is also a good educational tool.

APPLICATION AT THE BUSINESS EXCELLENCE MODEL ELEMENTS IN THE GARDENER UNIT

Although the Gardener Unit has not used the business excellence model explicitly to support its clinical governance agenda, it has highlighted many of the elements included in it for attention.

Leadership

Over the last 20 years there has been increasing attention to the area of leadership within the NHS, with two distinct schools of thought emerging. The choice might therefore appear to be between an efficient organizational structure or one that develops its human resources. But it is becoming increasingly clear from the empirical literature that this is a false dichotomy (Bryman 1976).

Leadership functions within the team are varied. In addition to the structuring of tasks there are other important dimensions to effective leadership. House (1976) identified them as:

- demonstrating effective involvement with patients
- communicating high expectations of other staff and showing confidence that they can be met
- articulating a grasp of the overall goals of the team and providing a broad view of the nature and significance of the role a service has.

None of the leadership functions needs to be carried out by one person. When leaders are allowed to emerge in groups it often happens that leadership functions are shared between two or more people (Secord and Blackman 1964). In the team there is usually more than one person who has the experience and ability to exercise some degree of leadership. Normally a team will function better if there is more than one person who is prepared to carry out a leadership function.

There are many ways in which leadership functions can be distributed, but it can be said that the more people are able to make a contribution to the leadership functions, the better integrated the team will be.

There are leadership functions which are required outside the service. Usually this will be the responsibility of one person. It involves representing the service to the organization and explaining why it may want to operate in a particular way even when the organization has very little knowledge of the complex environment in which the service operates. Likewise the leader needs to have the ability to interpret decisions made by the organization which maintains the confidence of the service and the organization. The most important objective is to secure the maximum amount of autonomy for the service whilst at the same time respecting that it is a component part of a wider organization.

Leadership needs to be seen at a number of levels: organizational, service, clinically and professionally. Structures need to be clear but at the same time sufficiently flexible to accommodate the tensions that subsequently arise. There needs to be a maturity in the service that recognizes that at times leaders outside the direct service may make decisions that impact on the service.

Policy and strategy

The National Service Framework (NSF) for mental health published in September 1999 is the most recent national guidance in respect of mental health services. It focuses on the needs of adults of working age up to 65. It sets national standards, service models and action for implementation towards the achievement of an appropriate range of services to meet needs. Integration and closer collaboration of specialist secure services into mainstream mental health and learning-disability services is an important feature in the expected outcomes of the NSF.

Policy guidance on care coordination in mental health services is contained in *The Care Programme Approach* (CPA; DoH 1990) and is accepted as a standard requirement.

Whilst specialist and secure services are clearly part of the NSF, the principles and requirements set out in the Reed Report (DoH 1992) continue to be a key guidance for the range of secure services.

The Health Act 1999 brought two further key policy initiatives together, namely the establishment of specialist commissioning and the development of new provider configurations around primary care and mental health/ learning disability specialties. Specialized commissioning devolves the strategic planning and procurement of highly secure psychiatric care to the National Health Service Executive regional offices, while incorporating the existing medium- and low-secure responsibilities.

The impact of the Fallon enquiry has made high secure services increasingly uneasy about providing services for adolescents. It is clear that over the past few years a growing percentage of adolescents who would have previously been cared for by highly secure services are now in the Gardener Unit – estimates indicate that this figure is in the region of 25%. The service is increasingly providing high levels of 'special observation', sometimes by three staff for long periods, often for several weeks. Patients are also being nursed for long periods in areas away from the main inpatient group. Higher levels of assaultative behaviour are being contained and managed. Anecdotal evidence suggests an inability to provide such intense nursing input, and that often adult services would be able to manage such behaviours only through long periods of seclusion.

The inability of Tier 4 services (see Chapter 23) to manage adolescents with intensive care needs are increasing resulting in inappropriate referrals to the service. This is not to say that adolescents do not need periods in a secure environment, but one would seriously have to question if their needs are best met in a forensic service. However, the service has much to offer through consultation and advice on the management of disturbed or challenging behaviours.

At a local level the Gardener Unit is required to produce an annual business plan. This serves as an opportunity to articulate the principal functions of the service, what its mission and aims are. It addresses other strategic considerations such as:

- a SWOT (strengths, weaknesses, opportunities, threats) analysis
- an environmental scanning exercise looking at the demographic, epidemiological, economic, political, ethical and legal, social and technical influences on the service
- a strategic direction statement of the service
- a human resource agenda including training and staff planning
- the financial framework
- service relationships/networks
- the clinical effectiveness agenda and monitoring arrangements
- a review of the previous year's objectives
- a list of the service objectives for the forthcoming year (these objectives are in line with the Trust's objectives of clinical governance and national priorities as well as including service specific objectives).

Most of the strategic aspirations of the service are driven from within. The service had to establish mutually supportive working relationships with a range of stakeholders, including commissioners, the criminal justice system, other adult secure services, educational establishments, adolescent services and the voluntary sector. In order to keep staff at all levels involved in the strategic development process, a range of communication systems are required.

People working in the service

ROLES AND RESPONSIBILITIES

A service is only as good as the people who work in it. Adolescent forensic services need to take a broad and comprehensive view of their patients so we should not be surprised that we need a broad and comprehensive range of staff to provide the service. This raises issues of coordination. How can different professions be engaged with a patient without working at cross purposes?

There are arguments for the development of clearly defined roles and responsibilities within a multidisciplinary team and demands to be clear about what is core to the identity of a profession or discipline. This may be an appropriate avenue to go down, but it does not provide all the answers. When staff are regularly required to find innovative clinical solutions, a network of control in which roles are adjusted through mutual interaction is more effective. Wilkinson (1973) found that resistance to innovations is less likely if there is a high level of interaction amongst staff. A further argument for having a flexible distribution of tasks is that it is easier for staff to deputize for one another.

Members of staff are not just important for the professional contribution they make, but also for their social backgrounds and life experiences. In dealing with problems of social adjustment, the varied social backgrounds and attitudes of the team are a considerable asset in planning realistic programmes of care. Between them the members of the team often provide a good cross-section of ages, sexes, races, social classes and educational attainment (Watts and Bennett 1983).

SKILLS

For most staff working in an adolescent forensic service, their basic training is inadequate. In his work on nursing in adolescent forensic services, McDougall (2000) highlights the importance of appropriate training. He writes:

> 'providing young people with a safe, secure and caring environment requires an awareness of fundamental issues related to security, safety and control and how they impact on the delivery of quality nursing care.'

In an attempt to meet the training needs of staff working in the Gardener Unit, a comprehensive training needs analysis was conducted. It involved gathering information from three perspectives:

1 an audit of patient needs as outlined in the care plan
2 an identification of the skills required to work in the service
3 a skills and needs questionnaire.

Stage 1

The identification of patient needs was seen as an imperative. It was intended that by using case conference reports and information from individual care plans an adequate baseline of patient needs could be identified.

Stage 2

Two multi-disciplinary focus groups were held. The purpose of the first focus group was to identify the 'core skills' that were required by all staff in the service. The purpose of the second was to identify the 'advanced skills' required

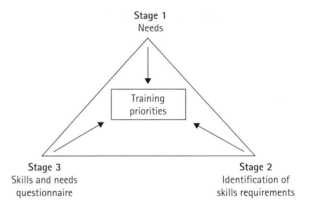

Figure 26.2 *Identification of patient needs.*

by the service. The rationale was that in identifying the skills required, comparisons could then be made against a list of skills already available in the service, and this would then identify priority training areas.

The focus groups took the format of a brainstorming session whereby consideration was given to the problem profile of the patients, family and parent needs, the needs of other agencies, and the clinical framework for care planning. This activity also included a literature review of relevant clinically effective interventions.

Stage 3

Questionnaires were distributed to all qualified staff, support workers and auxiliary staff (housekeepers, catering, administration and clerical), and to teachers at Cloughside School. The questionnaires were initially completed by staff on their own, but there was a requirement that all staff then meet with their appraiser to verify the information. The intention of the questionnaires was to identify:

- training undertaken and being undertaken
- qualifications of staff
- skills available
- performance in relation to completion of mandatory training.

The recommendations of the analysis were:

- to develop a mandatory in-house training programme to produce the core skills for the identified priority training needs
- to develop an appraisal system that further encompassed analysis of skills
- to review the preceptorship and induction package to ensure it reflected development of priority training needs
- to ensure the availability of 'advanced skills' in all priority training need areas
- to ensure all staff have access to clinical supervision training
- to develop a skills register
- to develop an improved database for training undertaken

- to prioritize training in the following areas: understanding of adolescents and adolescent development, conditions of serious mental disorder, risk assessment and management of violence and antisocial behaviour, self-harm, relevant clinical frameworks (CPA) and mandatory training.

STAFF APPRAISAL

As stated earlier, a service is only as good as the people who work in it. This statement implies that staff are aware of what is expected of them and that they get feedback on their performance.

In the Gardener Unit there has been an attempt to develop competency-based job descriptions for all staff, irrespective of profession or grade. The competencies required are used as a framework for appraisal; that is, staff's performance is baselined against the competency criteria. The gap that is identified is addressed throughout the development of a Personal Development Plan (PDP) for each member of staff. Fundamental to this is the core competencies as described in the training needs analysis. This process needs to be supported by a sound and comprehensive induction.

When staff start in the service they are allocated an appraiser. There is a core induction programme for all staff, but it is then tailored to meet the personal and professional needs of the staff. The core induction cover all aspects of health and safety, management of the physical security of the unit, awareness of relevant policies and procedures for operational and clinical security, policies on management of incidents, introduction to the clinical decision frameworks of the service, introduction to the client group in terms of the needs of adolescents with severe mental illness, introduction to all members of the multi-disciplinary team and awareness of the management and clinical structures within the service.

Upon completion of induction a formal appraisal takes place. This is when staff review their performance against the competency-based job description. PDPs are then structured and timetabled for review.

A variety of methods are used to address development needs. They include formal training, attendance at courses, shadowing, exposure to new clinical and/or management situations, secondments, visits to other services, involvement in project work, teaching, involvement in research, audit and other service developments – this list is not exhaustive.

CLINICAL SUPERVISION

Clinical supervision is quite distinct from appraisal. Appraisal is the formal (usually line management) review of performance. Clinical supervision is a more reflective process whereby the impact of an individual practitioner's performance is reviewed.

A number of definitions have been offered, but perhaps the most comprehensive is (NHS Executive 1993):

'Clinical supervision is the term used to describe a formal process of professional support and learning which enables individual practitioners to develop knowledge and competence, assumes responsibility for their own practice and enhance consumer protection and the safety of care in complex clinical situations'

It is recognized that all professional groups require supervision. Within the service each professional group has identified what the specific professional requirements are. Consensus has then been developed about the essential requirements for all professionals in the service. A service standard was then developed which forms the basis for an annual clinical audit exercise.

Many staff have been suspicious of the introduction of clinical supervision, because they have confused it with the process of appraisal. Most of the literature about clinical supervision is for qualified members of staff, but the service is committed to exploring models of clinical supervision for unqualified staff, the rationale being that it is often unqualified staff who have the highest levels of client contact. Since one of the aims of clinical supervision is to ultimately improve patient care, clinical supervision has got to be available to all staff.

Clinical supervision has been described as an activity of examining one's practice with a more experienced and skilled professional in a formal relationship (Faugier 1994). Although one would expect these 'more experienced' professionals to be within the service, the service allows staff the opportunity to approach people from outside the service who may have relevant expertise to offer. All nursing staff within the service have an explicit requirement to both receive and provide clinical supervision – this is included in all job descriptions. Each member of staff is expected to meet with his or her clinical supervisor to agree a contract for their relationship. The contract involves specifying: the frequency of their meetings, the duration of the meetings, arrangements for facilitating the meetings, respective understanding of confidentiality, the educational objectives, the method of recording the meetings, the method of evaluating the process, and options for conflict resolution. It is clear that the specific content of the clinical supervision meeting is confidential, but each member of staff is required to confirm the contents of the contract with his or her appraiser. All staff have different development needs at different points in their careers, so they are encouraged to regularly review the appropriateness of their supervisor over a period of time.

STAFF SUPPORT

Appreciating that individuals have different needs, it follows that staff need to have a range of support models.

The service recognized the part clinical supervision and appraisal have to play, but in addition there is a contract with the regional psychotherapy service to provide sessional input for individual and group supervision, and psychodynamic supervision is also available for staff. If staff are uncomfortable with support from within the service there is an opportunity to access a staff counselling service which is offered on a confidential basis through the Trust's personnel department.

Although there is need for formal systems of staff support, many of the staff report that a genuine supportive management culture is more important. There are specific policies in place that offer support, including carer and special leave arrangements. Carers' leave is a facility whereby staff can request time from the service in the event of a domestic or family issue arising; previously staff would have been left in a position of taking sick leave. Special leave is given at the discretion of the line manager. When the Gardener Unit first opened many staff took sick leave following serious traumatic incidents, including assaults, but staff now report that pressure has been greatly lessened as they feel managers within the service are more sensitive to the management of personal distress.

Increased access to training, opportunities for involvement in decision-making, and secondments are also recognized as opportunities for demonstrating staff support.

The development of a comprehensive system for reviewing serious incidents and debriefing are now well established within the service. The serious-incident reviews are seen as an opportunity to reflect on the management of incidents in a context of learning and improving practice, not as a management tool for apportioning criticism and blame. Debriefing is seen as a distinct part of the process. It is usually facilitated as soon as possible after the incident and is not seen as part of the formal management review. This allows staff the opportunity to express their thoughts and feeling in a safe environment.

Team development

Teams are about human relationships and the behaviour within them. We are all members of a variety of teams both in and outside work. What is common is that we play a variety of roles given the task of the team. Teams are established to achieve particular tasks and teams are a mechanism for controlling and coordinating activities. It should not be assumed that cooperation is normal, healthy and proper, neither should there be an assumption that conflict arises out of error or confusion. Successful teams contain both cooperation and conflict at the same time. Attempts to manage teams are only successful once the behaviour in the team is understood, and it needs to be acknowledged that different people have different realities and may have different goals and objectives.

There need to be opportunities for team development, not least because staff are a precious commodity. At the Gardener Unit each year a series of Away Days are externally facilitated for the staff. There are inevitable problems with covering shifts, which means it is impossible for the whole multi-disciplinary team to be together at once. Therefore the events are spread over a number of days and each member is required to participate in some identified activities. The Away Days are an opportunity to reflect on the highs and lows of the previous year, to reflect on the aims and objectives of the service, to reset tasks for the improvement of the service over the next year in a safe environment, and to talk about the challenges and stresses in the unit. Each member of the service is involved; ground-rules regarding confidentiality, need for openness and respect for all opinions are always established. The Away Days are held away from the Trust, usually at a venue which also provides an opportunity for socializing and eating together. Activities are designed which examine the various team functions, including setting objectives, sharing information, making decisions, allocating tasks, achieving objectives, evaluating performance, planning, communication, analysing problems and solving them. Following the Away Days action plans with timescales are drawn up. A small working group is then established which monitors progress against the plan; this is included also in the service's business plan. A regular report is provided to each member of the team.

A demonstrable outcome of the success of these team-building exercises has been measured through sickness levels in the service. Before the implementation of the review of the service, sickness levels were in the region of 12%; some four years later this had reduced to 4%.

Alongside the formal Away Days, support has now been given for the facilitation of what the service calls 'fun away days'. This is where the team have identified time for socializing in a setting away from the unit, with the specific objective of enjoying quality time together. Staff report this as one of the most effective means of getting to know each other without the restriction of professional roles and boundaries. It has added to team cohesion and communication in a particularly effective way. The service has provided the finances required to facilitate such activities.

The multi-disciplinary team

For the 10-bed inpatient unit the complement of staff is as shown in Table 26.1.

Having a rich multi-disciplinary team not only brings together different skills and interventions, it also allows for a range of perspectives. Much has been written about the often negative cultures that exist within secure services, namely the development of restrictive clinical and managerial practices. The availability of multi-disciplinary

Table 26.1 *Multi-disciplinary team for a ten-bed unit*

Medical	Nursing	Therapists	A&C
1 WTE Consultant	0.5 WTE Clinical Manager	1 WTE Grade 1 OT	0.5 Administrator
Level 2 SHO	2.5 WTE Grade H	1 WTE Basic Grade OT	1 Assistant Administrator A&C 4
Speciality Training SpR Post	3 WTE Grade F	0.5 WTE Art Therapist	1.6 Secretary A&C 3
	11 WTE Grade E	0.5 Music Teacher	1 Administration Assistant A&C 2
	6 WTE Grade B	0.8 WTE Social Worker	1 Ward Clerk A&C 2
	18 WTE Grade A		Receptionist/Clerk A&C 2
	3.8 Housekeepers		
	1.5 Chefs		

perspectives allows the opportunity for challenge and review. The fact that the service is able to facilitate the placement of students again brings a questioning perspective which is refreshing.

MEDICAL STAFF

Consultants who work in the service are required to be dual trained in the specialty of child and adolescents plus forensic. Whilst there are specific sessions required for direct work with the inpatient group, it is acknowledged that job plans also need to include other special interests, such as in areas of education and training, research, management, etc. This significantly reduces the potential for burnout and assists with longer-term recruitment and retention.

The service recognizes the value of trainees not only as a means for succession planning but as a method of increasing the knowledge base of other services as to the role and function of the service. The recent changes in the curriculum for medical trainees has also challenged some of the traditional roles previously carried out by junior doctors, in particular in the area of primary care. New roles have been examined to address this need. One preferred model is to establish a role for a nurse with specific training who can monitor the physical health needs of the patients; this role would also incorporate a health promotion perspective.

NURSING STAFF

Nurses are the only profession who provide care 24 hours a day, seven days a week. Investment is therefore needed to develop the range of tasks undertaken by nurses on the unit. The nursing structure needs to clearly identify the individuals who are responsible for the operational management of the unit, who takes on the lead for practice development and training, and the place of clinical nurse specialists. This provides clear distinctive career pathways for nurses.

Senior nurses still need to retain clinical credibility and recognize how professional clinical leadership can be provided. In the early days of the service the most senior nurses were encouraged to spend all their time in the clinical setting – they were often seen as a 'safe pair of hands'. Whilst there is no argument that they have a significant role to play in the delivery of direct patient care, junior qualified staff need to be exposed to clinical situations which increase their competency in the area of clinical decision-making and thus increase their autonomy as individual practitioners. This allows the senior nurses to develop a more strategic approach to the management of the nursing workforce.

Just like qualified nurses, untrained staff need career pathways. The service has developed the role of a senior support worker. There is a requirement to undertake formal accredited training for the role. They have a specific responsibility of promoting a positive residential philosophy and assisting in the feedback and monitoring of performance.

SOCIAL WORKERS

The unit has dedicated social work input to oversee the legal framework in which care is provided. By the very nature of the service admission criteria, the majority of patients are detained under sections of the Mental Health Act 1983. The social worker also has high levels of contact with many of the families, so needs formal training in this area. The social worker is often the conduit which provides the service with information from a range of other statutory agencies. There need to be clear lines of professional accountability in order to provide support. As a lone professional in the service the social worker can have an opinion which is different from that of healthcare professionals. Support to retain professional integrity is essential.

PSYCHOLOGY SERVICE

It is extremely difficult to recruit staff who have both adolescent and forensic experience. The Gardener Unit has addressed this by contracting psychology services from the local district Child and Adolescent Acute Trust. The service has devised a programme of personal development and a career pathway for the staff which particularly enhances the forensic perspective of their work. The psychologists are seen not only as a resource for direct clinical work, their time is also spent providing clinical supervision and training, particularly to nurses.

OCCUPATIONAL THERAPY

The senior occupational therapist in the service is essentially responsible for overseeing the programme of the therapeutic day. This is negotiated with the nursing staff who have responsibility for ensuring the residential management of the unit, and with the teaching staff who provide a programme of full-time education for those adolescents who are both below and above the school leaving age. All group work is coordinated by the development of terms of reference and aims and objectives.

CREATIVE THERAPIES

The unit has part-time art and music therapy staff. Their psychodynamic approach provides an alternative perspective to the assessment and treatment of the patients (see Chapter 21). It provides an alternative medium for the patients to express themselves, particularly as many of them have serious limitations with verbal communication. The opinions offered by these staff often provides a unique viewpoint not expressed by the rest of the multi-disciplinary team.

SPEECH AND LANGUAGE THERAPY

A needs assessment was undertaken which identified that almost 80% of the patients had speech and language difficulties. A contract was established with a neighbouring Trust for dedicated sessional input.

TEACHERS

The unit is obliged to provide a dedicated educational facility. The facility is bound by the same philosophy as that of a mainstream school, but it needs to provide a flexible approach which best meets the needs of the patients. The school has its own board of governors and is subject to statutory inspection. The teaching staff require detailed information on the patients which assists in their formulation of an education programme. Alternatives to examinations need to be available which reflect the patients' abilities to achieve academic accreditation. The teaching staff are an intrinsic part of the multi-disciplinary team and regularly co-work as part of care teams.

The teachers are again able to bring a unique perspective to the assessment of the patients. They make comparisons from their experience of providing education for 'normal pupils' and do not provide opinions from a medicalized health perspective and therefore do not make the same allowances in interpreting behaviour and conduct. The clinical staff appraise the teachers of the patients' mental health conditions and how this will impact on their ability to take part in formal academic tasks. For those patients over the age of 16 there is no legal requirement to take part in formal education, so alternative models of vocational training are required. The structure of the school day also needs to be negotiated in line with clinical activity and those routine aspects of the residential philosophy, such as attendance at community meetings.

ADMINISTRATION AND CLERICAL STAFF, AND ANCILLARY STAFF

Administration and clerical staff are essential members of the team who have variable degrees of contact with patients. It is not everyone who can work in a secure environment, and their education and training needs should not be under-estimated. It is often secretaries who have to type very detailed reports, which regularly include graphic and distressing accounts of index offences. Appropriate support and supervision is therefore necessary.

The unit employs its own catering and housekeeping staff. They often have high levels of patient contact and accordingly need to have appropriate support and supervision to carry out their duties.

Partnership and resources

It would be very easy for a secure service to become insular in its thinking and practices. The adolescent forensic service is unlike most other services in the Trust and is only a small exclusive part of both mainstream adolescent or forensic services, so it needs to work very hard at developing mutually supportive networks. These networks provide stimulation, challenge and opportunities. Networks need not just be with other clinical services but include relationships with education establishments, commissioners, interest groups, other statutory and non-statutory agencies.

The service needs to nurture relationships with commissioners who can facilitate opportunities for service and practice development. Commissioners in the context of the Gardener Unit includes those at local, regional and national levels. Investment also needs to be made with those who influence policy, not just in health but in local government and other providers of secure accommodation, including the criminal justice system. Increasingly the expertise of the service is being called upon from other providers, in particular in the prison system. The service has much to offer not just by way of direct clinical input but also through consultation and liaison, education and training and in the provision of clinical supervision for other professionals.

Strong links with an educational establishment provides opportunities for recruitment and retention of staff by way of students and trainees. Joint or honorary appointments with local universities does much to raise the profile of the service and provides avenues for influencing course curriculums for a range of professional roles. Links with professional organizations can facilitate a means of influencing policy and potential service developments.

Establishing links with other clinical services is essential. The experience of the Gardener Unit is that it has provided a means of transferring skills into the service as well as allowing staff secondments to occur. This can be in response to burnout and stress or a mechanism for appraising alternative practice which may be brought back to the service. Joint work on research, practice development, audit, training, and sharing of resources have be significantly beneficial. Time out from the service has also been a means of exposing staff to new cultures and ways of working. In particular, relationships with services providing adult forensic care and rehabilitation, and adolescent care, have served as means of facilitating more timely discharge and transfer of patients – which is clearly to the advantage of the patient. There has been an increase in comorbidity, which indicates the value of developing links with services for substance misuse and learning disabilities.

Positive working relationships with support services in the Trust can expedite service objectives. Canvassing the support of senior staff within the Trust should be encouraged, spending time with them to inform them about the service – the more informed they are, the more sympathetic they might be when support is required.

One of the most significant resources the service has is its extensive experience in this particular clinical speciality. The service has much to offer in the way of training to others. There is expertise in the treatment approaches required for adolescents with severe mental illness who present with high-risk behaviours. Advice on the physical environment required by such a service is also available.

The building in itself is a resource. The review team in 1994 accessed a budget of £1.8 million which was used to refurbish the building. Significant improvements to the facilities at Cloughside School were made, and much of the therapy space was converted. Dedicated administration and office accommodation was also developed. On reflection there was an under-estimation of the residential space required. Clients with serious mental illness need lots of space and a low-stimulus environment. The high levels of staff on duty and 10 patients need sufficient space so as to avoid potentially volatile and stressful situations. More creative solutions to maintaining security could have been considered, which have now developed as a consequence of advances in technology. Lessons have been learnt which on reflection would have been better addressed with the provision of a new purpose-built facility.

Processes

The main framework for clinical decision-making is facilitated through the care programme approach (CPA). This requires the assessment of both health and social needs, involving the patient in the formulation of an individual care plan, evaluating the effectiveness of the care plan, and having a care coordinator who is competent to manage the care plan. Appropriate operational systems are organized around this function.

The service has a number of initiatives to enhance the quality of care in the unit. Clinical audit is well established. Each year specific areas for attention are identified. Trust resources are available to support the programme of audit in the form of an audit assistant. The audit assistant is able to collect the relevant data and is able to provide objective interpretations of results.

It is true to say that the service has struggled to develop an effective agenda for measuring clinical outcomes. As in other adolescent services there is a requirement to use the national tool, Health of the Nation Outcomes Scales for Adolescents (Gowers 1998). Through negotiations with the commissioners of the service we have tried to identify a battery of measures which could demonstrate the effectiveness of treatment on the unit. In lay terms, they want to know:

1 Has there been an impact on the patient's mental state?
2 Has the individual's level of function altered?
3 Has there been an impact on risk behaviours?
4 Has there been a positive experience whilst receiving care?

Many of the measures which may assist in answering these questions lie in outcome tools from adult services. With permission from their authors we have been working on modifications of these tools.

Owing to the nature of the client group and their associated problems with concentration, choosing a tool which measures mental state has been difficult. The unit has decided to choose a short tool with the ability to measure change. To measure change in functioning, the service is working with Max Birchwood on the development of an adolescent version of his Social Functioning Scale (SFS; Birchwood 1990). Consideration is also being given to the Social Behaviour Rating Scale (SBRS; Wykes and Sturt 1986). Risk assessment is high on all mental health agendas, no more so than in secure settings, so the HCR-20 (Webster et al. 1997) is being appraised by the service.

The final perspective which the service is anxious to examine is the experience the patients have of their time on the unit. Many of the more common tools available are from adult general settings. Trying to measure the subjective experience of a patient in a secure setting is difficult, given that they rarely have a choice about being there. The nature of a secure unit may be interpreted as infringing on basic liberties, such as the freedom to come and go, and choosing to be involved in treatment whether that be pharmacological, interpersonal therapies or rehabilitation. The Lancashire Quality of Life Scale does provide a framework, and the service is in dialogue with Mark Swinton at Ashworth High Security Hospital who is researching the modification of the tool for secure settings; again, refinement is likely to be required for an adolescent population.

The hope of the service is to develop this initial battery of measures that will be administered at intervals during the patient's stay. There is recognition that secondary tools will need to be available that address specific challenging behaviours.

In advance of the development of a validated tool to measure the experience of the patients in the service, a patient survey has been developed which addresses the many facets of their experience in hospital. On discharge patients are asked to complete a confidential questionnaire. The questionnaires are collected over a period of time and are collectively summarized. The results of these surveys are then presented to the management group within the service; copies are also sent to the commissioners and to the Independent Representative within the service. The latter is a person who is commissioned to provide independent support and advocacy where appropriate to each of the patients. The Independent Representative belongs to a national charitable organization, The Voice of the Child in Care. This organization provides input to the majority of local authority secure accommodation establishments in the country. The Gardener Unit is unique in that it is the only health facility in the country with this provision.

In 1998, an audit of the ethnic backgrounds of 32 admissions was undertaken. Of these a total of 20 patients (16 males, 4 female) came from ethnic-minority communities. The ethnic origin was determined as black-Caribbean (7), Asian (5), Indian (5), Indonesian (1), Arabic (1) and black-African (1). Clearly patients from black and ethnic minorities are over-represented, something which is consistent with surveys in adult secure services. Local population profiles do not explain this as the service is a national service, taking patients from all parts of Great Britain.

To assist with improving the services for patients from ethnic backgrounds, the service commissioned the African Caribbean Mental Health Group to undertake an evaluation of the service. They were given a broad remit to look at all aspects of provision within the unit (the environment, institutional racism, staff recruitment and selection, culture and family, religion, food, access to appropriate clothes, skin and hair products) and general observations about the unit. Their report identified several specific recommendations for the service, and a small working group has responsibility for implementing them. Whilst many of the principles of good practice are common to all patients, the Afro-Caribbean audit provides a particular cultural perspective (see Chapter 14).

A community meeting takes place about three times a week on the unit, and there is an expectation that patients and staff will attend. The running of the meetings is shared between the patients and staff. The meetings are seen as part of the school programme and a substitute for morning assembly that would be found in mainstream schools. The service is also committed to exploring the development of a patients' council but needs to be reassured as to the appropriateness of the model.

The service is reviewed regularly by the Mental Health Act Commission. The service attempts to engage the Social Service Inspectorate in this work, thus giving a broader perspective than just the implementation of the Mental Health Act.

Societal expectations

There is still stigma attached to mental health, due in many respects to ignorance. At the same time the patients who are admitted to the Gardener Unit have often committed very serious offences. The public is not always sympathetic to the need to provide care and treatment to the most vulnerable individuals, particularly when they believe that there should be an element of punishment and natural justice in the total response to such crimes. Likewise, because of the public perception that mentally ill patients are dangerous, there is even more pressure on secure services to manage risk behaviour appropriately. The service has a duty to protect the public.

Changes in legislation, in particular the Crime and Disorder Bill 1998, could easily be interpreted as a response to the public's desire to 'lock up and throw away the key' for adolescents who offend. The means by which adolescents can now be placed in secure settings is easier than ever. Managers and clinicians working in adolescent forensic services have an increasing responsibility to lobby for the appropriate assessment, treatment and resources for these very vulnerable individuals. It is incumbent on such services to contribute to the evidence base that will provide some answers to the questions about why adolescents commit crime, what the effective treatment responses consist of, and the responsibilities of respective agencies to ensure that the wishes of society can be best met in a way that ensures the best outcome for the adolescent.

REFERENCES

Birchwood, M. *et al.* 1990: The Social Functioning Scale: development and validation of a new scale of social adjustment for use in family intervention programmes with schizophrenic patients. *British Journal of Psychiatry* **157**: 853–9.

Bryman, A. 1976: Structures in organisations: a reconsideration. *Journal of Occupational Psychology* **49**: 1–9.

DoH (Department of Health) 1990: *The Care Programme Approach for People with a Mental Illness Referred to Specialist Psychiatric Services*. HC(00)23, LASSL(00)11. London: HMSO.

DoH (Department of Health/Home Office) 1992: *Review of Health and Social Services for Mentally Disordered Offenders and Others Requiring Similar Services*. London: HMSO.

DoH (Department of Health) 1997a: *The New NHS: Modern and Dependable*. HMSO: London.

DoH (Department of Health) 1997b: *Health Service Guidance (HSG) 97/17*. London: HMSO.

DoH (Department of Health) 1998: *A First Class Service: Quality in the NHS.* London: HMSO.

Faugier, J. 1994: Thin on the ground. *Nursing Times* **90**(20): 18 May.

Gowers, S.G., Harrington, R.C. and Whitton, A. 1998: Health of the Nation Outcome Scale for Adolescents. *British Journal of Psychiatry* **174**: 413–16.

House, R.J. 1976: A 1976 theory of charismatic leadership. In Hunt, J.G. and Larson, L.L. (eds), *Leadership: the Cutting Edge.* Carbondale: Southern Illiois University Press.

McDougall, T. 2000: *Forensic Mental Health Nursing: Current Approaches.* Oxford: Blackwell Science.

NHS Executive 1993: *A Vision for the Future: the Nursing, Midwifery and Health Visiting Contribution to Health and Health Care.* London: NHS Executive.

NHS (NHS Health Advisory Service, Mental Health Act Commission, Department of Health) 1994: *Review of the Adolescent Forensic Psychiatry Services Based on the Gardener Unit, Prestwich Hospital, Salford, Manchester.* London: DoH.

Secord, P.F. and Backman, C.W. 1964: *Social Psychology.* New York: McGraw-Hill.

Watts, F.F. and Bennett, D.H. 1993: *Theory and Practice of Psychiatric Rehabilitation.* Chichester: John Wiley.

Webster, C., Douglas, K., Eaves, D. and Hart, S. 1997: *HCR-20 in Assessing Risk for Violence – Version 2.* British Columbia, Canada: Simon Fraser University.

Wilkinson, G.S. 1973: Interaction patterns and staff responses to psychiatric innovation. *Journal of Health and Social Behaviour* **14**: 422–5.

Wykes, T. and Sturt, E. 1986: The measure of social behaviour in psychiatric patients: an assessment of reliability and validity of the social behaviour rating schedule. *British Journal of Psychiatry* **148**: 1–11.

27

Growing up in prison

JULIET LYON AND DAVID WAPLINGTON

INTRODUCTION

Is it possible to create a healthy institution for children and young people? Young offenders are arguably both the most volatile and the most vulnerable group within the prison population. Staff in young-offender institutions are faced with the challenge of building an environment which at the least does no further damage and at the most offers young people a genuine opportunity to stop and think.

The characteristics of young offenders have been well documented (Boswell 1995; Emler and Reicher 1995; Farrington 1996; Graham and Bowling 1995; Rutter *et al.* 1998). Along with the fractured family relationships, lack of parental supervision, low income, poor health and interrupted schooling which so many share, all young people in prison have in common the fact that they are in transition from childhood to adulthood. They are growing up in an institution.

The experience of incarceration will not be a neutral one. Imprisonment is bound to have a profound effect on young people who, at this stage in their development, are most open to influence, both positive and negative. Knowing this, we are faced with two imperatives. The first is to use prison as a place of absolute last resort for the young, if we are to avoid the confirmation of criminal identities at an early age. The second is to ensure that young-offender institutions operate to the highest possible quality and standards if we are to avoid further alienation and more disordered lives.

It is never easy to care for children and young people away from home. But it is possible to learn from an analysis of social care settings (Bullock *et al.* 1998; Davies *et al.* 1998; Hagell *et al.* 2000; Utting 1997). There are some basic tenets of good-quality care which hold true across a range of institutional settings. These are:

- the creation of a safe, healthy environment with clear objectives and firm boundaries
- the maintenance of family ties and links with education, employment, outside agencies and friends
- a purposeful and active regime which provides opportunities for young people to confront their offending behaviour and to plan for the future
- stable, consistent leadership and professional staff committed to the respectful treatment of young people coupled with a belief in their capacity to change.

In summary, a place which holds young people should be designed for young people. It must be underpinned by what is known about adolescent development, needs and behaviour.

On 1 April 2000, under the Crime and Disorder Act, the Detention and Training Order (DTO) replaced the sentences of Detention in a Young Offenders Institution (DYOI) for 15- to 17-year-olds and the Secure Training Order for 12- to 15-year-olds. These changes were wide-ranging and affected every aspect of the custody of children. Substantial funding was allocated by the Youth Justice Board to ensure that each establishment holding juveniles (aged under 18) would have an active, reformative and adequately staffed regime. New standards were set initially by the Prison Service and subsequently by the Youth Justice Board, for work with this age group.

The Youth Justice Board manages and monitors the new arrangements for individuals aged under 18 years.

It commissions and purchases juvenile secure accommodation from three main sources. These are the prison service, local authority secure units and secure training centres. Many of the secure training centres are run by private contractors and it is anticipated that they will increase their investment and consequently the number of places they provide. It remains to be seen whether the voluntary sector is prepared to engage in running such institutions. The intention of the whole model is to improve standards, to create a coherent system, and to provide better value for money. For the foreseeable future the prison service will continue to be the major accommodation provider, but not all existing young-offender institutions have been developed as part or wholly under-18 establishments. These remaining young-offender institutions continue to hold 18- to 21-year-olds in separate accommodation.

The Youth Justice Board made a commitment to remove all girls under the age of 18 from Prison Service custody in 2002. Initially the commitment was to do so by April 2001. This proved not to be possible owing to increasing numbers being sentenced to custody and the lack of available secure alternatives. A regrettable and unintended consequence of the introduction of the Detention and Training Orders appears to have been a lowering of the custody threshold for this age group. Over the first year there was a 7% increase in the number of children held in prison.

AGE–APPROPRIATE REGIMES

The main principles of the regimes for under-18s are those which experience has shown to be successful in young-offender institutions. These are:

- a full, purposeful and active day
- rigorous assessment of health, social, educational and vocational needs
- education and training to meet these needs
- regular progress reviews against each individual's plan
- support of a personal officer
- inter-agency cooperation and support.

The latter principle is helped by the fact that half of the Detention and Training Order sentence is served in custody while the other half is served under supervision in the community.

The other main features are:

- the involvement of external agencies, particularly Youth Offending Teams (YOTs) and, where possible, the family of the young person
- education for those who are under school leaving age, and an emphasis on improving numeracy, literacy and

preparation for further training and employment for the others
- accredited vocational skills and personal development
- a structured day providing activities relevant to the energy, needs and attention span of young people
- systems and staff behaviour which emphasize the rewards and benefits of good behaviour
- tackling the causes of offending behaviour.

It is probable that all regimes for young prisoners will be enhanced, but it is also likely that legislation will lead to all prisoners aged 18 and over being considered as adults. Consideration is currently being given to creating an estate for young adults in prison. For the present, however, YOIs continue to exist and young offenders constitute a significant and separate group in terms of policy, research and provision. Their reconviction rates are much higher than the reconviction rates for older prisoners, at 75% within two years for young men and something slightly less for young women. Their behaviour in prison is also generally more challenging than that of older adult prisoners. They are responsible for a disproportionately high percentage of assaults. Self-harm is much more common among this group, as is cell damage and 'smash ups'.

Recognizing these difficulties, the prison service has introduced a training course for staff on understanding and handling adolescents in custody. This training programme was developed and used as a cornerstone for the creation of a healthy regime for young people at HM YOI Lancaster Farms (Lyon and Coleman 1998; Sparks 1997). The course identifies key features and some of the challenges involved for staff working with adolescent prisoners. Understanding that adolescence is a time of transition from child to adult helps prison staff to respond to different and apparently inconsistent behaviour from individual prisoners. They are made aware of the importance of the peer group as a source of both inhibition and encouragement. Negative behaviour such as scapegoating and violence are particularly important for institution staff to spot and combat.

Young-offender institutions will vary in their security. The strongest perimeters and cells will generally house the most serious longer-term offenders. Low-security prisoners may be housed in open or partially open conditions. However, there is a requirement for them all to be safe for staff and prisoners, health-promoting, disciplined and reformative. This is made clear in *Prison Service Order on Regimes* for under-18s. It states:

> Governors' consideration of security should not focus exclusively upon the quantitative measure of physical and procedural security. Although the height of walls and fences and the frequency of searches are of negligible importance (symbolically they have a profound effect), security, particularly dynamic security, depends much more upon the quality – how procedures are carried out,

how behaviour affects performance and how feeling safe is more important than being told you are safe.

SAFETY

Young people cannot be expected to learn or change if they are frightened or fear for their safety. The need to prevent bullying is a major task. If left unaddressed bullying leads to disorder, assaults, self-harm and occasionally suicide. Unpublished research has also indicated that a high percentage of escape attempts from young-offender institutions are the result of bullying. This is not the case with escapes and attempted escapes from adult establishments.

Bullying has adverse effects on the individual, the regime, security and order. An anti-bullying strategy is essential and to be effective it must be supported by the whole establishment. The best kind of anti-bullying strategies involve prisoners as well as staff as they have the most to gain from a safe community. This mirrors the whole school approach to tackling bullying which appears to have been successful in the education system.

The following principles are essential for an effective, safer prison strategy:

- management commitment to develop a safe environment for everyone
- respect for the humanity and individualism of every prisoner
- effective communications
- ensuring that no incident is allowed to go uninvestigated and action is taken which demonstrates the staff's attitude towards bullying
- involvement of the whole community – staff and prisoners
- continuous and imaginative monitoring
- development of a positive and supportive environment
- improved arrangements for reception and induction and the introduction of first night in custody centres.

A POSITIVE ENVIRONMENT

Experience has shown that young offender institutions that base their regimes predominantly upon sanctions and punishments are less successful than those that stress achievements and rewards for good behaviour.

A varied, purposeful and active regime is essential if staff and management are to fulfil this aim of reforming and training prisoners. As we have said, young-offender institutions are not neutral in their effect. Left to their own devices young prisoners will experience crime and bullying and there is the ever-present danger that the institution becomes a 'school of crime' where knowledge of how to commit crime is enhanced. In reality there is no

sensible alternative to an active reforming regime for those who need to be in prison. For those who do not, there needs to be robust community orders and intensive supervision and support.

The importance of a positive and supportive regime is also necessary for the success of anti-offending courses. Research into what works in reducing offending stresses the importance of staff–prisoner relationships and the regime generally. Where there is a supportive and positive culture there is likely to be a better outcome for accredited anti-offending courses. A supportive regime will also help to reduce levels of self-harm and help prevent suicides. Experience shows that it also helps to reduce violent incidents and the kind of problems that force staff into unproductive use of their time. Staff are very important to adolescents in prison and their influence can be crucial. It is important that they spend as much time as possible guiding and helping prisoners.

STAFF AS 'SIGNIFICANT ADULTS'

Staff who have been trained to understand and work successfully with adolescents in custody can influence and motivate them. They are important role models. Adolescence training teaches the importance of 'significant adults'. This description includes institutional staff like themselves. This training also provides staff with the knowledge that adolescents need a disciplined but purposeful environment. It asks staff to explore the concept of authoritative parenting and its implications for the core and control of young people in custody. The following is an extract from an evaluation sheet written by a YOI officer who attended a training course; it illustrates the value of such training in practice.

'I gained an understanding of why adolescents act and react in the ways they do. The course made me think back to my own youth and enabled me to project this forward to the inmates we have. I believe this will give a more positive attitude in my work on the wings.'

It is significant that in response to the open-ended question 'What is the best thing about Lancaster Farms?', 29% of young prisoners said it was the staff and the way in which they treated young prisoners with respect and trust. Unfortunately, similar surveys of prisoners' views of comparable institutions in the North West produced no such results. Staff are the most important asset of the institution. They should all direct their work towards influencing and encouraging prisoners. Their training stresses that they are dealing with adolescents who are growing up in prison and, unless staff create them, there are few opportunities for prisoners to contribute and 'do good'. To help counteract this, staff are encouraged to persuade prisoners to join problem-solving committees and peer-group support schemes and, in the most mature settings, to become advocates. These strategies, when successful, will bring staff and prisoners closer together and can help young prisoners to develop an honest and good self-image.

Of course, if the energy of the staff is to be directed towards the goal of influencing prisoners they themselves need support. This should include clear and visible leadership, regular communications, the knowledge that positive expectations are held of them, a chance to develop and contribute, recognition and a positive environment. Staff working in young-offender institutions are doing work of a high quality and they experience much stress and frustration working with a difficult and demanding group of young people. Initiating and maintaining good relationships with young people requires energy, enthusiasm and skill. It is difficult but also rewarding. Staff managers should recognize that humour, and even fun, are often very useful indicators that things are going well. The prison service is struggling to develop consistent stable leadership. The high turnover and rapid movement of governors is particularly damaging to young people who need to know who is in charge.

THE HEALTHY INSTITUTION

Health has always been an issue in institutions, and the task of keeping the environment clean and hygienic is well understood. Lately it has been realized that young-offender institutions contain a high proportion of people who have special health needs. Many of them have histories which include damaging experiences in childhood, abuse and loss, experimentation with drugs or alcohol, truancy and sleeping rough. Their lives have been characterized by change and disruption. As one young woman in custody said (Lyon *et al.* 2000):

> 'We've all been through social services, foster, children's homes, getting kicked out of school, secure unit ... I'm sure we've all been through that road. It's like a journey and we've all collected our tickets along the way.'

These young people are also particularly vulnerable to mental health problems (Lader *et al.* 2000). Imprisonment itself is usually a stressful experience often accompanied by feelings of guilt, shame and low self-worth. Young prisoners are cut off from their families and other supportive relationships.

For all of these reasons, young offender institutions must have a policy to support the health needs of their population. Awareness of the possibility of a secure custodial environment providing a good opportunity for health education and health interventions has also been realized. As a result, a major government initiative has seen drug-prevention workers introduced into every YOI and there have been other initiatives to improve awareness of the risks of HIV/AIDS. A World Health Organization initiative to improve mental health has been promoted in all young-offender institutions in England and Wales.

It is instructive to discover that some of the ways of improving the well-being of prisoners include activities which attract some criticism because they are enjoyable – such as drama, art and music. Prisons are not meant to be 'enjoyable', and in reality they are not. Loss of liberty is a grave punishment. The pain of imprisonment should not, however, be extended to exclude even some constructive activities. Other regime activities necessary in a 'healthy prison' are regular physical exercise, participation in education, work and training, and effective anti-bullying strategies. Health research also suggests that 'whole prison' approaches to anti-bullying were the most effective; and that where the culture was one of respect, care and trust between staff and prisoners and between prisoners also, a healthy setting was more likely.

RESETTLEMENT

Resettlement is probably the most difficult area of work for a young-offender institution. The high rate of reconviction amongst young offenders is alarming. Many of them leave prison well-intentioned but ill-prepared. They lack support in the community and are heavily influenced by a criminal peer group. Drug taking and the presence of drugs generally has exacerbated these problems.

Recently several institutions have opened branches of the YMCA inside the prisons. These give prisoners access to YMCA hostels, job-search and youth employment schemes. Some YMCA schemes target young offenders who were sleeping rough prior to reception. Outside drug workers have also been helpful in obtaining treatment support for prisoners on release. Unfortunately this is an area where, until recently, demand outstripped provision.

The most successful resettlement initiatives for young offenders have involved some form of mentoring support on discharge. One of the most successful of these was the 'high-intensity regime' at Thorne Cross which provided a mentor for each discharged young offender, from the Society of Voluntary Associates (SOVA). These are all volunteers who provide informal support during the crucial early stages of resettlement. Research into the success of this in improving reconviction rates has been most encouraging. It is hoped that such initiatives will continue and grow. The fact is that good regimes for children and young people are costly, well managed and small in scale.

Other recent initiatives in YOIs include the introduction of the government's Welfare to Work scheme. This has provided many young offenders with specific and relevant training, leading on release to access to further training, voluntary work or employment. It has also seen the introduction of career services working alongside young offenders prior to their release. This too has been beneficial and seems to be a most promising initiative.

Of course the ultimate measure of the success of a young-offender institution remains a reduced rate of reconviction. However, there are some very real difficulties in obtaining results about the impact of specific regimes. This is especially true of young-offender remand centres with their rapid throughput of prisoners and short period of imprisonment. The transition period following release is particularly difficult, and often success is dependent upon the support available to the young person in the community. Many have little family support that they can rely on. The Social Exclusion Unit has reviewed how to reduce re-offending and the needs of short-term prisoners. It is clear that a reduction in the use of custodial remand, an improvement in remand conditions and a sustained focus on resettlement would all make a positive difference. It is difficult, but possible, to create healthy secure conditions for children and young people, particularly if prison can be reserved as an absolute place of last resort and if institutions for young people are run to the highest possible quality and standard, with the needs of the adolescents they contain maintained firmly at the centre of the work that is done.

REFERENCES

Boswell, J. 1995: *Violent Victims: the Prevalence of Abuse and Loss in the Lives of Section 53 Offenders*. London: Prince's Trust.

Bullock, R., Little, M. and Millham, S. 1998: *Secure Treatment Outcomes: the Care Careers of Very Difficult Adolescents*. Aldershot: Ashgate.

Davies, C., Archer, S., Hicks, L. and Little, M. (eds) 1998: *Caring for Children Away from Home: Messages from Research*. Chichester: John Wiley/DoH.

Emler, N. and Reicher, S. 1995: *Adolescence and Delinquency*. Oxford: Blackwell.

Graham, J. and Bowling, B. 1995: *Young People and Crime*. Research Study 145. London: Home Office.

Hagell, A., Hazell, N. and Shaw, C. 2000: *Evaluation of Medway Secure Training Centre*. London: Home Office.

Lader, D., Singleton, N. and Meltzer, H. 2000: *Psychiatric Morbidity among Young Offenders in England and Wales*. Norwich: TSO.

Lyon, J. and Coleman, J. 1998: *The Nature of Adolescence: Working with Young People in Custody*. Brighton: Trust for the Study of Adolescence.

Lyon, J., Dennison, C. and Wilson, A. 2000: *Tell Them So They Listen: Messages from Young People in Custody*. Home Office Research Study 201. London: Home Office.

Rutter, M., Giller, H. and Hagell, A. 1998: *Antisocial Behaviour by Young People*. Cambridge: Cambridge University Press.

Social Exclusion Unit 2002: *Reducing Offending by Ex-prisoners*. London: HMSO.

Sparks, C. 1997: *Lancaster Farms: Preventing the Next Victim*. London: Prison Reform Trust.

Utting, W. 1997: *People Like Us*. London: Department of Health and the Welsh Office.

BIBLIOGRAPHY

Farrington, D. 1996: *Understanding and Preventing Youth Crime*. York: Joseph Rowntree Foundation.

HM Chief Inspector of Prisons 1997: *Young Prisoners: a Thematic Review*. London: HMSO.

HM Chief Inspector of Prisons 1999: *Suicide is Everyone's Concern: a Thematic Review*. London: HMSO.

HM Chief Inspector of Prisons 2000: *Unjust Deserts: a Thematic Review. The Treatment and Conditions for Unsentenced Prisoners in England and Wales*. Norwich: TSO.

Youth Justice Board 2002: *ASSET*. Annual Report. London: Youth Justice Board.

28

Prison psychiatry

CLAIRE DIMOND AND PETER MISCH

INTRODUCTION

By their very nature, prisons, particularly those that contain children or young people, evoke powerful emotions in both those held within them and the public at large. Despite the dismally high rates of reconviction for adolescents leaving prison, custody remains a popular disposal for the British Courts, resulting in the UK having one of the highest rates of imprisonment per capita population in Europe. The large size of this population, combined with its high level of risk factors for mental disorder and the shortfall in psychiatric resources for this population outside of prison, inevitably results in prisons acting as reservoirs of mental disorder.

From a psychiatric perspective, prisons, with all their inherent problems, and which for some children is the place where they grow up, present both a massive challenge and also one of the most varied, interesting, psychiatric populations. A study of these populations, which at first sight appear to be clearly demarcated from the rest of the community by the surrounding prison wall or fence, leads not just to an understanding of the institution but also a viewing point or perspective on the community outside of its walls.

Society imposes two, at times contradictory, demands on prisons and those working within them:

- deprivation of liberty, the sanctioned punishment for serious or persistent offending

- that prisoners be held humanely and be given the opportunity of reform in order that they may lead law-abiding lives on their release.

This contradiction is highlighted when a significant proportion of the general population and some politicians extol the virtues of ever-longer sentences and harsh and austere regimes. Psychiatry has an important contribution to make to the second of these aims in the promotion of the 'healthy prison' concept as discussed in Chapter 27.

HISTORICAL PERSPECTIVE

Up to the end of the eighteenth century, imprisonment was not in itself a penalty for crime; prisons were mainly places where persons either awaited trial, or they awaited a punishment – which for major offences was death or transportation, and for minor offences fines and corporal punishments. When transportation to America finished as a consequence of the American War of Independence, legislation was introduced allowing convicts, who would otherwise have been transported, to be confined. The prison building programme, which resulted in some of the prisons still used today, was embarked on between 1840 and 1850.

Under common law, the age of criminal responsibility in England and Wales was 7 years. Accordingly, juveniles accused of crimes were treated as adults at both trial and disposition stages and they could be executed, transported or imprisoned. Whilst the need for special jurisdiction over juvenile offenders was first noted in the early nineteenth century, it was not until 1879 that the number of juveniles in prisons was substantially reduced by trying most juveniles at magistrates Courts. Despite the introduction of reformatory and industrial schools resulting in an overall reduction in the use of prisons for juveniles, children were still required to serve 14 days in prison before moving on to these institutions.

The Children Act of 1908 marked the beginning of a welfare perspective by establishing the Juvenile Court and viewing parents as having some responsibility in relation to their children's wrongdoings. Imprisonment under the age of 14 was ended in 1908, but a new institution with rigid discipline and work in a secure environment was set up as an alternative. The first of these was in Borstal in Kent, subsequently giving its name to numerous similar establishments. The Children and Young Persons Act 1933 saw a further move towards a welfare focus. The age of criminal responsibility was raised from 7 to 8 years and magistrates were to have regard to the 'welfare of the child'. The Act replaced the reformatory and industrial schools by approved schools and introduced remand homes providing a place of custody for criminally remanded juveniles and those alleged to be in need of care, protection or control.

In 1963, the age of criminal responsibility was raised to 10 years, where it remains today. Borstals changed their name to Youth Custody Centres in 1982 and subsequently Young Offender Institutions (YOIs) in 1988. Boys aged between 15 and 21 years were held in young-offender institutions and remand centres which, in all but name, have been similar to those holding adult offenders (the terms 'YOIs' and 'prison' will be used interchangeably in the text).

Many YOIs have repeatedly been the focus of ever-increasing critical reports, particularly by successive Chief Inspectors of Prisons and non-statutory pressure groups who have repeatedly highlighted the often appalling conditions for young people in these institutions. Particular concern was raised for the 15- and 16-year-old boys who faced conditions vastly inferior to those of similar age in local authority secure units. Criticism about the poor quality or lack of healthcare particularly for vulnerable or mentally disordered offenders has been equally prominent. The increased rate of deaths of young offenders by suicide has augmented these criticisms, building up political pressures that undoubtedly have resulted in reforms to both the young-offender institutions and healthcare provision to prisons that are due to be implemented in the coming years. Whilst not prison service establishments, secure training centres are the latest in the line of custodial institutions and hold boys and girls between the ages of 14 and 17 years, with plans to remove all girls under the age of 18 years from prison and to increase the number of secure training centre beds to over 500.

THE HISTORY OF HEALTHCARE IN PRISON

The Prison Medical Service is the oldest civilian medical service in England and Wales, it has its roots in the legislative result of the prison reformer John Howard's investigation into the state of English prisons. The appalling conditions he described led to the passing of the Health of Prisoners Act 1774. This Act required prisons to appoint 'an experienced doctor or apothecary in order to preserve the health of prisoners in gaol'. The idea that doctors subsequently acted as a force for positive change is challenged by sociologist Joe Sims in *Medical Power in Prisons*, which notes the prolonged plunging of prisoners into cold baths being advocated by doctors in 1796 in order to detect prisoners who were feigning madness (Sim 1990). In 1873 the medical commissioner to prisons supported the use of the notorious treadwheel.

In 1879, the new prison commissioner, Dr Glover, drew attention to the continuing large number of mentally disordered in prison and to the high suicide rate. The year 1877, when the administration of 'local prisons' was taken over by the government, marked the birth of the Prison Medical Service.

Although the integration of the Prison Medical Service with the National Health Service was mooted at the latter's birth in 1948, the two systems remained separate. Most prisons by this time had a 'hospital wing' based on the military sick-bay concept, staffed by a medical officer and hospital officers, a brand of prison discipline staff who received a brief training in nursing orderly duties.

In the last 40 years prison healthcare has continued to be the subject of much comment and criticism. The 'Efficiency Scrutiny' report in 1990 resulted in the renaming of the Prison Medical Service as the Health Care Service for Prisoners, which now aimed to be a purchaser rather than provider of healthcare and form a closer alignment with the NHS. Fundamental structural problems remained unresolved, and in 1996 after little progress the Chief Inspector of Prisons, Sir David Ramsbotham, published an influential report entitled *Patient or Prisoner?* (HM Chief Inspector of Prisons 1996). This report advocated, as part of resolving these problems, that the NHS should take over responsibility for the healthcare of prisoners. A subsequent joint prison service and NHS working group (HM Prison Service and NHS Executive 1999) did not go so far as advocating fusion of the two services, but did implement structural changes that included for the first time a joint Home Office–NHS Policy Unit and Task Force. An agenda for change over 3–5 years on the basis of this formal partnership includes comprehensive health needs assessment and prison health improvement programmes for the entire prison estate (Grounds 2000). It remains to be seen how effective these reforms will be in improving mental healthcare for prisoners.

MODELS OF PSYCHIATRIC CARE FOR ADOLESCENTS IN PRISON

In the traditional model of medical provision within the prison healthcare service, primary care was provided by medical officers, doctors directly employed by the prison service, and more recently visiting general practitioners. Specialist psychiatric care is provided by visiting psychiatrists, although primary-care doctors provide the majority of assessment and the day-to-day management of mentally disturbed prisoners. Nursing input was traditionally provided by a grade of prison officers with no professional nursing qualification, known as a Health Care Officer who receive a brief training; fully trained nurses are now taking over this role. Many prison psychologists are not clinically trained. The healthcare officers and nurses control access to the general practitioner.

Prison 'hospitals' are graded 1 to 3 according to whether they contain a sick-bay with a few cells used for observation to a large wing with 24-hour healthcare cover. Hospital wings generally contain a diverse mixture of prisoners: those who are physically ill, those who are vulnerable or self-harming, the floridly mentally ill, and sometimes healthy prisoners 'lodging' in the hospital when the prison is full. Some prison hospital wings built for young offenders as late as the 1980s continued to contain cells designated for the mentally ill without any direct access to toilets, thus necessitating 'slopping out'. This archaic and unhygienic practice no doubt reflected the underlying institutional prejudice and stigma about mentally ill prisoners.

An investigation into the facilities for inpatient care of mentally disordered people in prison (Reed and Lyne 2000), which surveyed 13 inpatient units comprising 20% of all beds in prison, highlighted the following facts:

- No doctor in charge of inpatients had completed specialist psychiatric training.
- Twenty-four per cent of nursing staff had mental health training; 32% were non-nursing trained health-care officers.
- Only one prison had occupational therapy input; two had input from a clinical psychologist.
- Most patients were locked in their cells for about 21.5 hours a day.
- The average length of a period of seclusion was 50 hours.
- Healthcare standards for prison which are outlined in several documents were frequently not being met.

A developmentally appropriate model of prison mental healthcare that has been proposed as a template for healthcare provision in a YOI will now be described (Misch 1998). Young prisoners, especially those who spend long periods in prison, present the same range of mental healthcare needs as young people in the general community where mental healthcare is provided on a tiered level.

When this model of care is applied to a young-offender institution, the relationship between the prison officer and inmate comes into sharp focus and dictates that the personal (prison) officer shares a degree of parental care with the young person's parents or carers, and should to some extent act as the young person's advocate in prison, as is the case in secure units run by social services (Rutter *et al.* 1998, pp. 364–5). The first tier of care should in essence be similar to that provided in the general community, allowing direct access and confidential consultation with a general practitioner.

The next tier of care (equivalent of CAMHS outpatient) should be provided by a multi-disciplinary adolescent mental health team which incorporates a mechanism to allow confidential referrals directly from either young prisoners or by prison officers and others caring for them. The 'community' within a prison setting can be regarded as the ordinary 'wings', also called 'ordinary location.' The disciplines within this team should include psychiatry, psychology, nursing and individual/family therapy. It is also desirable to have representation from other agencies working within the prison such as the drug project team, chaplaincy and probation.

In principle, the requirement for the next, inpatient tier of mental healthcare for young prisoners should be small and reserved for crisis intervention or a brief period of assessment. This level of care requires specialist adolescent nursing, consultant adolescent forensic psychiatry, clinical psychology, occupational therapy, family and individual therapies (including creative non-verbal therapies). Specialist educational input is also essential for this age group.

Patients identified as being acutely psychotic or severely depressed, and some patients with a severe personality disorder, should be swiftly transferred to outside hospitals. In practice, however, the lack of appropriate NHS resources (which is particularly acute for this age group), and disagreements between catchment area psychiatrists about responsibility and disposal, all conspire to result in many mentally disordered patients spending very long periods in prison hospitals. The Mental Health Act 1983 does not apply to prisons; that is, no healthcare facility within prison is regarded as a 'hospital' for the purposes of the Mental Health Act 1983. Thus in prison medication can be administered without consent only in an emergency under the provisions of common law.

It is essential that a continuum of care be provided such that when a young person leaves prison he or she has access to appropriate psychiatric care. The Care Plan Approach (CPA) should be applied both for adolescents coming into prison with established mental health problems and also for those leaving. In practice there is often little or no contact between CPA key-workers or CAMHS staff and prison healthcare staff (Health Advisory Committee 1997). Continuity of care requires close liaison between prison health services and the NHS team with ongoing responsibility for the person's care.

Currently there is a paucity of child and adolescent psychiatric input, both general and forensic, into young-offender institutions.

PREVALENCE OF PSYCHIATRIC DISORDER IN YOUNG PRISONERS

Adolescents in prison have a very high prevalence of psychosocial stresses and adversities known to be associated with psychiatric disorder. A stark indicator of this is that over a third of adolescents in prison have been 'looked after' by the local authority. As a group, they report high levels of previous physical, sexual and emotional abuse, have high rates of school exclusion, poor academic attainments and high levels of unemployment; many are also teenage parents. For some, placement in prison will be the first time they have been separated for any considerable period of time from parents or carers. For many, the circumstances leading to their placement in prison will have been significantly traumatic. Many young people will be exposed to further psychological and physical victimization and trauma whilst in prison. (HM Chief Inspector of Prisons 1997a; Lader et al. 2000). The presence of large numbers of people with serious mental illness in prison has been recognized for over 200 years.

The Reed Report (DoH 1992) argued in relation to young offenders that 'assessments should always take account of developmental factors affecting adolescents' and that 'assessment by adult criteria should be avoided'. Adolescents in prison should be interviewed with age-appropriate instruments and assigned age-appropriate diagnoses.

Two issues arise from the several recent large-scale studies aimed at ascertaining the prevalence of psychiatric disorder in the prison population, including adolescents, in the UK.

1 These studies did not screen for the ICD-10 category of 'behavioural and emotional disorders with onset usually occurring in childhood or adolescence' (equivalent to the DSM-IV category of 'disorders usually first evident in infancy, childhood or adolescence').

2 Children aged 16 years were assigned diagnoses of personality disorder. ICD-10 states that 'personality disorder tends to appear in late childhood or adolescence and continues to be manifest into adulthood. It is therefore unlikely that the diagnosis of personality disorder will be appropriate before the age of 16 or 17 years.' A DSM-IV diagnosis of antisocial

Table 28.1 *Institute of Psychiatry prison surveys in England and Wales*[a]

	Remanded (n = 206)	Sentenced (n = 404)
Psychosis	1.9	0.2
Neuroses	18.9	5.7
Personality disorders	11.7	14.1
Sexual deviations	0	0.2
Substance misuse	36.4	18.6
Organic	1.5	0.5
Mental retardation	2.0	0.2
Any diagnosis	53.0	33.0

[a] Percentages of specific diagnoses in samples of male youths aged 16–20 years (combining primary with additional diagnoses).

personality disorder requires that persons must be 18 years or older.

Given the caveats described above, the large-scale studies of the prison population to be described provide an indication of the prevalence of psychiatric disorder in adolescents in prison (Table 28.1).

Gunn et al. (1991) surveyed 5% of the population of sentenced male youths, and Maden et al. (1995) surveyed 10% of the population of unconvicted male youths in their studies of the prevalence of psychiatric disorder in the prison population in England and Wales. Psychiatrists administered semi-structured interviews designed for the studies. In both of these studies the prevalence of personality disorder was reportedly under-diagnosed as the assessment was not sufficiently detailed and there was a lack of informant information. In these studies, comorbidity was common, with 17% having dual diagnosis and 7% having three or more diagnoses in the study by Maden et al. (1995).

Several factors have been proposed to result in an increase in psychiatric morbidity among remand prisoners. The remanded period is a particularly stressful time for many young prisoners who have to cope with the stress of reception into prison, including separation from home, friends and relatives, the uncertainty regarding the eventual outcome of their case, and for many a sudden cessation and unsupported withdrawal from drugs and alcohol. In many establishments, the prison regime is particularly deprived for remand prisoners with even longer periods of time being spent locked up in cells, less exercise and opportunities for education, and a faster movement of prisoners within the estate, which erodes the opportunity for positive inmate–officer relationships.

In a recent study by the Office for National Statistics, which surveyed the psychiatric morbidity among prisoners in England and Wales (Singleton et al. 1998), 590 young offenders aged 16–20 were interviewed (Table 28.2). Lay interviewers using various assessment instruments conducted interviews. One hundred received a follow-up

Table 28.2 *Psychiatric morbidity in young offenders aged 16–20 years in England and Wales: ONS survey (percentages)*

Diagnosis	Male		Female	
	Remanded (n = 314)	Sentenced (n = 169)	Remanded (n = 26)	Sentenced (n = 81)
Psychosis (from clinical interview)	8	10	Too small	Too small
Neuroses	52	41	[20]	67
Personality disorder (any) (from clinical interview)	84	88	Too small	Too small
Antisocial personality (from clinical interview)	76	81	Too small	Too small
Alcohol misuse	62	70	[13]	51
Substance dependence	57	52	[13]	58

Note: In view of the small number of female remand prisoners, actual numbers are given in square brackets.

interview with a psychiatrist or psychologist, who administered interview instruments to assess psychotic disorder and personality disorder. Data from the prisoners who had both interviews were used to estimate the 'probable' prevalence of personality disorder and psychotic disorders in the population as a whole (Lader *et al.* 2000). In all sample groups, at least 95% were assessed as having one or more disorders, and a very large proportion, about 80%, were assessed as having more than one. The higher prevalence rates obtained in the ONS study as compared to the Gunn and Maden studies may reflect the use of different study designs.

Nicol *et al.* (2000), as part of a health needs study, used the Kiddie SADS-E to interview 56 adolescents, aged under 18, in a young-offender institution. In this sample, 30% were diagnosed with anxiety, 13% with depression, 2% with a past history of psychosis, 86% with an externalizing disorder (conduct disorder and/or hyperactivity), and 53% with substance misuse. There was a high level of comorbidity. Only eight of the young people interviewed did not receive a diagnosis.

Kazdin (2000), in a review of the literature on the prevalence of psychiatric disorders in 'incarcerated adolescents' in the USA, noted that the available research is sparse and highlighted that many of the studies used small groups restricted to a given facility and did not use standard diagnostic assessment methods. Gross prevalence rates were: conduct disorder 41–49%, attention-deficit hyperactivity disorder (ADHD) 19–46%, substance abuse and dependence 25–50%, mood disorders 19–78%, anxiety disorders 6–41%, psychoses 1–6%, and mental retardation 7–15%. However, one study of over 1200 youths in a juvenile detention facility used the Diagnostic Interview Schedule for Children; the prevalence rates fell within those given and 80% of the youths were found to have at least one disorder. Comorbidity was common in these studies.

In summary, studies indicate that there is extensive psychiatric morbidity among adolescents in prison. Studies consistently show that adolescents in prison have high

rates of affective disorder, alcohol and substance misuse. The prevalence of conduct disorder and ADHD, when assessed, in adolescents in prison has been found to be high, but this is expected given the definition of conduct disorder and its comorbidity. In those studies in which adolescents were assessed for a personality disorder, the prevalence of antisocial personality disorder was high. The rates of reported psychotic disorders have varied widely. The prevalence of mental retardation and pervasive developmental disorders in adolescents in prison in England and Wales is unknown. It is important that future studies further elucidate any gender differences and the relationships between offences and psychiatric disorder. Further studies of young people in prison are required, using appropriate instruments and diagnostic criteria, to provide valid estimates of their treatment needs.

TREATMENT NEEDS OF PRISONERS

Evidently the treatment needs of prisoners need to be viewed within the context of their environment and the emerging literature on evidence-based medicine. The studies on sentenced and remand prisoners (Gunn *et al.* 1991; Maden *et al.* 1995) give estimates of the treatment needs of young male prisoners according to clinical judgement (Table 28.3).

Table 28.3 *Treatment needs of young male prisoners*

	Youths (%)	
	Sentenced	Remanded
Transfer to NHS inpatient	1	3
Prison hospital/outpatient care	9	15
Therapeutic community	4	11
Further assessment	5	1.5
Substance misuse	–	12

Gunn and associates estimated that 20% of the young people interviewed in their study required treatment and that only 4% were receiving it. Maden and associates estimated that 42% of their sample required psychiatric intervention or treatment. When these (conservative) estimates are extrapolated to a large YOI such as Feltham, at any one point in time 21 inmates require either NHS transfer or prison hospital and 225 inmates require some sort of outpatient intervention. In practice the need has been demonstrated to be even higher than this. As a local prison serving the London and surrounding Courts, this prison has a very high throughput, receiving 12,000 new prisoners per year (Misch 1998). The national needs assessments which are being conducted by the Prison Service–NHS partnership at the time of writing aim to provide more specific data on which services should be planned.

'OFFENDING BEHAVIOUR' PROGRAMMES PROVIDED WITHIN YOUNG-OFFENDER INSTITUTIONS

There are a number of different programmes run within YOIs that are aimed at addressing offending behaviour. The following prison service programmes have been accredited by an independent body and are run within YOIs:

- enhanced thinking skills
- reasoning and rehabilitation
- reasoning and reacting (pilot)
- sex-offender treatment programme.

These are group programmes based on a cognitive–behavioural framework. Whilst these programmes are available for motivated prisoners, they might well exclude those who have learning difficulties, or display behavioural problems of, for example, an autistic type, or have other psychiatric problems that make their inclusion in a group programme difficult.

A new prison drug initiative called CARAT (counselling, assessment, referral, advice and through-care) aims to ensure effective delivery of drug programmes in prisons which link with both prison health and community drug programmes. The provision is delivered on a contracted-out basis.

SCREENING FOR PSYCHIATRIC DISORDER

In order to prevent mentally disordered offenders entering prison unnecessarily and to facilitate early interventions for those who do, a number of Court diversion schemes have been set up which provide rapid psychiatric assessments for magistrates' Courts. In a recent study, Shaw et al. (1999) found a poor detection rate, which resulted in only 14 of 96 adult defendants from overnight custody with serious psychiatric disorder being identified by Court staff and referred for psychiatric assessment.

'ASSET' (assessment profile) – a screening protocol recently introduced by the Youth Justice Board to be completed on all offenders under the age of 18 years subject to a Court order or final warning – includes some screening questions about psychiatric disorder and vulnerability factors and should be completed before a sentenced and, at latest, within a few days after a remanded young person enters prison.

Screening on reception into prison is usually carried out by healthcare officers or nurses followed by a clinical examination by the prison doctor. Bearing in mind the almost total lack of any social or medical background information accompanying many prisoners, and the large number of over 50 new prisoners who may enter a young-offender institution in an evening, the findings by Birmingham et al. (1996) that less than a quarter of the mentally disordered adult prisoners were identified at reception screening is not unexpected. The same study found that only two out of five patients requiring urgent treatment were placed in the prison healthcare centre. As a result of a study aimed at evaluating the prison screening process (Birmingham et al. 2000), the authors concluded that the health screen for new prisoners needs revision and improvement. Improvement of reception screening is now a priority of both the Prison Service Health Taskforce and Safer Custody (suicide) group (HM Chief Inspector of Prisons 1999).

ASSESSMENTS IN PRISON

Practical issues

Many mental healthcare professionals will have little or no experience of working within the prison environment. The lack of familiarity with practical issues can cause considerable uncertainty, frustration or anxiety about visiting or commencing work within these closed confines. It is helpful for the mental health worker to have some familiarity with the system (see also Chapter 27). The practical arrangements for carrying out a visiting mental health assessment can be organized by contacting the prison's healthcare manager. Prisons generally have fixed visiting times. The professional visitor should be prepared for routine bag searches and, depending on the establishment's security level, body searches. If commencing regular contracted prison work, a prison pass should be applied for well in advance; it requires checks and a formal security induction and results in allocation of keys and thus unaccompanied movement around the prison.

Contextual issues

Whilst the developmental and systemic principles that apply to child and adolescent psychiatric assessment in the community apply equally in the custodial context, it is easy to forget this. Many adolescents in custody are 'looked after', others may have been dislodged or rejected from their family of origin because of their challenging behaviour or as a consequence of the offence they are charged with. When these issues are combined with the physical (and symbolic) barrier of the perimeter fence, it is easy for the psychiatrist to be 'organized' by these factors and fail to contact family members or arrange family interviews according to usual practice in the community. Depending on the particular circumstances, contact may also be made with the person's youth justice worker or probation officer and any allocated social worker.

The assessor will need to be aware of the great variation of environments in British young-offender institutions, from the appalling where 23-hour 'bang up' and gross deficiencies in educational placements have been shown to be the norm (HM Chief Inspector of Prisons 1997a), to the few good establishments which meet the standards set out by the prison service.

Most psychiatrists will see adolescents in prison as a visiting psychiatrist to do a 'one-off' assessment. The following discussion particularly applies to this situation. Consideration must always be given to risk management prior to any direct contact with prisoners. As well as considering any potential risk of assault, it is important to be mindful that episodes of hostage taking in prison in England and Wales occur every year. Enquiry should be made to prison staff about the risk status of the individual prisoner and, on occasions, a balance stuck between the rights of a prisoner to have a consultation in privacy and the level of observation necessary to ensure safety. Usually, the young person will be brought to the healthcare centre. For example, it is not acceptable to see a young person in 'legal visits', a large room filled with tables and chairs. Sometimes the person may be seen on the 'wings' or 'ordinary location'. This may well be informative and provide an opportunity to assess the quality of care being provided to the young person. Some areas of the prison may pose particular problems such as when the young person is in 'segregation'. Whilst one may decide to defer the assessment until another time, it is worth bearing in mind the possibility that an undetected mental illness may be driving the behaviour that led the prisoner to be placed in the segregation unit or the behaviour that prolongs the stay in the segregation unit.

It is important to inform the adolescent as to whether the assessment is being carried out on the instructions of person's solicitor, the Court or CPS, or the prison authorities, and to explain to the young person the destination and potential use and limits of confidentiality of the psychiatric assessment. Throughout the interview one should be aware that the young person might be feeling particularly powerless and dealing with a lot of stress and uncertainties. The style and content of the interview will be guided by its purpose. It is important to be aware that after the interview the young person is probably returning to a locked cell, possibly alone and for a long period of time. Thus, one has to make judgements regarding discussion around sensitive issues such as abuse.

Prior to or after an assessment, the IMR (inmate medical record), including any medical notes and the medication chart, should be reviewed. Discussion with the staff (prison officers or healthcare staff) can usefully include the following:

- the staffs' general observations and view of the adolescent, including observations about mood and behaviour, particularly any concerns about self-harm
- the adolescent's relationships with both staff and inmates, including whether to their knowledge the adolescent has been involved in bullying, either as a perpetrator or victim, or episodes in the segregation (punishment) wing.

Enquiries should be made as to attendance at education/training and association (the time when inmates are allowed to watch television or play pool in a group, colloquially referred to as 'soc') and their understanding of the reasons for any non-attendance; and whether the adolescent has a job (e.g. as a cleaner), as these are allocated on a graded basis to 'trusted prisoners'. After the assessment any concerns about the adolescent's safety are appropriately discussed with the prison officers and/or prison medical staff.

Reports to court

Psychiatrists working within a prison may prepare reports for a number of reasons. The prison governor is responsible for obtaining medical reports regarding prisoners whose ill-health may affect their ability to attend or appropriately participate in Court proceedings. A mentally disordered prisoner may be considered 'unfit to attend Court' where his or her behaviour may 'constitute a public scandal'. A floridly psychotic and disinhibited patient may be such a person. Alternatively a prisoner may be found fit to attend Court but not fit to plead or to attend trial. It is appropriate for a psychiatrist working on behalf of a prison to submit a voluntary report to the Court in these circumstances even where such a report has not been requested. Where a prisoner is not as yet tried, it is wise to avoid comment on issues other than the patient's immediate mental health problems as this could compromise the criminal case. The Court should, however, be advised against the informal release of a mentally disordered defendant back into the community without appropriate psychiatric care where it is believed that the person's behaviour may constitute a serious risk to self or others. The Court can be advised to consider a psychiatric disposal or return to prison. There is a statutory requirement that all defendants facing murder charges must have a psychiatric assessment, and the Crown Prosecution Service instructs these reports. A psychiatric report may be requested to be submitted to the Court in order to provide an opinion about whether a young defendant in prison under the age of 18 years should be deemed to be 'vulnerable' by virtue of 'emotional immaturity or propensity to self-harm' and thus warrant transfer to a local authority secure unit.

CLINICAL ISSUES

In this section a number of clinical issues particularly relevant to prison psychiatry are discussed.

Post-traumatic stress disorder

One could hypothesize that the prevalence of post-traumatic stress disorder (PTSD) in adolescents in prison is high. They have been exposed to high levels of trauma in their childhood, there is extensive victimization within prison, and in addition they may develop PTSD symptoms as a direct consequence of their offence. It is a subject that is only beginning to be explored. The prevalence rates found in different studies have varied greatly. In the ONS study (Lader *et al.* 2000), 4% of young male remand and sentenced and 7% of female sentenced young offenders were diagnosed with PTSD. In studies in the USA, 32.3% of incarcerated young males (Steiner *et al.* 1997) and 48.9% of incarcerated young females (Cauffman *et al.* 1998) had a current diagnosis of PTSD. These differences may reflect different diagnostic practices in England and the USA. In addition, the American studies were specifically examining rates of PTSD.

The most commonly reported antecedent traumas in young prisoners are being a victim of a violent act, witnessing a violent act, and participating in a violent act (Steiner *et al.* 1997; Cauffman *et al.* 1998). Further studies investigating the prevalence, antecedent trauma and comorbidity of PTSD in young prisoners are required.

General and specific learning difficulties

Gunn *et al.* (1991) estimated the levels of mental retardation using clinical criteria. Maden *et al.* (1995) screened for low IQ using the Quick Test. They noted that this does not assess social competence and that it should only be regarded as a tool that brings attention to a group with vulnerability who require further assessment. In their study the diagnosis of mental retardation was given to 2% of youths; these scored below the cut-off of 70 and had evidence of impaired social functioning. Interestingly, 7.8% of the sample of male youths gave a history of attending a school for those with mental retardation.

In the ONS survey (Lader *et al.* 2000), the Quick Test was used. The median score for all the different sample groups was 31, the published norm for 16-year-olds being 37. However, the scores were not converted to IQ scores because of a number of potential biases: cultural and social biases, the inclusion of subjects for whom English was not the first language, the fact that the test was developed in the 1950s, and the way in which the test was administered.

What is indisputable is that a significant proportion of young prisoners have poor literacy and educational attainments.

Paranoia and voices

Young prisoners frequently are referred to a psychiatrist complaining of 'paranoia' and 'voices'. There are numerous difficulties in ascribing a diagnosis to this presentation within a prison context, in particular the differentiation between an evolving psychotic mental illness or an evolving personality disorder of the paranoid or borderline types. The early recognition of schizophrenia in the adolescent population in general can be particularly difficult as the onset is frequently insidious with premorbid cognitive and social impairments gradually shading into prodromal symptoms before the onset of positive psychotic symptoms (Hollis 2000). The following factors should be considered during an assessment:

- Feigning symptoms is unusual and is usually easily detected.
- There may be genuine reasons to feel under threat within a prison.
- Illicit substances are frequently available within the particular prison.
- The prison environment can accentuate paranoid symptoms in adolescents who have pre-existing paranoid traits to their personalities.

Initially, the adolescent can be assessed within a prison healthcare centre; this may necessitate transfer to a YOI with a healthcare centre with 24-hour cover. This measure leads to resolution of the symptoms in some adolescents. If the disorder is not transient the adolescent should be transferred to an NHS hospital for a fuller assessment.

Suicide and deliberate self-harm

COMPLETED SUICIDE

Many people in prison have multiple risk factors associated with an increased risk of suicide. The rate of suicide within prison is reflected by the number of government publications on the issue, including *Suicide is Everyone's Concern* (HM Chief Inspector of Prisons 1999) and

Prevention of Suicide and Self Harm in the Prison Service: an Internal Review (2001). The reduction of suicide and self-harm in prisoners is currently a 'top ministerial priority'.

Studies examining deliberate self-harm and suicides in prison have had different focuses. Some have investigated completed prison suicide (Dooley 1990; Towl and Crighton 1998; Liebling 1995). In some studies a random sample of prisoners have been interviewed regarding current and past thoughts about self-harm and suicide and their past history of self-harm and suicide attempts (Maden *et al.* 1995; Lader *et al.* 2000). Other studies have involved interviewing people in prison who are known to have self-harmed in prison. Liebling (1992, 1995; Liebling and Krarup 1993) has conducted three major, overlapping and complementary studies.

It has been argued that it is not useful to differentiate between those who complete suicide, those who attempt suicide and those who engage in self-harm within the prison context (Inch *et al.* 1995; Liebling 1995). Others have argued for further examination of the relationship between self-injury and suicide (Towl and Crighton 1998).

Data on prison suicide and self-harm within prisons are collected by the Prison Service Safer Custody Group. The prison service category of self-inflicted death includes all suicide and open verdicts where the harm was self-inflicted but there was insufficient evidence to prove that the intention was death. This is consistent with the definition used by the Office for National Statistics and thus allows comparison with community rates. We will use the term 'suicide' to include this broader definition and use it interchangeably with 'self-inflicted death'.

The rate of self-inflicted deaths in prison has increased dramatically in recent years. Figures per 100,000 of the average annual prison population rose from 54 in 1982 to 128 in 1998, representing in 1998 a total of 82 deaths in prison custody. The rate of male suicide in the community was 17.4 per 100,000 in 1996. Between 1990 and 1998 there were no self-inflicted deaths in girls aged 15–17 and two in the age range 18–20. However, there were 14 suicides of boys aged 15–17 and 63 of young men aged 18–20. Towl and Crighton (1998), in their study of prison suicides between 1988 and 1995, concluded that young prisoners aged 15–17 appear to be at increased risk of suicide compared to other age groups. This was not supported by the thematic review (HM Chief Inspector of Prisons 1999), which found that the percentage of self-inflicted deaths occurring in each age group was broadly in proportion with that of the prison population as a whole. The number of female suicides in prison is in accordance with their proportion of the prison population.

The suicide rate in prison can be measured either per 100,000 receptions or per 100,000 of the average daily population (ADP). When rates are calculated using the ADP, rates for remand prisoners are extremely high. When rates are calculated using the former method rates

for remand prisoners are similar to sentenced prisoners given short sentences and lower than for those given longer or indeterminate sentences. Thus, Towl and Crighton (1998) have argued that remand status as an individual marker for an increased risk of suicide has perhaps been over-emphasized. Prisoners serving life sentences are a high-risk group.

Whatever their status, 10% of suicides occur within the first 24 hours of imprisonment, 40% within the first month and 80% within the first year. Those charged with or convicted of a violent offence, particularly homicide, or a sexual offence are at a significantly higher risk of suicide. The vast majority of deaths, around 90%, occur by hanging (Dooley 1990; HM Chief Inspector of Prisons 1999).

Studies on prison suicide have highlighted the importance of both individual and systemic/institutional factors. In studies of completed suicides in prisons in England and Wales (Dooley 1990; HM Chief Inspector of Prisons 1999), risk factors identified included mental illness, a history of psychiatric contact (around 40%), a history of single or multiple substance misuse (30–70%), a history of self-harm (around 50%), loss of social contact and relationship difficulties, victimization by other inmates, and difficulties coping with the prison regime.

Liebling (1995), in a review of 177 prison suicides, discusses a 'typology' of prison suicides with three groups: the 'psychiatrically ill', life/long-sentence prisoners, and 'poor copers'. The 'poor copers' were described as aged 16–25, often having a history of self-harm and motivated by fear, helplessness, distress and isolation.

ATTEMPTED SUICIDE AND DELIBERATE SELF-HARM

Data on attempted suicide and deliberate self-harm are collected together by the prison sevice. The number of people for whom there were recorded incidents of attempted suicide or deliberate self-harm during the two years 1996–97 was recorded as 73 in the age group 15–17 years and 277 in the age group 18–20 years. Those aged 21–29 years account for a disproportionate number of incidents (HM Chief Inspector of Prisons 1999). These reported incidents increased by 50% between 1999 and 2000. The recorded rates are certainly a huge under-estimate brought about by poor recording; it is one of the present author's experience that up to 20 separate incidents of deliberate self-harm could occur in one YOI in one day! In an epidemiological study on the nature and extent of suicide attempts and self-injury in prison, Liebling (1995) recorded that despite considerable effort and time invested in the task, there were major problems relating to the effective and consistent recording of suicide attempts and self-injury and that the picture obtained was incomplete.

Liebling (1992, 1995) conducted a study between 1988 and 1990 in four YOIs, two for boys and two for girls. Interviews were carried out with 50 prisoners who had attempted suicide and 50 drawn randomly from the same establishments. A second similar study was carried out across the age range. In these studies it was noted that all the prisoners had backgrounds with multiple disadvantages. However, the differences to emerge between suicide attempters and the comparison group were differences of 'degree'. Suicide attempters were more likely to report multiple family breakdown, frequent violence leading to hospitalization, local authority placement as a result of family breakdown (as opposed to offending), truancy as a result of bullying (as opposed to boredom or peer pressure), experiences of sexual abuse, and previous episodes of self-harm. They are more likely to report family and relationship difficulties, including being isolated from families once in prison. The suicide attempters found prison life more difficult in most respects.

Aspects of the prison regime which have been reported to be important triggering factors to self-harm include bullying, being locked in a cell for long periods, and a lack of supportive relationships with staff. Liebling referred to this group of prisoners as 'poor copers' and argues that this group matches the 'poor copers' identified in prison suicides (see earlier).

A study by Inch et al. (1995) supported these findings and also showed that adolescents who self-harm in prison have higher scores on the General Health questionnaire. These results are also supported by the thematic review of the HM Chief Inspector of Prisons for England and Wales (1999).

Studies have consistently shown that thoughts of self-harm and a previous history of self-harm are very prevalent among adolescents in prison. Maden et al. (1995) reported that 17% of their sample of young offenders had a history of self-harm prior to the current remand and that for the vast majority the first episode of self-harm had occurred in the community. In the ONS survey (Lader et al. 2000), 38% of young male remand prisoners reported having thoughts of suicide in their lifetime, 30% in the past year and 10% in the week prior to interview. The equivalent figures for suicide attempts were 20%, 17% and 3% respectively. For all time periods, male remand young offenders had a slightly higher prevalence of both suicidal thoughts and suicide attempts than did male sentenced young offenders. Young women reported higher rates of suicidal thoughts and suicide attempts than their male counterparts. Male and female, remand and sentenced adolescents reported similar rates of self-harming without the intention of suicide during their current period of detention, varying from 7% for male remand young offenders to 11% for female sentenced young offenders.

MANAGEMENT OF SUICIDE RISK

Within the prison system, psychiatrists have a role in the management of deliberate self-harm and attempted suicide. This includes the assessment of suicidal intent, the identification of psychiatric disorder (it is recognized that deliberate self-harm can be an indicator of psychiatric morbidity), and the formulation of a management plan. It has been argued that those with psychiatric disorder and assessed as a persistent suicide risk in the prison setting should be referred for urgent hospital transfer (Gunn et al. 1991).

Reducing the prevalence of self-harm and suicide attempts in young people in prison will require both screening, identification and management of high-risk cases and, much more importantly, changes in the prison regime. All of these aspects, including current practices, are discussed in the thematic review by HM Chief Inspector of Prisons for England and Wales (1999), which introduces the concept of a 'healthy prison'.

RACE AND CULTURE

Issues around race, culture and racism in forensic psychiatry are of paramount importance. The reader is referred elsewhere for a detailed discussion of them (Fernando et al. 1998; Kaye and Lingiah 2000). The criminal justice system does not exist in isolation and the experience of young black people within it needs to be seen within both an historical and the current context.

The massive over-representation of black people, both adults and adolescents, males and females, in the prison system has been documented for many years. In 1991, black males aged 17–19 were six times as likely as white males to be imprisoned (Rutter et al. 1998). In mid-1999, there were 8329 young offenders (aged under 21) serving a sentence in prison custody in England and Wales, and 13.4% of these were described as of black ethnic origin (Home Office 1999). Their over-representation in the remand population is even higher. In 1998, 17.5% of 15- and 16-year-olds remanded into prison custody were described as of black ethnic origin. The ethnic variations vary according to offence, being greatest for drug offences and robbery. Adolescents from South Asia are not over-represented in prison.

The reasons for the over-representation of black people within the prison system have been explored by a number of reviewers. The consensus is that cumulative biases (many as a result of direct discrimination) in processing are operating, but cannot account for the huge disparities in imprisonment and that there are differences in offending patterns. Authors do not agree on the extent of the effects of the processing biases (Hood 1992; Tonry 1994; Fernando et al. 1998; Rutter et al. 1998). Tonry (1994) concluded that racial disparities in offending 'will abate substantially only when social arrangements are recast to provide equal life chances to all citizens of every racial and ethnic group'.

Black people are under-represented among those who commit suicide in prison. They are also under-represented among the recorded incidents of attempted suicide or deliberate self-harm (HM Chief Inspector of Prisons 1999). The differential rates of reported self-harm might partly account for the fact that within young-offender institutions young black people are less likely, experience suggests, to be placed on wings designated for 'vulnerable' prisoners. This subject, although complex, requires further study, otherwise it is likely that young black people in prison who are depressed and/or distressed will go unnoticed by a predominantly white system.

The issue of racism within the prison system is being increasingly acknowledged. At the time of writing, the Commission for Racial Equality (CRE) announced a formal investigation into racial discrimination in the prison service. CRE chairperson Gurbux Singh commented:

'CRE commissioners are deeply concerned at some incidents of proven racial discrimination in the prison service. ... The decision [to launch an inquiry] follows serious concerns about the murder of Zahid Mubarek whilst in prison service custody [at HM YOI Feltham] and the belief that the murder was racially aggravated, and circumstances surrounding the treatment of a prison officer serving at HMP Brixton.'

It was also noted that the prison service director had requested the CRE to carry out a formal investigation to clarify problem areas and develop an action plan for change.

The needs (including mental health needs) of asylum seekers are beyond the scope of this chapter. However, within the prison system they are likely to be an especially vulnerable group. They have suffered extensive losses and are coping with enormous uncertainty.

GIRLS IN PRISON

Girls account for a relatively small amount of the young prison population. Girls aged 15 or 16 cannot be remanded into prison custody unless they are convicted and awaiting reports. There has been an increasing focus on the needs of women in prison custody, evidenced by a thematic review devoted to the topic (HM Chief Inspector of Prisons 1997b).

Girls in prison complain of similarly high levels of childhood deprivation as boys, reporting high levels of being 'in care'. They report higher levels of childhood sexual abuse. Within prison, young women are more likely to report being the victim of unwanted sexual attention or forced sexual attention and of bullying in general. They are much more likely to be taking medication acting on the central nervous system than are men, particularly hypnotics, anxiolytics and antidepressants. However, they do not spend as much time locked in their cells as their male counterparts (HM Chief Inspector of Prisons 1997b; Lader et al. 2000).

In terms of psychiatric morbidity, small numbers of girls have been interviewed in some of the studies described in this chapter. Ulzen et al. (1998), in their sample of 11 females, commented that they presented with a higher level of psychiatric morbidity for some disorders (including depression) and a distinct pattern of comorbidity. They report higher rates of suicidal thoughts and suicide attempts than in male counterparts (Lader et al. 2000). It is important that future studies elucidate any gender differences with respect to the prevalence and comorbidity of psychiatric disorders, because this has treatment implications.

ETHICAL CONSIDERATIONS

General issues

The complexity of ethical practice within a prison environment is highlighted by the fact that the Royal College of Psychiatrists (RCP 1992) produced a document devoted to the topic that is currently under review.

The healthcare of prisoners requires a sound ethical framework. The quality of care provided should not be dependent upon the vagaries of prevailing social and political attitudes towards crime and punishment. A number of international ethical frameworks inform policy on the psychiatric care of prisoners. Loss of liberty does not imply the loss of a right to medical treatment or of a proper ethical standard, and the central principle in ethical statements is the concept of equivalence of care – the provision of equivalent treatment to that available outside prison. This in turn rests upon the principle that imprisonment should be used 'as a punishment, not for punishment'.

Achieving equitable care for prisoners requires sustained effort by, and exceptional cooperation of, health professionals working in the community and in prison, prison staff and the government, and is a long way from being achieved. In the interim period clinicians will need to apply ethical guidelines for professional practice in clinical settings falling short of what is expected of a comprehensive psychiatric service.

In order to work effectively in prisons, health professionals need to understand the needs of a prison and of the wider organization, yet must not allow their ethical standards to be compromised. Discussion with colleagues who are working outside the prison system is advocated.

Health professionals who visit and work in prisons have a responsibility to act as advocates for adequate healthcare for mentally disordered prisoners by drawing the attention of the prison governor and the local health authority to the need to improve services. There is also an ethical obligation on psychiatrists outside the prison to respond promptly to requests for urgent assessment.

Consent

Issues of consent and capacity in relation to adolescents and the mentally disordered are discussed elsewhere in this volume. As mentioned previously, prior to interviewing a prisoner for a report a psychiatrist has the ethical responsibility to obtain the informed consent of the prisoner, after explaining to him or her the purpose of the assessment and to whom the report will be sent. However, within the prison context there are two particular restraints on consent.

Firstly, prisoners have no real choice in relation to medical and psychiatric services. In this respect they are extremely vulnerable. In addition, an adolescent in prison does not have much of an opportunity to discuss any problems or proposed assessment or treatment with friends or relatives.

Secondly, an adolescent in prison may feel that a refusal to see a psychiatrist or accept medication will jeopardize his or her overall position.

Confidentiality

Maintaining confidentiality of health information is one of the keystones of the patient–clinician relationship. Guidance regarding confidentiality is provided by the General Medical Council (GMC 2000) and the Royal College of Psychiatrists (RCP 2000). Whilst these principles apply in prisons, a number of issues need to be borne in mind.

Some particular groups of inmates (e.g. asylum seekers detained under the Immigration Act 1971) may require considerable reassurance before they are able to trust professionals. Maintaining confidentiality, however, is particularly difficult in a prison. Prisons are closed societies and prison officers and other inmates alike may surmise something about an individual's health simply by observing which professional a prisoner is going to see or which drug he or she is taking. A prisoner scheduled to see a psychiatrist might be seen as crazy. This, in turn, may discourage individuals from seeking or accepting psychiatric help.

There are occasions when it is in the best interest of the patient, or is essential for the safety of others, that information be shared with others. These include the following:

1 Information and advice may be necessary for non-healthcare staff (wing manager, personal officers, teachers or workshop supervisors) about the best way to manage and support a particular patient on ordinary location. It will frequently be appropriate for health professionals to act as advocates, for example to promote family contact, extra visits or telephone calls, influence appropriate location, support suitable work placements or the acquisition or appropriate reading or art materials. In some ways this is analogous to giving information to relatives and carers in the community.

2 Information needs to be shared when participating in the multi-disciplinary processes set up to plan the individual's 'through care' in prison and aftercare in the community. In some ways this is analogous to participating in multi-disciplinary Care Programme Approach meetings in the community. It is essential to share information outside healthcare in order to facilitate creative solutions such as moves between wings and the healthcare centre, 'respite' stays in the healthcare centre, mixed locations (e.g. education centre or sheltered work during the day, healthcare centre at night), and a planned response to crisis – for example in the case of chronic self-injury in the presence of personality disorder, where several disciplines may be involved.

3 When the health professional becomes aware that the patient is planning self-harm or harm to some other individual or group of individuals, or that a person under the age of 18 is at risk of serious harm (including abuse), obviously this information must be shared with the appropriate prison officer.

There are several ways to maximize the sharing of information that is required for multi-disciplinary care while maintaining the requirements of confidentiality and the trust of the patient. These include the following:

1 *Agreements allowing confidentiality to be held within a designated team.* This is what occurs within general practice teams and within multi-disciplinary mental health teams (usually consisting of doctors, nurses, social workers, occupational therapists, psychologists and non-professional 'support workers').

2 *Asking the patient for permission to share certain information with others.* Emphasize that the purpose is to ensure that the patient is treated as well as possible on ordinary location and receives appropriate aftercare when he or she is released. Permission should be written if possible.

Maintaining healthcare standards

Delivering healthcare within a prison involves particular challenges. Even at its best, it can be argued that the environment is intrinsically conducive to the development of depression, anxiety and paranoia – for example, separation from loved ones and friends, the inability to make decisions for oneself, inactivity, and lack of access to normal ways of coping. Health professionals, both those visiting and those working within prisons, have the difficult job of deciding at what point prison conditions (such as overcrowding and lack of activity) have deteriorated to such an extent that protest is no longer sufficient and further action of some sort is ethically compelling.

Ultimately no health professional should work in any environment in which the leadership attempts to force him or her to do what the professional believes is wrong or unethical. All health professionals are not only entitled but have a duty to disclose situations which they believe to be damaging to the standards of care for their patients.

If such a situation arises, health professionals should make a contemporaneous record in writing detailing the event and pass on the information as soon as is practically possible. Doctors working in prison should forge a working alliance with members of the prison's senior management team and ensure there is clarity as to how particular issues are addressed. If local and central channels of disclosure are exhausted and concerns remain about practices they regard as unethical, they are entitled to voice these concerns with the Board of Visitors, NHS management and professional organizations. Doctors should follow GMC guidance in relation to concerns about the medical practice of colleagues. All healthcare workers should be aware of the provisions of the Public Interests Disclosure Act 1998.

Use of segregation

Individuals who are mentally ill and who can only be safely contained within the prison by use of seclusion or segregation should be transferred immediately (within 24 hours) to an NHS hospital. Where paranoid features of the illness mean that the individual refuses the limited access to exercise that is available, transfer is even more urgent.

Individuals who are not transferred to the NHS and who are at increased risk of spending frequent or extended periods of time in segregation present complex challenges (Coid 1998; Crassian and Friedman 1986). Frequent or extended use of segregation, especially but not exclusively transfer from the segregation unit in one prison to that in another in order to provide respite to staff, should trigger a multi-disciplinary assessment and the development of appropriate multi-disciplinary care plans.

REFERENCES

Birmingham, L., Mason, D. and Grubin, D. 1996: Prevalence of mental disorder in remand prisoners: consecutive case study. *British Medical Journal* **313**: 1521–4.

Birmingham, L., Gray, J., Mason, D. and Grubin, D. 2000: Mental illness at reception into prison. *Criminal Behaviour and Mental Health* **10**: 77–87.

Cauffman, E., Feldman, S., Waterman, J. and Steiner, H. 1998: Post-traumatic stress disorder among female juvenile offenders. *Journal of the American Academy of Child and Adolescent Psychiatry* **37**: 1209–16.

Coid, J. 1998: The management of dangerous psychopaths in prison. In Millon, T., Simonsen, E., Mirket-Smith, M. and Davis, R.D. (eds), *Psychopathy, Antisocial, Criminal and Violent Behaviour*. New York: Guilford Press.

Crassian, S. and Friedman, N. 1986: Effects of sensory deprivation in psychiatric seclusion and solitary confinement. *International Journal of Law and Psychiatry* **8**: 49–65.

DoH (Department of Health/Home Office) 1992: *Review of Health and Social Services for Mentally Disordered Offenders and Others Requiring Similar Services*. London: HMSO.

Dooley, E. 1990: Prison suicide in England and Wales 1972–87. *British Journal of Psychiatry* **156**: 40–5.

Fernando, S., Ndegwa, D. and Wilson, M. 1998: *Forensic Psychiatry, Race and Culture*. London: Routledge.

GMC (General Medical Council) 2000: *Confidentiality: Providing and Protecting Information*. London: GMC.

Grounds, A. 2000: The future of prison health care. *Journal of Forensic Psychiatry* **11**(2): 260–7.

Gunn, J., Maden, A. and Swinton, M. 1991: *Mentally Disordered Prisoners*. London: Institute of Psychiatry and Home Office.

HM Chief Inspector of Prisons for England and Wales 1996: Patient or Prisoner?: New Strategy for Health Care in Prisons. London: Home Office.

HM Chief Inspector of Prisons for England and Wales 1997a: *Young Prisoners: a Thematic Review*. London: Home Office.

HM Chief Inspector of Prisons for England and Wales 1997b: *Women in Prison: a Thematic Review*. London: Home Office.

HM Chief Inspector of Prisons for England and Wales 1999: *Suicide is Everyone's Concern: a Thematic Review*. London: Home Office.

HM Prison Service and NHS Executive 1999: *The Future Organisation of Prison Health Care*. London: DoH.

Hollis, C. 2000: Adolescent schizophrenia. *Advances in Psychiatric Treatment* **6**: 83–92.

Home Office 2000: *Prison Statistics in England and Wales 1999*. London: Home Office.

Hood, R. 1992: *Race and Sentencing: a Study in the Crown Court*. Oxford: Oxford University Press.

Inch, H., Rowlands, P. and Soliman, A. 1995: Deliberate self-harm in a young-offenders institution. *Journal of Forensic Psychiatry* **6**: 161–71.

Kaye, C. and Lingiah, T. (eds) 2000: *Race, Culture and Ethnicity in Secure Psychiatric Practice*. London: Jessica Kingsley.

Kazdin, A. 2000: Adolescent development, mental disorders and decision making of delinquent youths. In Grisso, T. and Schwartz, R. (eds), *Youth on Trial*. Chicago: University of Chicago Press, 33–65.

Lader, D., Singleton, N. and Meltzer, H. 2000: *Psychiatric Morbidity among Young Offenders in England and Wales*. London: Office for National Statistics.

Liebling, A. 1992: *Suicides in Prison*. London: Routledge.

Liebling, A. 1995: Vulnerability and prison suicide. *British Journal of Criminology* **35**(2): 173–87.

Liebling, A. and Krarup, H. 1993: *Suicide Attempts in Male Prisons*. London: Home Office.

Maden, A., Taylor, C., Brooke, D. and Gunn, J. 1995: *Mental Disorder in Remand Prisoners*. London: Institute of Psychiatry and Home Office.

Misch, P. 1998: Proceedings of the Annual Prison Health Conference. HM Prison Service.

Nicol, R., Stretch, D., Whitney, I. *et al.* 2000: Mental health needs and services for severely troubled and troubling young people including young offenders in an NHS region. *Journal of Adolescence* **23**: 243–61.

Reed, J. and Lyne 2000: Inpatient care of mentally disordered ill people in prison: results of a year's programme of semi-structured inspections. *British Medical Journal* **320**: 1031–4.

Rutter, M., Giller, H. and Hagell, A. 1998: *Antisocial behaviour by adolescents.* Cambridge: Cambridge University Press.

Shaw, J., Creed, F., Price, J., Huxley, P. and Tomenson, B. 1999: Prevalence and detection of serious psychiatric disorder in defendants attending court. *Lancet* **353**: 1053–6.

Sim, J. 1990: *Medical Power in Prisons.* Milton Keynes: Open University Press.

Singleton, N., Meltzer, H. and Gatward, R. 1998: *Psychiatric Morbidity among Prisoners in England and Wales.* London: Office for National statistics.

Steiner, H., Garcia and Matthews, Z. 1997: Post-traumatic stress disorder in incarcerated juvenile delinquents. *Journal of the American Academy of Child and Adolescent Psychiatry* **36**: 357–65.

RCP (Royal College of Psychiatrists) 1992: *Ethical Issues in Psychiatric Practice in Prisons.* Council Report CR15. London: RCP.

RCP (Royal College of Psychiatrists) 2000: *Good Psychiatric Practice: Confidentiality.* Council Report CR85. London: RCP.

Tonry, M. 1994: Racial disparities in courts and prisons. *Criminal Behaviour and Mental Health* **4**: 158–62.

Towl, G. and Crighton, D. 1998: Suicide in prison in England and Wales 1988–95. *Criminal Behaviour and Mental Health* **8**: 184–92.

29

Inter-agency management of children and young people who sexually abuse

DAVID O'CALLAGHAN AND MARIE CORRAN

INTRODUCTION

This chapter aims to explore the context, particularly at an inter-agency level, in which practice with young sexual abusers is located. Young people who sexually abuse could be said to straddle a number of ideological, legal and structural systems. Services have not developed to the extent that many working in the area a decade ago would have hoped. A significant reason for this has been the general failure of agencies to work cooperatively and share responsibility. Certain of the key philosophical questions as to the basic approach remain in contention and we have yet to invest in the detailed studies which would assist in identifying which forms of intervention are the most effective, for which groups of young people. Examples of good practice are, however, to be seen and a number of areas have developed systematic procedures and services. Perhaps most significantly, the issue of problematic sexual behaviour is now widely recognized as an unavoidable topic for all whose practice involves work with young people.

PROFESSIONAL RECOGNITION OF YOUNG PEOPLE WHO SEXUALLY ABUSE

The 1990s saw a dramatic growth in awareness, at an academic and clinical level, of young sexual abusers. One stimulus was provided by research, primarily from North America, which identified a significant proportion of *adult* sex offenders beginning their sexually abusive career in adolescence, the most influential and frequently quoted being that of Gene Abel and colleagues (Abel *et al.* 1987). This study identified that a significant proportion of serious adult sex offenders had a history of, frequently undisclosed, sexual offending dating back to adolescence. An inference drawn from this research was that intervention at the start of young peoples 'careers' of sexual aggression may offer a more positive prospect for change. More debatably, the research was used to support a contention that young sexual offenders, compared with the generality of young people who offend, were more likely to continue and develop in their offending pattern than 'grow out of it'.

An important stimulus to the recognition of young sexual abusers was victim surveys which found that a significant proportion of respondents identified their abuser as an adolescent (e.g. Finkelhor 1979; Havgaard and Tilley 1988; Fromuth *et al.* 1991). Such studies have continued to highlight the role of young people in the perpetration of sexual assault, for example the Rhode Island survey of 1700 adolescents reporting sexually abusive experiences (Kikuchi 1995), in which 57% of respondents identified the abuser as aged 13–17 years at the time of the assault. A number of UK studies, published in the early 1990s (Northern Ireland Research Team 1990; Kelly *et al.* 1991; Glasgow *et al.* 1994) explored the demographic characteristics of perpetrators and victims of child sexual abuse within this country. They found adolescents identified as perpetrators in approximately one-third of cases, thus echoing the North American research.

Official records have also highlighted the role of young people in the commission of offences. Masson and Morrison (1999) reviewed UK crime statistics which identified that a total of 23% of total convictions and cautions for sexual offences was by offenders aged between 10 and 20 years. Of those offenders cautioned for sexual offences, 45% were in this age group (35% under 17 years).

In 1990 the National Children's Home published a survey of treatment facilities for child victims of sexual abuse and young abusers (NCH 1990). Fewer than half of local authorities surveyed considered they had any services available for young abusers and there was little evidence of consensus as to the organization and delivery of such services. Subsequently NCH established a commission of enquiry to explore the development of a coherent response to young sexual abusers. Reporting in 1992, the commission stressed the need for a multi-agency response coordinated through the Child Protection System. The phrase 'continuum of care' was a key concept within the commission's report (NCH 1992) in relation to how the system responds to young people who sexually abuse. It was recognized that, given the diversity of young sexual abusers as a group, there was a need to develop a broad range of services for assessment, placement and treatment, relevant to specific therapeutic needs and the appropriate management of risk. Over the period since the publication of the NCH report, services for young abusers have developed, though perhaps not to the extent and diversity recommended.

CENTRAL GOVERNMENT GUIDANCE

Throughout the 1980s, stimulated by a number of critical enquiry reports, agencies were prompted to develop more comprehensive local guidelines concerning multi-agency cooperation in child protection. As the focus shifted from physical to sexual abuse, there was little formal acknowledgement of children and young people who sexually abused prior to the 1990s when some recognition of this client group began to be reflected in the guidance from central government. The Department of Health's *Working Together under the Children Act 1989* (DoH 1991) recommended that there should be a consistent professional response in all cases where the abuser is alleged to be a child or young person, recommending a child protection conference should be held in respect of the young alleged abuser. The conference should be presented with an initial assessment of the situation based on the details of the offence together with the alleged abuser's family circumstances and his or her level of understanding of the offence. The conference could then

recommend that a comprehensive assessment of the young person be undertaken and conference reconvened to consider and coordinate any further professional involvement considered necessary. The *Working Together* guidance was an important stimulus for Area Child Protection Committees (ACPCs) to draft local inter-agency procedures concerning children and young people who display abusive sexual behaviours.

As Masson (1995, 1997) has found, whilst such inter-agency procedures have become common there is considerable local variation in the specific arrangements. Many areas have highly proscriptive approaches, linked to the presence of a specialist team, project or clearly identified staff responsible for assessment and intervention. In other areas the response is more variable and lines of responsibility for provision of service unclear.

Despite such local variations, *Working Together* did establish the principles of an inter-agency and multi-disciplinary response to young abusers, and that the lead responsibility for coordinating this lay with the Area Child Protection Committee. The revised *Working Together to Safeguard Children* (DoH 2000a) continues this approach, although with the changes introduced in the Crime and Disorder Act 1998 it now highlights the joint responsibility of Area Child Protection Committees and Youth Offending Teams. *Working Together 2000* continues to advocate the convening of a child protection conference in cases where the young person is thought to be at risk of significant harm, and the need for inter-agency coordination where a young abuser's needs are particularly complex. It stresses the potential value of early intervention in that it may divert individuals from a pathway into sexual offending in adult life. It advocates three principles which should guide the provision of services:

- Ensure a coordinated approach between youth justice and child welfare agencies (including education and child and adolescent mental health service).
- The needs of young people who abuse should be considered separately from their victims.
- An assessment should be carried out in every case which should explore any unmet developmental needs in addition to specific needs arising from the individual's behaviour.

This assessment should be undertaken under s17 of the Children Act 1989, using the *Framework for the Assessment of Children in Need and their Families* (DoH 2000b). The framework stresses the importance of holistic assessments which give consideration to the personal, familial, professional and environmental strengths and resources which can be harnessed in order to formulate a comprehensive intervention and protection strategy. Print and Erooga (2000) have provided an outline of how this assessment framework can be applied specifically to young people who sexually abuse.

THE CONTEXT OF PUBLIC OPINION AND POLITICAL RHETORIC

For those whose daily work concerns young people who sexually abuse, we bring together two figures – that of the 'young offender' and that of the 'sex offender' – who have been increasingly demonized over recent years. Soothill (1997) notes how the media and parliamentary debate concerning the changes introduced by the Criminal Justice and Public Order Act 1994, which enabled 10- to 13-year-olds to be charged with rape, was 'both selective and vivid' and took its tone from a series of high-profile accounts in newspapers. It is notable that the Crime and Disorder Act 1998 has major elements concerned with youth crime and sexual offences. In the Home Secretary's preface to the guidance notes regarding the Sex Offender Orders introduced by the Act, he comments:

> 'Sex offenders prey on other people, particularly those unable to defend themselves, and their actions leave their victims scarred for life. This cannot be tolerated.' (Home Office 1989a)

The rhetoric of media and politicians can generalize from a handful of atypical cases, contributing to a public reaction such as seen when groups of local people have besieged police stations, hostels and homes where its is thought or rumoured that sexual offenders are resident. There have been examples of young people or their families being subjected to similar instances of violence or intimidation, including those provoked by unofficial 'community alerts' (Campbell 1998). Wyre (1997) has suggested that this climate serves only to promote myths concerning sex offenders as dangerous outsiders, and distracts from the broader and more complex issues of developing a range of provisions for the diversity of those who sexually offend.

Chaffin and Bonner (1998) have criticized the 'punitive, aversive and absolutist tone' of many programmes for young sexual offenders in the USA, noting that this response has now been generalized to much younger children who display inappropriate sexual behaviours. Laws (1998) has argued for professionals in this field to be more proactive and less defensive in engaging with the public. He suggests this offers many opportunities to counter myths concerning sexual offending and ultimately engenders a climate in which more victims *and offenders* will come forward for services.

CHANGES IN THE CRIMINAL JUSTICE SYSTEM DURING THE 1990s

Prins (1996) suggests that the two major criminal justice Acts of the early 1990s promoted a significant shift in philosophy, emphasizing the issue of 'public protection', which has now become the commonplace of political rhetoric. This has continued throughout the period, with both young offenders and sexual offenders being singled out as a particular cause of concern.

THE CRIMINAL JUSTICE ACT 1990

This Act introduced Youth Courts to deal with all offenders up to the age of 17 years. Probation Orders became available as a disposal for those aged 16 years or over at the time of the offence, although the use of Supervision Orders continues to be most likely form of disposal for this age group.

THE CRIMINAL JUSTICE ACT 1991

A central theme of the Act is the treatment of offenders after conviction. One of the most important changes brought about by the Act concerns the sentencing procedures and practices. In principle, the severity of an individual's sentence should reflect the severity of the crime that has been committed, or the need to protect the public from the offender. There is also a sharp distinction made between property offences and offences of a violent or sexual nature committed against the person. The Act suggests that additional restrictions may need to be placed on violent and/or sexual offenders to protect the public, and provides Courts with powers both to impose longer custodial sentences for such offenders and to direct longer periods of post-sentence supervision. It also enabled the Courts to make additional requirements to probation orders, for longer periods than was previously the case.

Another change within the 1991 Act, of major importance for practitioners, is the way in which children and young people are dealt with under the criminal law. The basic standpoint taken by the Act is that the criminal justice system must deal with young offenders in a way that reflects both their age and their development. As with the Children Act 1989, the Criminal Justice Act 1991 also seeks to include the principle of parental responsibility for the behaviour of their children. For example, parents are expected to attend Court hearings, and the Court can consider whether parents can be bound over to exercise proper control and care of their children.

The Act changed to the way in which young people are dealt with both before and after their cases are heard. Firstly, remand to prison custody for 15- to 16-year-olds is abolished; instead the Courts have been given new powers to decide whether any young person of this age should be held in local-authority secure accommodation. To make such a decision the Court must be satisfied that there is a need to protect the public from serious harm. The Act further provides new powers to impose conditions when remanding any juvenile to local-authority accommodation.

Under the Act, 16- and 17-year-olds are seen to be nearing adulthood and are dealt with as a distinct group. It is argued that some young offenders will need to be dealt with as young adults and sentenced accordingly;

for example, 16-year-olds can now receive either a Probation or a Supervision Order.

THE CRIMINAL JUSTICE AND PUBLIC ORDER ACT 1994

The most significant changes made in this Act concerning sexual offending relate to the law in respect of rape. The Act for the first time it made it possible to charge children aged 10–13 with rape. It also revised the law regarding rape within marriage, and created the category of 'male rape'.

THE SEX OFFENDER ACT 1997

This Act arose during a period of intense media and seeming public interest in the subject of sex offenders. Prior to the Act campaigners were calling for a register, a system of community notification on the whereabouts of sex offenders. In the USA this system is known as 'Megan's Law'. There, community notification is popularly understood to be a system whereby local people will be alerted to the whereabouts of a convicted sex offender. In the USA this can mean leafleting, door-to-door announcement or community meeting, around the close vicinity of the offender's home.

The concept of a sex offender register was incorporated into the 1997 Act, as well as provisions relating to sex offenders who commit sexual offences abroad (inappropriately known as 'sex tourism').

The sex offender register

The Act imposes requirements on sex offenders – including those aged under 18 – to notify the police of their name and address, and any subsequent changes to these. The information given to the police is held on the police's national computer. The terms of the Act affect those who were subject to the terms of a sentence from 1 September 1997, including community sentences, and to those who are subsequently convicted or formally cautioned for a relevant offence.

A comprehensive range of sexual offences determines which offenders need to go on the register. These range from offences such as rape and violent sexual assault, to offences connected with child pornography. The Act applies also to people who are subject to detention in hospital or guardianship orders under the Mental Health Act 1983 following conviction *or* cautioning for a relevant offence. The provisions also apply to young sex offenders aged under 18 years who are sentenced under s53 of the Children and Young Persons Act 1983 and are detained in local-authority secure accommodation. Offenders are not required to register whilst they are detained, but must do so within 14 days of release from detention.

The length of time someone stays on the register is determined by the length of the original punishment either in prison or under a community sentence. The minimum period of registration is five years, and for the most serious offences registration is for life. For young offenders,

those under 18, the registration period is halved. Under the legislation it is the responsibility of offender to make sure their details are on the register and are correct. This includes changes of name, as well as changes of address and temporary addresses (if more than 14 days from the home address). If the offender fails to comply with the requirements laid down in the Act, or gives misleading information, he or she is liable to a fine (£5000) or imprisonment (a maximum of six months) or both.

In relation to people under the age of 18, the duty of notification is the responsibility of the parent or individuals with parental responsibility. The penalty for failing to notify is financial only and the 'responsible parent' is liable.

Currently the key agencies – police, probation and social services, health and education services – are working to interim guidance. The importance of arrangements that are agreed with all agencies at a national level is acknowledged and work is progressing toward a substantive protocol to be issued by central government.

THE CRIME AND DISORDER ACT 1998

The Act's central provisions relate to young offenders, and it amounts to a complete overhaul of the youth justice system. The Act contains provisions that create new duties on local authorities and the police to lead local partnerships of organizations and communities to reduce crime and disorder. It explicitly creates a system based on multi-agency working and the expectation of strategic direction and oversight.

Two key duties that will be placed on local authorities are the production and implementation of Crime and Disorder Strategies and the establishment of local Youth Offending Teams.

Crime and disorder strategies

The Home Office required the first three-year Crime and Disorder Strategy to commence in April 1999. The strategy is drawn up by the police and the local authority and they are required to cooperate with other specified agencies, such as health, voluntary agencies and community groups. The strategies are to be formulated by:

- a review of the level and patterns of crime and disorder
- an analysis of results of the review
- published reports and consultation with local bodies.

The strategies will include:

- objectives to be pursued by the responsible authority in partnership with other agencies
- long- and short-term performance targets to measure the extent to which objectives are achieved.

Youth Offending Teams

The second duty placed upon a local authority is the creation of Youth Offending Teams (YOTs), comprised of social workers, probation officers, police officers, education and health staff. Youth Offending Teams will take a lead role in the provision of services to young sexual abusers, in terms of its staff either working with young people directly or acting as commissioners of specialist services. In doing so the YOTs are exhorted to have regard to the new principle of the youth justice system – to prevent offending by children and young people. In addition to the provision of direct services these teams will be required to formulate a *youth justice plan*, based on audits of the types and needs of young offenders and available services. The Home Office (1998b) guidance specifically mentions young sexual offenders as amongst the type of offenders who could be included in this audit. The guidance also mentions the need to develop effective information systems to monitor the outcomes of interventions.

Youth Justice Board

The Act also establishes a Youth Justice Board for England and Wales. Its function will be to:

- monitor the performance of the Youth Court, Young Offender Teams and the delivery of secure accommodation
- advise on standards, and monitor and publish results
- identify and disseminate good practice
- advise the Home Secretary on the operation of the youth justice system.

Reprimands and final warnings

A system of reprimands and final warnings have replaced police cautions for young offenders. Police can refer to the local Youth Offending Team for assessment prior to delivering a final warning. The primary role of this assessment is to explore the young person's attitude to intervention and the likelihood of the individual engaging in an appropriate programme of work – termed a 'rehabilitation programme'. When the offence in question is one that would lead to registration under the Sex Offender Act, the YOT are required to offer particular guidance to the young person and parents as to the implications of this.

Sex-offender orders

The police may apply to a magistrates' Court for such an Order, on the basis that a particular sex offender (as defined in the Sex Offender Act 1997) has given reasonable cause for concern that he or she poses a risk of serious harm to the public. The Order stipulates that the individual has to register with the police under the Sex Offender Register and may make certain specific prohibitions (e.g. not frequenting areas close to certain schools or approaching a particular household). The *Guidance Circular* (Home Office 1998a) notes that, whilst Sex Offender Orders do apply to 10- to 18-year-olds, they should be sought only under exceptional circumstances and in consultation with social services and other relevant agencies.

Further significant elements of the 1997 Act

- The abolition of *doli incapax* removes the presumption that a child age 10–14 may not know that his or her criminal actions were seriously wrong and is thus incapable of committing a criminal offence.
- New Youth Panels will deal with first-time offenders.
- New sentences available include: *Parenting Orders* requiring parents to attend counselling and guidance to help supervise their children; *Child Safety Orders* requiring children under 10 years to comply with arrangements aimed at ensuring that they receive appropriate care, protection and support and are subject to proper control (e.g. to be home at a certain time or to avoid a certain area); *Child Curfew Schemes* enabling local authorities to operate temporary curfews prohibiting children of specified ages (under 10) from being in a public place during specified hours, unless they are under the control of a responsible person aged 18 or over; *Reparation Orders* requiring young offenders to make reparation to the victim of the offence or the community at large; *Action Plan Orders*, a short (three months' duration) community penalty requiring a young offender to address their offending behaviour.
- Detention and Training Orders provide for a single new custodial sentence for 10- to 17-year-olds. Secure accommodation means a Secure Training Centre, a Young Offender Institution or local-authority secure accommodation
- Extended post-release supervision for sexual and violent offenders can be up to a maximum of ten years for sexual offenders.

THE INTER-AGENCY SYSTEM

Before exploring the evidence on how agencies have in fact responded to the challenge of providing services to young sexual abusers, to it may it worth while to briefly review the key responsibilities of the main agencies in this area.

AREA CHILD PROTECTION COMMITTEES

The current structure of Area Child Protection Committees was established following a string of child abuse inquiries during the 1980s, most significantly the Cleveland Report (DoH 1988). Their membership is drawn from senior staff from the main agencies who hold statutory powers and responsibilities concerning the protection of children. Area Child Protection Committees will usually include representation from social and health services, probation service, police, education, the NSPCC and legal representatives. Amongst the main tasks of the Area Child Protection Committees are:

- to establish, maintain and review local inter-agency guidelines and procedures

- to monitor the implementation of such procedures
- to review and make recommendations to the responsible agencies in respect of work required to prevent, respond to and manage child maltreatment
- to ensure a relevant programme of inter-agency training.

Most Area Child Protection Committees delegate specific areas of work to subcommittees, to which additional specialist representatives can be co-opted. In many areas there will be a subcommittee to consider the inter-agency management of sexual offenders. With the establishment of Youth Offending Teams from April 2000, Area Child Protection Committees now share a responsibility to formulate a clear operational framework in which assessment, decision-making and case management take place.

SOCIAL SERVICE DEPARTMENTS

Social services are predominantly the lead agency for child protection matters and will be concerned with the investigation, assessment and management of cases concerning young abusers, particularly when:

- other children are considered to be at risk
- the young person is thought to have been abused or at risk of abuse
- the young abuser is considered a 'Child in Need'.

Young abusers may require removal to a substitute care setting should they present a risk to others, be themselves at risk or possibly due to bail/remand conditions or family rejection.

YOUTH OFFENDING TEAMS

Established under the Crime and Disorder Act 1998, Youth Offending Teams have a lead responsibility in providing services for young people who sexually abuse, including:

- the assessment prior to or subsequent to a final warning, to establish suitability for an offence-related programme of work
- providing the Courts with pre-sentence reports
- providing offence-specific programmes to young people on community orders
- care for young people subject to custodial sentences, including post-release supervision.

YOTs have a broader remit to develop crime prevention initiatives through coordinating corporate and inter-agency strategies.

THE PROBATION SERVICE

Allam and Browne (1998) note that 97% of regional probation services report they now have provision for sex offender treatment. However, this relates primarily to community-based groups run for adult offenders – as identified in the recent Thematic Inspection (IoP 1998)

which commented on the absence of systematic services to young sexual offenders. Prior to the establishment of YOTs there was a lack of clarity as to which agency had lead responsibility for the provision of therapeutic services. Whilst clearly viewing YOTs as having this role for young sexual offenders, the recently revised probation guidance (Home Office 1999) on the management and supervision of sex offenders stresses the need for probation staff to work in close liaison with child protection and child welfare services in the case of younger sexual offenders.

THE PRISON SERVICE

In the UK the prison service provides an extensive multi-site Sex Offender Treatment Programme (SOTP) run in 25 prisons and primarily available to offenders sentenced to more than four years' imprisonment. SOTP is a group-work based programme delivered by prison officers, probation officers and psychologists employed within the prison service (Mann and Thornton 1998). At the time of writing only two Young Offender Institutions have SOTP provision available to young offenders.

THE HEALTH SERVICE

Children and young people who sexually abuse may be referred to a variety of psychologists or psychiatrists within the National Health Service. Accessibility to clinicians who are willing and able to provide assessment or therapeutic services is variable, with adolescent forensic services in particular being available only in a limited number of regions. It is increasingly recognized that the most damaged and difficult young people who sexually abuse are likely to present with a constellation of behavioural and emotional/psychological problems which require a multi-disciplinary approach – including child mental health professionals.

THE POLICE

The police have responsibility for the investigation of crime and share a requirement with social services to undertake such jointly in cases of child sexual abuse. The *Memorandum of Good Practice* (DoH 1992) provides a structure for the joint interviewing of children and other vulnerable witnesses. The Sex Offender Act 1997 places new responsibilities upon the police for the management of sex offenders in the community, including adolescents.

EDUCATION SERVICES

Within the UK the role of the education system has not been stressed in relation to work with young people who sexually abuse. In North America, considerable resources have been invested in 'primary prevention' strategies with both children and adolescents. These involve integrating into the school curriculum teaching programmes addressed at increasing awareness of rights and responsibilities involved in sexual behaviour, and in particular identifying to children the appropriate boundaries to sexual activity. One of the most influential of such programmes is that developed by Ryan (1996).

Schools are, however, a vital component of the multi-agency management of young abusers. Fellow pupils are not infrequently victims of sexually aggressive young people. Even when this is not the case, schools are understandably anxious with the presence of an abusive adolescent within the school setting and may respond by excluding the pupil. Recent guidance for schools concerning the 'social inclusion' of problematic, vulnerable and under-achieving pupils (DfEE 1999) stresses the role of schools as part of the multi-disciplinary network, and includes specific comment on schools' responsibility to address 'sexual harassment' directed by male pupils at female peers.

VOLUNTARY AGENCIES

As statutory agencies have moved towards an environment of greater partnership with the voluntary sector, this has led to an increase in the quasi-statutory work undertaken by voluntary agencies. Frequently the voluntary sector is seen as being more able to develop innovative responses to new areas of identified need. The role of the voluntary sector has been significant in the provision of therapeutic services to young abusers and there are now a number of specialist projects nationally, most frequently established on the basis of joint resources or funding. Voluntary sector agencies particularly active in this area have been the NSPCC, Barnardo's and NCH's Action for Children.

THE PRIVATE SECTOR

Independent providers have been particularly active within the area of residential care for sexually abusive young people, with a number of group care providers identifying themselves as specializing in this area.

INTER-AGENCY WORKING IN PRACTICE

HOW SERVICES FOR YOUNG ABUSERS HAVE DEVELOPED

Masson's (1995, 1998) research into the experiences of practitioners involved with young abusers identified a set of concerns relating to the systems, cooperation and communication that existed between agencies. Lack of clarity as to responsibility, lack of specialist services for assessment and treatment, problems in the placement of young abusers, and inadequate training, supervision and managerial support were amongst the main issues reported by staff. Masson identified a number of models for the delivery of services but found that these were rarely fully multi-professional, with a low level of health service participation. Unless the local arrangement was delivered via

a dedicated project then practitioners reported a relatively low degree of time allocated and a limited amount of clinical experience gained.

Many of these themes have recently been echoed by the Thematic Inspection undertaken by the Probation Inspectorate into services for sex offenders (IoP 1998). Whilst praising the extensive development of services for *adult* offenders that occurred almost entirely during the 1990s, the report found that:

> 'The largest and most worrying gap in provision was for adolescent sex offenders, responsibility for whom did not lie solely or principally with the probation service. There appeared to be no coherent national strategic approach and in many of the areas inspected no provision specifically designed to tackle sexual offending by adolescents.'

Indeed, in eight out of the ten areas inspected there existed either a fragmentary and *ad hoc* service for young abusers or no specific provision whatsoever. It appeared that in the competition for resources, certainly within the probation service, adolescent abusers were judged to be a low-priority area. The report makes the following recommendation:

> 'The Home Office should collaborate with the Department of Health to ensure sexual offending by adolescents is effectively addressed through the development of systematic assessment, intervention and relapse prevention services and ensure this matter is included in the current review of the youth justice system.'

Calder (1999) advocates a 'consortium approach', in which agencies on regional level pool resources to offer a service is this specialized area. McGarvey and Peyton (1999) provide an account of the development of such a multi-agency project in Northern Ireland. Such projects remain the exception, and Margetts (1998) suggests that a number of factors influence the resistance of agencies to such collaborative ventures:

- a wish to define responsibilities as narrowly as possible
- a fear that new projects will identify unmet need
- a wish by agencies to remain in control and avoid the scrutiny of their practice by others
- historic myths and misunderstandings as to other agencies and professional groups.

ORGANIZATIONAL COMPETENCE IN THE DELIVERY OF SERVICES

Reflecting on organizational theory, Morrison (1995) identifies a number of key building blocks for delivering a quality service to young people who sexually abuse. These could be divided into three tiers:

- *Strategic.* At this level, agencies must accept the validity of such provision, agree inter-agency procedures and allocate adequate resources.

- *Managerial.* Staff concerned with this area of work require adequate training, supervision and consultation.
- *Practice.* Clinical work should be based upon a written and accepted philosophy of intervention and reflect a holistic view of the young person and his or her developmental needs.

Morrison (1997) has also discussed the concept of 'emotional competence' to consider whether organizations provide practitioners with a safe structure to engage with the complex issues arising in the field of sexual aggression. Without such organizations, workers may drift into mirroring the distorted dynamics of young people and their families. Ladwa-Thomas and Sanders' (1999) survey of social workers involved with young abusers found that most felt immobilized by a lack of specific knowledge, skills and clear procedural framework. Hughes (1998) suggests that agencies must be prepared to challenge their own assumptions in order to work effectively with others and resolve internal tensions rather than use inter-agency activity as 'mere displacement activity'. Furthermore they must be willing to share responsibility and control as circumstances require. Margetts (1998) suggests that the potential benefits of inter-agency working include:

- shared information
- shared responsibility
- avoiding duplication of services
- providing a 'seamless' service
- developing the practice base.

The need for a shared philosophy is also relevant to effective inter-agency practice. Sanders and Ladwa-Thomas (1997) surveyed staff in various agencies with regard to perspectives on young abusers. They identified a substantial agreement in relation to many of the perspectives across the *social work* groups (child protection, child and family, youth justice and probation). The police officers surveyed, however, had a strikingly different theoretical perspective. A wider spread of opinion was found on a set of specific questions related to practice issues with young abusers. The statements which produced the greatest diversity of views concerned:

- whether young abusers should be seen as victims first and offenders second
- whether local authorities should have a register of children and young people who abuse others
- to what extent children under the age of 10 understand their own sexuality.

PROVISION OF SERVICES

Identifying those most likely to continue in sexually aggressive behaviour

There have been only a small number of relevant recidivism studies relating to adolescents. Of studies currently available, a consistent feature is the low base rate of identified re-offending, of 3–14% , and the fact that young sexual offenders appear at much greater risk for the commission of non-sexual offences (Rasmussen 1999; Hagan *et al.* 1994).

Studies have suggested that clinical judgements are frequently flawed and biased towards 'false positives' – i.e. an over-estimate of risk (Kahn and Chambers 1991; Lab *et al.* 1993). Current evidence would point to actuarial models such as the SACJ (Grubin 1998), used within the UK to assess adult sexual offenders, as offering a more reliable predictive instrument. Prentky *et al.* (2000) have produced a tentative model addressing risk factors in adolescents, including both pre- and post-treatment variables. Although at an early stage in this process, we do appear to have some primary signposts to factors associated with the persistence of sexual re-offending (see also Rasmussen 1999; Figueredo and Hunter 1999; Skuse *et al.* 1998; Knight and Prentky 1993), most significantly:

- a general pattern of conduct disorder and other non-sexual offending
- poor social functioning
- discontinuity of care
- trauma and neglect
- high levels of family dysfunction
- evidence of offence planning or sexual preoccupation
- early dropout from treatment programmes.

We have seen a conjunction between research interests in sexual offending and that exploring life-course persistent antisocial behavior more generally, with a developing consensus that the focus should be on the interactive process between early experience, particularly attachment, and subsequent life experiences (Ward *et al.* 2000).

NEEDS-LED ASSESSMENTS

Whilst issues of risk and community safety may dominate considerations of sexually abusive youth, it is vital that the importance of a needs-led assessment is not lost. As identified in the Framework for Assessment (DoH 2000b) and applied specifically to young abusers by Print and Erooga (2000), this should be multi-disciplinary in nature and aim to identify the global needs of the young person in terms of health, development and community safety. Access to services for young people is dependent upon locally defined eligibility criteria and related to their assessed level of vulnerability. A needs-led assessment is central to a young person being viewed holistically as opposed to an exclusive focus on sexual behavior. For example, young people who are sexually aggressive continue to have rights with regard to education, albeit that some may not be safely placed within a school setting for a brief or extended period. We would suggest the main aims of any comprehensive assessment of a young abuser should address the following:

- problem formation – what do we understand about the factors influential to the development and maintenance of this behavior
- risk analysis and management strategy – including placement and supervision issues
- care and developmental needs
- identified goals and targets for change – these should be specific and achievable
- factors impacting upon the young person's ability to participate in a therapeutic process (e.g. motivation; disability; trauma)
- a clearly articulated intervention strategy.

CULTURALLY AND DEVELOPMENTALLY SENSITIVE PRACTICE

Sexual aggression fundamentally reflects an abuse of interpersonal power. The wider societal context forms the background and often underpins the vulnerability of group or individuals to exploitation or abuse. The increasing recognition of the abuse of children and adults with disabilities is a case in point (Cooke and Sinason 1998). Young abusers may at one and the same time come from the most disadvantaged and powerless in our society, whilst on an interpersonal level have exploited power over those weaker then themselves. Practitioners have frequently struggled to resolve these tensions, which may in part explain the relative paucity of provision or even discussion of services for sexually aggressive young people with learning disabilities (O'Callaghan 1998), those from ethnic minorities (Lewis 1999) or young women who abuse (Blues et al. 1999).

Hackett (1999) argues that practitioners need to explore and critically appraise their own beliefs and attitudes in order to engage with young people who sexually abuse, in ways that empower change.

YOUNG PEOPLE WITH PROBLEMATIC SEXUAL BEHAVIOURS IN SUBSTITUTE CARE

Farmer and Pollock's (1998) research highlighted the specific needs of young people in the care system who display sexually abusive behaviours. They found that in comparison with the wider sample this group presented with multiple disadvantages and were more likely to display the following characteristics:

- to be assessed as having a learning disability
- to have a history of severe behavioural problems
- to have witnessed sexual activity
- to have been victimized by multiple abusers
- to have suffered chronic neglect
- to have a longer history of professional concerns.

Farmer and Pollock identified significant problems in planning for and managing these young people, and

highlighted the ongoing vulnerability of other children in shared placements to victimization by these young abusers. The crucial role of care staff was evident, with the best outcomes for young people being in placements in which carers were actively involved and committed to the therapeutic process.

EVIDENCE-BASED PRACTICE

An increasing consensus has been emerging that treatment interventions with sexually aggressive young people needs to be multi-systemic and located within that young person's developmental process (Bourke and Donohue 1996). To date the only randomized comparative study published in relation to young sexual offenders has been that evaluating the impact of multi-systemic therapy compared with a traditional individual counselling approach (Borduin et al. 1990). The study concluded that multi-systemic therapy had a significantly greater impact in reducing risk of sexual re-offending. As Brown and Kolko's (1998) recent review identifies, we have a limited number of outcome studies from which to inform the development of practice. Latterly figures in the field have questioned the extent to which interventions with young sexual offenders should be considered as a specialized area, distinct from programmes aimed at the wider population of chronically offending youth (Ryan 1999). From the richer research available from these programmes, and from outcome data available with regard to adult sex-offender programmes, we can draw certain tentative conclusions as to the principal features of effective interventions.

1 Interventions should be ecologically orientated, promote systemic change and employ a variety of methods (e.g. individual; family and group work) (e.g. Hollin 1999; Swenson et al. 1998; Chapman and Hough 1998).
2 Interventions should promote skill development, behavioural and attitudinal change (Hollin 1999; Beech et al. 1999; Chapman and Hough 1998).
3 Programmes should be structured to address factors that contribute to the maintenance of all forms of criminal and antisocial behaviour (Rasmussen 1999).
4 Treatment for more problematic and deviant clients requires significant intensity and duration (Beech et al. 1999).
5 Programmes should actively involve families and carers (Sheridin et al. 1998; Farmer and Pollock 1998).
6 The design of interventions should be informed by those factors seen to promote resilience and positive outcomes for young people (Rutter et al. 1998; Rutter 1999; Daniel et al. 1999).
7 Services need to consider how to engage non-cooperative and poorly motivated clients (O'Reilly et al. 2001; Figueredo and Hunter 1999).
8 The most effective programmes are characterized by high treatment integrity (Hollin 1999; Beech et al. 1998; Chapman and Hough 1998; Allam and Browne 1998).

DESIGNING INTERVENTIONS

To date, relapse prevention (Pithers 1990) has been the primary treatment model for sex-offender programmes across the UK and North America and is predicated on the individual being able to transfer knowledge and skills from the therapeutic setting to external community situations. This approach has been critiqued, and more pathways into re-offending than identified in the original model have been articulated (Ward and Hudson 1998), along with an emphasis on the need to develop social competence (Marshall et al. 1999) and provide individuals with positive life goals as apposed to simply avoiding risky behaviours (Schofield and Mann 1999). Barber (1992), writing more generally on relapse prevention, has suggested that the quality of an individual's social network is the primary factor influencing whether skills and knowledge are maintained post-treatment.

Rich (1998), addressing young abusers specifically, proposes a developmental framework in which the constellation of possible services needs to be tailored to the needs of the young person and coordinated and cross-referenced, such that evaluation is based on the young person's overall global functioning. Suggesting that the 'treatment of adolescent sexual offenders may be more similar than different to the treatment of adolescent with other types of serious emotional and social dysfunction', Rich proposes four features of an integrated approach to interventions with this client group:

1 There should be flexibility of treatment, attuned to the specific needs of the individual.
2 Treatment should address general behaviour patterns in the young person's life which parallel sexual offending patterns.
3 Interventions should be comprehensive and promote positive adaptive behaviours.
4 Treatment should be integrated into the young person's everyday care setting.

G-MAP

The first author of this chapter is co-director of G-MAP (Greater Manchester Adolescent Programme), an independent sector provider working with children and young people who display sexually aggressive behaviours (Print and O'Callaghan 1999; O'Callaghan 1999). G-MAP provides individual, group and family work and provides a residential service in conjunction with a local authority provider. The majority of the young people who attend G-MAP for therapeutic work are resident in a substitute care setting of some form. Attempting to integrate the components of effective interventions described in the above sections, we have designed a service delivery framework structured around six key areas:

• offence-specific problems
• family issues

• the young person's sexuality
• influences on the young person's participation
• social functioning
• non-sexual conduct problems.

The role of carers is central to such an approach, to monitor progress, to reinforce key messages and to assist the young person to identify areas of risk. Young people in our programme have both concurrent individual group work and progress review sessions, undertaken jointly with their residential keyworker. These sessions have three broad themes:

• progress within the residential setting on key goals/identified targets
• review of treatment issues and performance in therapeutic work and expanding/reinforcing work undertaken
• specific decisions concerning individual care plans (e.g. allied developmental needs, supervision and community access).

FAMILY PARTICIPATION

Even when the young person is not currently resident at home, family participation can prove an invaluable motivator and source of information. Longer-term families may also take on a more direct role in support and supervision of young people. An evaluation of the Dublin-based Northside Inter-Agency Project (Sheridan et al. 1998) found a correlation between positive treatment outcomes and degree of familial support and participation. We have found involving families to be a powerful force, particularly when young people can bring from the treatment context issues to share with families. Families usually find it empowering to learn more of the nature of the work being undertaken and respond to being approached as allies. As Bentovim (1998) addresses in his work on family systemic approaches, a number of families do need intensive concurrent therapy if they are to make changes to become safe environments for victims or abusers.

EVALUATION OF SERVICES

In their survey of a number of treatment services for sexually abused children and young abusers, as part of the Messages from Research initiative, Monk and New (1996) found that services failed to build in systems that would facilitate an evaluation of their effectiveness. In particular, poor assessment and problem formation, and poor record-keeping, hindered a consideration of the specific needs of the young person as judged on intake. Services generally failed to provide a description of the treatment provided and evaluation of the young person's functioning at the conclusion or at key points of involvement with the service. Monk and New argue that clarity of assessment and integrated evaluation processes are essential, both to effective decision-making concerning an individual young person and to programme evaluation and development. Allam and Browne (1998) suggest that whilst 'in-house' evaluation systems are of some value, professional understanding of the effectively of various interventions with specific subgroups of sex offenders will be only achieved through large-scale independent research. The Home Office-sponsored STEP research in the UK (Beech *et al.* 1999) is an ongoing project to evaluate the effectiveness of adult sex offender treatment programmes in community and prison settings, though we await a similar initiative with adolescents.

REFERENCES

Abel, G.G., Becker, J.V., Mittleman, M. *et al.* 1987: Self-reported crimes of non-incarcerated paraphiliacs. *Journal of Interpersonal Violence* **2**(6): 3–25.

Allam, J.A. and Browne, K.D. 1998: Evaluating community-based treatment programmes for men who sexually abuse children. *Child Abuse Review* **7**: 13–29.

Barber, J.G. 1992: Relapse prevention and the need for brief social interventions. *Journal of Substance Abuse Treatment* **9**:157–168.

Beech, A., Fisher, D. and Beckett, R. 1999: *STEP3: An Evaluation of the Prison Sex Offender Treatment Programme.* London: Home Office.

Bentovim, A. 1998: Family systematic approach to work with young sex offenders. *Irish Journal of Psychology* **19**(1): 119–25.

Blues, A., Moffat, C. and Telford, P. 1999: Work with adolescent females who sexually abuse: Similarities and differences. In: Erooga, M. and Masson, H.C. (eds), *Children and Young People who Sexually Abuse Others: Challenges and Responses.* London: Routledge. xxii, 168–82, 278.

Borduin, C.M., Henggeler, S.W., Blaske, D.M. and Stein, R.J. 1990: Multisystemic treatment of adolescent sexual offenders. *International Journal of Offender Therapy and Comparative Criminology* **34**: 105–13.

Bourke, M.L. and Donohue, B. 1996: Assessment and treatment of juvenile sex offenders: an empirical review. *Journal of Child Sexual Abuse* **5**(1): 47–70.

Brown, E.J. and Kolko, D.J. 1998: Treatment efficacy and program evaluation with juvenile sexual abusers: a critique with directions for service delivery and research. *Child Maltreatment* **3**: 362–73.

Calder, M. (ed.), *Working with Young People who Sexually Abuse: New Pieces of the Jigsaw.* Russell House Publishing.

Campbell, D. 1998: Branded. *The Guardian,* 11th August 1998.

Chaffin, M. and Bonner, B. 1998: Don't shoot, we're your children: have we gone too far in our response to adolescent sexual abusers and children with sexual behaviour problems? *Child Maltreatment* **3**: 314–16.

Chapman, T. and Hough, M. for HM Inspectorate of Probation 1998: *Evidence Based Practice: a Guide to Effective Practice.* London: Home Office.

Cooke, L.B. and Sinason, V. 1998: Abuse of people with learning disabilities and other vunerable adults. *Advances in Psychiatric Treatment* **4**: 119–25.

Daniel, B., Wassell, S. and Gilligan, R. 1999: It's just common sense isnt it? Exploring ways of putting the theory of resilience into action. *Adoption and Fostering* **23**(2): 6–15.

DfEE (Department for Education and Employment) 1999: *Social Inclusion: Pupil Support.* Circular 10/99. London: DfEE Publications.

DoH (Department of Health) 1991: *Working Together Under The Children Act 1989.* London: HMSO.

DoH (Department of Health; Home Office) 1992: *Memorandum of Good Practice on Video Recorded Interviews with Child Witnesses for Criminal Proceedings.* London: HMSO.

DoH (Department of Health) 1998: *Report of the Inquiry into Child Abuse in Cleveland 1987.* London: HMSO.

DoH (Department of Health; Home Office; Department for Education and Employment) 2000a: *Working Together to Safeguard Children.* Norwich: Stationery Office.

DoH (Department of Health) 2000b: *Framework for the Assessment of Children in Need and their Families.* Norwich: Stationery Office.

Farmer, E. and Pollock, S. 1998: *Sexually Abused and Abusing Children in Substitute Care.* Chichester: John Wiley.

Figueredo, J. and Hunter, J.A. 1999: Factors associated with treatment compliance in a population of juvenile sexual offenders. *Sexual Abuse: a Journal of Research and Treatment* **11**(1): 49–67.

Finkelhor, D. 1979: *Sexually Victimised Children.* New York: Free Press.

Fromuth, M.E., Jones, C.W. and Burkhart, B.R. 1991: Hidden child molestation: an investigation of perpetrators in a nonclinical sample. *Journal of Interpersonal Violence* **6**: 376–84.

Glasgow, D., Horne, L. *et al.* 1994: Evidence, incidence, gender and age in sexual abuse of children perpetrated by children: towards a developmental analysis of child sexual abuse. *Child Abuse Review* **3**: 196–210.

Grubin, D. 1998: *Sex Offending Against Children: Understanding the Risk.* Police Research Unit Series Paper 99. London: Home Office.

Hackett, S. 1999: Empowered practice with young people who sexually abuse. In Erooga, M. and Masson, H (eds), *Children and Young People who Sexually Abuse Others: Challenges and Responses.* London: Routledge.

Hagen, M., King, R. and Patros, R. 1994: Recidivism among adolescent perpetrators of sexual assault against children. In *Young Victims, Young Offenders.* New York: Haworth Press, 127–37.

Havgaard, J.J. and Tilly, C. 1988: Characteristics predicting children's responses to sexual encounters with other children. *Child Abuse and Neglect* **12**: 209–18.

Hollin, C. 1999: Treatment programs for offenders: meta-analysis, what works, and beyond. *International Journal of Law and Psychiatry* **22**: 361–72.

Home Office 1998a: *Draft Guidance on Establishing Youth Offending Teams.* Circular 122/98, Task Force on Youth Justice. London: Home Office.

Home Office 1998b: *The Crime and Disorder Act: Sex Offender Orders – Guidance.* London: Home Office.

Home Office 1999: *The Work of Probation Services with Sex Offenders.* London: Home Office.

Hughes, G. 1998: *Understanding Crime Prevention: Social Control, Risk and Late Modernity,* Buckingham: Open University Press.

IoP (HM Inspectorate of Probation) 1998: *Exercising Constant Vigilance: the Role of the Probation Service in Protecting the*

Public from Sex Offenders. Report of a Thematic Inspection. London: Home Office.

Kahn, T.J. and Chambers, H. 1991: Assessing re-offence risk with juvenile sexual offenders. *Child Welfare* LXX(3).

Kelly, L., Regan, L. and Burton, S. 1991: *An Exploratory Study of the Prevalence of Sexual Abuse in a Sample of 16–21 Year Olds.* London: Child Abuse Studies Unit, Polytechnic of North London.

Kikuchi, J. 1995: When the offender is a juvenile: identifying and responding to juvenile sexual abuse in offenders. In Hunter, M. (ed.), *Child Survivors and Perpetrators of Sexual Abuse.* Beverly Hills, CA: Sage.

Knight, R.A. and Prentky, R.A. 1993: Exploring characteristics for classifying juvenile sex offenders. In Barbaree H.E., Marshall, W.L. and Hudson, S.E. (eds), *The Juvenile Sex Offender,* New York: Guilford Press. 45–103.

Lab, S.P., Shiels, G. and Schondel, C. 1993: Research note: an evaluation of juvenile sexual offender treatment. *Crime and Delinquency* **39**(4).

Ladwa-Thomas, U. and Sanders, R. 1999: Juvenile sex abusers: perceptions of social work practitioners. *Child Abuse Review* **8**: 55–62.

Laws, R.D. 1998: Sexual offending as a public health problem. Paper presented at the Conference of the National Association for the Development of Work with Sex Offenders (NOTA), Glasgow, UK.

Lewis, A.D. 1999: *Cultural Diversity in Sexual Abuser Treatment: Issues and Approaches.* Safer Society Press.

Mann, R. and Thornton, D. 1998: The evolution of a multi-site offender treatment program. In Marshall, W.,Fernandez, Y., Hudson, S. and Ward, T. (eds), *Sourcebook of Treatment Programs for Sexual Offenders.* New York: Plenum Press.

Margetts, T. 1998: Establishing multi-agency working with sex offenders: setting up to succeed. *NOTA News* **25**: 27–38.

Marshall, W., Anderson, D. and Fernandez, Y. 1999: *Cognitive Behavioural Treatment of Sexual Offenders.* Chichester: John Wiley.

Masson, H. 1995: Children and adolescents who sexually abuse other children: responses to an emerging problem. *Journal of Social Welfare and Family Law* **17**: 325–6.

Masson, H 1997: Researching policy and practice in relation to children and young people who sexually abuse. *Research, Policy and Planning,* **15**(3): 8–16.

Masson, H. 1998: Issues in relation to children and young people who sexually abuse other children: a survey of practitioners' views. *Journal of Sexual Aggression* **3**(2): 101–18.

Masson, H. and Morrison, T. 1999: Young sexual abusers: conceptual frameworks, issues and imperatives. *Children and Society* **13**: 203–15.

McGarvey, J. and Peyton, L. 1999: A framework for a multi-agency approach to working with young people who sexually abuse. In Calder, M.C. (ed), *Working with young people who sexually abuse: new pieces of the jigsaw.* Lyme Regis, Dorset: Russell House Publishing.

Monk, E. and New, M. for the Department of Health 1996: *Report of a Study of Sexually Abused Children and Adolescents, and of Young Perpetrators of Sexual Abuse who were Treated in Voluntary Agency Community Facilities.* London: HMSO.

Morrison, J. 1995: *DSM-IV Made Easy: The Clinician's Guide to Diagnosis.* New York: Guilford Press.

Morrison, T. 1997: Emotionally competent child protection organisations: fallacy, fiction or necessity? In Bates, J., Pugh, R.

and Thompson, N. (eds), *Protecting Children: Challenges and Change.* London: Arena.

NCH (National Children's Home) 1990: *Survey of Treatment Facilities for Abused Children and of Treatment Facilities for Young Sexual Abusers of Children.* London: NCH.

NCH (National Children's Home) 1992: *The Report of the Committee of Enquiry into Children and Young People who Sexually Abuse Other Children.* London: NCH.

Northern Ireland Research Team 1990: *Child Sexual Abuse in Northern Ireland: a Research Study of Incidence.* Antrim: Greystone Books.

O'Callaghan, D. 1998: Practice issues in working with young abusers who have learning disabilities. *Child Abuse Review* **7**: 435–48.

O'Callaghan, D. 1999: Young abusers with learning disabilities: towards better understanding and positive intervention. In Calder, M. (ed.), *Working with Young People who Sexually Abuse: New Pieces of the Jigsaw.* Russell House Publishing.

O'Reilly, G., Morrison, T., Sheerin, D. and Carr, A. 2001. A group-based module for adolescents to improve motivation to change sexually abusive behavior. *Child Abuse Review* **10**: 150–69.

Pithers, W. 1990: Relapse prevention with sexual aggressors. In Marshall, W., Laws, D. and Barbaree, H. (eds), *Handbook of Sexual Aggression.* New York: Plenum Press.

Prentky, R., Harris, B. *et al.* 2000: An actuarial procedure for assessing risk with juvenile sex offenders. *Sexual Abuse: a Journal of Research and Treatment* **12**(2): 71–93.

Prins, H. 1996: Risk assessment and management in criminal justice and psychiatry. *Journal of Forensic Psychiatry* **7**(1): 42–62.

Print, B. and Erooga, M. 2000: Young people who sexually abuse: implications for assessment. In Horwath, J. (ed.), *The Child's World: the Reader.* Department of Health, NSPCC and University of Sheffield.

Print, B. and O'Callaghan, D. 1999: Working in groups with young men who have sexually abused others. In Erooga, M. and Masson, H. *Children and Young People who Sexually Abuse Others: Challenges and Responses.* London: Routledge.

Rasmussen, L.A. 1999: Factors related to recidivism among juvenile sexual offenders. *Sexual Abuse: a Journal of Research and Treatment* **11**(1): 69–85.

Rich, S.A. 1998: The developmental approach to the treatment of adolescent sexual offenders. *Irish Journal of Psychology* **19**(1): 102–18.

Rutter, M. 1999: Resilience concepts and findings: implications for family therapy. *Journal of Family Therapy* **21**: 119–144.

Rutter, M., Giller, H. and Hagel, A. 1998: *Antisocial Behaviour by Young People.* Cambridge: Cambridge University Press.

Ryan, G. 1996. *Goals of group process; the struggle for safety.* Presentation given at NOTA Conference, Chester, UK.

Ryan, G. 1999: Treatment of sexually abusive youth: the evolving consensus. *Journal of Interpersonal Violence* **14**: 422–36.

Sanders, R.M. and Ladwa-Thomas, U. 1997: Interagency perspectives on child sexual abuse. *Child Maltreatment* **2**(3): 264–71.

Schofield, C. and Mann, R. 1999: An approach goal oriented intervention. Paper presented at the Conference of National Organization for the Treatment of Abusers, University of York, October 1999.

Sheridan, A., McKeown, K., Cherry, J. *et al.* 1998: Perspectives on treatment outcome in adolescent sexual offending: a study of a community-based treatment programme. *Irish Journal of Psychology* **19**(1): 168–80.

Skuse, D., Bentovim, A., Hodges, J. *et al.* 1998: Risk factors for development of sexually abusive behaviour in sexually victimised adolescent boys: cross sectional study. *British Medical Journal* **317**: 175–9.

Soothill, K. 1997: Rapists under 14 in the news. *Howard Journal* **36**: 367–77.

Soothill, K. and Francis, B. 1998: Poisoned chalice or just deserts? (The Sex Offenders Act 1997). *Journal of Forensic Psychiatry* **9**(2): 281–93.

Swenson, C., Henggeler, S.W., Schoenwald, S., Kaufman, K. and Randall, J. 1998: Changing the social ecologies of adolescent sexual offenders: implications of the success of multi-systemic therapy in treating serious antisocial behaviour in adolescents. *Child Maltreatment* **3**: 330–8.

Ward, T. and Hudson, S. 1998: A model of the relapse process in sexual offenders. *Journal of Interpersonal Violence* **13**: 700–25.

Ward, T., Nathan, P., Drake, C.R. *et al.* 2000. The role of formulation-based treatment for sexual offenders. *Behaviour Change* **17**: 251–64.

Wyre, R. 1997: A matter of conviction. *Community Care*, 30th October 1997.

PART 7

Legal frameworks, national and international

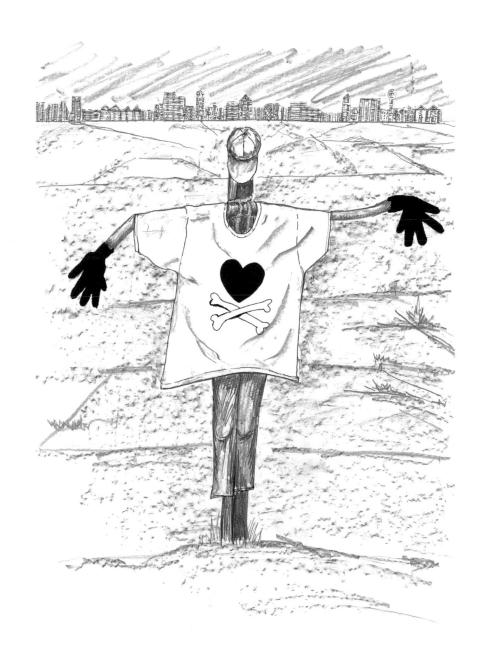

30

Children, psychiatric treatment and compulsion

ANTHONY HARBOUR

INTRODUCTION

Children accused of, or sentenced for, criminal offences may require and benefit from psychiatric treatment. This chapter deals with the law relating to the provision of this treatment. Children who are imprisoned are entitled to have their choices in relation to medical, including psychiatric, treatment respected in exactly the same way as young people living in the community or receiving in-patient medical or psychiatric treatment.

SOURCES OF LAW

The sources of law in this field are found in the common law and statute. The phrase 'the common law' is used to describe the 'rules which are extrapolated from the practice of the judges in deciding cases' (Montgomery 2003). In general, the law relating to children accused of crime is silent in relation to medical treatment. The Children Act is not a statute that deals comprehensively with issues around medical treatment. The Mental Health Act is not a child-centred jurisdiction. Common law principles, particularly as applied to the capable child who is refusing medical treatment, may appear out of date.

In addition, human rights law must be taken into consideration. This means the Human Rights Act 1998, which incorporates the European Convention of Human Rights into domestic law, and international conventions including the United Nations Convention on the Rights of the Child.

THE AGE OF THE CHILD

Although the age of 16 years is legally significant for some purposes, full adult status is not reached until the age of

18. Chapter 31 of the *Mental Health Act 1983 Code of Practice* applies to 'children and young people under the age of 18', and s105 of the Children Act 1989 defines a 'child' as meaning a person under the age of 18. These legal definitions do not necessarily coincide with professional boundaries between child/adolescent psychiatry and adult psychiatry.

TREATMENT AND THE COMMON LAW

CONSENT AND CAPACITY: ADULTS

In general, valid consent is required from a patient – of whatever age – before medical treatment can be given. There is a legal presumption that, in relation to medical treatment issues, all adults have capacity to make their own medical decisions.

Treatment which involves touching without consent can constitute an assault. For consent to be valid the patient must be capable of consenting, the consent must be freely given, and the patient consenting must be given suitable information. The exceptions to this general proposition include the giving of treatment in emergency circumstances where the patient lacks capacity (for example where the patient is unconscious and did not make a valid advance refusal of treatment before losing consciousness), and where statute allows for treatment to be given without consent (e.g. Part IV of the Mental Health Act 1983).

DEFINING CAPACITY: ADULTS

The courts in a number of cases have developed 'tests' to be used in assessing capacity. These tests are essentially aids to analysing medical evidence. In the case of person

MB (Re MB [Medical Treatment] (1997) 2 FLR 426) the Court had to decide whether a pregnant woman had the capacity to refuse consent to a caesarean section. The evidence before the Court was that her needle phobia made her incapable of making a decision. The Court applied the following principles in assessing her capacity. The patient is presumed to have the capacity to make a treatment decision unless she is *unable*:

- to comprehend and retain the information which is material to the decision, especially as to the likely consequences of having or not having the treatment in question
- to believe the information
- to use the information and weigh it in the balance as part of the process of arriving at the decision.

Where a child is regarded as 'Gillick competent' (see below) alternative tests and guidance can be developed (BMA/Law Society 1996). In particular, the MB questions were not devised for children and more detailed guidance as to good practice in assessing capacity/competence in children could be developed.

INCAPACITY: ADULTS

If an adult is regarded as lacking capacity then medical treatment can be provided on the following basis, which is known as the 'principle of necessity':

> '[A doctor] can lawfully operate on or give other treatment to adult patients who are incapable of consenting to [the doctor] doing so, provided that the operation or treatment is in the best interests of such patients. The operation or treatment will be in their best interests only if it is carried out in order either to save their lives or to ensure improvement or prevent deterioration in their physical or mental health.' (Re F (1989) 2 All ER 545)

TREATMENT DECISIONS: CHILDREN

THE CHILD WHO LACKS CAPACITY

Where children are incapable of consenting to medical treatment themselves, the consent of a person with 'parental responsibility' must be obtained except in emergencies. This will usually be one of the parents: mothers have parental responsibilty automatically when the child is born; fathers also obtain parental responsibility automatically if they were married to the mother at the time of the birth of the child, or if they marry the mother after the birth of the child. Fathers will also obtain parental responsibility if they make a 'parental responsibility agreement' with the mother, or obtain a parental responsibility order from the Court. Non-parents may also obtain parental responsibility; for example, a local authority obtains parental responsibility if a care order is granted in its favour.

Where more than one person has parental responsibility, s2(6) of the Children Act 1989 states that it is not necessary to seek consent from them all. Valid consent may be obtained from any person with parental responsibility. Application to the Court may be necessary to proceed to provide treatment if consultation with the parent is thought not to be in the interests of the child (e.g. if abuse by the parent is alleged). This may mean the service providers initiating such an application, or participating in applications brought by social services. In circumstances where parents refuse consent for treatment of their child which is thought by a doctor to be necessary, the use of Court proceedings must also be considered.

LIMITS ON THE RIGHT OF THE PARENT TO BE CONSULTED

The 'Gillick case' established that advice and treatment by a doctor could be given to a competent minor in certain circumstances without the child's parents being consulted or consenting (Gillick *v* West Norfolk & Wisbech Area Health Authority (1985) 3 All ER 402). The circumstances included:

- the child understanding the doctor's advice
- the doctor not being able to persuade the child to inform her parents or authorize the doctor to inform her parents
- the patient's best interests required the advice and treatment to be given.

Although this case referred to contraceptive advice, the principles are nevertheless applicable to other forms of medical treatment including psychiatric treatment.

EMERGENCY TREATMENT

Under common law a doctor may lawfully treat a child in an emergency even though he is unable to obtain a valid consent. In exceptional cases, emergency treatment can be provided in the face of parental opposition. Per Lord Templeman in the Gillick case, above at 432:

> 'I accept that where there is no time to obtain a decision from the court, a doctor may safely carry out treatment in an emergency if the doctor believes the treatment to be vital to the survival or health of an infant and notwithstanding the opposition of a parent or the impossibility of alerting the parent before the treatment is carried out.' (Quoted in Jones 2003)

TREATMENT DECISIONS BY CHILDREN

The law separates a child's decision-making about medical treatment into two components – *consent* and *refusal*. These appear to be artificial categories but have been adopted by lawyers in analysing the legal consequences of certain decisions. At one time it was assumed that the right of a child with capacity to consent to be treated covered both agreements to be treated as well as refusal. This assumption is not correct. The legal position, as set down in a number of cases, is that the refusal of a child to be medically treated can be overridden by the courts or by those exercising parental responsibility, even where the child has the capacity to consent (Re R (a minor) Wardship [Medical Treatment] 1992 1 FLR 190; and Re W 1993 1 FLR 1; and Re K, W & H (minors) [Medical Treatment] 1993 1 FLR 854).

Consent and the over-16s

Where a child is aged 16 or over and is capable of 'effective consent' to 'surgical, medical and dental treatment' the child has the legal right to consent on their own behalf (Family Law Reform Act 1969 s8(1)).

If the child aged 16 years or over is regarded as incapable of consenting to treatment, because, for example, he or she is severely disabled, then a parent's consent must be obtained (except in emergencies – see above).

Consent and the under-16s

The Gillick case, noted above, established that if a child has 'sufficient understanding and intelligence', then she or he can consent to medical treatment. The Court rejected a rigid age limit in favour of the more flexible concept of an individual assessment of the child's ability to understand.

Therefore 'Gillick competent' children can consent to medical treatment without their consent being overridden by their parents. However, good practice guidance underlines the need for consensus in evaluating consent. Where a child has given valid consent, this does not require a clinician to provide any treatment which he or she considers to be contrary to the child's best interests.

REFUSAL OF MEDICAL TREATMENT BY THE UNDER-18s

The courts have decided that a child's refusal to be treated can be overridden, even where the child is 'Gillick competent' and regardless of the child's age or capacity. Medical treatment which a child is refusing can be given with the consent of a person with parental responsibility, be it parent or local authority holding a care order.

THE MENTAL HEALTH ACT 1983

The Mental Health Act is not age-specific, so persons of any age can be detained under the Act. The Act covers patients who are civilly detained (Part II) and those who fall within Part III of the Mental Health Act, that is mentally disordered offenders.

If a child is detained under either or both of Parts II and III of the Mental Health Act, certain forms of treatment, most commonly medication and ECT, can be provided only either with the consent of the patient or on the authority of a second-opinion doctor. (An important qualification to this statement is that for the first three months of a patient's detention medication can be given without consent or the necessity of a second opinion.)

Section 63 of the Act states that the child's consent is not required for any medical treatment for mental disorder which falls within Part IV. 'Treatment' under this section has been given a wide meaning, including tube feeding where the patient's refusal of food is the result of mental disorder (B v Croydon Health Authority (1995) 2 WLR 294).

Detention under s3(2)(c) of the Mental Health Act requires that:

> 'it is necessary for the health or safety of the patient or for the protection of other persons that he should receive such treatment and *it cannot be provided unless he is detained under this section* [emphasis added]'.

This provision may not always be easy to satisfy for children. It may be argued that, in cases where there is no dispute between those who hold parental responsibility and those treating the child, the child could be detained and treated on the basis of parental consent, and so detention under s3 of the Act would be unnecessary.

The Courts have not yet considered this argument in an application for discharge. However, the requirement imposed on public bodies under the Human Rights Act to construe legislation in a way which is compatible with the individual's human rights, plus a positive analysis of the benefits conferred by detention under mental health legislation, would mean that the outcome of such argument is uncertain. Arguably the statutory detention of a child, even though the person with parental responsibility is in agreement with all aspects of the child's psychiatric treatment, best protects the child's Convention rights. The particular right in question is Article 5 which provides that a person (including a child) has a right to have his or her detention speedily reviewed by a Court.

THE CHILDREN ACT 1989

PARENTAL RESPONSIBILITY

Parental responsibility is defined in s3 of the Children Act as meaning 'all the rights, duties, powers, responsibilities and authority which by law a parent of a child has in relation to the child and his property'. Parental responsibility includes decisions about medical treatment, and also decisions about where the child lives, and who the child sees.

In any dealings with a child, whether in relation to outpatient assessment or inpatient treatment, staff must identify who has parental responsibility for the child. The person, or body, with parental responsibility can provide consent to treatment being undertaken which the child may be refusing. If the child lacks capacity, treatment cannot be provided to a child, except in emergencies, without the consent of the person with parental responsibility, or a Court order.

Under s33(3)(b) of the Act, if a child is subject to a care order, the local authority has parental responsibility for the child, and the power to determine the extent to which a parent of the child may meet his or her parental responsibility for the child.

THE STATUTORY RIGHT TO REFUSE TO BE ASSESSED/TREATED

The Children Act refers to various circumstances in which a child can refuse assessment or examination. These circumstances include the following:

- an emergency protection order (s43)
- a child assessment order (s44)
- an interim care order (s38(6))
- a supervision order (s35).

The provisions in the Children Act state that, notwithstanding any Court direction, a child who is of sufficient understanding to make an informed decision can refuse to submit to the examination or assessment. However, a judge, exercising the High Court's 'inherent jurisdiction', may override such a refusal.

The 'Glamorgan case' involved a 15-year-old girl who, by the time legal proceedings had commenced, had confined herself in the front room of her father's house for 11 months (South Glamorgan CC v W & B (1993) 1 FLR 574). By the time the High Court had made a decision, there had been 22 previous Court appearances. The local authority commenced care proceedings and the issue to be determined was whether she could be treated in a specialist psychiatric inpatient unit without her consent. She was regarded as having sufficient understanding to refuse to be assessed. It was decided that the Court could override a child's statutory right to refuse to be assessed and direct that steps be taken to assess and treat the child against her wishes.

EMERGENCY INTERVENTION IN CHILD-PROTECTION CASES

The authority to consent to treatment on behalf of a child may be limited by statute, particularly where local authorities have obtained short-term child-protection powers. Under s44(5)(b) of the Act, emergency protection orders empower the applicants only to take such action in meeting his or her parental responsibility as is reasonably required to safeguard and promote the welfare of the child. A welfare provision in s46(9)(b) deals with children removed by police in cases of emergency: 'The designated officer shall do what is reasonable in all the circumstances of the case for the purpose of safeguarding or promoting the child's welfare.'

SECURE ACCOMMODATION

The vast majority of children who require inpatient treatment for mental disorder are either treated on the authority of the person with parental responsibility or detained under the Mental Health Act. Secure-accommodation orders are very occasionally used, typically for young people with learning difficulties who are exhibiting challenging behaviours.

There are two distinct routes into secure accommodation. The first, considered in Chapter 31, is via the criminal Courts under a Court-imposed security requirement. The other route is via s25 of the Children Act 1989 where no criminal offence is alleged but the order may be sought because the child may be, for example, behaviourally disturbed.

Under s25 of the Children Act, a child who is being looked after by a local authority may not be placed in 'accommodation provided for the purpose of restricting liberty' (secure accommodation) for more than 72 hours in any 28 days, unless the local authority obtains a secure-accommodation order. Section 25 has been extended by regulations to children being provided with accommodation by health authorities and in residential care homes, nursing homes and mental nursing homes. A social service authority, health authority, health provider, local education authority or person carrying on the home may apply for a s25 order.

Restricting the liberty of a child in these forms of accommodation requires a secure-accommodation order, or an order under the High Court's inherent jurisdiction. These orders are available only if the Court is satisfied: (a) that the child has a history of absconding and is likely to abscond from any other description of accommodation, and if he or she absconds, is likely to suffer significant harm; or (b) that if the child is kept in any other description of accommodation he or she is likely to suffer injury or injure other persons.

A secure-accommodation order provides the legal justification for detaining the child in a therapeutic setting. However, it does not provide legal justification for compulsory treatment of the child. It is still necessary to seek the consent of the child (if 'Gillick competent' – see earlier), or a person with parental responsibility, or (in exceptional cases) a Court order authorizing treatment. If the child is detained under mental health legislation, this provides a legal justification for both detention and treatment. Therefore, it is not necessary to apply for a secure-accommodation order for a child who is detained under the Mental Health Act.

There is also some doubt as to what exactly constitutes 'secure accommodation': a maternity unit was regarded as 'secure accommodation', but an eating-disorder clinic was not (respectively: A Metropolitan Borough Council v DB [1997] 1 FLR 767; and Re C [Detention: Medical Treatment] [1997] 2 FLR 180).

THE HUMAN RIGHTS ACT 1998

The Human Rights Act incorporates the rights and freedoms set out in the European Convention of Human Rights (hereafter, 'the Convention') into UK law. It applies in England, Wales, Scotland and Northern Ireland. Any person who is involved in the delivery of mental health services, be they user, carer or professional, will be affected.

The Convention does not deal expressly with the rights of children. Like the Mental Health Act, the Convention is not age-specific.

Under s1 of the Human Rights Act it is unlawful for a 'public authority' to act in a way which is incompatible with a Convention right. 'Public authority' is very widely defined, to include Courts and 'any person certain of whose functions are functions of a public nature'. Taking this section of the Act into account, clinicians will be required to act in ways which recognize the basic human rights of all the children under their care.

The rights protected under the Act include the following:

- the right to life (Article 2)
- protection from torture and inhuman or degrading treatment or punishment (Article 3)
- protection from slavery and forced or compulsory labour (Article 4)
- the right to liberty and security of person (Article 5)
- the right to fair trial (Article 6)
- protection from retrospective criminal offences (Article 7)
- protection of private and family life (Article 8)
- freedom of thought and conscience and religion (Article 9)
- freedom of association and assembly (Article 11)
- the right to marry and found a family (Article 12)
- freedom from discrimination (Article 14).

The articles that are most relevant to children who are being treated against their will, either under the Mental Health Act or with the agreement of the person with parental responsibility, will be 5 and 8.

The Human Rights Act should be regarded as a human-rights code which should be used alongside, and complementing, existing statute and common law. For example, if a child is being treated against his or her wishes outside the Mental Health Act, the child's Article 5 rights must be considered alongside the Article 8 rights of the parent to seek medical treatment on the child's behalf. The new language of human rights is a very important development, but does not necessarily threaten existing standards of good practice. This is because the 'Convention rights' are not usually absolute rights, and it is possible to balance different rights against each other. For example, the parents' right to make decisions must be balanced against the child's own rights to privacy, and the need to protect the child's health. Similarly, the child's right to liberty is not absolute.

Recent BMA guidance suggests that the Human Rights Act will require a reconsideration of the power of parents to authorize the compulsory treatment of children:

'... while uncertainty remains regarding the extent to which practice will change in relation to minor's rights as a result of the Human Rights Act, such rights are increasingly seen as an important matter for debate and re-evaluation. ... It is conceivable therefore that as we become more accustomed to looking at a range of issues, such as healthcare, through the prism of human rights, views about parental authority over competent children will also undergo significant changes'. (BMA 2001)

PARTICULAR PROBLEM AREAS

When should the Mental Health Act be used, as opposed to relying on parental consent?

Factors to be taken into account are:

- the age of the child
- whether the parents are making decisions in the best interests of the child
- the stigmatizing consequences of detention
- the advantage of external review and legal representation conferred by the Mental Health Act
- the statutory framework of the Act aimed at protecting the interests of the detained patient.
- protection under the Act for the interests of the treatment providers.

When is Court involvement still appropriate?

The Courts have sought to discourage applications by treatment providers who are concerned about the ethics of overriding the refusal of treatment by, in particular, the older child. Circumstances still clearly exist where reference to Court is still justified; for example:

- where treatment decisions need to be made and the person with parental responsibility is incapacitated, again for example in dealing with the accommodated child
- where the person with parental responsibility may not be acting in the interests of the child both in consenting, or refusing to consent, to medical treatment on behalf of the child
- where the local authority does not wish to refer treatment decisions to the parent, for example in cases of suspected abuse
- where the treatment is particularly controversial.

What is the scope of parental consent to treatment, where the child is refusing treatment and the Mental Health Act is not being used?

Particular questions are:

- Can we use force?

- Can we restrict liberty?
- Can we compulsorily treat?
- Does 'common law' intervention have to be confined to emergencies?

Unfortunately, the Courts have not provided clear answers to these questions.

As discussed above, the Courts have said that treatment can be given to a child who is refusing, provided that a person with parental responsibility has given consent. It might be argued that this also justifies the use of force, and the restriction of liberty, to the degree necessary to carry out the treatment. Relying upon parental authority, or 'common law' powers, is problematic because there are no legal safeguards for the children concerned, or for the staff carrying out the treatment:

> 'Although case law has achieved a situation whereby those responsible for the health care of adolescents can ensure that they received essential treatment, the methods adopted enabling this to happen are often unnecessarily insensitive and ignore the basic human rights accorded to adults forced to undergo medical treatment against their will.' (Fortin 2003)

What registration requirements/formalities need to be complied with when children are being detained?

This is to deal with the practicalities of detention. If the Mental Health Act is to be used then the place of detention must be a hospital as defined by the Act, or a registered private mental nursing home. If the child is subject to secure accommodation then the detaining unit will have to be subject to the registration requirements imposed by the Children Act.

If the treatment providers wish to treat with the agreement of the parents, what happens if there is a disagreement between those who have parental responsibility for a child?

As discussed above, only one valid consent is required from a 'Gillick competent' child, or one person with parental responsibility. Treatment may be given if there is valid consent, but there is no obligation to provide treatment which is not considered to be in the child's interests. If there is a valid consent, and a person with parental responsibility wishes to prevent the treatment, that person could apply for a Court order to resolve the dispute.

It is usually good practice to attempt to resolve disagreements informally, but if this is not possible, it might be appropriate for the dispute to be referred to the Court by the professionals responsible for the child's treatment. This may be particularly important to protect staff in cases where the parent who disagrees with treatment would take legal action if it was carried out against his or her wishes.

What does 'de facto' detention mean?

'Detention' is a matter of fact. A child who is not formally detained under the Mental Health Act, or a secure-accommodation order, may be detained in fact if steps have been taken to prevent him or her from leaving a particular place. Locked doors do not automatically indicate that the patient is detained, if the doors are unlocked if he or she requests this. Similarly, even if the doors are unlocked, the child may be detained in fact (for example, if clothing or footwear has been removed).

If a child is de facto detained on the authority of the person with parental responsibility in an inpatient psychiatric unit, must a s25 application be made?

A secure-accommodation order may be necessary if the child is not formally detained under the Mental Health Act, and is held in 'accommodation provided for the purpose of restricting liberty' for more than 72 hours in a period of 28 days. A secure-accommodation order is not necessary if the child is being looked after by a local authority or accommodated by a health authority, or in a residential care home, nursing home or mental nursing home. A secure-accommodation order is also unnecessary if the child's detention is authorized by a judge under the High Court's inherent jurisdiction.

What are the child's rights to confidentiality?

The psychiatrist's duty of confidentiality owed to a child patient is as great as that owed to any other person. There is, however, no absolute right to confidentiality and there may be circumstances where a breach of confidentiality may be justified. Current guidance states that 'children's rights to confidentiality should be strictly observed' (*Mental Health Act 1983 Code of Practice*, paragraph 15.25).

REFERENCES

BMA/Law Society 1996: *Assessment of Mental Capacity: Guidance for Doctors and Lawyers.* London: BMA/LS, 66.

BMA 2001: *Consent, Rights and Choices in Health Care for Children and Young People.* London: BMJ Books.

Fortin, J. 2003: *Children's Rights and the Developing Law*, 2nd edition. London: LexiNexis UK: 122.

Jones, R. 2003: *Mental Health Act Manual*, 8th edition. London: Sweet & Maxwell.

Montgomery, J. 2003: *Health Care Law.* Oxford: Oxford University Press, 7.

31

The youth justice system in England and Wales

MARK ASHFORD AND SUSAN BAILEY

INTRODUCTION

ACTS AND CONVENTIONS

The law relating to children accused of crime is to be found in a series of statutes spanning more than 60 years. As well as having detailed rules passed by parliament, the youth justice system is increasingly influenced by general human-rights principles contained in international conventions.

The most important human-rights document is the European Convention on Human Rights. Since 2 October 2000, the principles of this convention have been incorporated into domestic law by the Human Rights Act 1998. Every public body and Court of law is required to make decisions in compliance with the principles of the European convention. In the field of youth justice the most important guarantees are as set out in Chapter 30.

The UK is also a signatory to the United Nations Convention on the Right of the Child. This establishes general principles that, in any decision involving a child, his or her best interests shall be a primary consideration (Article 3) and that a child has the right to express views in all matters affecting his or her life (Article 12). The UN convention also deals specifically with the youth justice process in Articles 37 and 40. The United Nations Minimum Standards for the Administration of Juvenile Justice (commonly referred to as the 'Beijing rules') provide more detailed guidelines.

AIMS OF THE SYSTEM

The principal aim of the youth justice system is to prevent offending by children and young persons, as stated in s37 of the Crime and Disorder Act 1998. A Court must also have regard to the welfare of any child or young person who appears before it, as stated in s44 of the Children and Young Persons Act 1933.

The Youth Justice Board for England and Wales (established in September 1998) monitors the operation of the youth justice system and also manages the juvenile secure estate – institutions contracted to provide places of detention for young people aged 10–17 years.

THE ROLE OF LOCAL AUTHORITIES

Since April 2000, all local authorities in England and Wales have coordinated their work with young offenders in a multi-disciplinary agency called a Youth Offending Team (YOT). Under s39(5) of the Crime and Disorder Act 1998, the team is required to include at least one of the following:

- a social worker
- a probation officer
- a representative of the local education authority
- a police officer
- a representative of the local health authority.

The health worker is often a drugs worker or a community psychiatric nurse, but in some areas the team may include a clinical psychologist.

YOTs provide a range of services which include:

- schemes to divert young offenders from the Courts
- bail supervision and support schemes to reduce offending whilst on bail
- reports for the Courts regarding convicted defendants
- implementation of community sentences
- supervision of young offenders released from custody.

The YOT is required to assess each child who has contact with the team. This assessment is carried out with the aid of a standardized questionnaire called ASSET. The questionnaire concentrates on factors which affect the likelihood of further offending, but there is a supplementary assessment which examines the child's vulnerability in custody.

Under s17 of the Children Act, the local authority also has a duty to safeguard and promote the welfare of children who are in need. The main agency which will carry out this duty is the social services department. Where a child is considered to have suffered or to be at risk of suffering significant harm, and that harm is attributable to the care given by his or her parents, the local authority may institute care proceedings.

THE YOUTH COURT

The Youth Court is the main criminal Court dealing with children. The Court's procedures are designed to be minimally formal and the proceedings are held in private. The magistrates who sit in the youth Court receive special training.

Before 1991, a single Court – the Juvenile Court – dealt with children accused of crime and children subject to care proceedings. Since then the hearing of care proceedings has been dealt with by the Family Proceedings Court. The Youth Court has no power to refer a child to the latter even if there are considerable concerns regarding his or her welfare.

DEFENCE LAWYERS

A child accused of a crime may be represented by a defence lawyer who could be a solicitor or a barrister. There is no specialist accreditation of lawyers who represent children in the criminal Courts.

CRIMINAL RESPONSIBILITY

Article 40(3)(a) of the UN convention states that every criminal jurisdiction should have a minimum age below which children shall be presumed not to have the capacity to infringe the penal law. This minimum age 'shall not be fixed at too low an age level, bearing in mind the facts of emotional, mental and intellectual maturity' (Beijing rule 4.1).

In England and Wales, the age of criminal responsibility is set at 10 years in s50 of the Children and Young Persons Act 1933. As a child under that age is presumed to be incapable of committing a crime, he or she can neither be arrested nor prosecuted in the criminal Courts for an act committed before the tenth birthday. The age of 10 years is not remarkable in comparison with other jurisdictions in the British Isles (8 years in Scotland and

7 years in the Republic of Ireland), but it is low in comparison with other countries in the Council of Europe where the median age is 14 or 15.

After a child has attained the age of 10 years, he or she is subject to the full rigours of the criminal law. Until 1998 there was a presumption that a child under the age of 14 was incapable of forming the necessary criminal intent. This presumption – known by the Latin phrase *doli incapax* – could be rebutted if the prosecuting authorities could prove that the child knew that the criminal act was seriously wrong as opposed to merely naughty. With the abolition of the presumption of *doli incapax* in the Crime and Disorder Act, there is no longer any assessment of the child's moral understanding before attributing criminal culpability (see Chapter 5).

THE INVESTIGATIVE STAGE

ARREST AND DETENTION

When police officers investigating a crime identify a suspect they will normally arrest that person. A suspect may be held without charge for 24 hours (longer in the case of serious offences). This applies to young suspects as it does to adults.

Responsibility for a suspect whilst in police detention rests with the custody sergeant. The sergeant is independent of the investigation and must decide whether there is sufficient evidence to charge the suspect immediately or whether further detention is necessary whilst the investigation continues. The custody sergeant is responsible for the suspect's well-being whilst in custody. All suspects are entitled to regular meals and refreshment whilst in custody. Juveniles should not be held in a cell unless no other accommodation is available and it is not possible to supervise them otherwise. If there are any health concerns the custody sergeant will ask the police doctor (sometimes referred to as the 'forensic medical examiner') to attend the police station to examine the suspect.

APPROPRIATE ADULT

In the case of suspects under the age of 17 years, the police are required under s34(2) of the Children and Young Persons Act 1933 to notify a parent or guardian of the child's arrest. They are also required to arrange for the attendance of an 'appropriate adult' (*Police and Criminal Evidence Act 1984 Code of Practice*, code C paragraph 1). The appropriate adult will normally be a parent but may in some cases be a member of a YOT or a volunteer acting on the team's behalf. There is no formal requirement that an appropriate adult be present in the case of a 17-year-old suspect, unless he or she is mentally disordered, in which case there is a separate requirement to arrange for an appropriate adult.

LEGAL ADVICE

A child or young person under arrest has a right to free legal advice while in the police station. Most firms of solicitors who are contracted to do criminal defence work operate 24-hour emergency services for clients who have been arrested. If the child or young person is not able to nominate a particular solicitor, there is a duty solicitor scheme which means legal advice is available 24 hours a day, 365 days a year.

INTERROGATION

An important means of evidence gathering is the questioning of the suspect by the police. A suspect under the age of 17 years may not normally be interviewed unless an appropriate adult is present. The appropriate adult is expected to facilitate communication with the child and ensure that the interview is conducted fairly. The interview will be recorded, usually on audiotape, but increasingly on videotape.

A suspect of any age has a right not to self-incriminate. This is often referred to as the 'right to silence'. Following the passing of the Criminal Justice and Public Order Act in 1994, since 1995 there has been a limitation on the right to silence in that Courts are now permitted to draw adverse inferences from a suspect's failure to:

- explain his/her presence at the scene of a crime
- explain his/her possession of incriminating articles
- to mention when questioned a fact later relied upon in his/her defence which s/he could reasonably have been expected to have mentioned at the time.

Before the interview starts the interviewing officers are required to advise the suspect of the right to silence and the possibility of adverse inferences being drawn from remaining silent. This warning is usually referred to as 'the caution' and the suggested wording is as follows:

'You do not have to say anything. But it may harm your defence if you do not mention when questioned something which you rely upon later at Court. Anything you do say may be given in evidence.'

DISPOSAL

Where the police consider that there is sufficient evidence to prove that a child suspect has committed a crime, they can send the individual to Court. If the public interest does not require Court action, the child may be diverted by the police administering a reprimand or, in more serious cases, a warning under s65 of the Crime and Disorder Act 1998. A child receiving a warning will also be referred to the Youth Offending Team who may work with the child and parents to prevent further offending. This is called a 'rehabilitation programme'.

THE ADJUDICATIVE STAGE

When a child is charged, the police will normally send the individual to a Youth Court. If an adult is jointly accused of being involved in the crime, the child will be sent to a magistrates' Court along with the adult defendant.

In the case of certain 'grave crimes' (e.g. robbery, residential burglary, wounding with intent to cause grievous bodily harm), the Youth Court may send the child to the Crown Court for trial. This decision is based upon the seriousness of the alleged crime and the adequacy of the sentencing powers of the Youth Court (see R v Inner London Youth Courts *ex parte* Director of Public Prosecutions [1996] Crim LR 834; and (1997) 161 JP 178).

In the Youth Court there are automatic restrictions on the news media reporting the name, address or any other particulars which would lead to the identification of the young accused. In the adult magistrates' Court and in the Crown Court, there is a power to impose similar conditions. In practice such an order will be made at the first appearance; but if the child is convicted, the Court may lift the reporting restrictions if it considers that it would be in the public interest to do so.

LEGAL REPRESENTATION

Article 6 of the European Convention on Human Rights guarantees a right to legal representation if the interests of justice so require. In England and Wales such representation will be funded by the Criminal Defence Service (part of the Legal Services Commission). The defence lawyer will either be from a private firm which is contracted to provide publicly funded representation or be a salaried employee of the Public Defender Service.

The fact that a right to legal representation exists does not mean that the child will have the intellectual and emotional ability to instruct a lawyer adequately. In civil and care proceedings a child is presumed to be *unable* to instruct a lawyer, being considered too young to assume the responsibility for making decisions. To deal with this problem, an adult is appointed to make decisions in the best interests of the child. This adult is referred to as a 'litigation friend'. The exception is where the Court is satisfied the child is of sufficient age and understanding to instruct the lawyer directly. No such concept exists in criminal proceedings; instead the defence lawyer is expected to act on the instructions of the young client without any adult intermediary.

BAIL AND REMANDS

Under s4 of the Bail Act 1976 and Article 5 of the European Convention on Human Rights, any person accused of a crime has a right to liberty whilst the case is being considered before the criminal Court. Whether released by the police or the Courts, the accused person is on bail. Bail may be refused by the police or the Courts for a number of reasons specified in the Bail Act. The most common reasons for refusal are that there are substantial grounds for believing that the accused person will:

- fail to return to Court for future hearings
- commit further offences whilst on bail
- interfere with the course of justice (e.g. intimidating a witness or disposing of potential evidence).

A juvenile may be refused bail if the Court is satisfied that he or she should be kept in custody for the individual's own welfare (Bail Act, Schedule 1, paragraph 3).

Under s3(6) of the Bail Act the Court may grant bail with conditions which are considered necessary to deal with the concerns outlined above. Common conditions include:

- a requirement to sleep every night at a particular address
- a curfew
- a condition of reporting to the local police station on a regular basis.

Before the accused is released on bail, the Court may require that money be paid into Court (a security) or another person guarantees the accused will answer to bail (a surety).

A 17-year-old who is refused bail will be sent to a prison or remand centre. When a juvenile is not released on bail, he or she will normally be remanded to local authority accommodation under s23(1) of the Children and Young Persons Act 1969. Where the accused is aged between 12 and 16 years, remand may be to local authority accommodation with a security requirement. This will mean that the young accused is placed in a local authority secure unit. Under s23(5) of the same Act, the Court may impose a security requirement only if:

- the defendant is *either* (a) charged with, or has been convicted of, a violent or sexual offence, or an offence punishable in the case of an adult with imprisonment for a term of 14 years of more, *or* (b) has a recent history of absconding while remanded to local authority accommodation and is charged with, or has been convicted of, an imprisonable offence alleged or found to have been committed while he or she was so remanded
- *and* the Court is of the opinion that only remand with a security requirement would be adequate to protect the public from serious harm.

As there are not enough secure units to meet demand, there are special provisions for 15- and 16-year-old boys under s23(5) of the foregoing Act (as modified by the Crime and Disorder Act 1998). For this group, if the Court considers that the above criteria are satisfied, the remand will be to a prison or remand centre unless the Court:

- is notified that a secure bed is available

- is satisfied that, by reason of his physical or emotional immaturity or a propensity of his to harm himself, it would be undesirable for him to be remanded to a remand centre.

RIGHT TO A FAIR TRIAL

Article 6 of the European Convention on Human Rights provides a number of procedural guarantees for the child accused of crime. These include the presumption of innocence, the right to be informed of the nature of the charges, the right to be legally represented, and the right to examine witnesses and call witnesses in defence. Read as a whole, Article 6 guarantees the right of an accused to participate effectively in his or her own trial. With child defendants, the European Court of Human Rights has emphasized that this includes a developmental perspective:

'[It] is essential that a child charged with an offence is dealt with in a manner which takes full account of his age, level of maturity and intellectual and emotional capacities, and that steps are taken to promote his ability to understand and participate in the proceedings.' (T & V v United Kingdom (1999) 30 EHRR 121; and [2000] 2 All ER 1024)

In response to this Court ruling, a *Practice Direction* has been issued which suggests ways in which the trial procedure may be modified for a child defendant to promote understanding and participation (*Practice Direction*: Trial of Children and Young Persons in the Crown Court [2000] 1 WLR 659; and [2000] 1 Cr App R 483). The suggestions include allowing the child to sit with his or her family and legal advisers, removal of wigs and gowns, simplification of the language used in Court, and regular breaks. Psychologists and psychiatrists may be involved in advising the Court on the child defendant's capacities and suitable modifications that are required to ensure effective participation. Where there is doubt that the child accused is able to participate effectively in the trial, the question of fitness to plead may be raised (see Chapter 30).

TRIAL

The criminal justice process in England and Wales is an adversarial one. This means that the prosecution and defence present to the Court their opposing versions of what happened. The Court itself does not take an active part in the discovery of the relevant facts but instead relies almost totally on the evidence presented to it by the opposing parties. The accused person is presumed innocent until proven guilty and the burden of proving guilt must be discharged by the prosecution beyond reasonable doubt.

In the Youth Court or adult magistrates' Court, the trial is before either a district judge (formerly a stipendiary magistrate) or three lay magistrates. The district judge or the lay magistrates hear all the evidence and also rule on the admissibility of any disputed evidence. In the Crown Court the trial is before a judge and jury. The judge's role is restricted to managing the trial and ruling on the admissibility of evidence. The jury hears only factual evidence admitted by the judge. The jury alone decides on the innocence or guilt of the accused, although they hear a summary of the evidence from the judge and an explanation of the relevant law.

DISPOSAL

A criminal Court is required to sentence any offender on the basis of the seriousness of the offence. In deciding on the appropriate disposal, the Court will also consider the offender's:

- previous criminal convictions
- compliance with previous orders of the Court
- personal mitigation.

In the case of a child, a significant mitigating factor will be the age of the defendant. The Courts have demonstrated a willingness to reduce a sentence to reflect the lesser responsibility for wrong-doing and the lesser awareness of the consequences of the offence; nevertheless, in the case of serious offences, the Courts are prepared to pass long sentences to protect the public and to act as a deterrent to others (e.g. respectively: R v Pritchard (1989) 11 Cr App R (S) 421; and R v Ford (1976) 82 Cr App R 303).

INFORMATION ABOUT THE YOUNG OFFENDER

Before sentencing, the Court will usually wish to obtain information about the child offender's family and education. This will normally be provided by the youth offending team in the form of a pre-sentence report. A report may be requested from a psychologist or psychiatrist, but this is unusual.

CHOICE OF CRIMINAL SENTENCE

Having considered information about the offence and the young offender as well as any mitigation by a defence lawyer, the Court will decide on the appropriate sentence. The sentence will be commensurate with the seriousness of the offence.

Discharge

The Court may discharge the young offender if it is not considered expedient to impose any punishment. The discharge may be *absolute* or *conditional*. In the latter case the offender may be resentenced if he or she commits another offence in the period of the discharge. Under s66(4) of the Crime and Disorder Act 1998, a conditional discharge may not be imposed if the young offender received a warning in the previous two years, save in exceptional circumstances.

Financial penalty

The Court may punish the young offender by ordering a fine. The Court is also under a duty to consider ordering financial reparation by means of a compensation order. If the offender is aged under 18 years, the Court may order the parent or guardian to pay. The Court is also under a duty to consider imposing a reparation order, which would involve reparation directly to the victim of the crime or unpaid work which would benefit the community at large, to a maximum of 24 hours.

Community sentence

The Courts have a range of sentences specially designed for young people. These include orders designed to address the child's offending by individual sessions or group work (supervision order) and orders which are designed to punish by depriving the child of free time (attendance-centre orders). The new action plan order combines elements of both types of order as well as providing a means by which the child offender may make reparation to the victim or the community at large. In the case of 16- and 17-year-olds the Courts may also make use of the ordinary adult community sentences.

Where the child has mental health problems, the Court can impose a supervision order or probation order with a requirement to receive psychiatric treatment. Before such a sentence may be imposed the Court must consider a report from a doctor approved under s12 of the Mental Health Act 1983.

Custodial sentence

The youth Court may sentence 12- to 17-year-olds to a detention and training order for between four and 24 months. Half of this sentence is served in custody; the other half under supervision in the community.

As well as the detention and training order, the Crown Court has the option, in the case of grave crimes, of imposing a longer period of detention under s91 of the Powers of Criminal Courts (Sentencing) Act 2000. This is the only custodial option for a 10- or 11-year-old.

In the case of violent or sexual offences, the Crown Court judge may pass a longer than normal sentence where she or he considers that the young offender poses a risk of serious harm to the public. This could be a life sentence if the maximum penalty for the offence so permits. Frequently, before a longer than normal sentence is imposed, the Court would obtain and consider a psychiatric report.

The mandatory sentence for a child convicted of murder is detention during Her Majesty's pleasure. This is an indeterminate sentence. The trial judge will announce in Court a minimum period the child will serve before being considered for release. This tariff period is intended to reflect the punishment element of the sentence. The offender will be released until after the expiry of this tariff period but even then only if the Parole Board considers that the person no longer presents a risk to the public.

A custodial sentence may be served in a prison service establishment, a local authority secure unit or a privately run secure training centre. The decision where to place the child offender is made by the Youth Justice Board, following an assessment of the child by the YOT.

Orders made in relation to parents

When a child is convicted of a criminal offence, the parent or guardian may be bound over to exercise proper care and control of the child. The Court may also impose a parenting order which includes a requirement to attend parenting classes for up to three months and may include other conditions (under s8 of the Crime and Disorder Act 1998) such as a requirement to take the child to school every morning.

MENTAL HEALTH ACT DISPOSALS

In the case of a mentally disordered young offender, the Court may also make an order under the Mental Health Act 1983.

Hospital order

This order may be made either by a Youth Court or the Crown Court. The order transfers the offender to a psychiatric hospital where he or she is treated as being detained under the Mental Health Act in the same way as civil patients.

Under s37(2) of the Act, the Court may make a hospital order if:

- the Court is satisfied, on the written or oral evidence of two registered medical practitioners, that the offender is suffering from mental illness, psychopathic disorder, severe mental impairment or mental impairment
- the mental disorder from which the offender is suffering is of a nature or degree which makes it appropriate for him or her to be detained in a hospital for medical treatment and, in the case of psychopathic disorder or mental impairment, that such treatment is likely to alleviate or prevent a deterioration of the person's condition
- the Court is of the opinion, having regard to all the circumstances including the nature of the offence and the character and antecedents of the offender, and to the other available methods of dealing with the person, that the most suitable method of disposing of the case is by means of a hospital order.

When a Court is considering making a hospital order, the defendant should, except in the rarest circumstances, be legally represented.

Restriction order

A restriction order is a hospital order where the Court decides that the offender's release shall be subject to special restrictions, under s41(1) of the Mental Health Act. A restriction order may be made only by a Crown Court judge. The order may be made only when making a hospital order if it appears to the Court, having regard to the nature of the offence, the antecedents of the offender and the risk of the person committing further offences if set at large, that it is necessary for the protection of the public from serious harm. Before the order can be made, s41(2) of the Act stipulates that at least one of the medical practitioners must give evidence orally before the Court.

A Youth Court or adult magistrates' Court which has convicted a defendant may under s43(1) of the Act commit him or her to the Crown Court with a view to a restriction order being made, but only if:

- the person has attained the age of 14 years by the date of conviction
- the offence is imprisonable in the case of an adult
- the conditions for a hospital order are satisfied (see above)
- it appears to the Court, having regard to the nature of the offence, the antecedents of the offender and the risk of the person committing further offences if set at large, that if a hospital order is made a restriction order should also be made.

If committal is made under this power, the offender shall be committed in custody to the Crown Court. If the offender has not attained the age of 17 years, it is submitted that committal to custody should be construed subject to the provisions of s23 of the Children and Young Persons Act 1969.

Guardianship order

A guardianship order may be made by either a Youth Court or a Crown Court. The offender must have attained the age of 16 years. Under s37(2)(a)(ii) of the Mental Health Act, the Court may make the order only if it is satisfied that the relevant social services department or other person is willing to receive the offender into guardianship.

The preconditions for the making of a guardianship order are as for a hospital order, except that there is no requirement that the mental disorder must be treatable. A guardianship order gives the local-authority social services department or other person nominated in the order the power to determine the young person's place of residence, education or training. The young person may also be required to attend for treatment.

HAVING A CRIMINAL CONVICTION

Once a child has a conviction, he or she has a criminal record which will be stored on the police national computer (PNC). Although the conviction will remain on the PNC indefinitely, the Rehabilitation of Offenders Act 1974 provides a mechanism by which convictions may be wiped from a person's record ('spent' in the wording of the Act) after the passage of time. Once a conviction is spent, the conviction need not be disclosed to an employer or to a financial institution from whom a loan or insurance is being sought. The period of time required before a conviction is spent depends on the sentence passed, not on the offence. The required period is halved if the offender was aged under 18 years at the date of conviction. The Act does not apply to certain types of employment (see Rehabilitation of Offenders Act 1974 (Exceptions) 1975).

A person convicted of a sexual offence specified in the Sexual Offences Act 1997 is required to notify the police of his or her address. Any change of address for a period of more than 14 days must also be notified to the police. This requirement lasts for a term which depends on the penalty imposed for the offence. The minimum term is two and a half years; the maximum term is for life. It is a criminal offence not to notify the police of the current address.

A DEVELOPMENTAL APPROACH TO MEDICO-LEGAL ASSESSMENTS

GENERAL ISSUES

There are common core principles that should be applied to medico-legal assessments of juveniles. Key questions concern the young person's 'fitness to plead' and capacity to 'effectively participate in the proceedings' (Grisso and Schwartz 2000). The European Court of Human Rights has made explicit that the right of an accused to a fair trial has to include children. Two key suggestions for practice emerge from a review of international practice.

1 All young defendants, including those charged with serious offences, should be tried in Youth Courts (with permission for adult sanctions for older youths if certain conditions are met). This should enable a mode of trial for young defendants to be subject to safeguards that can enhance understanding and participation.
2 The maturity of young defendants' cognitive and emotional capacities should be assessed before a decision is taken about venue and mode of trial.

One fundamental distinction in the criminal law is between conditions that negate criminal liability and those that might mitigate the punishment deserved under particular circumstances. Very young children and the profoundly mentally ill may lack the minimum capacity necessary to justify punishment. Those exhibiting less profound impairments of the same kind may qualify for a lesser level of deserved punishment even though they meet the minimum conditions for some punishment. Immaturity, like mental disorder, can serve both as an excuse and as a mitigation in the determination of just punishment. Capacity is sometimes thought of as a generic skill that a person either

has or lacks. However, that is not so. To begin with, it is multi-faceted, with four key elements:

• the capacity to understand information relevant to the specific decision at issue (understanding)
• the capacity to appreciate one's situation as the defendant is confronted with a specific legal decision (appreciation)
• the capacity to think rationally about alternative courses of action (reasoning)
• the capacity to express a choice among alternatives (choice).

The second key point is that capacity is a feature that is both situation-specific and open to influence – as brought out in discussions of the assessment in relation to children's consent to treatment (BMA 2000), participation in research (RCP 2000), and criminal responsibility (Justice 1996). Young children may well appreciate the difference between right and wrong but yet not understand the seriousness of some forms of irresponsible behaviour. With respect to their ability to understand legal procedures (as distinct from their crime), much can be done to aid their understanding (Ashford and Chard 2000).

EVALUATION OF COMPETENCE

Any evaluation of competence (Grisso 1997) should include assessment of possibly relevant psychopathology, emotional understanding as well as cognitive level, the child's experiences and appreciation of situations comparable to the one relevant to the crime and to the trial, and any particular features that may be pertinent in this individual and this set of circumstances. The clinician should also be alert to possible treatment needs, and should be aware of how these might be met for this individual, given the forensic situation. Before the evaluation it is important to be sure that the rules and limits of confidentiality for the evaluation are clear and that the child and the family understand them (Bailey 2000). The appropriate level of clinical thoroughness and detail will vary with the intrinsic clinical complexity of the case, with the specific legal context and with the consultant's role in the legal system. The general principles to be used in the assessment are broadly comparable to those employed in any clinical evaluation (see Chapters 1, 2 and 3). However, particular attention needs to be paid to developmental background, emotional and cognitive maturity, trauma exposure and substance misuse. The likely appropriate sources for obtaining clinical data relevant to assessment of a juvenile's competence to stand trial will include a variety of historical records, a range of interviews and other observations and, in some cases, specialized tests.

Records of the child's school functioning, past clinical assessment, treatment history and previous legal involvements need to be obtained. In coming to an overall formulation, there should be a particular focus on how both developmental and psychopathological features may be relevant to the forensic issues that have to be addressed.

EVALUATION OF FUNCTIONAL CAPACITIES

Here the main focus is on the youth's ability to understand and cope with the legal process. This comes from three sources:

- direct questioning of the defendant
- inferences from functioning in other areas
- direct observation of the defendant's behaviour and interaction with others.

It is useful to enquire about the youth's expectations about what the consequences of the Court involvement might prove to be. Because the course of juvenile proceedings can vary so widely, with consequences ranging from the extremely aversive to extremely beneficial, rational understanding will necessarily involve a high degree of uncertainty.

Potentially relevant problems include: inattention, depression, disorganization of thought processes that interferes with the ability to consider alternatives, hopelessness such that the decision is felt not to matter, delusions or other fixed beliefs that distort the understanding of options (or their likely outcomes), immaturity of judgement, and the developmental challenges of adolescence.

Gudjonsson (1992; Gudjonsson and Singh 1984) found that adolescents were more prone than adults to offer inaccurate information to persons in authority when they were pressured. Younger adolescents were significantly more likely to change their stories to give answers that were less accurate than their original descriptions. This has practical implications for interviewing by police and lawyers. The ability to take another person's perspective is important for effective communication, an ability that has matured by middle adolescence but is less reliably found in early adolescence.

Sometimes concerns about a young person's conduct may be raised as potentially significant to his or her competence (Barnum 2000). A youth may be impulsive, loud, angry or disruptive during trial and it may be suggested that these tendencies may undermine the formality or integrity of the proceedings. In addressing this question, it is important to be clear about the general clinical basis for any expected functional problems, and even more important to be clear about specific implications of potential disruptiveness for the relevant features of competence. If a young person's impulsiveness may be expected to interfere with his or her attention to the proceedings in the courtroom, and if the individual's attention to the proceedings actually matters for effective collaboration with council, then it will be important to characterize these expectations or implications. For instance, if a youth is so angry and disruptive that he seems unable to sit and confer with council,

this may have important implications for his ability to understand the issues and respond helpfully to them. The clinician therefore needs to attend to these issues and show how they stem or do not stem from clinical disorder or developmental deficit.

In providing information to the Court, written reports have the advantage of a standard format that helps the consultant to consider all the relevant questions; it also provides a familiar structure for readers. In essence, for the sake of consistency and clarity, competence reports need to cover the following areas:

- identifying information and referral questions
- the description of the structure of the evaluation including sources and a notation of the confidentiality expectations
- the provision of clinical and forensic data
- discussion and presentations of opinions.

The assessment of competence to stand trial presents challenging questions. Consultants need to appreciate the systems implications of competence questions and must be able to provide opinions and recommendations that match the legal and systems circumstances of individual cases. This area is full of uncertainty and the complexity of these challenges can sometimes seem overwhelming. However, in responding carefully and thoughtfully to questions posed, consultants can contribute to the development of a potentially important aspect of legal and clinical practice (Zimring 2000).

REFERENCES

Ashford, M. and Chard, A. 2000: *Defending Young People in the Criminal Justice System*, 2nd edn. Glasgow: Legal Action Groups.

Bailey, S. 2000: Confidentiality. In Cordess, C. (ed.), *Myths and Realities in Confidentiality*. London: Jessica Kingsley.

Barnum, R. 2000: Clinical and forensic evaluation of competence to stand trial in juvenile defendants. In Grisso, T. and Schwartz, R.G. (eds), *Youth on Trial: a Developmental Perspective in Juvenile Justice*. Chicago: University of Chicago Press, 199–224.

BMA (British Medical Association) 2001: *Health Care for Children and Young People: Consent Rights and Choices*. London: BMA.

Grisso, T. 1997: The competence of adolescents as trial defendants. *Psychology, Public Policy and Law* **3**: 3–32.

Grisso, T. and Schwartz, R.G. 2000: *Youth on Trial: a Developmental Perspective on Juvenile Justice*. Chicago: University of Chicago Press.

Gudjonsson, G. 1992: *The Psychology of Interrogations, Confessions and Testimony*. New York: John Wiley.

Gudjonsson, G. and Singh, K. 1984: Interrogative suggestibility and delinquent boys: an empirical validation study. *Personality and Individual Differences* **5**: 425–30.

Zimring, F.E. 1998: *The Challenge of Youth Violence*. New York: Cambridge University Press.

32

Scottish juvenile justice and forensic adolescent services

PARAG SHAH

JUVENILE JUSTICE: THE CHILDREN'S PANEL

Much as in North America, where state legislative independence is the norm, Scotland has many of its own policies, statutes and legislative systems. This independence has been further enhanced by the Scottish Parliament's legislative powers introduced in recent years. Arguably, there is no more striking difference than that between the Scottish juvenile justice system – the Children's Panel – and the youth justice system in England and Wales.

The Children's Panel system places its emphasis on welfare as opposed to penal measures when dealing with juveniles. The ground for referral to the Panel is laid out in s52 of the Children's Act (Scotland) 1995. The three 'overarching principles' the Panel works to are:

- the welfare of the child is paramount
- the child's view must be taken into account
- no order should be made unless it is better to make the order than to do nothing (see www.childrens-hearing.co.uk/background.htm).

Over the years there have been various attempts to dilute this emphasis to bring it more in line with the English/Welsh system, but the system remains essentially intact (Lockyer and Stone 1998). There is thus a recognition that a juvenile in the legal system in Scotland has more needs than just those addressed by legislative provision. Disposals and interventions are orientated to the welfare needs of the child. Index offences are relevant only as they relate to the needs of the child.

The Children's Panel has been in existence since the late 1960s, when it was brought in by the Social Work (Scotland) Act of 1968. It runs in parallel with the criminal justice system of Sheriff's Courts (roughly equivalent to English and Welsh Magistrate Courts) and the High Courts. The powers of the Children's Panel can be limited, with serious crime (e.g. murder) being dealt with within the criminal justice system.

Entry into the Panel system is gate-kept by the Reporters, who can recommend that any one case be dealt with within the Children's Panel system, ask for informal social work intervention (without resorting to the Panel hearing), or take the matter no further.

The Panel itself is made up of three lay members who are representative of the community in terms of age, ethnicity and occupation. Both sexes are represented on each individual Panel. They will hear the case, look at available reports (possibly request additional reports), and then decide on appropriate interventions. Every intervention has to be justified on welfare grounds. There are no powers for penal detention. Supervision orders with residential requirements (including secure accommodation) can be made, so long as it is in the interests of the child's welfare. Re-attendance to the Panel can also be required to assess progress in the form of a Review Hearing. The criminal justice system can also access the Panel system to assess the needs of a child, and to ensure his or her needs are being met.

The age of criminal responsibility is 8 years in Scotland. The Panel system remit extends to dealing with those aged under 16, but should the child come into the system before 16 he or she can remain in it until reaching 18.

There is a heavy emphasis on inter-agency cooperation. Social services, of which the Children's Panel is an integral part, need to work together with other agencies to provide adequate resources to meet the needs of an individual case. This would in certain circumstances include health services. It is nonetheless important to note that compliance on the family and child's part with interventions is on a voluntary basis – the Panel has no powers to enforce compliance with any recommendations. The decisions are legally binding but are open to appeal.

As with any system, the Panel system is not without its problems. Criticisms have included under-intervention, over-intervention (e.g. overuse of residential placements – Scotland having 30% more such placements than England; Whyte 1998), problems with inter-agency cooperation and support (Lobley and Smith 1999), and the lack of compulsion powers leading to problems of compliance with interventions. Encouragingly, nonetheless, there is evidence that the system does have a positive effect, with Scottish figures on juvenile crime rates being lower than in England and Wales, and recidivism being lower. Admittedly this cannot be totally attributed to the Children's Panel system.

ADOLESCENT FORENSIC SERVICES

Psychiatric services can potentially be a part of the initial process of the Panel (e.g. in providing reports), or be a part of the interventions. For example, mental state review and psychiatric treatment could be an integral part of meeting the needs of the child.

Psychiatric services should be focused on the overall, as well as the psychiatric, welfare of the child. Child and adolescent psychiatry work best with inter-agency cooperation, both similar to the Panel system. Having such a system in place should be seen as an opportunity for psychiatric services to effect a positive change for a vulnerable adolescent.

Scotland currently has one developing adolescent forensic service in Glasgow, potentially available to the Panel or criminal justice systems, comparable to the adult forensic services for adults in the criminal justice system. There are no immediate plans for secure psychiatric beds within the NHS in Scotland at the time of writing. A recent survey has highlighted a lack of skills and a perceived need of forensic psychiatry expertise within the child and adolescent psychiatrists in Scotland (Shah 2001). In an unpublished work, Parry-Jones and associates instigated a multi-agency survey into the perceived need of an adolescent forensic service. The survey showed general support for the service and identified referrals for it (amounting to 444 referrals in five years). There was less support for multi-agency funding of it. The national UK units (Newcastle, Manchester and Birmingham) do provide 'cover' for Scotland, but cannot be considered ideally placed to provide the service, either geographically or legislatively.

Finally it must be noted that, in 1999, fifteen people aged under 21 (no definite figures for under-18s are available) were made subject to hospital orders under the Mental Health Act (Scotland) 1984. When over the age of 18 these individuals can be placed in the State Hospital at Carstairs or under local adult psychiatric provisions, whichever is most appropriate. The under-18s have no such provision in Scotland. Adolescents are potentially made subject to compulsive detention in Scotland under criminal proceedings and mental health legislation. By definition, such children require a degree of security within a hospital provision. Generic adolescent inpatient units are rarely equipped, either physically or in having the skills base, to deal with a psychiatrically disordered juvenile offender. There is no place that could fully offer adequate provision for such children in Scotland. Private provisions could be used (with substantial resource implications) and at times children could be placed inappropriately in adult provisions.

CONCLUSIONS

In short, the Scottish legislative provision of a welfare-orientated juvenile justice system offers a potential for psychiatric services to effect a positive change in an adolescent's life, without the legal problems that are sometimes associated with penal systems. This potential is currently not being exploited fully. There is multi-agency perceived need to develop an adolescent forensic service in Scotland, but there is a lack of expertise in the field within the country.

REFERENCES

Lobley, D. and Smith, D. 1999: *Working with Persistent Juvenile Offenders: an Evaluation of the Apex Cue Ten Project.* Edinburgh: Scottish Office.

Lockyer, A. and Stone, D. (eds) 1998: *Juvenile Justice in Scotland: Twenty-Five Years of the Welfare Approach.* Edinburgh: T. & T. Clark.

Scottish Office 1999: *Statistical Bulletin.* Criminal Justice Series. HMSO.

Shah, P. 2001: Child and adolescent forensic psychiatry survey in Scotland. *Scottish Health Bulletin* **59**(1): 54–6.

Whyte, B. 1998: Rediscovering juvenile delinquency. In Lockyer, A. and Stone, D. (eds), *Juvenile Justice in Scotland: Twenty-Five Years of the Welfare Approach.* Edinburgh: T. & T. Clark, 209.

33

Developments in youth care and the justice system in the Netherlands

THEO DORELEIJERS

INTRODUCTION

In the Netherlands in the course of the twentieth century, child and adolescent mental healthcare, welfare and protection have split up considerably. This fragmentation was caused by the fact that the institutions responsible for youth care come under three to four different ministries: the Ministry of Health, Welfare and Sports, the Ministry of Justice, and the Ministry of Education. There is not a separate Ministry of Juvenile Affairs as in countries like Germany. In the Netherlands, child and adolescent mental healthcare is administered by the healthcare section of the first ministry mentioned above and youth welfare by the welfare section of this ministry. The Ministry of Justice administers care provided as a part of civil or criminal law measures. The Ministry of Education is in charge of the psychologists and social workers employed at schools and by educational advisory services.

Unfortunately, the source of the funding of the various sectors is different as well. Educational institutions are centrally funded by the state and that also holds good for judicial institutions. Welfare agencies are funded by the provinces (except for the four largest cities which act as provinces in this respect). While mental healthcare is funded by the Exceptional Medical Expenses Act, the health insurers – private commercial bodies that they are – serve as intermediaries and responsible parties.

In addition to this fragmentation, sectarian compartmentalization has taken place for more than a hundred years. The remains of the sectarian struggle which once was fought physically in the Netherlands can still be found in the multiplicity of organizations active in politics, education, healthcare, broadcasting, sports, theatre, etc. For instance, in addition to Roman Catholic schools there are Jewish and Moslem schools as well as a wide variety of Protestant schools in the major cities. Comparable alternatives could and still can be found here and there when turning to healthcare organizations or joining a sports club or subscribing to a broadcasting corporation. For years, sectarianism could be encountered in the jurisdictions of mental healthcare and public welfare services as well. Public facilities have always existed alongside these sectarian institutions. They are funded by cities, provinces or the state and are accessible to everyone.

In larger cities like the Hague (with a population of 400,000) there were in the 1980s, all in all, about 50 facilities for youth care: crisis centres, runaway shelters for girls, medical day-care centres, child and adolescent psychiatric facilities, juvenile probation agencies, family guardianship agencies, etc. Each of these facilities was under the auspices of the Catholic, Protestant and other groups. Client referral was a disaster, as was finding the right place for aftercare. Furthermore, each of the 50 facilities had its own director, with its own executive secretary office and boardroom, its own logo, administrators, accountants and lawyers – in short, an expensive reminder of the 1960s and 70s.

In 1994, the then State Secretaries of Justice and Health, Welfare and Sports made a clean sweep of this kaleidoscope of agencies and initiated a mega project, called Direction in Youth Care. The broad aim of Direction in Youth Care is a double-barrelled reorganization. In the first place there is easy access to youth care with protocols for intake and diagnostic procedures. Then, after the indication is made and the care assigned it is the turn of the second part of Direction in Youth Care: care programming.

ACCESS TO YOUTH CARE

To prevent children and their parents from being sent from pillar to post, an 'open door' was developed to which they could be referred and to which clients could also refer themselves. In smaller towns or regions there should literally be one physical entrance to care facilities; in larger cities and regions the entries can be spread over a number of facilities. In these so-called 'youth-care agencies', intake teams have been designed, consisting of professionals from various disciplines all of whom are experienced enough to gain a proper diagnostic impression after an initial (screening) contact. This impression should particularly differentiate between a request for help for which a short-term intervention (at most five sessions) is indicated and one for which a more specialized diagnostic assessment is indicated. Specialist diagnostics like this, provided by highly qualified multi-disciplinary teams (also organized on a regional basis), can yield an indication for more intensive care such as psychotherapy and semi-residential care, which can be distinguished from the short-term 'open-access' care. Different regions have experimented with such youth-care agencies, that by definition bring with them teething problems. For example, social workers from the family guardianship agencies, psychologists from mental healthcare facilities, juvenile probation officers and youth welfare workers together have to form intake teams and specialized diagnostic teams together.

About twenty years ago the facilities for outpatient mental healthcare – most of which had been established on a sectarian basis in the course of the twentieth century – were merged together into regional institutes for outpatient mental healthcare (the so-called Riaggs). The traditional conviction that two religions stand in each other's way was gradually resolved in the 1980s, but welfare work proceeding from different ministerial sectors has brought new hindrances that have to be battled against fiercely.

Nor have the lawmakers solved the problems: parliamentary delay in the ratification of the new youth-care Act has been considerable. One of the objects of this Act was to enable all services to be funded under one law; however, child and adolescent psychiatrists have stubbornly opposed this and these professionals have succeeded in retaining separate funding.

CARE PROGRAMMING

The Direction in Youth Care project has two main ingredients: access to youth care discussed above, and care programming. The object is for care programming to be much more centrally administered, for care allocation to be simplified to ensure all the knowledge in a certain field matches better the needs of the children and families. Formerly an autistic child, for example, would be (inadequately) diagnosed and treated in the child welfare system, followed by the public mental healthcare system (where child psychiatrists are not always employed), only in the third stage reaching a child and adolescent psychiatrist. Juvenile delinquents with psychiatric disturbances ended up at the forensic youth psychiatrist by way of the police station, the child welfare council, the juvenile probation office and sometimes prison. Years of welfare work could pass without a psychologist or psychiatrist being involved. In this way many diagnoses have been missed and it often took much too long for adequate treatment to be instituted.

Care programming provides a solution to this. Groups around nosological units are being formed in many cities. For example, in the Hague welfare workers from various fields (justice, youth welfare and mental healthcare) are working together to initiate a care programme for disordered juvenile delinquents, for youths with attention-deficit hyperactivity disorder (ADHD), and for autistic children.

Care programme coordination – personified by an experienced jack-of-all-trades – is to be funded by the participating institutions. This coordinator is the head of a care programme committee, whose other members come from the various disciplines within the different participating institutions. The programme coordinator is backed up by a board whose members represent the directors of the participating institution. Clients, who have gone through an extensive diagnostic work-up, can – with an indication – be presented to the programme committee, which draws up a tailor-made care plan. The various elements of this plan – called modules – are provided by the providing institutions. Daily management is in the hands of a case manager who maintains good relations with the client and his or her family as well as with the various caregivers involved.

The following is an example of an actual case. Steven, aged 15, has ADHD and uses marijuana excessively as a self-medication. He comes from a somewhat chaotic family as his father also has ADHD and his mother cannot cope with her impulsive and domineering husband. Steven commits ever more serious burglaries to obtain the money he needs for his drugs. The magistrate ordered a forensic diagnostic assessment, that recommended Steven be put on probation under the condition and that he seeks treatment in the care programme. In addition, the juvenile probation officer has to report regularly to the public prosecutor. The care programme team has drawn up the following treatment plan:

- medication contacts with a psychiatrist in the local child and adolescent psychiatric centre

- group therapy for his marijuana habit and to improve his social skills
- parent counselling alternating with family intervention sessions.

Steven has his group therapy in the local regional institute for outpatient mental healthcare (Riagg). The parental counselling is facilitated by the family guardianship agency also responsible for juvenile probation. The case manager regularly liaises with Steven's school as well as with his caregivers.

The success of such an undertaking is strongly dependent on the commitment from the management of the various institutions as well as bonuses offered to caregivers for good teamwork. Regular evaluations of the experiences of the clients involved and the client system give the programme commission and the caregivers accurate feedback. On balance, the governmental funders must be good managers so that the budgets are tailored to the care offered without risk of discontinuity.

DEVELOPMENTS IN YOUTH JUSTICE: JUVENILE DETENTION CENTRES

In the Netherlands, the juvenile criminal law concerns minors aged between 12 and 18 years. Children below 12 years of age are not prosecutable; in cases of criminal acts committed by these children the Council of Child Protection requests the Juvenile Court to take a civil measure. The juvenile criminal law is marked by its pedagogical character: it is not so much the conflict between the suspect and society that is stressed, but rather priority is given to finding a solution for the psychosocial troubles experienced by the youngster in order to benefit him or her.

In 1995, the revised juvenile criminal law came into force. It was designed to meet the emancipation of youths and the political cry for a more consistent approach to juvenile crime. Under the new law, the maximum punishment by imprisonment has been increased from 6 to 12 months for 12- to 15-year-olds, and to 24 months for 16- to 17-year-olds. The maximum fine has been raised from 502 to 2500 euros ($3300). A complex system of alternative forms of sanctions has also been worked out. The revised law no longer allows judges in juvenile cases to impose a civil measure on delinquents over the age of 12.

Some 70% of youngsters who are arrested by the police are seen by the public prosecutor because of the seriousness of their offences. Only in 15% of all arrests is the youngster brought before the Juvenile Court at the request of the prosecutor. The Court tends to be used only for young people well advanced in their criminal behaviour. Young delinquents might be sent to a detention centre for three reasons, and therefore these centres have three functions:

- custody for young people on remand pending sentencing, who sometimes have to undergo a diagnostic examination

- custody for young people with unconditional prison sentences imposed by a judge
- treatment (in some centres) for young people who, in addition to or instead of detention, have a Court order to undergo coercive treatment based on a diagnosis of mental disorder or mental deficiency or an indication for rehabilitation.

Passionate debates are taking place in the Netherlands as to what kind of care these young people in detention centres should be receiving. The following notes some of the points under discussion.

DIAGNOSTIC EXAMINATION

The public prosecutor and/or the magistrate calls for a diagnostic examination during or right after arraignment. They do this on their own authority but they can also obtain advice from the Child Welfare Council which visits all youths as soon as they are locked up by the police on suspicion of having committed a serious offence.

The Court authorities can request a diagnostic examination from psychologists and/or psychiatrists who are in private practice or who are employed by (semi)-governmental ambulatory agencies. If the youths are on remand, these judicial authorities can ask the diagnosticians to examine them in prison. But also the prison staff itself can be asked to have an – internal – report made up by a team of psychiatrists, psychologists and social workers employed by the prison. The first approach provides a speedy report, reasonably inexpensive, but usually produced from only one single discipline with only a limited view (a snapshot). The second approach allows a longer observation period (usually several weeks); such a report is multi-disciplinary and also provides comments on the progress in the course of these weeks (so not a snapshot, but rather a video recording). The final approach is five to ten times as expensive as the former external one.

But it is not only a question of which is better, but also how one can standardize the indications for one type of report or the other. Sometimes the nature of the crime will be indicative (serious violent crimes and sexual offences mostly necessitate internal reporting; for misdemeanours external reporting will do). The question remains: Who determines the indications when the psychopathology is not made clear by the type of crime committed?

However, other problems play a role in this debate as well. For example, for both types of reporting the question remains whether, apart from advising the judicial authorities, the report can also be used to draw up a treatment plan when treatment is indicated in the post-trial period. Diagnostics for the purposes of a Court-ordered report make different demands on methods for the purposes of welfare work. Different parties commission the reports: Juvenile Court magistrates on the one hand and parents and caregivers on the other.

RESPONSIBILITY FOR CARE

There is a debate concerning who is responsible in daily practice for the direct care of juveniles in prison. If a psychologist is responsible for reporting to the judicial authorities, she or he cannot at the same time be responsible for the care that the juvenile requires in daily life. The proponents of reporting by external observers argue for total externalization of the entire reporting procedure. The advocates of reporting by the prison's own staff disagree with this because a wealth of information will be lost when observers pay only a flying visit once a week without participating in daily team conferences.

To cope with this problem, a 'flying team' has been installed in one of the prisons. This team operates independently of the units and does not have a caregiving relationship with those they report on. They can easily participate in observation conferences, provided the juveniles concerned and their parents give permission.

There is also the problem between the therapist in the institution where a juvenile is being treated and the general practitioner and nurses. The former is on the treatment team (responsible for modifying the juvenile's behaviour and putting an end to symptoms and offending disturbances). The latter are on the medical team in the same institution, responsible for daily healthcare. What does one do with a juvenile suffering from somatization whose symptoms are receiving attention from the treatment team, but who still regularly checks in during the office hours of a general practitioner who feels a different type of responsibility?

NEW FACILITIES

It is increasingly recognized that traditional detention, no matter how much education and training are given in the detention centres, is not helping to prevent recidivism, let alone getting the stagnated development moving again. While we are continuing to meet society's clamour for retribution – that is 'imposed distress' – we are beginning to realize that this type of punishment cannot prevent recidivism.

We are trying to invest much more in:

- the early recognition of signals leading to criminal behaviour
- putting an end to psychiatric disturbances which co-occur with criminal behaviour
- remedying family problems and learning and behavioural difficulties at school
- coaching in job-seeking and improving social skills.

When these aims make it necessary to restrict the length of detention to a few months or to a number of hours daily, alternative forms of detention such as night detention or alternative forms of treatment such as coercive outpatient treatment, if necessary, in combination with night detention are possible. The drawback to this latter form of combined detention and treatment is that it is a double provision: the justice system has to set aside and pay for a cell, and the health authorities have to reserve and budget a treatment slot.

Every effort is being made to prevent criminal behaviour or to counter changes for the worse in minor criminal behaviour. All sorts of projects are being developed locally. The SPRINT project in Amsterdam is one of the few scientifically evaluated projects. we have. As part of this project, schoolteachers of 10-year-olds are being asked to designate high-risk children. These children are screened and, if their high-risk status is confirmed by the screening instruments, their parents are approached for a meeting in which the matter is explained and they are then offered the possibility of participating in a controlled therapeutic study. The aim of this treatment is of course to turn the children away from the criminal path.

The difficulty with most of the innovative projects in the Netherlands is that only a very small proportion are scientifically evaluated. Consequently, it is a tricky matter for policymakers to decide whether to continue a project after the experimental phase has ended.

CIRCUITS AND TRAJECTORIES

The aim of the Direction in Youth Care projects is to fine-tune the work of the various caregivers so that we prevent some clients from being driven from pillar to post and others from falling between two stools. One of the aims of forensic care that should be most striven for in the near future will be the development of circuits so that treatment trajectories will be characterized by continuity. The circuits are organized regionally and all welfare sectors participate in them. Moreover, one circuit will provide both outpatient and residential care. Care programming will oversee the continuity and this will be aided by the fact that funding will also be oriented towards continuity. It is not the individual institutions or units any more that will be funded, but care programmes that can annually demonstrate their efficacy. Evaluation studies in the Dutch juvenile detention centres have indicated that, in the past few years especially, a total lack of aftercare has been responsible for the high recidivism rate. Thus, in trajectory supervision, particular attention must be paid to intensive counselling of juveniles about to be released from prison, starting several months before their discharge and extending to many months afterwards.

BOTTLENECKS

On the face of it these developments seem to be very positive. The Netherlands are innovators in trying to cope with increasing violence, increasing criminality and increasing alienation among our young people. There is a great deal still to do in order to achieve the ideal state of affairs.

Imagine a juvenile admitted to our 'ideal' forensic day-care clinic, where the therapy is successful owing to the umbrella of the Court-ordered probationary (involuntary) treatment. Then he is arrested for shoplifting, so he may have to serve his time anyway – however much we consider this to be anti-therapeutic, and however much the juvenile probation office or the boy's lawyer tries to make this clear to the Court. In short, the legal and judicial framework is absent while the modern facilities are already operational. On the other hand, the Court finds that caregivers are doing their work without sufficient awareness of all the legal and judicial ins and outs.

One more problem deserves mention. Involving families in the treatment of their children is in general an uphill battle. Parents may be too disturbed to be compliant, they may be living abroad or be in prison. Sometimes the treatment of the juvenile may itself be the major issue in a conflict between the parents. Our system still does not provide the tools and the insights to tackle these problems. We are also regularly plagued by the fact that the authority rests with parents who may refuse to cooperate. Juveniles are then often too old to have civil measures taken against them. When they reach the age of 17 years the Court often finds it a waste of time to place them in custody.

CONCLUSIONS

This chapter has provided an outline of what is currently happening in the criminological and forensic world of juveniles in the Netherlands. Recapitulating, the gist of it is that the efforts proceeding from various disciplines, ministries and financiers are becoming geared to one another. In any event, there is an increasing recognition that effective control of criminality and effective care for vulnerable young people place high demands on teamwork, rapport, innovation and scientific research. The time is ripe for it. In the Netherlands there even seems to be available funding, so what's to stop it?

Appendix: Post-basic, multi-disciplinary training for child and adolescent forensic mental health workers

KNOWLEDGE BASE

1 **Normal child development**
   Developmental stages
   Parent–child relationships: nurture and growth
   Attachment theory
   Autonomy and separation

2 **Family as context of development**
   Systems theory
   Family lifecycle
   Family scripts: integrated processes
   Family within wider social systems
   Cross-cultural issues

3 **Impacts of adversity on development**
   Concepts and definitions of abuse and neglect
   Consequences of childhood abuse trauma
   Dysfunctional family: cycles of abuse
   Psychology of victimisation
   Pathways from dysfunctional attachment to
      disturbed behaviour
   Gender differences

4 **Developmental psychopathology**
   Classification of child and adolescent mental disorders
   Multi-axial classification system
   Adolescent disturbance in family and social context
   Adaptation, accommodation and motivational context
   Dissociation, post-traumatic stress disorder (PTSD)
      and 'avoidance behaviours'
   Borderline states and personality disorders
   Deliberate self-harm; suicidal and self-injuring
      behaviour
   Depression, self-esteem and disorders of mood
   Psychosis
   Anorexia and bulimia

5 **Forensic presentations and mental disorder**
   Conduct disorder
   Psychotic mentally disordered offender
   Disorders of sexual development and offending
      behaviour
   Substance abuse and offending behaviour
   Prodromal personality disorder and offending
      behaviour
   PTSD in relation to offences

6 **Legal framework in England**
   Mental Health Act 1983
   Crime and Disorder Act 1998
   Children Act 1989
   Education Act 1996
   Child protection procedures – The Children Bill 2004
   Care programme approach (CPA)
   European Human Rights Act 1998

CLINICAL PRACTICE

1 **Assessment**
   Psychopathology with special reference to multi-
   morbidity
      application of ICD 10/DSM IV
      use of checklists
   Needs assessment
      Salford needs assessment schedule for adolescents
      (SNASA)
   Risk assessment
      agreed multi-agency definitions
      risk assessment tools, e.g. EARL 20-B, SAVRY
   User and carer perspective
   Formulation and agreed multi-agency tasks

2   Contexts
Community
Specialist day units
Residential
   open
      social care
      health
      education
   secure
      prisons
      social care
      health
      other

3   Therapeutic environments
Safe environments
   achieving appropriate adolescent–professional and
      adolescent–adolescent relationships
   individual and group dynamics
   nurture and care; stimulation and education
   emotional containment
   maintaining safe limits, boundaries and authority,
      e.g. anti-bullying policies and practice
         responding to disclosure of abuse
   ongoing needs assessment, review of mental
      health needs
   family and user active involvement

4   Integrated therapeutic approaches
Interviewing skills
   motivational interviewing
Psychological treatments
   individual and group
Cognitive behavioural therapies
   dialectical behavioural therapies
   multi-systemic therapies
Psychodynamic therapies
Non-verbal therapies
   art
   music
   drama
Physical treatments
Use of medication

Care and responsibility
   physical restraint
   single separation
Exceptional treatments, e.g. ECT

**5   Care Programme Approach: integrated process
through assessment and transitions**
Developing an integrated care plan
   health
   education
   social care
   justice
Links between treatment for forensic behaviours and
   mental health problems
Risk reduction interventions
   offence behaviour
   mental illness
   harm to self
Understanding roles, e.g. key worker
Review processes
Addressing unmet and new needs

SPECIAL ISSUES

- Skills base for mental health consultation
- Liaison and staff support in residential, secure and community youth justice settings
- Working with adolescent sex offenders
- Working with adolescent substance misusers
- Working with adolescent arsonists
- Working with adolescents' violent behaviours
- Working with traumatised adolescent offenders
- Working with adolescent offenders with learning disabilities and autism spectrum disorder
- Research methodology in forensic practice

CLINICAL GOVERNANCE

- Working within statutory frameworks
- Setting, monitoring standards for practice
- Outcomes for health and offence reduction
- Applying research knowledge to practice.

Index